Research
in Nursing

Second Edition

HOLLY SKODOL WILSON
RN, PhD, FAAN

Addison-Wesley Publishing Company
Health Sciences, Redwood City, California
Reading, Massachusetts / Menlo Park, California
New York / Don Mills Ontario / Wokingham, England
Amsterdam / Bonn / Sydney / Singapore
Tokyo / Madrid / San Juan

For my three daughters: Molly, Hillary, and Emily

Executive editor: Debra Hunter
Sponsoring editor: Armando Parcés Enríquez
Production supervisor: Judith Johnstone
Cover designer: Rudy Zehntner
Interior designer: Michael Rogondino
Art coordinator: Sue Gemmell
Copyeditor: Antonio Padial
Proofreader: Merry Finley
Indexer: Steven Sorensen

Wilson, Holly Skodol.
    Research in nursing.

    Bibliography: p.
    Includes index.
    1. Nursings—Research—Methodology.
I. Title.
RT81.5.W55   1989   610.73′072   88–8062
ISBN 0–201–05946–0

BCDEFGHIJ—DO—89109

ISBN 0-201-05946-0

Addison-Wesley Publishing Company
Health Sciences
390 Bridge Parkway
Redwood City, California 94065

Preface

The first edition of this textbook and its accompanying supplements was based on a straightforward but potentially revolutionary premise: If nursing is to build a scientific body of knowledge and if nursing practice is to be shaped by research findings rather than tradition, intuition, or habit, then the investigative skills of all nurses, regardless of their educational level, must be as integral to their repertoire as communication skills and sterile technique. All nurses must be prepared to know *something*, if not a good deal, about how to read, comprehend, evaluate, apply, participate in, and conduct research in nursing. Nursing science and nursing research must become as interesting and accessible to every nurse clinician as they are to a career nurse scientist.

Changes in the Second Edition of *Research in Nursing*

This book has been revised in keeping with the spirit and style of the first edition. However, some important new information and improvements are included. (1) The relationship of nursing theory to the research process has been expanded and updated. (2) The chapter on qualitative analysis includes contemporary use of the phenomenologic interpretive method in nursing research. (3) An entirely new chapter on advanced statistics has been added. (4) Examples, references, and information have all been updated, particularly in areas of rapid growth like computers.

Content and Features

The original premise of this text may have been revolutionary, but it is not original. As discussed in Chapter 1 and reflected throughout this book, it is a goal stated formally and informally at every level of the nursing profession. *Research in Nursing* addresses this goal by:

- Challenging the traditional assumption that to become an informed consumer of research in nursing a nurse must first be trained to conduct independent research. Appreciating a fine painting or a gourmet meal, after all, does not require you to become an artist or a chef. In our profession the research degree is earned at the doctoral level, but we cannot afford to rely solely on doctorally prepared nurses to bridge the research-practice gap. Research consumership can and must be learned early in a nursing student's educational career. This text, therefore, discusses the skills of intelligent research consumership after presenting an introduction to science and the research process that highlights relevance to nursing practice and ethical concerns crucial to health care and nursing research.

■ Demonstrating the application of research to all aspects of the nursing profession, but particularly to clinical nursing practice. Students usually choose nursing as a career because they want to help, care, support, and comfort, not because they want to analyze, conceptualize, theorize, or criticize. Failure to show the important relationship between the two sets of activities, however, has been a major stumbling block to the integration of research as a value for every practicing nurse. In specific chapters devoted to the topic of application, as well as through a kind of textual "role modeling" on virtually every page, *Research in Nursing* makes the case that knowing how we know is essential to doing what we do.

■ Choosing an informed, conversational tone and writing style. By demystifying research terminology, the text presents scholarship not as the dry, esoteric, and pretentious exercise it is sometimes reputed to be, but as the lively, engaging, and sometimes humorous enterprise it often is.

■ Emphasizing the qualities of discovery and creativity, as well as precision and rigor, that underlie the best in nursing research. Scientific imagination is given its proper place alongside scientific accuracy and technique.

■ Presenting, in two chapters, the methodologies of qualitative research. In our early stage of scientific maturity, description and generating theory are as vital to our development as testing hypotheses and verifying theory. Numerous examples of field studies and qualitative analyses are therefore discussed to show the power and promise that these methodologies can offer research in nursing. Examples of qualitative studies can be found in other chapters as well.

■ Reinforcing information through clear pedagogical devices. **Chapter objectives, lists, boxes, tables, figures, critique guidelines, annotated examples, summaries of key ideas and terms, further readings, a research glossary, and appendices of research resources** enrich the content, making it easier on the eye and more accessible to the mind.

■ Offering a package of supplements that assist the instructor and motivate the student. The **Instructor's Manual** is keyed to the text chapter by chapter and includes topical lecture outlines, transparency masters, and activities for individual, small-group, and full-class learning. The extensive bank of **NCLEX test questions** addresses the learning objectives for each chapter.

Audience

This comprehensive introductory text provides the nursing student with the knowledge and skills required of nurses in investigative roles, ranging from research consumer to scientific investigator. It is therefore **appropriate as a reference** for an issues or professionalism course in diploma or associate-degree curricula, where research in nursing is covered as a unit or topic; as **a required text** in an introductory course in nursing research, whether at the baccalaureate or beginning master's level; or as **a resource** for more advanced graduate students and practitioners seeking a book that conveys the fascination and scope of this growing field in an easy to understand style. Nurses employed in health care settings, where research is emerging as a significant aspect of leadership, will find this text a worthwhile addition to their personal and institutional libraries.

Organization

Research in Nursing is organized into four parts. Part 1 introduces the reader to science as a way of knowing and the research process as the tool of science. It advances values and attitudes that foster an appreciation of the significance of science and research to nursing practice and patient care. It also addresses the nurse's role in respecting and advocating research ethics.

Part 2 focuses on the skills of research consumership, from acquiring a research vocabulary to preparing a complete, formal research critique.

Part 3 is devoted to the steps actually taken when conducting a scientific investigation. It gives equal attention to qualitative data collection techniques such as observation and interviewing and to quantitative data collection using psychosocial and biological instrumentation. Analysis procedures for qualitative data and descriptive and advanced statistical procedures, along with a full chapter of current information on the use of computers in nursing research, conclude this part.

Part 4 provides the developing nurse scholar with specific guidelines and strategies for communicating the methods and findings of scientific work through journal articles, books, scientific papers, and talks at professional meetings. Planning and writing a research proposal are also covered in Part 4.

All chapters need not be assigned, nor is adhering to a single sequence necessary to make the text a coherent learning tool. The extensive glossary of research terminology, research resources, and samples in the appendixes, as well as statistical tables and symbols, add to the reference utility of this text.

Building the scientific basis for clinical nursing practice is a top priority for nursing research in the 1990s. While each chapter of this text sustains the importance of nursing research directed toward the promotion, maintenance, and restoration of human health, the values of studies in nursing administration, nursing education, nursing history, and nursing philosophy are also underscored. Thus the title *Research in Nursing* reflects scientific diversity rather than an exclusive focus on clinical nursing research.

Acknowledgements

Writing this book reminded me that an author's work requires a long encounter with solitude. Sustaining my energy and enthusiasm for the project would have been impossible without the support, help, inspiration, and contributions of certain key people. I acknowledge them here with my warmest thanks.

- The nursing students at Sonoma State University and the University of California, San Francisco, to whom I've taught the required introductory nursing research courses since 1974, and whose responses convinced me of the worth of this book's contents. Also the doctoral students at UCSF, who generously shared their in-progress work for examples and illustrations.

- My colleagues and friends Sandra Ferketich, Sally Hutchinson, Diane La-Rochelle, Ada Lindsey, Linda Moody, Sandra Scheetz, Nancy Stotts, and Joyce Verran, who contributed their expertise by writing chapters on "Getting Started," "The Theoretical Context," "Psychosocial Instruments," "Biophysiologic Variables," "Applying Statistics," "Multivariate and Advanced Statistics," and "Computers."

- The executive editor at Addison-Wesley, Debra Hunter, whose support and patience were essential; and my new sponsoring editor, Armando Parcés Enríquez, who courageously saw this book through to completion. The production supervisor, Judith Johnstone, whose skills have served me in earlier books as well.

- The following authorities who reviewed and critiqued chapters in this book during its development: Victoria Champion, MSN, DNS, Indiana University; Carole Chenitz, RN, EdD, Veteran's Administration Medical Center, San Francisco, California; Sherry Gevedon, MS, PhD, Columbia Union College; Marion Good, RN, PhD, Medical College of Ohio; Karen Haller, RN, PhD, Loyola University, Chicago; Carolyn Kee, MN, PhD, Georgia State University; Brighid Kelley, MSN, PhD, University of Cincinnati; Virginia Knowlden, RN, EdD, St. Joseph College, West Hartford, Connecticut; Violet Malinsky, RN, PhD, Hunter College-Bellevue School of Nursing; Barbara Munro, RN, PhD, University of Pennsylvania; Judy Ozboldt, MS, PhD, University of Michigan.

Holly Skodol Wilson

Biographical Notes

About the Author

Holly Skodol Wilson, RN, PhD, FAAN, is a professor in the Department of Mental Health, Community, and Administrative Nursing, School of Nursing, at the University of California, San Francisco, where she teaches the required introductory research course for registered nurse students in the articulated BS/MS program. It was for this course that she was awarded the Outstanding Teacher of the Year Award by students at their 1983, 1984, and 1986 commencements. Her clinical and research interests focus on the severely and chronically mentally disordered, family caregivers, psychogerontology, and psychiatric nursing diagnosis. She has authored and co-authored eleven books and contributed over 50 articles to scholarly journals. She is active nationally and internationally as a speaker and consultant and has taught in Japan, The People's Republic of China, Kenya, East Africa, Australia, New Zealand, Hong Kong, Argentina, and Israel. Her honors include Distinguished Alumni, Duke University, School of Nursing; Distinguished Dissertation of the Year, U.C. Berkeley; and the American Nurses' Foundation Scholar Citation. During the writing of the first edition of this text and its supplements, she was awarded a Kellogg National Leadership Fellowship to study international models of care for the mentally disordered elderly.

About the Contributors

Sandra L. Ferketich, RN, PhD, is an associate professor and Division Head for Family and Community Health Nursing at the College of Nursing, University of Arizona in Tucson. Her research focus is on the reproductive and childrearing family when a member has a catastrophic illness. She has published numerous research articles on family function and individual member health. Her advanced preparation in nursing research methodology and statistics has resulted in publications on graphic residual analysis and model building with Dr. Joyce Verran. She has served as a member of local, regional and national grant review sections.

Sally A. Hutchinson, RN, PhD, is an associate professor in the College of Nursing, University of Florida. She teaches qualitative research methods to master's and doctoral students and a course on cultural influences in nursing care. A recipient of Division of Nursing pre- and post-doctoral research fellowships, she presently is studying nurses who are chemically dependent. She has published in numerous nursing journals and contributed chapters to several nursing research texts. She was a seminar leader and a co-leader of Professional Seminar Consultants' study tours to China and Africa. Her scholarly interests are in anthropology, qualitative research methods, and psychiatric nursing.

Diane R. LaRochelle, RN, PhD, is a professor in the College of Nursing, University of Florida, where she teaches courses in nursing administration and health policy. She has developed and taught courses in quantitative research methods to master's students at two universities, and has extensive experience as a research proposal reviewer for professional organizations, including two chapters of Sigma Theta Tau and the American Educational Research Association. She has just designed a research instrument with M. Challela, DNSc, to assess the level of development of interdisciplinary teams. Her current research focuses on career patterns in nursing. She has written numerous articles, serves on the editorial/review boards of the *Journal of Ambulatory Case Management* and *Image*, and is the co-editor of the *Florida Nursing Review*. She has presented her work at national and international meetings and was a leader for Professional Seminar Consultants on a study tour to Japan, Thailand, and Hong Kong, and co-leader on a study tour to Russia.

Ada M. Lindsey, RN, PhD, FAAN, is a professor and dean, School of Nursing, at the University of California, Los Angeles. Her more recent major contributions have been to graduate nursing education. She has been an active member of the Oncology Nursing Society, the American Association of Critical Care Nurses, and has been elected a Fellow in the American Academy of Nursing. The focus of her clinical and research interests has included cachexia and anorexia in cancer patients and the influence of moderator variables, such as social support, on health outcomes. She has authored and coauthored a number of book chapters and journal articles and has presented her work at national and international meetings.

Linda E. Moody, RNC, PhD, FAAN, is a professor at the College of Nursing, University of Florida at Gainesville. She holds a PhD in educational research from the University of Florida, as well as master's and baccalaureate degrees in nursing. She also has a master's degree in health policy and administration from the University of North Carolina at Chapel Hill. She has done postgraduate work at the University of Arizona, focusing on pulmonary research; at Johns Hopkins University in health program evaluation; and, at the University of Edinburgh, a summer course in English studies and linguistics. Additional coursework includes philosophy of science and the sociology of knowledge. Dr. Moody has taught theory analysis and theory-building through research in the doctoral program at the University of Florida since 1984. She has published many research articles in health and nursing periodicals. She has been the PI or Co-PI on a number of grants funded by National Institutes of Health, Center for Nursing Research, Robert Wood Johnson Foundation, and other government and private foundations.

Sandra L. Scheetz, RN, DNSc, recently completed an NIMH postdoctorate training program in clinical services research through the Department of Psychiatry, University of California, San Francisco. Her research there focused on utilization patterns of clients seeking services in a county hospital psychiatric emergency service. She completed her doctorate at UCSF in 1986. Her Chapter, "Computers and Data Processing in Nursing Research," flowed out of her own experiences in completing her graduate research studies and in teaching computer courses to nursing graduate students for over five years as a staff member of the nationally known Computer Resource Center, School of Nursing, UCSF. She has taught and consulted widely regarding applications of computers in nursing education, administration and practice as well as research, and has shared her expertise at national conferences.

Nancy A. Stotts, RN, EdD, is an associate professor and coordinator of the graduate specialty "Adult Nursing: Surgical," in the Department of Physiological Nursing, School of Nursing at the University of California, San Francisco. Her clinical expertise and research are focused in the area of surgical nursing, including wound healing, nutrition, and nursing education. She has been active in the American Association of Critical Care Nurses and currently serves as the chairman of the Program Committee. She has authored and co-authored a number of journal articles and book chapters.

Joyce A. Verran, RN, PhD, is an associate professor and Division Head for Adult Health Nursing at the College of Nursing, University of Arizona in Tucson. Her advanced education in clinical nursing research and statistics has led to joint authorship on several articles with Dr. Sandra Ferketich. She is a statistical consultant for *Nursing Research* and on the editorial board for the *Journal of Neuroscience Nursing.* Her research interests involve subjective estimation of sleep of hospitalized and healthy adults and nursing technology as it relates to organizational functioning.

Contents

P A R T

I

Scientific Research,
the Nursing Profession,
and You

CHAPTER

1

What Is Nursing Research?

HOLLY SKODOL WILSON

Chapter Objectives

After reading this chapter, the student should be able to:

- Appreciate the meaning and usefulness of the scientific method of problem solving and decision making in nursing practice

- Compare the scientific approach with (1) trial and error and common sense. (2) authority and tradition, (3) inspiration and intuition, and (4) logical reasoning

- Identify the assumptions, characteristics, and aims of the scientific approach

- Compare the positivist philosophy with the symbolic interactionist philosophy

- Locate a nursing study on a continuum based on its relevance to nursing practice

- Recognize types of nursing studies through identification of study purpose and design

- Explain ten typical steps in the deductive research process

- Trace the major landmarks in the developmental history of nursing research, specifying one significant outcome for each

- Interpret the implications of past trends for the future of nursing research

In This Chapter . . .

The August night was hot and sticky despite the hum of the hospital's antiquated air conditioning system. The man tossed in his narrow bed as the other three figures in the ward lay sleeping. He groaned and opened his eyes to the darkness. His body felt prickly, and his heart was pounding harder than usual. He searched for the dab of light emanating from the nurses' station down the hall. The patient tried to settle back into his sleeping position, but a peculiar sensation inside his abdomen brought him wide awake, and he was overcome with the feeling that something terrible was about to happen. It felt like a mouse running up and down inside of him. His heart was swelling, filling his chest and forcing its way up into his throat. The mouse increased its frantic run and began to spin inside, scratching his guts with its claws. A wave of nausea swept over him, and a veil of sweat covered his face. Trying not to disturb the others, the man reached for his call bell and rang for the nurse. "I'm sick, I'm sick as hell," he whispered to her. Two months later this man, who had been admitted to the hospital for cartilage repair associated with an old soccer injury, died of acute adult leukemia.

That same August night, five floors higher in the hospital, an eager pair of mothers watched as a nurse walked into their room with two pink babies balanced carefully in her arms. The babies were yelling with open, hungry mouths. Their waiting mothers gathered them in, and the nurse moved between the sucking infants, gently adjusting a position here, offering a word of encouragement there, and feeling a sense of satisfaction and tenderness about her work.

Panger, Daniel. *The Dance of the Wild Mouse.* Glen Ellen, Calif.: Entwhistle Books, 1979. Reprinted by permission of the author and the publisher.

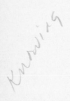

The realities of human suffering and joy challenge and enrich our practice of the scientific, professional discipline of nursing. Each day you may carry out tasks that are viewed by others as rewarding, frightening, or even distasteful. You will often have to rely on your own judgment in the absence of complete information. Your work may arouse in you feelings of compassion, outrage, guilt, pity, anxiety, confusion, or curiosity. Confronting these experiences requires both the *engaged* and the *analytic* ways of knowing (Ackerman 1969):

> The Engaged style of knowing demands effective human contact between the individual and the object of his/her attention. The Analytic style gives the individual precision tools with which to manipulate the environment (p. 855).

The engaged study of humanities, according to Prior (1962), "includes types of learning that are directly concerned with human responses to all forms of experience" (p. 11). This conception strongly resembles the definition of nursing in the American Nurses' Association's social policy statement (1980): "Nursing is the diagnosis and treatment of human responses to actual or potential health problems" (p. 9). From studies that emphasize the engaged style we derive our notions of freedom, justice, imagination, commitment, loyalty, beauty, and compassion. Yet professional nursing also requires nurses to have at their command:

> a large body of knowledge that is theoretical as well as empirical, extends beyond practical and established nursing knowledge, [and] includes a large selection of alternative explanations and predictions for nursing problems . . . some of which are abstract, complex, and not clearly understood, and require nursing actions which may be innovative and probabilistic (Waters et al 1972).

In short, nursing competence requires mastery of analytic knowing as well as engaged knowing.

Although some philosophers argue that the engaged style of knowing is dramatically different from the analytic style in its language, content, and goals, Bronowski (1956) sums up the approach to science that you will learn about in this chapter:

> The discoveries of science and the works of art . . . are explorations of a hidden likeness or unity. . . . This is the act of creation in which an original thought is born and the act is the same in . . . science and in art (p. 30).

Science and research are indeed keystones in the edifice of professional nursing practice, but they do not stand alone. Nursing's goals of wisdom, vision, social significance, accountability, fulfillment, collegiality, and excellence can be achieved only when we synthesize the engaged with the analytic—the humanities with the sciences. Nursing research at its best captures this synthesis.

The scientific approach, when conceived of as a process of learning about patients of the sort whose stories began this chapter, has been defined by Jacox (1974) as:

> The systematic attempt to understand and comprehend the world, . . . to enter deeply into the world, not just superficially, but to achieve a rational expression in language and mathematical symbolism of the order and beauty of operation that lies behind the external world (p. 6).

Not everyone writing about research shares my judgments and biases, which include the following ideas:

1. Scientific research does not pretend that the knowledge conveyed is literal and irrevocable truth. Many research textbooks and courses inhibit genuine inquiry by their dogmatic methodological pretensions and mechanical procedures. Such an approach simply obscures good ideas and fails to inspire students.

2. Science does, of course, involve a process of proof, but it also involves a spirit of *discovery*.

3. Knowledge won through research is not just knowledge of facts, but of *facts interpreted*; good scientists realize that such knowledge is fragile, open to doubt, and subject to change.

4. Most of the principles of scientific research are applied in thoughtful nursing practice, and the substance of much research exists in everyday nursing practice.

Read on if you are a nurse or nursing student who believes that research is more than the meticulous application of given procedures to relatively insignificant questions, and if you wish to penetrate the mystique of research methods so that you will know

- what to look for in research studies
- what meanings to assign their findings
- how to put findings into practice
- how to use your curiosity, imagination, and reasoning to adapt the technology of science to acquiring fresh knowledge and solutions to practical problems

The aim of Chapter 1 is to define the meaning of science and research for nurses who will be conducting studies themselves or applying study findings in their clinical practice. In this chapter you will learn about the scientific way of knowing as contrasted with the alternatives of common sense, tradition, intuition, and logical reasoning. We will also consider two major philosophies of science, several types of nursing study, the typical steps in the research process itself, and the historical evolution and the future directions of nursing research. Finally, the chapter aims to help you learn how nursing research can foster your own intellectual development, advance the nursing profession, and improve the quality of care given to patients.

Chapter 1 opens the door to a rich adventure in the world of discovery and scientific competence. Take a stand when you read it. Argue about the ideas. Be opinionated. Later, soften your attitude to one, in Kerlinger's (1966) terms, of "intelligent conviction and emotional commitment." Technical competence is empty without a basic understanding of the nature and promise of research in nursing.

Why Do Research?

Nurses make decisions and solve problems each day in the process of delivering care to patients. This section encourages you to pause and consider the basis on which you answer clinical questions. Imagine the following situation:

A mother-to-be was admitted to a California hospital at 3:40 A.M. in active labor. An external monitor was applied, and her membranes broke about 20 minutes later. When her physician's associate checked in at 5:00 A.M., the obstetrical nurse expressed concern about the monitor tracing and asked him to check it. After he did so and did a pelvic exam on the laboring mother, he *suggested* that the nurse call the patient's primary obstetrician. Unknown to him, however, was the fact that the obstetrician had left standing orders not to be disturbed between 10:00 P.M. and 7:00 A.M., "except in an emergency." Because the associate did not *declare* this case to be an emergency, the nurse followed the standing orders. By 7:30 the monitor was exhibiting a marked late deceleration, and by 10:00 the obstetrician had come to the hospital and performed an emergency caesarean section. The newborn exhibited signs of brain damage. Now, at 3½ years of age, he is a spastic quadriplegic with mental retardation (Snyder 1983).

How does a nurse decide what to do in such a situation? Should he or she follow the standing instruction of an authority and abide by the institution's traditions? Or is there an independent accountability to the patient that requires the nurse to recognize the seriousness of the situation from the monitor tracings and make judgments on some other basis?

If you are inclined to favor the latter alternative, consider another situation. Imagine that you have taught prenatal classes to expectant parents for five years. One of your patients has been complaining of severe nausea and vomiting and is taking Bendectin left over from a previous pregnancy (a combination of doxylamine and pyridoxin). She reads in the local paper that the drug's manufacturer is no longer making and distributing the drug but that it has not been withdrawn from the market and will continue to be available until supplies in the hands of drug distributors, wholesalers, and pharmacies are exhausted. She asks *you* whether it is true that taking this drug will cause pyloric stenosis in her infant. Or will nausea and vomiting, without treatment, themselves increase the same risk? Would she be better off taking a different drug, even though it has not been so well studied as Bendectin? The mother-to-be seeks your counsel. On what basis do you respond?

Questions in everyday nursing practice as well as health-care planning surround you. Are old women "sicker" than men when it comes to the incidence of chronic diseases, or do they just outlive men and thus become more susceptible? If you were planning a prevention program targeted to the reports that older women get osteoporosis three to five times more often than men and therefore have more bone fractures in later life, would you recommend calcium supplements, high-protein diets, exercise, or supplemental estrogen? On what bases would you decide? Should women over the age of 47 be taught breast self-examination for cancer despite the fact that the incidence peaks in women between 42 and 47 (McKeever 1983)? Should elderly women have a pelvic exam as part of a usual physical assessment? What is the risk to young children of electrically powered beds with automatic bed-lowering controls, or "walkaway switches"? Do most patients know the names of the drugs they take? their purpose? how and when to take them? when to stop? what food, drinks, and other drugs to avoid? what side effects can occur? The scientific approach as reflected in nursing research offers you important resources for answering difficult clinical and health-related questions.

Ways of Knowing

Although this text advocates the scientific method as the way to address the questions posed in the last section, there are alternative ways of knowing:

- *You can use trial and error combined with common sense.* If the other patients in your prenatal class who took Bendectin did not have babies with pyloric stenosis, then your common sense might compel you to say that the drug was safe.

- *You can use authority and tradition.* If you choose to follow the stated rules in procedure books and standing orders, you will not feel obligated to make an independent interpretation of the fetal monitor's tracings for evidence of an emergency.

- *You can use inspiration and intuition.* If your engaged style of knowing compels you to predict that elderly women are disadvantaged by the level of care they receive, you will be inspired to become an advocate for better care for the aged, minorities, and other disadvantaged groups and support teaching them self-care.

- *You can use logical reasoning.* If your own sense of logic alerts you to the ideas that (1) children and some adults are particularly curious about how mechanical beds operate, (2) the metal underparts of such a bed can have a scissors, or guillotine, action, and (3) being caught between the stationary portion of the bed and its moving frame could crush a child to death, you will conclude that removing or deactivating the "walkaway" down switches on these beds, at least in pediatric and psychiatric wards, is definitely indicated.

What Is the Scientific Approach?

The way of knowing developed in this book is that of scientific research blended with what Diers (1983) has defined as "clinical scholarship"—a stretching of one's mind for new insights. Let's begin with some basic assumptions that underpin the scientific approach:

1. It is better to be knowledgeable about the world than to be ignorant of it.

2. Scientists can use their senses to apprehend an external reality.

3. Observers of the world are able to relate observations conceptually and make meaning out of them.

4. It is possible to discern an underlying order in the psychosocial as well as the physical world.

5. Cause-and-effect relationships exist in the social *and* physical orders.

Given these assumptions, we can define **scientific inquiry** as a process in which observable, verifiable data are systematically collected from the world we know through our senses to describe, explain, or predict events. The scientific approach has two *characteristics* that the other ways of knowing do not: (1) *self-correction*, or **objectivity**, and (2) *the use of sensory*, or **empirical**, evidence.

This approach to knowing has built-in checks throughout the investigative process. If a scientist finds that a particular hypothesis is supported in an experiment, he or she will also test alternative hypotheses, and this testing must be open to the criticism of others. The quality of objectivity is what some authorities call the checks that attempt to distance the way of knowing as much as possible from the scientist's personal beliefs, values, and attitudes.

The second key characteristic is that the scientific approach appeals to evidence (called empirical data) in a systematic way.

The basic *aims* of scientific inquiry are to (1) develop explanations of the world (these explanations are called **theories**—see Chapter 9) and (2) find solutions to problems (see Chapter 2). The key features of the scientific approach are summarized in Table 1–1. Although these two aims in nursing science are related, some researchers emphasize the development of our general understanding of human beings interacting with their environment, whereas others emphasize the determination of effectiveness of specific nursing interventions in practice situations.

Now that we have examined the assumptions, characteristics, and aims of the scientific approach, we can contrast it with the commonsense way of knowing, in Table 1–2.

In sum, if as a clinician you began to wonder why some myocardial infarction patients were allowed to drink ice water and others were not, you could draw on books of procedure, your past experiences, trial and error, and common sense to

---

TABLE 1–1   *Summary of Basic Points about the Scientific Approach to Knowing*

Assumptions	Characteristics	Aims
The existence of underlying order in the universe	Built-in self correction for objectivity	Build a body of theories that describe, explain, and predict
The value of knowledge over ignorance	Reliance on empirical evidence	Solve practical problems
Use of empirical evidence		
Existence of causal relationships		
Conceptualizations are based on observation		

---

arrive at an explanation. *Or* you could try to use the tools of science to answer your question.

Despite the commonly accepted principles of the scientific approach just discussed, scientists themselves can differ in how they view this approach. To capture the subtle diversity here, we must think for a moment about the dominant perspectives on the philosophy of science.

Two Perspectives on Philosophy

Two schools of thought, or intellectual tradition, are reflected in nursing research questions and procedures. These schools of thought are sometimes called a researcher's **epistemology**. The first school of thought is called the **positivist** tradition, and the second, the **symbolic-interactionist**, or *neo-idealist*, tradition. The positivists, according to Sjoberg and Nett (1968), adhere to the following opinions about science:

1. Scientists can and do attain objective knowledge of both the physical and the psychosocial worlds.

2. The logic of inquiry and research procedures should be the same whether one is studying plants or people.

3. Social order in the universe is relatively mechanistic.

TABLE 1–2 *Scientific Knowing Versus Common Sense Knowing*

Scientific Approach	Common Sense
uses conceptual schemes that have been empirically tested	may accept fanciful explanations
acquires evidence to test theories according to systematic methods	selects evidence on the basis of personal experiences or preferences, usually to verify a personal position
uses a controlled method for ruling out other variables that might explain a phenomenon	makes little or no attempt to control variables
tends not to deal with metaphysical explanations that cannot be empirically tested	may be highly metaphysical or spiritual
has a built-in mechanism for self-correction	allows explanations to persist even if incorrect

4. Objectivity in research can be obtained by setting forth a formal research design.

The nonpositivists, or neo-idealists, subscribe to a different set of beliefs:

1. Fundamental differences exist between the natural, or physical, sciences and the psychosocial sciences, and different methods must be applied in the study of each.

2. Research that studies the whole person must take into account both the historical dimension of human action and the subjective aspects of human experience.

3. There is no one objective reality waiting to be measured.

4. If scientists are to comprehend people, they must come to understand each person's own definition of his or her reality.

5. Social order is constantly in a state of becoming. Therefore scientists cannot impose rigid categories on a social world that is constantly in the process of evolution.

For extensive illustrations of how the positivist philosophy is reflected in nursing research, see Chapters 14 and 15, on statistics. Likewise, see Chapter 12, on field methods, and Chapter 13 on the craft of qualitative analysis, to see how the symbolic-interactionist perspective influences research practices. The basic distinction is that positivists advocate methods dictated by rules of verification, whereas, symbolic interactionists emphasize being pragmatic and seeking whatever is meaningful and useful.

Types of Nursing Research

Earlier in this chapter I specified the two aims of scientific inquiry: (1) to develop theories that increase the state of knowledge and (2) to solve problems or make decisions for what are considered practical purposes. Research conducted with the first aim is often called **basic**, or *pure*, *research*. It is often compared to building blocks, on which increments in knowledge and further research are based. Research directed to the second aim is usually called **applied research**. It includes not only studies directed toward solving practical problems and making nursing decisions but also clinical trials aimed at developing and evaluating a new program, product, method, or procedure.

This somewhat dated distinction becomes a bit fuzzy when used to categorize research conducted in a practice discipline such as nursing. Suppose you were to do a study of the health care needs of elderly Hispanic-American women. Your study's purpose and design might be limited to building a data base and thereby contributing to a body of knowledge in an area where there has been a paucity of research. In this sense, by the standard definition your research would be basic—knowledge for knowledge's sake. Someone else, however, might subsequently use your findings to alter aspects of nursing care for this population of patients, thus transforming a basic study into an applied study by using the findings to reform the ills of practice.

Diers (1979) sees virtually *all* nursing research as applied research when she enumerates three distinguishing properties of research problems in nursing:

1. The potential nursing research problem must involve "a difference that matters" in terms of its consequences for improving patient care.

2. The nursing research problem also has a relationship to more conceptual issues and therefore has the potential for contributing to theory development and our body of scientific nursing knowledge.

3. Finally, a research problem is a nursing research problem when nurses have access to and control over the phenomenon being studied.

According to these criteria, all nursing research is **clinical research**—a blend of pure and applied research—and the critical point is its *clinical relevance* for nursing practice and our knowledge about that practice. Research topics that really make no difference to patients, that are not instances of a class of related problems, or that are not in nursing's domain do not fall within the scope of Diers's definition of nursing research.

In sum, according to Diers and many of her colleagues at the Yale University School of Nursing, as well as researchers at other centers, knowledge in practice professions is *for something*; specifically, in nursing, it is for improving the services given to the consumers of nursing services. If a nurse studies factors that contribute to the success of integrating the education and practice roles in nursing, by Diers's definition the study would probably be classified as research in administration! If another nurse studies how baccalaureate nursing students learn to care for terminally ill patients in the context of routine clinical instruction, the nurse is conducting a study in the field of education. But a nurse who studies the effects of rate of injection on intensity and duration of first and second pain of intramuscular injection is conducting a nursing research study.

The Pure-Applied Continuum

An alternative to the old basic-applied distinction that is probably more useful in classifying types of nursing studies is a *pure-applied continuum* based on *how relevant* (1) the subjects, (2) the content, and (3) the conditions are to real-world nursing problems and decisions (Cooperative Graduate Education in Nursing 1975). (See Figure 1–1.) This continuum can be divided into five stages.

Stage 1. Not Directly Relevant Consider a nurse physiologist interested in the mechanisms of skin healing and studying the optimum time and temperature of wet soaks on guinea pigs' wounds in a laboratory. This research is an example of a Stage 1 study on the pure-applied continuum in Figure 1–1. Such a study is not directly relevant to the practice of nursing.

Stage 2. Relevant Topic or Subjects Now consider a researcher interested in the concept of hunger and conducting a laboratory study with college students who drank Metrecal through a tube from behind a screen with no visual cues to how

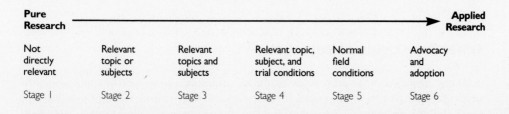

Pure Research					Applied Research
Not directly relevant	Relevant topic or subjects	Relevant topics and subjects	Relevant topic, subject, and trial conditions	Normal field conditions	Advocacy and adoption
Stage 1	Stage 2	Stage 3	Stage 4	Stage 5	Stage 6

Figure 1–1 Pure-applied continuum based on relevance to Nursing Practices

much they had consumed. This research, designed to determine if a natural factor influences feeling satisfied, is a Stage 2 study because it is being conducted with people instead of animals but the topics of hunger and satiation are not specifically related to a nursing activity.

Stage 3. Relevant Topic and Subjects   A study to determine whether premature infants placed in different body positions consumed different amounts of energy is a Stage 3 study because it involves people as subjects and compares different positioning choices, a topic of direct concern to nursing practice.

Stage 4. Relevant Topic, Subjects, and Trial Conditions   Now consider a study of hospitalized children that investigates how incorporating the parents' needs in the nursing care plan affects the children's recovery rates. This is an example of researching a nursing intervention under special conditions, a Stage 4 study. (Of course, one of the problems with a study under special conditions is that the conditions themselves may account for the results.)

Stage 5. Normal Field Conditions   Studying the quality of nursing care for chronically ill patients with different staffing patterns under normal hospital conditions would quality as a Stage 5 study.

Stage 6. Advocacy and Adoption   Research that demonstrates the applicability of primary nursing—in which one nurse is totally responsible for a case load of patients—to a diverse array of practice settings would be at the extreme "applied" end of the continuum, or at Stage 6.

Classification by Purpose and Design

Nursing research can also be classified by its purposes and related study designs. Table 1–3 summarizes five of the major purposes of research—to explore, to describe, to explain, to experiment, and to test a method—and cites illustrative contemporary nursing studies for each.

Other Typologies of Research

Nursing studies can also be categorized as primarily inductive (moving from observation to explanation to general theory) or deductive (testing hypotheses deduced from theory). Ot they can be described as *factor-isolating*, *factor-relating*, *situation-relating*, or *situation-producing*. These subjects are taken up in detail in subsequent chapters on design and theory (Chapters 5 and 9).

TABLE 1–3   *Types of Nursing Study According to Purpose or Design*

Type	Purpose	Methods	Examples
Exploratory	To obtain a richer familiarity with a phenomenon and clarify concepts as a basis for further research	Interviewing, participant observation, document analysis, case studies	Passage through hospitalization of severely burned, isolated school-age children (Kueffner 1976) An exploratory study of the meaning of current dance forms to adolescent girls (Wilson 1968)
Descriptive	To obtain complete and accurate information about a phenomenon	Interviews, questionnaires, direct observation, analysis of records	An epidemiologic study of psychiatric symptom pattern change (Nakagawa, Osborne, Hartmann 1972) Patient problems related to tube feeding (Walike et al 1975) Patient reaction to sound in an intensive coronary care unit (Marshall 1972)
Explanatory	To provide conceptual analyses grounded in observation of human behavior	Interviews, participant observation, constant comparative analysis	Fairing: Control of staff work in a healing community for schizophrenics (Wilson 1978) Three phases in the development of father involvement in pregnancy (May 1982)
Experimental and quasi-experimental	To test hypotheses about relationships	Experiments, quasi-experiments	A physiological, behavioral approach to understanding the mechanisms of obesity and anorexia (Walike 1973) Effect on postoperative recovery rate and comfort of four approaches to nursing care of dogs: A pilot study (Hadley et al 1970) The effect of stimulation on the sleep behavior of the premature infant (Barnard 1973)

TABLE 1–3   *Types of Nursing Study According to Purpose or Design (Continued)*

Type	Purpose	Methods	Examples
Methodological	To develop or refine a new research technique or procedure	Validity and reliability tests	Adjustment to widowhood after a sudden death: Suicide and nonsuicide survivors compared (Demi 1978)
			Developing a psychometric instrument for the use of children's drawings in cross-cultural research: Problems, procedures, and potentials (Schuster 1971)
			Development of a symptom distress scale (McCorkle and Young 1978)
			Quantification of self-report data from two-dimensional body diagrams (Voda et al 1980)

Steps in the Research Process

If the basic aim of science is to find general explanations of natural events so that we can describe and predict such events, scientific research is the systematic empirical investigation of presumed relations among these natural phenomena. *In other words, if developing theories and verifying them are the goals of science, the research process is the tool of science.* It represents one particular approach to coming to know that something is or is not true. The purpose of research is to discover solutions to problems and generate general principles and theory by applying scientific procedures designed to increase the chances that data collected will be reliable, relevant, and unbiased.

To increase the chance that any particular study meets the criteria of this definition, researchers customarily consider a sequence of phases, or steps, when planning the study. These steps may vary in their sequence and number depending on the purpose of the study and the style of the investigator. Abdellah and Levine (1965) list 12 major steps. Polit and Hungler (1987) describe 15 steps that "normally occur in sequence." Diers (1979) identifies nine "elements of all studies." Fox (1982) extends the list of stages to 20. Seaman and Verhonick (1982) cut the number of phases to 4. Treece and Treece (1982) group them into a list of 5. Sweeney and

Oliveri (1981) place the number of steps at 12, and Woods and Catanzaro (1988) specify eight steps in what they call the "linear sequence in positivist-empiricist research." All this goes to show that whether they are called steps, phases, or elements, parts of the process are likely to be expressed in different forms and numbers depending on the level of inquiry and type of study. In some cases the steps are rearranged, and in others some are omitted. Research, however, is a process, and by definition it has some number of steps that occur in relation to one another. This section is intended not to put forth a rigid set of steps but rather to use the metaphor of steps to describe the general thinking of most investigators who plan a deductive study. (The sequence is quite different in studies designed to generate theory rather than test it. See Chapters 12 and 13.) My list, for the purpose of clarity and comprehensiveness, has *ten* modular, mobile, and flexible steps. They are

1. stating a research problem

2. defining the purpose of the research

3. reviewing related literature

4. formulating hypotheses and defining variables

5. selecting the research design

6. selecting the population and sample

7. conducting a pilot study

8. collecting the data

9. analyzing the data

10. communicating conclusions

Each of these steps is taken up in comprehensive detail for the consumer of nursing research (in Part II), and for the conductor of research (in Part III). To give you a sense of the whole picture, however, I describe each step briefly here.

Step 1. Stating a Research Problem

An investigator's task initially involves moving from a broad area of interest to a more circumscribed problem that specifies exactly what he or she intends to study. Most investigators try to define their research problems as precisely as possible. A problem is often stated in the form of a question. Here are some examples from published nursing research studies:

■ How many different treatments for pressure sores are advocated by nurses, and what rationales are given for their use?

- Do mothers who are not given a prepartum enema have higher rates of contamination than mothers who are given an enema?

- Do different postoperative activity schedules affect the recovery of physical fitness among athletes?

- Is there a relationship between types of care of indwelling urethral catheters and the incidence of urinary tract infection?

- What is the optimal time needed to obtain an accurate oral temperature with a glass thermometer?

- What is the effect of low-frequency auditory and kinesthetic stimulation on neurological functioning of the premature infant?

If a study problem is too broad or vague, proceeding to subsequent stages of the process becomes very confusing. This is true even in the instance of field research and qualitative analysis, where the study problem per se may "emerge" from the data after a researcher enters the field (see chapters 12 and 13.) A research question, according to Brink and Wood (1988), p. 2), *"is an explicit query about a problem or issue that can be challenged, examined, analyzed, and will yield useful new information."*

Step 2. Defining the Purpose of the Research

The second step is sometimes called defining the rationale of the study. It is the researcher's statement of *why* the question is important and what use the answer will serve. It lets the reader or funding agency know what to expect from the study. If the investigator's purpose is highly expedient—that is, just to fulfill requirements for a course or promotion—most of your colleagues in the scientific community will perceive it. The purpose of a study also influences its review by an institutional review board (see Chapter 3). Many nursing studies are challenged on the basis that they seem to be exercises in methodology with no real or even conceivable benefit to anyone. A trivial purpose will influence judgments about the risk-benefit ratio if human subjects are involved. An excellent example of the statement of a study's purpose is the report of Kathryn Barnard's (1973) classic research on the effects of environmental stimulation on the sleep of premature infants:

> Previous work with full term neonates and older infants supports the general notion that particular kinds of stimulation assist in the regulation of sleep and arousal status. Given this evidence and the increasing evidence that quiet sleep in the immature infant can improve neurological development . . . *the purpose of the current investigation was to study the effect of regular, controlled stimulation on the neurological functioning in the infant born prematurely* (p. 15).

Step 3. Reviewing Related Literature

If researchers want their study to build on, confirm, or even transcend the existing knowledge in a discipline and thereby qualify as a real contribution to science, they must know what has already been done. A review of the literature provides the researcher with ideas for defining concepts and instruments for their measurement (see Chapter 8). A theoretical framework is an essay in which the investigator relates the existing concepts and theories and research methods and findings to his or her study question and purpose (Brink and Wood 1988). At the least, constructing such a framework provides relevant concepts for the research; at best, it can give the researcher a full awareness of facts, issues, prior findings, theories, and instruments that might be related to the study question (see Chapter 9).

Step 4. Formulating Hypotheses and Defining Variables

Hypotheses are statements of the relationship between two or more concepts, or variables (see Chapter 4). Some studies are intended to *develop* hypotheses (exploratory, descriptive, and grounded theory designs), and others are intended to *test* hypotheses using the statistical principles in Chapters 14 and 15. Stating hypotheses requires not only that there be sufficient knowledge on a topic to make a prediction about the outcome of a study but also that the researcher specify definitions for the variables under investigation in measurable terms. Finally, the investigator must articulate the relationship between or among the variables. Hypotheses can be explicitly stated, as Sitzman and her colleagues (1983) did in their study of biofeedback training:

HYPOTHESIS (H_I): Emphysema and chronic bronchitic patients who receive a biofeedback training program to decrease their respiratory rate will have a significantly decreased respiratory rate at the end of the training program and one-month follow-up.

HYPOTHESIS (H_{II}): Emphysema and chronic bronchitic patients who decreased their respiratory rate by the end of the biofeedback training program will have significantly increased their tidal volume at the end of the training program and at one-month follow-up (p. 219).

Hypotheses (H) may also be stated as null hypotheses (H_0) (see Chapter 8), which essentially test the idea that *there are no significant differences* in what it called the criterion, dependent, or outcome variable other than *what can be attributed to chance*. Because stating hypotheses requires the investigator to specify the concepts being studied, it is also important at this point to determine how these variables are going to be defined for the purpose of measuring them. For example, social support might be defined as a score on a written self-report scale, or inventory. This step is called **operational definition** of the variables. If you do a convincing job, your study is said to have construct, or concept, validity. The ideas of validity and measurement will be thoroughly discussed in subsequent chapters (see Chapters 4 and 10).

Step 5. Selecting the Research Design

A research design is a well-thought-out, systematic, and even controlled plan for finding answers to study questions. It offers a roadmap or blueprint for organizing a study, from methods of data collection through methods of data analysis. Chapter 5 covers the array of possibilities that are available for structuring the research plan.

Step 6. Selecting the Population and Sample

Once researchers have reduced a general idea of interest down to a specific study question, reviewed the related literature, and decided on a plan for designing their study, they must choose a study population and select a sample. A **population** is the group to be studied. To whom should the study's findings apply? Populations that have been the focus of recent nursing studies include divorced fathers, older persons, hospitalized children, disadvantaged minorities, depressed women, nursing mothers, patients with cancer, persons with AIDS, patients who have had surgery, and nursing students. The **sample** refers to those elements of a population from whom data will actually be collected and from whom generalizations to the population will be made. The details of various kinds of sample and procedures for selecting them are spelled out in Chapter 8.

Step 7. Conducting a Pilot Study

If you are an undergraduate student just venturing forth on your first attempt at using the method of scientific inquiry to solve a problem, answer a question, or make a decision, it may not be feasible or practical to do a small-scale practice run, called a **pilot study**. If you are working on a master's thesis, doctoral dissertation, or postgraduate research, however, you can learn a lot about the strengths and weaknesses of your larger project's intended design, sample size, and data-collection instrument by doing a pilot study. Such attempts have been so helpful in strengthening nursing studies by weeding out problems in advance that many funding agencies are not inclined to approve study proposals for which no pilot study has been conducted.

Step 8. Collecting the Data

The scientific method is characterized by a reliance on information collected from the empirical, or observable, world to make statements about what is true. Any study that goes beyond "armchair speculation" eventually requires the researcher to collect data. Data sources may be people, documents, or laboratory materials, and data-collection instruments may include interviews, questionnaires, physiological tests, and psychological tests. All of these possibilities are covered in depth in Chapters 10, 11, and 12. The basic point, however, is that by moving either from observation to idea (called *inductive theory*) or from idea to observation (called *deductive theory*), the scientific method relies on an *empirical* basis for discovering or testing knowledge. Data relevant to the variables being studied are collected using the researcher's senses and measurement tools. The amounts of time and energy required for this step in the process vary according to the research design. Field studies, historical research, surveys and most experiments all demand a lot of both during this phase.

Step 9. Analyzing the Data

The next step in the research process involves taking the data that have been collected apart and reorganizing them so that the researcher can make some sense of them in relation to the study question, research objectives, or stated hypotheses. Analyses of numerical data can be accomplished using the statistical procedures discussed in Chapters 14 and 15. Qualitative data such as open-ended questionnaire responses, observational field notes, interview transcripts, case studies, documents, and the like can be analyzed according to a variety of approaches explained in Chapter 13. The most important part about this step is to *have a plan in mind, the requisite skills for doing it, and the realization that this work is the source of answers to the original research questions.*

Step 10. Communicating Conclusions

The researcher's challenge at the final stage is to explain the results of the investigation and link them with the existing body of knowledge in the discipline. Whether published articles or books, spoken presentations, or both, are used, the study's real contribution cannot be judged unless the conclusions are communicated to colleagues and critics (see Chapter 18). As Polit and Hungler (1987) put it, "Even the most compelling hypothesis, the most careful and thorough study, and the most dramatic results are of no value to the scientific community if they are unknown." Communicating the conclusions, interpreting the real meaning and implications of the findings, recognizing the study's possible limitations, and suggesting directions for future lines of inquiry culminate the research process and provide the investigators with yet another chance to synthesize their imaginative, insightful, engaged style with their rigorous, systematic, analytical one.

Most researchers acknowledge these steps as conventions, or recipes, and then with creativity, imagination, and pragmatism vary and adapt them to the unique situation they are addressing.

The History of Nursing Research

In 1986 the National Center for Nursing Research (NCNR) was established as part of the National Institutes of Health (NIH) by congressional mandate. The mandate for the NCNR is to fund nursing research and research training related to:

- patient care
- promotion of health
- prevention of disease
- mitigation of effects of acute and chronic illness and disabilities

The NCNR is expected to place nursing research in the mainstream of scientific investigation focused on our nation's health. Nursing research has a history, which provides the backdrop for this step forward. Earlier landmarks are summarized in Box 1–1.

Nursing Research in the 1980s

As Box 1–1 illustrates, since at least the early 1950s nursing research has received increased federal funding and professional support. Centers for research have been developed, the number of doctorally prepared nurses engaged in the scientific enterprise has increased, and avenues for communicating research reports (journals, conferences, and meetings) have expanded. Nursing research is viewed as a legitimate field of interest not only for students at the entry level but also for *all nurses*. Spruck's 1980 National League For Nursing (NLN) survey of 286 accredited baccalaureate nursing programs revealed that research content was included as required coursework in 83% of the schools, and the remainder were moving toward incorporating a research component. A second survey, by Thomas and Price (1980), obtained usable responses from 205 of the 291 NLN-accredited baccalaureate nursing programs in the United States. Of them, 198 reported explicit provision for teaching nursing research in their programs; the remaining seven were in the process of developing research content. In sum, the question "Should nursing research be taught at all levels of nursing education?" has now become "What should be taught about nursing research, at what level, and how?"

Evidence abounds that our profession has reached a consensus that some involvement in research at all levels of educational preparation is necessary for the advancement of the nursing profession and the welfare of patients. With such an overpowering agreement, one would expect that nursing research in the 1980s and early 1990s would be an unquestionable success story. Unfortunately, this is not the case. McClure (1981) summarizes the problem:

Far too few practitioners are genuinely concerned about research process or outcomes. . . . The vast majority of active nurses are concerned about the professionalization of nursing . . . but they have little knowledge of and even less interest in nursing research. . . . Our practice is almost entirely founded on personal wisdom rather than scientific conclusions (p. 66).

"To do," not "to study," sums up a prevailing attitude that day-to-day clinical problems are too far removed from nursing research and that research seems esoteric, dull, or even meaningless to the practicing nurse.

Accounting for the Discrepancy

What accounts for such a dramatic discrepancy between what nursing leaders espouse as a value and the negative attitudes and avoidance behaviors many clinicians and nursing students express? McClure (1981) cites the need to create an environment in the service arena that supports research by nurses. She also notes what she calls the "faculty withdrawal syndrome," which has resulted in:

1. lack of patient-focused research

2. lack of interdisciplinary research with other health-care professionals

3. estrangement of service from education

4. devaluing by nurses of academic preparation

5. devaluing by others, both inside and outside the health-care delivery system, of academic preparation for nurses

6. isolation of nursing faculty from service settings

The following can be added to McClure's list:

7. lack of a cumulative knowledge base for nursing practice

8. lack of programmatically oriented research, as opposed to small, unimportant, independent studies

9. lack of replication of nursing studies

Finally, echoing authors who have lamented the substitution of "tenacity for inquiry" and an addiction to a "pseudotechnical mentality," Wilson (1982) cites the tendency to view research according to an overly dogmatic, "cookbook" approach as a block to nurses' full expression of their creative talent through scientific discoveries with relevance to practice.

Box 1–1   Historic Landmarks in Nursing Research (Continued)

Date	Event	Outcomes
1853–1856	Florence Nightingale records detailed observations about the impact of nursing care during the Crimean War.	She fosters the idea that nursing practice should be based on disciplined inquiry.
1923	The Goldmark Report is published, after a comprehensive study of nursing education sponsored by the Committee for the Study of Nursing Education and funded by the Rockefeller Foundation.	The report maintains that advanced preparation is essential for teachers, administrators, and public health nurses. It encourages the hiring of registered nurses for hospital care to free nursing students to study. Yale University's School of Nursing is established. The Vanderbilt University and Western Reserve University schools of nursing follow. The real pioneers had been Teachers' College, Columbia University (1899) and the University of Minnesota (1910), the first schools to emphasize the higher education of nurses.
1948	The Brown Report is published.	The report recommends studies of in-service education, nursing functions, nursing teams, practical nurses, roles and attitudes, nurse–patient relationships, hospital environments, and the economic security of nurses. The National Accrediting Service is begun in 1950 under Dr. Helen Nahm to establish a sound method of accrediting nursing education programs.

(Continued)

Box 1–1   Historic Landmarks in Nursing Research (Continued)

Date	Event	Outcomes
1952	*Nursing Research*, the first official journal for reporting studies related to nursing and health, is published.	Nursing investigators are provided with a means for communicating the results of their research.
1953	The Institute of Research and Service in Nursing Education is founded at Columbia University under the directorship of Dr. Helen Bunge.	It becomes the first formal structure within a university for conducting nursing studies.
1955	The American Nurses' Foundation, supported by the ANA, is established.	It serves as a receiver, administrator, and donor of grants for research in nursing.
1955	The nursing research grants and fellowship programs of the Division of Nursing of the U.S. Public Health Service are established.	Grants for research into causes, diagnosis, treatment, control, and prevention of physical and mental diseases are authorized.
1957	The Department of Nursing in The Walter Reed Army Institute of Research is established.	It parallels research by physicians and dentists into patient care; develops a core of nurse practitioners-researchers.
1963	The Surgeon General's Consultant Group on Nursing issues a report.	The report recommends a substantial increase in federal support for research in nursing and the training of nurse researchers.
1963	Lydia Hall conducts a classic study of care of the chronically ill patients at the Loeb Rehabilitation Center in New York.	Examples of research on patient care begin to influence the emergence of conceptual frameworks to define the nature of nursing practice.
1966	A team of nurse researchers collaborates with social scientists at the University of California at San Francisco on studies of death and dying.	Sociological methods and concepts begin to appear in the repertoire of nurse researchers.

(Continued)

Box 1–1   **Historic Landmarks in Nursing Research (Continued)**

Date	Event	Outcomes
1968	The Mugar Library at Boston University establishes a nursing archive.	It fosters nursing research and brings together a significant collection on the topic.
1970	The Lysaught Report is published by the National Commission for the study of Nursing.	The report urges that research in both nursing education and practice be financed.
1976	Elizabeth Carnegie reports a steady increase in the number of clinical investigations published in *Nursing Research*.	The value of clinical, or practice-related, research emerges as dominant over studies of nurses themselves or of education and administration.
1976	The Commission on Research of the ANA recommends that preparation for nursing research begin at the undergraduate level.	Courses and integrated objectives requiring some level of research competence appear in nursing curricula.
1968–present	The Western Interstate Commission for Higher Education in Nursing compiles data-collection instruments for practice and education; it sponsors conferences and workshops on conducting research and applying findings.	The visibility of nursing's growing involvement in research increases.
1970s	A number of refereed research journals for nursing are established, incuding *Advances in Nursing Science, Research in Nursing and Health*, and *The Western Journal of Research in Nursing*.	Nurse researchers have more vehicles for communicating their study findings to a growing community of nurse scientists.
1986	University of Colorado establishes Center for Human Caring in The School of Nursing.	Nontraditional methodologies from humanities are applied to nursing.

(Continued)

Box 1–1	Historic Landmarks in Nursing Research (Continued)	
Date	**Event**	**Outcomes**
1980s–present	Private and public agencies including the National Center for Nursing Research of NIH fund nursing research.	Nurse researchers have increased access to grant support to fund nursing studies.
1980s–present	Doctoral programs for nurses in the United States grow in numbers and quality.	By 1988 there were more than 35 doctoral programs and over 4,000 nurses with doctoral degrees.

Characteristics of the New Era of Nursing Research

The approach to science and research expounded in this text involves closing the gap between research and practice. Research does not become nursing research merely because it is done by a nurse. Many authors have distinguished between what they call nursing research and research in nursing. **Nursing research**, on the one hand, is research into the process of care and the clinical problems encountered in the practice of nursing. **Research in nursing**, on the other hand, is the broader study of people and the nursing profession, including historical, ethical, and policy studies. If we agree that the business of nursing is *practice* and also agree that the business of nursing research is answering questions and solving problems about that practice, then nursing practice and nursing research share the common goal of *improving nursing care*.

Carrying out this emphasis on nursing practice, the ANA Cabinet on Nursing Research (1985) has identified priorities for clinical nursing research during the 1980s. They are summarized in Box 1–2.

Research does not have to be complicated to be good and useful. We must be wary of trying at all cost to adhere rigidly to methods that were developed in the natural, or "hard," sciences. They may well be inappropriate for studying nursing phenomena in a natural setting. Emerging alternative methods are increasingly interesting to nurses involved in clinical research.

The shift in recent years toward describing nursing phenomena, evaluating outcomes of nursing intervention, and building empirically based theories that will be the cornerstones of a nursing science does not preclude the value of what Diers (1983) calls "clinical scholarship":

Scholarship is different from research. It implies . . . contemplation [and] the stretching of the mind for new insights. . . . Good research reporting may well fall into the definition of scholarship; mechanical reports which provide data but not insight, do not (p. 3).

Tomorrow's nursing will continue to emphasize studies of the interaction of physiological and psychosocial mechanisms in human experiences of stress and coping, evaluations of nursing interventions, the transfer of research findings into textbooks and practice, a focus on high-risk and underserved groups such as the elderly and minorities, and the creation of a body of scientific nursing knowledge. And today's student of research in nursing will be involved in its conduct and application.

Nursing Research and You

My own introductory course in nursing research is scheduled from 3:00 P.M. to 6:00 P.M. on Wednesdays in a huge, windowless lecture hall where the 52 RN students doze, having been in classes nonstop since 8:00 that morning. Almost without exception, students' initial reactions to the course are negative.

Student Reactions—Before

1. *Inadequacy*: "In every new nursing class, I'm ready to jump in and love it. But the thought of starting the research course evoked memories of my statistics instructor frantically scribbling statistical formulas and computations all over the blackboard that I just couldn't follow. I didn't understand all this validity and reliability language and, frankly, was afraid I might not even pass. Research is just not my level. Leave it to the scholars and nursing leaders."

2. *Resentment*: "I came back to get my degree because I want to be a head nurse in a CCU (critical care unit). I have absolutely no intention of becoming a teacher or of making research my career. I don't understand why our whole class is required to take the research course! My schedule is so packed that I can't take the elective in pharmacology that would really be practical to me in my clinical work."

3. *Boredom*: "I went into nursing because I find working with people exciting, interesting, and challenging. Research makes me think of cold, objective, eccentric scientists in laboratories, people who carried slide rules around in their pockets in high school, and pages of dull tables and charts full of numbers. My interests are music and play therapy for kids. Research with all its rigor, precision, and control sounds totally boring to me."

These unpleasant but normal feelings, if unchanged by teachers, textbooks, and experiences, probably account in part for why much of nursing practice relies

---

Box 1–2   American Nurses' Association Priorities for Nursing Research

Promote health, well-being, and ability to care for oneself among all age, social, and cultural groups.

Minimize or prevent behaviorally and environmentally induced health problems that compromise the quality of life and reduce productivity.

Minimize the negative effects of new health technologies on the adaptive abilities of individuals and families experiencing acute or chronic health problems.

Ensure that the care needs of particularly vulnerable groups, such as the elderly, children with congenital health problems, individuals from diverse cultures, the mentally ill, and the poor, are met in effective and acceptable ways.

Classify nursing practice phenomena.

Ensure that principles of ethics guide nursing research.

Develop instruments to measure nursing outcomes. Develop integrative methodologies for the holistic study of human beings as they relate to their families and life-styles.

Design and evaluate alternative models for delivering health care and for administering health-care systems so that nurses will be able to balance high quality and cost-effectiveness in meeting the nursing needs of identified populations.

Evaluate the effectiveness of alternative approaches to nursing education for the kind of practice that requires broad knowledge and a wide repertoire of skills, and for the kind of practice that requires specialized knowledge and a focused set of skills.

Identify and analyze historical and contemporary factors that influence the shaping of nursing professionals' involvement in national health policy development.

Source: American Nurses' Association, Cabinet on Nursing Research. *Directions for Nursing Research.* Kansas City, Mo.: 1985.

---

on conventional wisdom instead of a scientific basis for direction and guidance. If, however, research can be translated into the fascinating, versatile, funny, and powerful tool that it often is, students' attitudes and reactions can be transformed.

Student Reactions—After

1. *Identification:* "Researchers are human, interesting, flexible, and creative. What a great discovery! An intelligent, critical mind is a pleasure to behold, and to nurture. I think I'll be a better nurse because of it. I'd never thought of myself as a potential leader or writer. Now, I feel I've got the skills and motivation to try it. The pilot study I did for the research course has been accepted for

publication in the *Western Journal for Research in Nursing*! I've made scholarliness and intellectual craftmanship part of my definition of a truly professional nurse."

2. *Competence*: "My professional skills of using the library, reading, and writing clearly developed more in the research course than in the entire rest of the program. I've learned an entirely new way of approaching clinical questions, and I think the care and advice I give to patients will be better because of it."

3. *Demystification*: "Realizing that research isn't as rigid, structured, useless, and dogmatic as some would say decreased my anxieties about keeping up with it at least for applications to my practice. I'm no longer reluctant to pick up a copy of *Nursing Research* magazine."

4. *Enthusiasm*: "The subject of nursing research has become very important to me and I think it's critical to our profession's development. I have a new respect and enthusiasm about nursing's developing scientific basis and even hope to get my doctorate someday."

Learning about the scientific method and the research process is undoubtedly largely an intellectual task. But attitudes and values can be shaped as well. Nursing research allows you to bring the engaged and the analytic ways of knowing together in ways that make you a better nurse. A true scholar and scientist is not created by being taught technical methods, tools, or even a theoretical base. A true scholar and scientist transcends these tools and is the master of their use. You will learn the tools of research in the chapters that follow, and they will seem a lot less esoteric and formidable. But it is the wisdom acquired from using them in a spirit of inquiry that will make you a member of the scholarly and scientific community in nursing's future.

Guidelines for Critique

- What intellectual tradition underpins the study?

- Is the research basic, or is it applied?

- How relevant is the research to nursing practice? Determine at what stage it would fall on the pure-applied continuum.

- What type of research is it?
  exploratory
  descriptive
  explanatory
  experimental or quasi-experimental
  methodological

- Is it nursing research, or is it research in nursing?
- Does the study fall into a priority area for clinical nursing research?
- Has the study been influenced by one of nursings' historic landmarks?

SUMMARY OF KEY IDEAS AND TERMS

✓ The value and usefulness of the scientific approach for making real-world decisions about nursing practice are clearer if you realize that:

- Science doesn't have to be dogmatic and mechanistic.
- Science involves a process of discovery as well as a process of proof.
- Science requires interpretation of facts, and these interpretations can change.
- Most of the principles and topics for nursing research exist in the practice of clinical nursing.

✓ The *scientific approach* offers an alternative tool for making decisions and solving practical problems that can substitute for or augment trial and error and common sense, authority and tradition, inspiration and intuition, and logical reasoning.

✓ *Scientific inquiry* is based on specific assumptions about the existence of a basic natural order in the world. It has the characteristics of self-correction and empiricism. And it aims to develop explanations, called theories.

✓ The positivist and symbolic interactionist traditions are two distinctly different perspectives on the philosophy of science that influence the kinds of study a nurse might conduct.

✓ It is possible to classify types of nursing studies along a pure-applied continuum based on their relevance to nursing practice. Studies can also be classified according to their purpose and study design.

✓ The *research process* is the tool of science. It involves a series of progressive steps that usually include some version of the following:

- stating the study problem

- defining the purpose of the research

- reviewing related literature

- formulating hypotheses and defining variables

- selecting the research design

- selecting a population and a sample

- conducting a pilot study

- collecting data

- analyzing data

- communicating conclusions

✓ The history of nursing research dates back to the 1850s. Since then, landmark events have occurred to increase the amount, quality, and availability of nursing studies dramatically, particularly those studies dealing with nursing practice rather than nurses, nursing education, and administration.

✓ It is likely that at least understanding and using the results of nursing studies to improve practice will become an essential part of all nursing education programs.

✓ Bridging the gap between nursing research and nursing practice and avoiding an overly dogmatic approach can transform indifferent and negative attitudes toward research among clinicians and students.

References

Abdellah F, Levine E: *Better Patient Care Through Nursing Research*. New York: Macmillan, 1965.

Ackerman JS: Two styles: A challenge to higher education. *Daedalus* Summer 1969:855–868.

American Nurses' Association: *Nursing: A Social Policy Statement*. Kansas City, Mo.: 1980.

American Nurses' Association, Cabinet on Nursing Research: *Directions for Nursing Research*. Kansas City, Mo.: 1985.

Barnard K: The effect of stimulation on the sleep behavior of the premature infant. *Commun Nurs Res* 1973; 6:12–33.

Brink J, Wood MJ: *Basic Steps in Planning Nursing Research*, 3rd ed. Philadelphia: Lippincott, 1988.

Bronowski J: *Science and Human Values*. New York: Julian Messner, 1956.

Cooperative Graduate Education in Nursing: *Nursing Research Television Cassettes #1*. New

York: American Journal of Nursing Co., 1975.

Demand for nurses does a drastic turnaround. *Miami Herald* January 2, 1983.

Demi AS: Adjustment to widowhood after a sudden death: Suicide and nonsuicide survivors compared. *Commun Nurs Res* 1978; 11:91–99.

Diers D: *Research in Nursing Practice.* Philadelphia: Lippincott, 1979.

Diers D: Clinical scholarship. *Image* Winter 1983; 15:3.

Fox DJ: *Fundamentals of Research in Nursing*, 4th ed. Norwalk, Conn.: Appleton-Century-Crofts, 1982.

Hadley BJ et al: Effect on postoperative recovery rate and comfort of four approaches to nursing care of dogs: A pilot study. *Commun Nurs Res* 1970; 3:121–137.

Jacox A: Theory construction in nursing: An overview. *Nurs Res* January/February 1974; 23:4–13.

Kerlinger FN: *Foundations of Behavioral Research.* New York: Holt, Rinehart & Winston, 1966.

Kueffner M: Passage through hospitalization of severely burned, isolated school-aged children. *Commun Nurs Res* 1976; 7:181–197.

Marshall LA: Patient reaction to sound in a coronary care unit. *Commun Nurs Res* 1972; 5:93–97.

May KA: Three phases in the development of father involvement in pregnancy. *Nurs Res* November/December 1982; 31:337–342.

McClure ML: Promoting practice-based research: A critical need. *J Nurs Admin* November/December 1981; 11:66–70.

McCorkle R, Young K: Development of a symptom distress scale. *Commun Nurs Res* 1978; 11:5–6.

McKeever LC: Equality and quality of care for older women. *Calif Nurse* September 1983:5.

Nakagawa H et al: An epidemiological study of psychiatric symptom pattern change. *Commun Nurs Res* 1972; 5:9–27.

Panger D: *The Dance of the Wild Mouse.* Glen Ellen, Calif: Entwhistle Books, 1979.

Polit D, Hungler B: *Nursing Research*, 3rd ed. Philadelphia: Lippincott, 1987.

Prior ME: *Science and the Humanities.* Evanston, Ill.: Northwestern University Press, 1962.

Schuster HH: Developing a psychometric instrument for the use of children's drawing in cross-cultural research: Problems, procedures, and potentials. *Commun Nurs Res* 1971; 4:151–158.

Seaman C, Verhonick PJ: *Research Methods for Undergraduate Students in Nursing*, 2nd ed. New York: Appleton-Century-Crofts, 1982.

Sitzman J et al: Biofeedback training for reduced respiratory rate in chronic obstructive pulmonary disease: A preliminary study. *Nurs Res* July/August 1983; 32:218–223.

Sjoberg G, Nett R: *A Methodology for Social Research.* New York: Harper & Row, 1968.

Snyder MC: *Calif Nurse* September 1983:2.

Spruck M: Teaching research at the undergraduate level. *Nurs Res* July/August 1980; 29:257–259.

Sweeney MA, Oliveri P: *An Introduction to Nursing Research.* Philadelphia: Lippincott, 1981.

Thomas B, Price M: Research preparation in baccalaureate nursing education. *Nurs Res* July/August 1980; 29:259–261.

Treece EW, Treece JW: *Elements of Research in Nursing.* St. Louis: Mosby, 1982.

Voda AM et al: Quantification of self-report data from two-dimensional body diagrams. *West J Nurs Res* Fall 1980; 2:707–729.

Walike B: A physiological and behavioral approach to understanding the mechanisms of obesity and anorexia. *Commun Nurs Res* 1973; 6:201–211.

Walike B et al: Patient problems related to tube feeding. *Commun Nurs Res* 1975; 7:89–112.

Waters VH et al: Technical and professional nursing. *Nurs Res* December/January 1972; 21:124–131.

Wilson HS: The meaning of current dance forms to adolescent girls: An exploratory study. *Nurs Res* November/December 1969; 17:513–519.

Wilson HS: Fairing: Control of staff work in a healing community for schizophrenics. *J Psychiatr Nurs* March 1978; 16:24–38.

Wilson HS: Teaching research in nursing: Issues and strategies. *West J Nurs Res* 1982; 4:366–377.

Woods NF, Catanzaro M: *Nursing Research Theory and Practice.* St Louis: Mosby, 1988.

2

Using Research To Improve Nursing Practice

HOLLY SKODOL WILSON

Chapter Objectives

After reading this chapter, the student should be able to:

- Delineate investigative roles for nurses at all levels of educational preparation

- Describe progress made toward building a scientific base for clinical nursing practice

- Formulate directions for the future of the nursing research that will promote the goals of scientific inquiry

- Enumerate areas of consensus about research priorities for the 1980s and 1990s

- Compare and contrast four levels of reading

- Apply useful reading techniques

- Demonstrate skills of systematic skimming and analytic reading levels to comprehend a report of research findings

- Use indexes, periodical catalogs, and reference librarians to find research literature relevant to nursing

- Demonstrate familiarity with nursing's primary research journals

- Explain the significance of institutional and regional models for applying research findings to practice

- Realize the value and relevance of research in nursing to the development of the profession and to the quality of patient care

In This Chapter...

Voices in the vanguard of leadership in nursing call for bridging the gap between research and practice, a gap sometimes viewed as an abyss. This is a two-way process: making nursing practice (rather than education or administration) a more frequent focus for research, and increasing the application of research findings to practice. Editorials in nursing journals, officers in professional associations, and probably your own teachers all assert that without an empirically grounded body of scientific knowledge on which to base clinical practice, nursing's stance as a profession is weak. Everybody seems to agree that it is critical that nursing develop a scientific base and that research is the way to get it. Florence Downs (1981), editor of *Nursing Research*, writes: "We are and for some time have been a profession in a hurry. Yet, research is not something that can be brewed over night and ingested the next morning" (p. 332). Downs goes on to remind us that "premature consumption of findings certainly might be hazardous to someone's health."

Applying research to practice would be a lot easier if:

- the scientific community were closer to bringing some sense of order to the proliferating nursing research literature

- all nursing students were better prepared to find, read, and understand it

- service organizations were structured to foster such applications

On the first point, Gortner (1980) writes: "An onlooker might characterize most nursing research as discrete, nonaggregated studies of isolated empirical phenomena for which the underlying science or explanatory theory is not known or not yet well-defined" (p. 205). She adds: "Were we to dream about the vitality and credibility of our science 10 years hence, it would be that a number of well-defined, programmatic areas of research could be ongoing, each containing not one or two, but a dozen or more investigators" (p. 206). That leaves us, however, with the second and third points. Even if the quest to identify and build a scientific knowledge base that would replace traditions and habits is increasingly successful, practicing nurses, perhaps even you, will continue to experience frustration. For one thing, the knowledge base grounded in research findings that is needed to practice intelligently is hard to locate. For another, even when you do find it, its presentation in the traditional scientific format may be difficult for you to interpret. Finally, practice agencies are rarely structured to encourage change based on systematic appraisals of nursing research findings.

This chapter gives you some beginning tools essential to becoming an astute and unintimidated consumer of research findings. These tools can actually shape your future clinical nursing practice. In it you will find support for an investigative role of some kind for all nurses.

- It introduces you to a system for "active reading" that can be used on everything you read, including the most esoteric research protocol.

- It discusses solutions to problems you might have in finding and then becoming familiar with research literature.

- It shows you step by step how to comprehend a report of study findings and how to draw clinical implications from these findings.

- Finally, it summarizes characteristics that foster a research orientation in practice settings and tells some success stories about recent projects that have advanced the profession's commitment at long last to make research every nurse's business.

Basic Nursing on Research

Past Progress

The idea that research findings should be used to improve patient care is well-accepted among contemporary nurses. For at least ten years, nurses have shared the eagerness, expectation, and hope that nursing is at last about to achieve professional status. The strongest force in that direction has been nurses' growing progress in building a scientific base for nursing practice. We have witnessed the study of research, reserved in our not-so-distant past for the master's, doctoral, and postdoctoral levels, integrated into almost all basic entry-level programs in some form (see Box 2–1). Similarly, just as some degree of research competence is becoming part of every nurse's educational preparation, nursing research departments are springing up in hospitals and health care agencies. According to Parker and Labadie (1983), the functions of these departments include:

- providing leadership for nurses interested in designing and participating in a variety of scientific investigations

- providing consultation for nurses in investigative roles

- conducting seminars and workshops to help nurses learn research methods

- devising strategies to increase and intensify research activity within the agency

- participating in establishing guidelines for protection of the rights of human subjects (see Chapter 3)

- serving on research committees made up of staff nurses

- motivating nurses to become actively involved in seeking solutions to patient problems through scientific inquiry

- considering methods to share significant research findings

- coordinating research displays at appropriate occasions

- interacting with nurses employed in educational institutions to achieve shared goals

- seeking out available community resources for research

Dennis and Strickland (1987) studied the role of the clinical nurse researcher in inpatient settings. They discovered four major models for implementing the role all of which required organizational and colleague support for both visibility and viability. The National Center for Nursing Research at NIH serves to support and link together activities of existing nursing research and scientific organizations, such as the American Nurses' Foundation (ANF) and the American Academy of Nursing (AAN).

Present Barriers

Despite this rather impressive past progress, problems still arise when the means for integrating nursing research findings into practice decisions are explored. Unlike some disciplines, nursing has not yet systematically reviewed all of its important research reports and extracted the knowledge that is valid and relevant for practice. The *Annual Review of Nursing Research*, edited by Harriet Werley and Joyce Fitzpatrick and published in its first issue by the Springer Company in late 1983, is a move in the desired direction.

A second barrier is that, despite repeated acknowledgments that a scientist's responsibility includes *replicating work to establish the limits of a study's findings*, few examples of repeating prior scientific work can be found in either nursing literature or nursing practice. Isolated studies seldom offer findings that can be a direct and valid basis for making changes in practice, because the real world rarely matches conditions in a single study design.

Because nursing is not just a profession and not just a scientific discipline but *a professional discipline*, nurses can also assume responsibility for going beyond the

Box 2–1   Investigative Functions of a Nurse at Various Educational Levels

Associate Degree in Nursing

1. Demonstrates awareness of the value or relevance of research in nursing.

2. Assists in identifying problem areas in nursing practice.

3. Assists in collection of data within an established structured format.

Baccalaureate Degree in Nursing

1. Reads, interprets, and evaluates research for applicability to nursing practice.

2. Identifies nursing problems that need to be investigated and participates in the implementation of scientific studies.

3. Uses nursing practice as a means of gathering data for refining and extending practice.

4. Applies established findings of nursing and other health-related research to nursing practice.

5. Shares research findings with colleagues.

Master's Degree in Nursing

1. Analyzes and reformulates nursing practice problems so that scientific knowledge and scientific methods can be used to find solutions.

2. Enhances the quality and clinical relevance of nursing research by providing expertise in clinical problems and by providing knowledge about the way in which these clinical services are delivered.

3. Facilitates investigations of problems in clinical settings through such activities as contributing to a climate supportive of investigative activities, collaborating with others in investigations, and enhancing nursing's access to clients and data.

4. Conducts investigations for the purpose of monitoring the quality of the practice of nursing in a clinical setting.

5. Assists others to apply scientific knowledge in nursing practice.

Doctoral Degree in Nursing or a Related Discipline

1. Provides leadership for the integration of scientific knowledge with other sources of knowledge for the advancement of practice.

2. Conducts investigations to evaluate the contribution of nursing activities to the well-being of clients.

3. Develops methods to monitor the quality of the practice of nursing in a clinical setting and to evaluate contributions of nursing activities to the well-being of clients.

Graduate of a Research-Oriented Doctoral Program

1. Develops theoretical explanations of phenomena relevant to nursing by empirical research and analytic process.

2. Uses analytical and empirical methods to discover ways to modify or extend existing scientific knowledge so that it is relevant to nursing.

3. Develops methods for scientific inquiry of phenomena relevant to nursing.

Source: American Nurses' Association, Commission on Nursing Research, *Guidelines for the Investigative Function of Nurses*, Kansas City, Mo.: 1981.

traditional scientific dissemination of research in publications or paper presentations. They can translate the information gathered through research into professional practice. In Barnard's (1980) words, "Emphasis should be placed on getting researchers and clinicians to interact. New technologies exist to improve our ability to communicate. We must take them" (p. 212). Futurists predict that communication about research in the next decade will be not only through libraries, bookstores, and periodicals on computer but also through video monitors in individual nurses' offices, homes, and work places. Teleconferencing among investigators and health care agencies has already become common, diminishing the problem of communication delay. (The time lag in making new information available to clinicians is now estimated at two to three years for journals and up to ten years for books.)

Future Prospects

In June 1979 an invitational conference entitled "Knowledge for Practice: Directions for Research in Nursing" was convened by the then Division of Nursing, Bureau of Health Manpower, U.S. Department of Health, Education, and Welfare (now the Department of Health and Human Services). Its objective was to assess nursing research at the time and predict what it would be like in 1990. The conference participants attempted to delineate research topics that would have the greatest potential for improving nursing care. They also recommended strategies for applying nursing research to practice.

In considering the future, Gortner (1980) summarized the past by noting that most early research was commissioned by the nursing profession *to study itself*. Studies of nursing supply, distribution, job satisfaction, job turnover, and education seemed to be direct outgrowths of the need during World War II for an adequate number of nurses to serve both civilian and military demands. By 1970, however, the emphasis had shifted to practice-related nursing research (see Chapter 1). Federally funded studies were carried out at distinguished schools of nursing, including Case Western Reserve University, Ohio State, Wayne State, Yale, and the University of California at Los Angeles and at San Francisco. These studies dealt with topics such as maternal-infant attachment, death and dying, the care of patients with drug and psychiatric problems, and services for geriatric, maternity, pediatric, and surgical patients. Nursing research became a source of hope for establishing a science of health care through systematic study of the problems encountered in nursing practice, the characteristics and health care needs of patients, and the interpersonal interaction between nurses and patients. *In less than 20 years nursing research shifted from the study of the profession itself to the study of phenomena with which nursing is concerned.*

When it comes to the future, Gortner (1980) predicts the emergence of multiple clinical trials of standardized protocols for stress reduction, medication adherence, and care of decubitus ulcers, for example. As these shifts occur, participating in clinical research and using the findings as the basis for modifications in practice will become an important aspect of every nurse's role.

Clinical Research Priorities

In 1974 the Western Council on Higher Education for Nursing (WCHEN) and the Regional Program for Nursing Research Development surveyed 328 nursing faculty members to determine the future research priorities in nursing. What has become known as the *Delphi Survey of Clinical Research Priorities* (1974) revealed 150 priority items in three areas:

1. priorities important to the nursing profession

2. priorities for which nurses should have responsibility

3. priorities that would have the most influence on patient welfare

Box 2–2 lists the top 15 research priorities from the *Delphi Survey* that relate to patient welfare.

In 1980 the Commission on Nursing Research of the ANA highlighted the research-practice link when it issued its definitions, directions, and examples for research in the 1980s; these are presented in Box 2–3. The 1985 Cabinet on Nursing Research updated this original list (see Chapter 1).

The clinician and the researcher need to exchange expertise in order to benefit both patients and the profession. Many authorities, such as Jacox, writing in *Nursing Research* in 1980, believe that research programs that will receive funding in the next decade are most likely to be those that emphasize this collaboration because they:

1. focus on knowledge basic to providing clinical nursing care, such as pain assessment and alleviation or care of a specific population, for example, the frail elderly

2. involve nurses from both academic and practice settings working collaboratively

3. include testing or clinical trials of nursing interventions

4. are undertaken in settings or agencies where research is an integral part of every nurse's role

If you are among the growing number of nurses who are aware of the need to use research findings in your work but still find the idea somewhat intimidating because research reports are hard to find, the jargon is unfamiliar, and the benefits to practice are not easy to determine, the next section of this chapter should help.

Box 2–2   Results of WICHE Delphi Survey of Research Priorities

Rank   Item

1. Determine valid and reliable indicators of quality nursing care.

2. Determine and evaluate interventions by nurses that are most effective in reducing psychological stress of patients.

3. Find means of enhancing the quality of life for aged in institutions.

4. Determine factors that contribute to self-care education of patients with chronic disease.

5. Determine means for greater utilization of research in practice.

6. Determine effective means of communicating, evaluating, and implementing change in practice.

7. Discover effective nursing intervention for alleviating stress in patients with terminal disease.

8. Develop physical and psychological assessment procedures that provide information for improved patient care.

9. Study nursing intervention for the management of pain.

10. Clarify patients' rights and role as decision-makers in their own health care.

11. Explore ways to sensitize nurses to the needs of family members of critically ill patients.

12. Determine effective nursing intervention for reducing respiratory and circulatory complications for surgical patients.

13. Explore means of educating the public to optimize use of the health care system.

14. Establish relationship between clinical nursing research and quality care.

15. Find out which nursing behaviors and care settings are most likely to produce positive effects on individuals or families in a crisis-prone situation.

Source: Delphi Survey of Clinical Research Priorities. Boulder, Colo.: WICHE, 1984.

Box 2–3   ANA Commission on Nursing Research

**Directions for
Research**

Priority should be given
to nursing research that
would generate
knowledge to guide
practice in:

1. promoting health,
   well-being, and
   competency for
   personal care among
   all age groups

2. preventing health
   problems throughout
   the life span that
   have the potential to
   reduce productivity
   and satisfaction

3. decreasing the
   negative impact of
   health problems on
   coping abilities,
   productivity, and
   life satisfaction of
   individuals and
   families

4. ensuring that the
   care needs of
   particularly
   vulnerable groups
   are met through
   appropriate
   strategies

Examples

Examples of research consistent with these priorities
include the following:

1. Identification of determinants (personal and
   environmental, including social support networks)
   of wellness and health functioning in individuals
   and families, e.g., avoidance of abusive behavior
   such as alcoholism and drug use, successful
   adaptation to chronic illness, and coping with the
   last days of life.

2. Identification of phenomena that negatively
   influence the course of recovery and that may be
   alleviated by nursing practice, such as, for
   example, anorexia, diarrhea, sleep deprivation,
   deficiencies in nutrients, electrolyte imbalances,
   and infections.

3. Development and testing of care strategies to do
   the following:

   • Facilitate individuals' ability to adopt and
     maintain health enhancing behaviors (e.g.,
     alterations in diet and exercise).

   • Enhance patients' ability to manage acute and
     chronic illness in such a way as to minimize or
     eliminate the necessity of institutionalization
     and to maximize well-being.

   • Reduce stressful responses associated with the
     medical management of patients (e.g., surgical
     procedures, intrusive examination procedures or
     use of extensive monitoring devices).

   • Provide more effective care to high-risk
     populations (e.g., maternal and child care
     service to vulnerable mothers and infants,
     family planning services to young teenagers,
     services designed to enhance self-care in the
     chronically ill and the very old).

(Continued)

Box 2–3   ANA Commission on Nursing Research (Continued)

5. designing and
   developing health
   care systems that are
   cost-effective in
   meeting the nursing
   needs of the
   population

6. promoting health,
   well-being, and
   competency for
   personal health in
   all age groups

- Enhance the care of clients culturally different
  from the majority (e.g., Black Americans,
  Mexican-Americans, Native Americans) and
  clients with special problems (e.g., teenagers,
  prisoners, mentally ill), and the underserved
  (the elderly, poor, and the rural).

- Design and assess, in terms of effectiveness and
  cost, the models for delivering nursing care
  strategies found to be effective in clinical
  studies.

Source: American Nurses' Association, Commission on Nursing Research, *Research Priorities for the 1980's*, Kansas City, Mo.: 1981.

Understanding Research Findings

The Art of Active Reading

In 1940 Mortimer J. Adler and Charles Van Doren wrote a fantastic little volume called *How to Read a Book* (published by Simon & Schuster). It immediately became a best-seller and has since been translated into French, Swedish, German, Spanish, and Italian. The book hangs, as most good books do, on a single central idea: that *it is important for an intelligent reader to read different things better* (not necessarily faster, but with more comprehension). The Adler and Van Doren volume proceeds to introduce the reader to "the basic rules of the fine art of intelligent reading"—an essential skill if you are to apply research results from studies conducted by others to your clinical work. Regrettably this book is now out of print, but the essentials of its method and insights follow.

A piece of scientific writing is usually complex. How much of it you comprehend often depends on the amount of active thinking that you put into the process of reading it and the skill with which you perform the separate acts involved in good reading. Active-reading skills enable you to go beyond mere reading for information to *reading for understanding*. This level of understanding is possible when you know not only what a writer has to say but also what he or she means and why. According to Adler and Van Doren, "Being informed is a prerequisite to being enlightened. The point is, however, not to stop at being informed" (p. 11). The lessons that follow are as relevant to active listening as they are to active reading, and so they can be put to work by people attending conferences and symposia as well as readers of journal articles and books. Engaging in active reading is the opposite of passively dragging your way through seemingly endless pages of material that you don't understand. Instead, it is a process of actively questioning the material you read and of thinking about it according to an organized plan that allows you to make sense out of even the most difficult parts. **Active reading** lets you answer the question "What does this really say?" The effectiveness of your reading is determined by the amount of skill you put into it. Realizing the differences between levels of reading is basic to improving your reading skill. The four levels are elementary reading, systematic skimming, analytic reading, and comparative reading.

Elementary Reading   The first level of reading is also called initial, or rudimentary, reading. It refers to the kind of reading we do as children in passing from illiteracy to literacy. Because you are well into reading this text, we can assume that any problems you might have in reading nursing research literature are not at the elementary level.

Systematic Skimming   The second level of reading is called **systematic skimming**, or prereading. The aim of **systematic skimming** is to get the most out of a publication in a limited amount of time. When you read at this level, you examine the surface of the publication and learn everything that the surface can tell you, such as the structure, the qualifications of the author, the ingredients or parts, and the overall category of the article or book. Systematic skimming helps you decide what to read in a journal or book and in what sequence. Many of us become intimidated by research journals because we try to start at the beginning and plow through them from page one without even looking at the table of contents to see what might be relevant to our interests or work.

Analytic Reading   The third level of reading, **analytic reading**, makes somewhat heavier demands on you. Here is where you ask questions of what you are reading so that you can truly understand it. These questions can be asked in any order, but together they form the framework for active reading.

1.   *What is the book (journal or article) about as a whole?* You have to figure out what the fundamental theme or thesis of a piece is and how it is developed.

2.   *What is being said in detail, and how?* Here you need to discover the author's main ideas, assertions, and arguments.

3.   *Is the book, journal, or article true in whole or part?* If you have read something seriously, you must make up your own mind on this question. The strategies

for conducting a formal research critique offer you an approach to doing this in the case of a report of research findings (see Chapter 6).

4. *What of it?* If what you have read provides information, you ought to ask yourself about its significance. Here is where you can use your own scholarly talents to perceive clinical implications of a study even if the investigators themselves haven't done so.

Comparative Reading   The fourth and highest level, **comparative reading**, requires that you place what you are reading in relation to other things you have read that are related. The comparative reader can construct an analysis of a subject that doesn't appear in any single article or book. In short, this fourth level of reading is the most reliable way of *keeping up to date* on a topic or subject. It requires that you keep either a real or mental file of new ideas or findings in your area of clinical interest and always assess each new work that you read in light of that file of ideas. Are you reading a really new idea? a credible replication of a previously published idea? a contradiction to a prominent idea? Although this is the most difficult of the reading levels, Adler and Van Doren say about it, "The benefits are so great that it is well worth the trouble of learning how to do it" (p. 20). Let us turn to a few "how tos."

Reading Techniques Useful for All Levels

Active reading, as you can see, involves engaging in a mental dialogue with the authors of a book, article, or paper presentation. See Box 2–4 for some tips that can help you accomplish this fruitfully.

Guides to Systematic Skimming

1. Quickly read the title page and preface (or abstract, if it is a journal article). Get an idea of the subject, and place the article or book in the appropriate category in your mind. Is it a theoretical treatise, an article on methodology, or an actual report of findings? If you answered yes to the last question, is the problem under investigation of conceivable clinical relevance to the patients you are working with or might work with in the future?

2. Look carefully at the table of contents in a book or the headings in an article to get a general sense of the structure of the piece. They ought to act as a road map by letting you know in advance where you are headed.

3. Check the index. Make a quick estimate of the range of topics included to see which, if any, are relevant to your interests. You can use the index in this text to get some practice.

Box 2–4   Helpful Guides for Reading Comprehension

Underline or highlight. <u>Get in the habit of underlining or highlighting</u> points of major significance, particularly the central thesis of a book or article.

$\|$ *Use vertical lines in the margin.* This is just another way of emphasizing a key paragraph or section of a page that might be too long to underline.

✳ *Put stars or asterisks in the margin* to let you quickly locate the most important ideas in the piece.

4 *Write numbers in the margin* to indicate a sequence of points in the unfolding logic of an argument or to designate any other list.

35 cf *Write page numbers in the margin* to indicate where else in the book or article the author makes relevant or even contradictory points. Some readers use the abbreviation *cf*, which means compare, or refer to. For example, in reading a research report you might want to compare its findings to the list of original hypotheses to be sure that an investigator had not drawn unreasonable conclusions.

clarify ? *Write questions and reactions* in the margins or at the top or bottom of a page. Here is where you can quickly summarize your own personal understanding of what you have read and its relation to what else you have read.

---

4. Read the publisher's blurb or any boldface excerpts. It is common for authors to try to summarize their main points in these spots.

5. From your knowledge of the general nature of the book's or article's contents, look more carefully at chapters or sections that seem pivotal. For example, in the case of a report of research, read the section with the heading "Findings" or "Conclusions."

6. Finally, leaf through the whole piece, dipping in here and there to read a paragraph. Remember to read the last few lines, because most authors sum up important points at the end.

Systematic skimming requires that you become a detective actively looking for clues about a book's or article's major theme so that you can decide whether it deserves any more of your time. You should be able to place it in your mental card catalog (or computer file) and return to it later if necessary. All of this should take anywhere from a few moments to less than an hour, even with a full-length book.

A final suggestion about systematic skimming is not to try to understand every page of a research report or theoretical paper the first time through, particularly if it contains unfamiliar jargon or complicated statistics. This is the most important rule. Don't be afraid to seem to be superficial at first. Read quickly through even the hardest parts. You will be much better prepared *to read it well the second time through*.

Guides to Analytic Reading

There are nine rules for analytic reading:

1. Try to discern whether a book or journal article is reporting findings that have been reached according to the canons of science or whether it is essentially based on personal trial and error, or what is often called "conventional clinical wisdom." Examples of the former are more likely to be found in journals explicitly dedicated to research and nursing science. Major nursing research journals are examined later in this chapter.

2. Try to state in a sentence or two what an article or book's main theme is. Sociologists Glaser and Strauss, who have taught nurses, call this the "little logic" of a book or article. It is *little* because it can be expressed in a short space. It is *logic* because it is the hook, or central premise, that holds the piece together. In the case of a report of study findings, you often find the "little logic" in the statement of the study's purpose or the statement of the study problem.

3. Try to "x-ray" a book or article to uncover its structure and see how the major parts are organized. A study that tests a hypothesis probably follows a fairly typical format (see Chapter 18). If you are reading exploratory or descriptive studies or studies designed to develop rather than test hypotheses, or if you are reading historical or case study reports, you may encounter a wide variety of structures.

4. Find out what main questions or problems the article or book has set out to answer or solve. Determine which of them are primary and which are secondary. When reading a research article, you should be able to do this by comparing findings and conclusions to the study purposes, objectives, or hypotheses.

5. Find the important and unfamiliar words and determine their meaning. There may be a whole new vocabulary to digest. If you need help, see Chapter 4 and the glossary of research terms in this text.

6. Mark the most important sentences in an article or book, and uncover the propositions they contain. A good time to practice this step is when reading the conceptual framework for a study proposal or report (see Chapter 9).

7. Locate or construct the basic arguments or premises. This rule is more likely to apply to a theoretical analysis or an expository piece than to a report of empirical findings.

8. Find out what solutions or conclusions an author has come up with. Are there other solutions?

9. Be able to say with reasonable certainty "I understand it" before you begin to criticize it. The specifics of how to critique a research study are covered in detail in Chapter 6.

Guides to Comparative Reading

Comparative reading is designed to get a cumulative perspective on a question or topic. Follow these five steps when comparing more than one source to establish their relationship to one another and to your own understanding of the subject.

1. Find the passages that bear on your question, needs, or interests.

2. Translate the ideas of the various authors into your own terms.

3. Formulate your own set of questions, and read comparatively to determine how the respective authors do or do not address them.

4. Define any issues that emerge so that you can recognize, sort, and arrange controversies or contradictory findings in the literature.

5. Analyze the discussions you read by asking, "Are they true?" and "What of it?"

A Step-by-Step Example

The best way to learn the skills of systematic skimming and analytic reading is to practice them. As an example, we will try them out on an article from *Nursing Research* written by Lim-Levy.*

Systematic Skimming
1. Read the title and preface or abstract quickly to get an idea of what the article is about. In Lim-Levy's article, the following information appears in italics at the very beginning:

A study was conducted to determine the effect of oxygen inhalation by nasal cannula on oral temperature. One hundred healthy adult subjects were randomly assigned to

---

*Lim-Levy, F. "The Effects of Oxygen Inhalation on Oral Temperature." *Nurs Res* May/June 1982; 131:150–152.

a control and three experimental groups that received 2, 4, and 6 liters per minute of oxygen for 30 minutes. Oral temperatures were measured before and 30 minutes after oxygen treatment. The data analysis did not show any effect of the treatment (p. 150).

This is clearly a published report of an experimentally designed study. The report has implications for clinical practice—specifically, how to take the temperature of people who are getting oxygen.

2. What is the structure of the article? This article is relatively short. Its only headings are "Methods" and "Results and Discussion." We can assume that it roughly follows the typical format for presenting the results of research to test a hypothesis.

3. Because this article does not have an index, we will look instead at the references at the end (p. 152). They give us some ideas about what else we might want to read.

4. Read any boldface excerpts. We have already read an excerpt in italics.

5. Read the pivotal and final sections. In the next-to-last paragraph, the author sums up her study findings in straightforward clinical terms:

This study did not show a significant effect of oxygen inhalation on oral temperature (p. 152).

Analytic Reading   Having inspected the research report entitled "The Effect of Oxygen Inhalation on Oral Temperature" by Lim-Levy, we can now reread it more critically at the analytic level.

Rule 1 of analytic reading is to know what kind of piece you are reading. Because of its appearance in *Nursing Research* and its format, we know that we are reading the results of an empirical clinical study. We are further told that the study was conducted by a nurse clinical specialist in medical-surgical nursing.

Rule 2 is to locate the article's "little logic." We find it on page 150 in the fourth paragraph:

This study sought to determine how oxygen inhalation by nasal cannula affects oral temperature. If oral monitoring is not adversely affected, there is no need for rectal or axillary procedures.

Rule 3 is to identify the article's structure. We see by the format that it is a report of a hypothesis-testing study.

Rule 4 is to find out what the main problem or question was. We can see on page 150 that this study set out to test the following hypothesis: "Oxygen inhalation by nasal cannula of up to 6 LPM does not affect oral temperature taken with an electronic thermometer."

Rule 5 is to come to terms with the author's vocabulary. Some of the phrases that you would want to understand when reading this report would include:

- informed consent from subjects (see Chapter 3)

- random assignment to treatment groups (see Chapter 5)

- analysis of variance (see Chapter 14)

- statistical significance (see Chapter 14)

Rule 6 is to undercover the basic premises, propositions, and arguments. In this study we can extract the following line of argument.

1. Oxygen inhalation by nasal cannula is believed to affect oral temperature; in many instances, therefore, body temperature is taken by the rectal or axillary method rather than orally.

2. Many patients find that having their temperature taken rectally is uncomfortable, and nurses find that taking either rectal or axillary temperature is more time-consuming than the oral method.

3. This study of 100 healthy adult male and female volunteers ranging in age from 18 to 56 years was designed to determine whether oxygen inhalation by nasal cannula of up to 6 LPM does indeed affect oral temperature when measured with an electronic thermometer.

4. The study design controlled for some factors known to affect oral temperature and procedures for taking the temperature itself, in order to enhance the study's validity and reliability, respectively.

5. Findings indicated that there were no statistically significant changes between preoxygen temperatures and temperatures taken 30 minutes after the start of oxygen.

6. The clinical implication of this study is that changing from the oral method to the rectal or axillary method is unnecessary as well as inconvenient and inaccurate.

Rule 7 is to figure out what conclusions the author has reached and make sure you understand them. Based on F and p values that were not statistically significant (see Chapter 14), the author concludes that oxygen inhalation does not significantly affect oral temperature. But she recommends that further research using higher oxygen concentrations and longer treatment and febrile patients be conducted (p. 152).

If you wished to move on to the level of comparative reading, you would consult the *Cumulative Index to Nursing and Allied Health Literature* (CINAHL), discussed later in this chapter, for additional studies on the clinical topic of temperature taking by the oral route. Using the approach to reading research suggested above is one way of keeping up to date while using your reading time efficiently so that you really understand what you have read.

Finding Research Literature

Indexes, Abstracts, and Computer Searches

Literature that may be relevant to nursing practice often cuts across traditional disciplinary boundaries. Box 2–5 summarizes indexing and abstract resources that you may need to consult to locate literature in fields related to nursing.

Computerized searches also offer access to the literature on a designated subject (see Chapters 8 and 16). Some of the most commonly used computerized searches include MEDLINE/MEDLARS, HEIRS, PAIS, ERIC, and DATRIX.

Box 2–5   Indexing and Abstract Resources for Fields Related to Nursing

Abstracts for Social Workers

Bibliography of Reproduction (Cambridge, England)

Bibliography of Suicide and Suicide Prevention

Child Development Abstracts and Bibliographies

Dissertation Abstracts (microfilm from Ann Arbor, Michigan)

Excerpta Medica

Hospital Abstracts

Hospital Literature Index

Index Medicus

International Index

National Library of Medicine Catalogue (monthly holdings of the National Library of Medicine, Bethesda, Maryland)

Psychological Abstracts

Research Grants Index (U.S. Government Printing Office, Washington, D.C.).

Sociological Abstracts

Box 2–6 **Primary Computerized Literature Searches**

1. DATRIX (Direct Access to Reference Information)—Contains over 150,000 dissertation abstracts on University Microfilms

2. ERIC (Educational Resources Information Center)

3. HEIRS (Health Education Information Retrieval System)

4. MEDLINE/MEDLARS—Indexes over 2900 biomedical and nursing journals

5. National Clearing House for Mental Health Information of the National Institute of Mental Health

6. NEXUS—American Association for Higher Education's telephone information referral service

7. PAIS, PATELL, PADAT (Psychological Abstracts Information Services)—Available through tape leasing, direct access terminal, and printout

8. SSIE (Smithsonian Science Information Exchange)

9. U.S. Commerce Department's National Technical Information Service

---

MEDLINE/MEDLARS searches biomedical and nursing journals. HEIRS searches health education journals. PAIS searches psychology literature. ERIC searches education literature, and DATRIX searches dissertation abstracts. To use these computerized literature searches, identify from one to several topics for a search analyst, to whom you probably have access through the computer terminal in your university library or hospital. Computer searches not only are quicker and more efficient but also allow access to more current information than that published in indexes and abstracts. In most cases there is a fee for using these systems.* The primary computerized literature searches useful in nursing research are listed in Box 2–6.

Finally, the key sources for nursing literature itself are summarized in Box 2–7.

You now have a framework of questions for inspecting, analyzing, and accumulating ideas and conclusions from research that is published or presented. But in order to use these skills, of course, you must know where to start to find reports that are relevant to nursing practice. A good place to begin is the ***Cumulative Index to Nursing and Allied Health Literature*** in your school of nursing or hospital library, or with your reference librarian. These resources will probably lead

---

*To find out more about how to use them, see the *Encyclopedia of Information Systems and Services*, Detroit: Gale Research Company, 1978.

you to discover nursing's principal research-oriented journals. The next section of this chapter offers you an overview of each of them.

Nursing's Primary Research Journals

Locating reports of research that may be relevant to your clinical practice will become a lot easier once you are familiar with nursing's primary research journals. As of publication of this text the best known are *Nursing Research, Advances in Nursing Science*, the *Journal of Research in Nursing and Health*, and the *Western Journal of Nursing Research*. The *International Journal of Nursing Studies*, published by Pergamon Press in England, also disseminates nursing research. The newest journal (1988) is

---

Box 2–7   Abstracts, Indices, and Reviews of Nursing Literature

1. *Annual Review of Nursing Research*—Initiated in 1983 to critically review important works so that students, faculty, and other scholars can recognize the advances made, the existing gaps, and the areas that need further work.

2. *Cumulative Index to Nursing and Allied Health Literature*—Published quarterly with annual compilations since 1956 that draw from journals in nursing and related fields. Selectively indexes from over 2600 biomedical journals in *Index Medicus* as well as some popular journals.

3. Facts About Nursing—Published by the American Nurses' Association in Kansas City, Missouri. It includes information on numbers and distribution of nurses, their employment status, types of education programs, student characteristics, graduates, and the major nursing organizations.

4. *Indexes to Nursing Periodicals*—Published annually and in cumulative form.

5. *International Nursing Index to Periodical Literature*—Published by the American Journal of Nursing Company. In annual includes list of doctoral dissertations by nurses.

6. *Nursing Research Abstracts*—Began in 1959; a regular feature of *Nursing Research* between 1960–1978. Abstracts now appear in *Advances in Nursing Science*.

7. Nursing Studies Index—Published by J. B. Lippincott, Philadelphia, it contains an annotated guide to reported studies and methodology papers from more than 200 sources.

8. *Index Medicus*—Indexes over 2600 US and international biomedical journals, including nursing journals.

TABLE 2–1   *Characteristics of Selected American Nursing Research Journals*

Title	Circulation*	Subscription Cost	Issues per Year
Nursing Research	11,700	$23.00	6
Advances in Nursing Science	4,200	$49.50	4
Research in Nursing and Health	1,800	$60.00	6
Western Journal of Nursing Research	1,400	$45.00	6

*Source: Adapted from Swanson and McCloskey (1986).

Applying Nursing Research, edited by Joyce Fitzpatrick and published by W. B. Saunders. Its emphasis, like that of this text, is to present research clearly and directly for clinical application in nursing practice. Research studies are sometimes published in the general-practice and specialty nursing journals, and social science and medical literature also often contains information that can be useful to nursing. The *Cumulative Index to Nursing and Allied Health Literature*, mentioned above, as well as the *International Nursing Index*, the *Cumulative Medical Index*, and computerized biographical literature searches such as MEDLINE, help nurses keep up to date with these references.

Nursing Research   *Nursing Research* is nursing's oldest and most widely circulated professional journal whose "preferred subject content" is research (McCloskey and Swanson 1982) (see Table 2–1). It is published six times a year by the American Journal of Nursing Company in New York City. There are about ten full-length articles per issue.

Despite the fact that *Nursing Research* is nursing's oldest and most widely read source of research findings, its circulation of 8500 as of a 1981 survey is small when compared with that of nursing's most popular general-practice journals. In 1981, *Nursing 81* had 550,000 subscribers, The *American Journal of Nursing* had 385,000, and *RN* had 350,000. We can expect these numbers to change, though, as the value of nursing research in improving clinical practice is increasingly recognized. Investigators will be expected to make the practice implications of their research more explicit, service settings will benefit by developing systems for using research findings in practice, and nurses will need the skills required to read, understand, and interpret research-oriented literature.

Advances in Nursing Science (ANS)   *Advances in Nursing Science* is published quarterly by Aspen Systems in Maryland. The primary purpose of this journal is "to stimulate the development of nursing science." *ANS* focuses on empirical research, theory construction, concept analysis, practical application of research and theory, and investigation of values and ethics that influence the practice and research activities of nursing science. Since the first issue was published in October 1978, it has targeted all of its issues to specific topics. Each issue has approximately seven full-length articles. Notices of upcoming research or scientific conferences are included near the end.

Western Journal of Nursing Research (WJNR)   The *Western Journal of Nursing Research* was begun in 1979 by Phillips-Allen Publishers of Anaheim, California, and its first editor, Pamela Brink. *WJNR* was initiated to serve the growing need of nurses in the western United States to share information about what they are doing. It has a three-part editorial philosophy:

1. The communication and dissemination of nursing research can be practical.

2. Nursing research is good only if it is used.

3. Talking about research makes it more useful.

To these ends, *WJNR* serves three different functions:

1. It publishes completed research papers.

2. It disseminates information about research conferences, grants available, and developing research projects.

3. It provides "how-to" comments on the research process and its functions.

The journal is correspondingly divided into three distinct sections:

1. Three or four feature articles, each followed by at least two commentaries and an author's response.

2. The "Information Exchange," including meeting calendar, grant deadlines, brief news reports, brief conference reports, research briefs, requests for assistance, and book reviews.

3. Technical notes, problems in doing research, ethical issues, research utilization, and strategies for teaching research. Each is written by an expert in the area.

WJNR also publishes the proceedings of the annual conferences of the Western Society for Research in Nursing in its summer issue.

Research in Nursing and Health (RN&H)   *Research in Nursing and Health* is published quarterly by John Wiley and Sons of New York City. The titles of articles in this journal are indexed in the *Cumulative Index to Nursing and Allied Health Literature, Social and Behavioral Science Index, Index Medicus, International Nursing Index, Public Health Reviews, Social Science Citation Index*, and *Sociological Abstracts*. The first issue of *RN&H* was published in April 1978.

This journal's intent is to publish nursing theory, nursing research, and scholarly and analytic works that lead to improvement and refinement of both theory and research. *RN&H* also publishes significant inquiries into nursing administration and education, as well as inquiries into the nature of health. The journal's goal has always been to publish what is "new, true, and important." Each issue includes approximately five feature-length articles.

As of September 1983, *RN&H* announced an experimental program in the submission and publication of manuscripts that allows authors who have access to personal computers or word processors to submit manuscripts either on computer diskettes or electronically by telephone using a modem. Text files need to be prepared using either WordStar or Select word-processing programs.

International Journal of Nursing Studies (Int J Nurs Stud)   The *International Journal of Nursing Studies* is published quarterly in England by Pergamon Press. Its primary purpose is to enhance the practice of nursing through the promotion of international debate. It is supported by an editorial board comprising members from 11 different countries. In addition to refereed articles on subjects including nursing administration and education each issue contains a book review section.

Applied Nursing Research (ANR)   *Applied Nursing Research* was first published in May, 1988 by W. B. Saunders Co. of Philadelphia. It expressly emphasizes applications to practice of research studies across all clinical specialties and strives for a lively, readable style. Features include: Ask the Experts, Research Briefs, Clinical Methods, Book Reviews, news and announcements related to research conferences and funding opportunities and an editorial.

Using Research Findings in Practice

An Institutional Model

The emphasis of this chapter has been on helping the individual practicing nurse overcome barriers to applying research findings to his or her practice. Morse and Conrad (1983) have developed an eight-step process by which hospitals and health agencies can put research into practice on the institutional level. These steps are:

1. Identify a clinical need or problem by checking data sources such as management reports, audit scores, incident reports, and patient charts.

2. Use indexes to nursing literature and the help of a reference librarian to locate literature relevant to the problem or need identified in step 1.

3. Evaluate relevant research reports by critiquing them (see the questions in Chapter 6).

4. If the research study is relevant and scientifically sound, assess its applicability for achieving clinical objectives related to your original problem or need.

5. Prepare a written plan that includes:

■ a statement of the clinical problem

■ a list of clinical objectives for alleviating the problem

■ a description of the new procedures that will reduce or alleviate the problem

■ a detailed budget of labor and equipment costs

■ anticipation of any effects the change suggested in the research might have on hospital policy or procedure

■ a schedule that will help allocate time devoted to the project

6. Obtain cooperation and permission, which involves "selling" the plan to the hospital administration, the nursing staff, the physicians, and the patients.

7. Carry out the plan in an atmosphere of open communication and support.

8. Evaluate the process according to the four possible outcomes that can follow implementation of an innovative technique:

■ The innovation may actually be harmful and therefore should be stopped.

■ The outcome may be neutral, reflecting no change.

■ The outcome may be to realize the clinical goals.

■ The outcome may be positive or negative but, in either case, unexpected. For example, a program to teach self-care of wounds to the elderly may be so time-consuming that the stress of staff to complete other assignments may become overwhelming.

Whatever the outcome, the authors of this model urge clinicians who attempt to use it to communicate with the researcher who conducted the original study so that new problems can be identified and addressed. Interaction between clinicians and researchers is essential. Hinshaw and her associates (1981) acknowledge that research in the practice setting can bring forth major conflicts in the areas of risk taking, vested interests, the rights of research subjects, and the need to produce both scientific and practical knowledge. But they add that collaboration and negotiation between nursing staff and researchers can make it work.

A Regional Model: The WICHE Project

Under the auspices of the Western Interstate Commission for Higher Education (WICHE), the U.S. Department of Health, Education, and Welfare funded a six-year project that had as its original goal investigating the feasibility of increasing nursing research activities through a regional effort. An underlying assumption of the project was that research is necessary to develop a body of validated nursing knowledge on which to base improvements in the quality of nursing given to the public. Many believed that this project was the first large-scale attempt to link the knowledge producers with the practitioners in practice settings.

Part III of the final report of this project (Krueger et al 1978) is devoted to what its author called "research utilization." During the course of the project the participating nurses had an opportunity to identify problems that needed research-based solutions; this activity was not unlike the first step of the institutional model we just examined. The nurses then developed skills in reading and evaluating research for use in practice, learned more about how to locate usable research findings, and developed detailed plans for introducing change into their settings. Although its authors reported that the project was ultimately effective in helping nurses use research in clinical practice, the major problem was the difficulty experienced in finding valid, reliable nursing studies with clearly written implications for nursing care. The categories of clinical problem for which research findings were sought are summarized in Table 2–2.

The implications of the WICHE project were not only that nurses have the skills for evaluating research for possible application in the clinical area but also that *nurse researchers need to include implications for nursing practice in their reports of*

TABLE 2–2 *Categories of Nursing Problems Selected by Nurses in the WICHE Nursing Research Development, Collaboration and Utilization Project*

Nursing Problem	Percentage of Nurses
Clinical nursing	
Patient teaching	29.0
Patient assessment	21.3
Psychosocial problems	3.2
Primary care	4.9
Other direct care	14.7
Problem-oriented records	16.5
Continuity of care	14.7
Nonclinical nursing	4.9

findings. Researchers must assume some responsibility for putting the research report in a form that can be easily used by nurses in the practice setting (see Chapter 18).

Project participants offered a number of other recommendations based on their experiences. They expressed a need for a centralized index on nursing research (a research hot line), or "Index Nursicus," that would be similar to *Index Medicus* but specifically targeted to research literature. They agreed that research should be taught as part of all basic nursing education and that it should be followed up through continuing education. They urged researchers, in the meantime, to simplify the language used in research reports and to conduct more clinical studies. Participants and project staff alike concluded that:

> The use of research in nursing practice would be greatly accelerated by systematic identification, evaluation, and collation of generalizations in a form that is easily accessible to practitioners. Only then can the major difficulties of research utilization be diminished and valid research findings made available (Krueger et al 1978, p. 299).

In the final recommendation the following conclusions were drawn:

> Institutions must value and be committed to research in order to develop resources for its conduct. The value is institutionalized through its stated philosophy and goals. It is operationalized through job descriptions, recruitment policies, [and] retention and promotion criteria that reward nurses with research skills (p. 332).

It seems that the WICHE project's message is that nursing research will move forward only if skilled researchers collaborate with others who have clinical competence and ideas for clinically useful research problems.

A State Model

A more recent effort to apply research in practice was the five-year Conduct and Use of Research in Nursing (CURN) project, sponsored by the Michigan State Nurses' Association. This project attempted to stimulate the conduct of research in clinical settings and help nurses learn new ways of using research findings in their practice. It resulted in a set of nine volumes (Horsley 1981–1982), which earned the 1983 Book of the Year Award presented by the *American Journal of Nursing*. The volume titles give a sense of the range of clinical research conducted:

- *Mutual Goal Setting in Patient Care*
- *Closed Urinary Drainage Systems*
- *Distress Reduction through Sensory Preparation*
- *Pain*

- *Intravenous Cannula Change*
- *Preventing Decubitus Ulcers*
- *Preoperative Sensory Preparation to Promote Recovery*
- *Reducing Diarrhea in Tube-Fed Patients*
- *Structured Preoperative Teaching*

The project's principal investigator, Jo Anne Horsley, concluded from the project that research will be accepted by practicing nurses if it is relevant to practice and is communicated broadly through journals and conferences.

The Sigma Theta Tau Regional Research Conferences

The Sigma Theta Tau Regional Research Conferences put forth yet another prototype for exploring the dissemination and utilization of research in nursing practice. The primary goal of these conferences was to promote research-based nursing practice by identifying study findings that were ready to be used in practice. A second goal was to suggest further steps to be taken in research areas where the findings were not yet ready for clinical application.

Shaping Practice Through Nursing Studies

Part 2 of this text is devoted to reading, understanding, and evaluating nursing studies in depth. Chapter 6 offers you precise guidelines for conducting a formal study critique. In the meantime, however, it is crucial that you recognize that nursing research published to date has indeed shaped nursing practice and that you have the tools to make a preliminary assessment of a study's clinical potential. Here are two illustrations of the first point.

- As a result of a group of studies done in 1977–1978 by Barbara W. Hanson and her colleagues (Walike and Walike 1977), the undesirable effects of lactose intolerance in patients receiving tube feedings have been eliminated by the removal of lactose from these formulations. In consequence, tube-fed patients who are lactose intolerant need no longer experience the nausea, abdominal cramps, and distention caused by the inability to digest milk sugar.

- Because of work done by Ida Martinson et al (1977) with families of leukemic children in Minnesota, hundreds of children are now able to remain at home with their families during the terminal phase of their illness.

As far as the second point is concerned, you can begin your assessment of research by noting that good clinical studies, according to Fuller (1982), have the following characteristics in common:

1. They study a problem that occurs frequently in a definable population of patients.

2. The standard way the problem has been dealt with is unsatisfactory.

3. Some index of the problem can be measured.

4. The proposed solution alters patient care.

When you read or hear reports of clinical studies, use the following preliminary set of questions to help you consider their scientific merit and possible utility (Fawcett 1982):

1. Has the original study been replicated?

2. If so, are the findings similar in a variety of situations?

3. Have findings been corroborated in clinical situations with actual patients who receive nursing care?

4. What were the risks and benefits of the nursing action tested in the study?

5. Does the study focus on a significant problem in clinical practice?

6. Do nurses have clinical control over the study variables?

7. Is it feasible to carry out the nursing action in the real world?

8. What is the cost of implementing the nursing action?

9. What contribution to client health status does the nursing action make?

10. What overall contribution to nursing knowledge does the study make?

Valid, useful nursing research will help you improve the quality of life of patients in your care regardless of their health status. From nursing research, for example, we will learn better ways of intervening with the frail elderly, persons with AIDS, acutely ill children, the chronically ill, and the terminally ill. Research done by nurses includes both laboratory and clinical studies and may cut across traditional disciplines and methods. In the past, research-based nursing practice was more a litany being preached than a reality. But you are part of the tension and excitement of a new era in nursing research. In this era, all nurses, whether they make research a central part of their career or not, will need the skills to read, understand, and apply the expanding body of findings to their pratice, to participate in the clinical studies of others, and to safeguard the rights of human research subjects under their care. If practitioners collaborate in the entire research process, the outcomes will be used. Remember, the clinician and the researcher have an exchange to make and a profit to share.

Guidelines for Critique

- Does the study reflect nursing's clinical priorities?

- Can you actively read it analytically and comparatively?

- What strategies for systematic skimming do you use?

- Have you followed the nine rules for analytic reading?

- What is the relationship of this article to others on the topic or question?

- What indexes, abstracts and computer searches do you use?

- What nursing research journals do you read regularly and why?

- Can you locate an institutional, state or regional model for enhancing nursing research in your area?

SUMMARY OF KEY IDEAS AND TERMS

✓ Applying the growing number of findings from clinical nursing research to practice would be easier if (1) the scientific community were further along in bringing some order to the proliferating research literature; (2) all nursing students were better prepared to find, read, understand, and appreciate these findings; and (3) service organizations were structured to foster such applications.

✓ Evidence of progress toward establishing a *scientific basis* for nursing practice includes (1) a consensus about investigative roles for nurses at all levels of educational preparation; (2) the emergence of research departments in service agencies; and (3) the establishment of a national research center to coordinate, support, and disseminate nursing research.

✓ Although research conducted by nurses includes various types of study and cuts across traditional disciplines, priority is given today to clinical research directly related to developing the knowledge and information needed for the improvement of nursing practice.

✔   The art of *active reading* helps nurses assimilate research reports.

✔   Reading occurs at four levels: (1) elementary, (2) systematic skimming, (3) analytic, and (4) comparative. Nurses can use the last three to good effect.

✔   There are six well-known journals of nursing research and nursing science: *Advances in Nursing Science*, the *Journal of Research in Nursing and Health*, the *Western Journal of Research in Nursing*, *Nursing Research*, the oldest and most widely circulated of them, the *International Journal of Nursing Studies* and *Applied Nursing Research*.

✔   Systematic skimming of a journal such as *Nursing Research* makes its scientific style less intimidating and more accessible for the clinician.

✔   Systematically skimming and analytically reading a sample research report with clinical relevance can increase your ability to read and understand others like it.

✔   Applying research findings to clinical practice requires that investigators make their work more accessible to practitioners, that practitioners develop their skills of active reading and listening and keep up with research developments, and that service agencies adopt philosophies and strategies that reward putting research findings into practice.

References

Adler M, Van Doren C: *How to Read a Book*. New York: Simon & Schuster, 1940.

Barnard KE: Knowledge for practice: Directions for the future. *Nurs Res* July 1980; 29:208–212.

Delphi Survey of Clinical Research Priorities. Boulder, Colo.: WICHE, 1974.

Dennis KE, Strickland OL: "The clinical nurse researcher: Institutionalizing the role. *Int. J. Nurs. Stud.* 1987; 24:25–33.

Downs F: Editorial. *Nurs Res* November/December 1981; 30:332.

Fawcett J: Utilization of nursing research findings. *Image* June 1982; 14:57–59.

Fuller E: Selecting a clinical nursing problem for research. *Image* June 1982; 14:60–61.

Gortner S: Out of the past and into the future. *Nurs Res* July/August 1980; 29:204–207.

Hinshaw AS et al: Research in practice: A process of collaboration and negotiation. *J Nurs Adm* February 1981:33–38.

Horsley JA: *Using Research to Improve Nursing Practice* (Series of Clinical Protocols 9 vols). New York: Grune and Stratton, 1981.

Jacox A: Strategies to promote nursing research. *Nurs Res* July/August 1980; 29:213–217.

Krueger J et al: *Nursing Research: Development, Collaboration and Utilization*. Germantown, Md.: Aspen Systems, 1978.

Lim-Levy F: The effect of oxygen inhalation on oral temperature. *Nurs Res* May/June 1982; 31:150–152.

Martinson IM et al: When the patient is dying: Home care for the child. *Am J Nurs* November 1977; 77:1815–1817.

Morse JM, Conrad A: Putting research into practice. *Can Nurs* September 1983; 79:40–43.

Parker M, Labadie G: Demystifying research mystique. *Nurs Health Care* September 1983:383–386.

Swanson E, McClosky JC: Publishing opportunities for nurses. *Nursing Outlook* September/October 1986; 34:227–35.

Walike BC, Walike JW: Relative lactose intolerance: A clinical study of tube-fed patients. *JAMA* 1977; 238:948–951.

WICHE, Delphi Survey of Clinical Research Priorities. Boulder, Colo.: 1984.

3

Ethics and the Rights of Research Subjects

HOLLY SKODOL WILSON

Chapter Objectives

After reading this chapter, the students should be able to:

- Describe examples of historic cases of abuse of human subjects' rights

- Demonstrate awareness of the characteristics of ethical scientific research

- Compare the similarities between two existing codes of research ethics

- Recognize human subjects who are particularly vulnerable to risk in nursing research

- Analyze five categories of risk associated with research procedures

- Evaluate a research study's provisions for the protection of human rights: (1) to be free from harm, (2) to be given full disclosure, (3) to have self-determination, and (4) to have privacy, anonymity, and confidentiality

- Define *ethics, risk-benefit ratio, minimal risk, debriefing, informed consent,* and *institutional review board*

- Formulate a human subjects protocol and an informed consent form that comply with principles of research ethics and protect the rights of human subjects

(Continued)

- Appreciate the complexity involved in balancing individual rights with society's rights to the development of scientific knowledge

- Advocate the protection of human rights and the principles of ethical research in clinical and scientific activities according to a personal and professional ethical framework

In This Chapter . . .

A young teacher of bioethics in nursing once said: "Reasoning in ethics means bringing all one's faculties in a balanced way to bear on the sincere concern for human well-being in general and the meaning of human experience. . . . Being reasonable in ethics is more like having integrity than like being smart." **Ethics** is that branch of philosophy concerned with two basic questions: (1) "What is right or good?" and (2) "What should I do?" The moral judgments involved in answering such questions are most highly developed when the process of arriving at them and the reasons for believing in them are clear and convincing. At the heart of ethical judgments are the reasons for them. The goal of this chapter is to help participants in and consumers of nursing research develop a way of thinking about the complex ethical issues and dilemmas that are often associated with human science.

The ethics of research are the product of recent years, although they rest on long-honored moral traditions. In the not-so-distant past, violations of human rights under the guise of scientific advancement took place with shocking frequency. From 1932 to 1972 more than 400 black Alabama sharecroppers and day laborers were subjects in a government study designed to deliberately withhold treatment for syphilis to study the untreated disease. James H. Jones has recounted this sad tale in his book *Bad Blood: The Tuskegee Syphilis Experiment* (1981). In the early 1960s Timothy Leary and Richard Alpert (a lecturer and an assistant professor at Harvard University) stretched the tolerance of the scientific community with their use of human subjects in studying the effects of psilocybin and LSD. In 1963 a physician injected hospitalized elderly patients at the Jewish Chronic Disease Hospital in Brooklyn with live cancer cells without informing them. Yet another abuse of experimentation took place in the pneumonia, flu, and meningitis experiments conducted on incarcerated residents of two state mental hospitals in Pennsylvania. Accounts of research using the poor, destitute, and mentally retarded crowd the history books. Some of the most tragic and profoundly troubling violations were the Nazi "medical" experiments conducted by highly qualified scientists and physicians with appalling disregard for the rights of their captive subjects.

This chapter helps you to answer the question "How ethical is my research project?" It also provides you with a list of characteristics of ethical research and codes formulated to increase the likelihood that nursing's desire for scientific knowledge is compatible with the dignity and rights of individuals and social groups. It acquaints you with four fundamental rights of human research subjects and assists you step by step in developing a consent form and a protocol that might be required by your institutional review board. Such a board must conclude that the process of *informed consent* is adequately provided for in a research plan and that *an appropriate balance exists between potential benefits of the research and the risks assumed by the subjects.*

Making Science Ethical

Doctors regularly conduct research studies to identify a particular pathological process or to find out how effective an experimental medical regimen or surgical treatment is when compared with the "standard treatment." Examples of such studies include "Protein Utilization in Females with Glucose Intolerance during Pregnancy" or "Phase I/II Study of Hyperthermia Treatment Technique and Tolerance of Skin and Subcutaneous Tissues to a Temperature of 50–45°C," or "Experimental Fetal Therapy." Pharmacologists collaborate with others in drug trial studies in which the agents being investigated have names such as "BCNU-FU-HU-6MP" (used for the treatment of malignant brain tumors) and research questions include: "What is the optimal dose?" "Is it most effective when used alone or in combination with other treatment?" "What are the side effects?" "By what biochemical mechanisms does it work?" "Can less be given?" "For which patients is it most useful?" Dentists study procedures for improving dental hygiene, for dental surgery, or for the use of experimental oral devices. All of the above studies may be conducted with animals or with human subjects.

Nursing research, however, tends to focus more consistently on people—their health attitudes, experiences associated with illness, values, coping behaviors, support systems, community networks, and environmental stressors. Consequently, human subjects are almost always involved in nursing research. Being aware of the rights of human subjects is a major part of a nurse's responsibility when she or he plans a research project, assists in someone else's research, or evaluates a research article.

Characteristics of Ethical Research

Ethical research includes protecting the rights of human subjects but encompasses a broader list of characteristics (see Figure 3–1):

- *Scientific objectivity.* To be objective you (or any other investigator) must include all data points, including those that are unsupportive; try to be aware of personal values and biases; and don't preconceive a study's outcome or engage in any misconduct, fraud, or acts of bad faith in connection with the research.

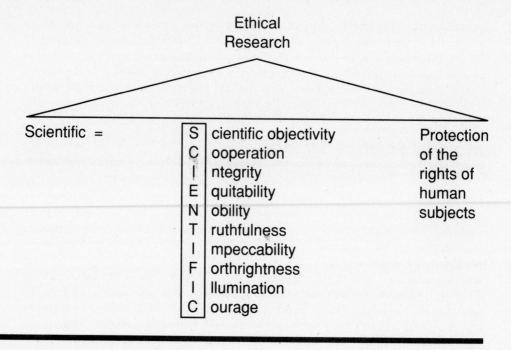

Figure 3–1 Making the scientific ethical

- *Cooperation* with duly authorized review groups, agencies, and institutional review boards. This means that you submit your proposed research to the appropriate committee in charge of reviewing provisions for the protection of subjects' rights and are willing to comply with their recommendations. Many journals require that study reports contain a statement that the research was approved from an ethical standpoint by the appropriate institutional committee.

- *Integrity* in representing the research enterprise. This means that you do not withhold information about your study's possible risks, discomforts, or benefits, nor do you intentionally deceive study subjects on these matters.

- *Equitability* in acknowledging the contributions of others. This means that you give credit where credit is due in publications, by listing coauthors, or in speeches and presentations, by acknowledging the work of others.

- *Nobility* in the application of processes and procedures to protect the rights of human subjects. This means that you actively assume responsibility for protecting subjects from harm, deceit, coercion, and invasions of privacy, even when your own study may be inconvenienced.

- *Truthfulness* about a study's purpose, procedure, methods, and findings. You do not attempt to disguise your research or conduct it "under cover."

- *Impeccability* in use of any privileges that may be associated with the researcher's role. You keep data anonymous and confidential. You are discrete about what you learn about people.

- *Forthrightness* about a study's funding sources and sponsorship. You disclose all sources of financial support as well as any special relationship between a study and its sponsors in publications and presentations of research findings.

- *Illumination* brought to your discipline's body of scientific knowledge through your publications and presentations of research findings. Research should yield fruitful results.

- *Courage* to publicly clarify any distortions that others make of your research findings.

Honor in Science

The Scientific Research Society, Sigma Xi, has published a 42-page book to give practical advice essential to beginning a lifelong habit of accuracy and integrity (Honor in Science 1986.) Awareness of the most tempting dishonest approaches to data ("trimming" to make data appear more precise, "cooking" to discard data that don't fit the theory, and "forging" or inventing data) should not prompt the conclusion that fraud and dishonesty are rampant in science. However, as we in nursing increase our scientific activity, sensitivity to potential ethical temptations is a critical part of our education.

Codes of Research Ethics

The preceding characteristics of ethical research are reflected in most professional codes of ethics for research. Box 3–1 presents the Code of Professional Ethics of the American Sociological Society, and Box 3–2 presents a summary of the American Nurses' Association's Human Rights Guidelines for Nursing in Clinical and Other Research. Conducting your research based on such codes will help you keep the *scientific, ethical.*

The Rights of Human Research Subjects

Protecting the rights of human subjects who are involved in research has become a high priority throughout all the professional and scientific communities. Nurse researchers are often among the most responsible and conscientious investigators when it comes to respecting the rights of subjects. The responsibility for ensuring that a study is ethical is no longer exclusively the investigator's. Recent guidelines such as those in Boxes 3–1 and 3–2 have been established to ensure an unbiased review. They rely on two historical documents.

The Nuremberg Code

The first internationally accepted effort to set up formal ethical standards governing human research subjects is now known as the **Nuremberg Code**, or *Nuremberg Articles*. When the U.S. secretary of state and secretary of war learned that the defense of the Nazi doctors during the trials of war criminals after World War II would center on justifying their atrocities on the ground that the doctors were "engaged in important research," the American Medical Association was asked to appoint a group to develop a code of ethics for research against which sadistic experiments on concentration camp prisoners would be judged. Box 3–3 contains the historic articles of the Nuremberg Tribunal.

The code requires informed consent in *all* cases and makes no provision for any special treatment of children, the elderly, or the mentally incompetent. Thus, its definitions of the terms *voluntary*, *legal capacity*, *sufficient understanding*, and *enlightened decision* have been the subjects of numerous court cases and the focus for several presidential commissions engaged in standard-setting. The code disallowed any research on subjects who were not capable of giving consent.

The Declaration of Helsinki

The **Helsinki Declaration** was issued in 1964 by the World Medical Association as a guide for physicians engaged in clinical research. Revised in 1974, the declaration differentiates between two major types of research: (1) that which is essentially therapeutic and (2) that which is essentially directed toward developing scientific knowledge and has no therapeutic value for the subject. The contemporary application of this document in nursing research emphasizes the requirement to inform research subjects when a clinical or nonclinical study will have no personal benefit to them and to avoid any subtle suggestion to the contrary. Both the Nuremberg Code and the Declaration of Helsinki served as the basis for the U.S. policies and regulations issued in 1966.

U.S. Policies and Procedures

The ethical protection of the rights of human subjects in research studies is no longer left solely to the judgment of the individual investigator, nor is the researcher's need to know something or even the benefit of society considered adequate justification for any and all research practices. The previous abuses of human beings

Box 3–1   Code of Ethics of Sociological Research and Practice

A. Objectivity and integrity

Sociologists should strive to maintain objectivity and integrity in the conduct of sociological and research practice.

1. Sociologists should adhere to the highest possible technical standards in their research. When findings may have direct implications for public policy or for the well-being of subjects, research should not be undertaken unless the requisite skills and resources are available to accomplish the research adequately.

2. Since individual sociologists vary in their research modes, skills and experience, sociologists should always set forth *ex ante* the disciplinary and personal limitations that condition whether or not a research project can be successfully completed and condition the validity of findings.

3. Regardless of work settings, sociologists are obligated to report findings fully and without omission of significant data. Sociologists should also disclose details of their theories, methods and research designs that might bear upon interpretation of research findings.

4. Sociologists must report fully all sources of financial support in their publications and must note any special relations to any sponsor.

5. Sociologists should not make any guarantees to subjects—individuals, groups or organizations—unless there is full intention and ability to honor such commitments. All such guarantees, once made, must be honored unless there is a clear, compelling and overriding reason not to do so.

6. Consistent with the spirit of full disclosure of method and analysis, sociologists should make their data available to other qualified social scientists, at reasonable cost, after they have completed their own analyses, except in cases where confidentiality or the claims of a fieldworker to the privacy of personal notes necessarily would be violated in doing so. The timeliness of this obligation is especially critical where the research is perceived to have policy implications.

7. Sociologists must not accept grants, contracts or research assignments that appear likely to require violation of the principles above, and should dissociate themselves from research when they discover a violation and are unable to achieve its correction.

(Continued)

Box 3–1   Code of Ethics of Sociological Research and Practice (Continued)

8. When financial support for a project has been accepted, sociologists must make every reasonable effort to complete the proposed work, including reports to the funding source.

9. When several sociologists, including students, are involved in joint projects, there should be mutually accepted explicit agreements, preferably written, at the outset with respect to division of work, compensation, access to data, rights of authorship, and other rights and responsibilities. Of course, such agreements may need to be modified as the project evolves.

10. When it is likely that research findings will bear on public policy or debate, sociologists should take particular care to state all significant qualifications on the findings and interpretations of their research.

B. Sociologists must not knowingly use their disciplinary roles as covers to obtain information for other than disciplinary purposes.

C. National research

Research conducted in foreign countries raises special ethical issues for the investigator and the professional. Disparities in wealth, power, and political systems between the researcher's country and the host country may create problems of equity in research collaboration and conflicts of interest for the visiting scholar. Also, to follow the precepts of the scientific method—such as those requiring full disclosure—may entail adverse consequences or personal risks for individuals and groups in the host country. Finally, irresponsible actions by a single researcher or research team can eliminate or reduce future access to a country by the entire profession and its allied fields.

1. Sociologists should not use their research or consulting roles as covers to gather intelligence for any government.

2. Sociologists should not act as agents for any organization or government without disclosing that role.

3. Research should take culturally appropriate steps to secure informed consent and to avoid invasions of privacy. Special actions may be necessary where the individuals studied are illiterate, of very low social status, and are unfamiliar with social research.

(Continued)

Box 3–1   Code of Ethics of Sociological Research and Practice (Continued)

4. While generally adhering to the norm of acknowledging the contributions of all collaborators, sociologists working in foreign areas should be sensitive to harm that may arise from disclosure, and respect a collaborator's wish or need for anonymity. Full disclosure may be made later if circumstances permit.

5. All research findings, except those likely to cause harm to collaborators and participants, should be made available in the host country, ideally in the language of that country. Where feasible, raw data stripped of identifiers should also be made available. With repressive governments and in situations of armed conflict, researchers should take particular care to avoid inflicting harm.

6. Because research and/or findings may have important political repercussions, sociologists must weigh carefully the political effects of conducting research or disclosure of findings on international tensions or domestic conflicts. It can be anticipated that there are some circumstances where disclosure would be desirable despite possible adverse effects; however, ordinarily research should not be undertaken or findings released when they can be expected to exacerbate international tensions or domestic conflicts.

D. Work outside of academic settings

Sociologists who work in organizations providing a lesser degree of autonomy than academic settings may face special problems. In satisfying their obligations to employers, sociologists in such settings must make every effort to adhere to the professional obligations contained in the code. Those accepting employment as sociologists in business, government, and other non-academic settings should be aware of possible constraints on research and publication in those settings and should negotiate clear understandings about such conditions accompanying their research and scholarly activity.

E. Respect for the rights of research populations

1. Individuals, families, households, kin and friendship groups that are subjects of research are entitled to rights of biographical anonymity. Organizations, large collectivities such as neighborhoods, ethnic groups, or religious denominations, corporations, governments, public agencies, public

(Continued)

Box 3–1   Code of Ethics of Sociological Research and Practice (Continued)

officials, persons in the public eye, are not entitled automatically to privacy and need not be extended routinely guarantees of privacy and confidentiality. However, if any guarantees are made, they must be honored unless there are clear and compelling reasons not to do so.

2. Information about persons obtained from records that are open to public scrutiny cannot be protected by guarantees of privacy or confidentiality.

3. The process of conducting sociological research must not expose subjects to substantial risk of personal harm. Where modest risk or harm is anticipated, informed consent must be obtained.

4. To the extent possible in a given study, researchers should anticipate potential threats to confidentiality. Such means as the removal of identifiers, the use of randomized responses, and other statistical solutions to problems of privacy should be used where appropriate.

5. Confidential information provided by research participants must be treated as such by sociologists, even when this information enjoys no legal protection or privilege and legal force is applied. The obligation to respect confidentiality also applies to members of research organizations (interviewers, coders, clerical staff, etc.) who have access to the information. It is the responsiblity of the chief investigator to instruct staff members on this point.

Source: Excerpted from "Toward a Code of Ethics for Sociologists," *The American Sociologist*, July 1984. Reprinted with permission of the American Sociological Society.

---

in the interest of science have resulted in insistence by the government agencies that support nursing, medical, biological, and social research that ethical standards be followed if a project is to be funded. In fact, the U.S. surgeon general, in 1966, and subsequent secretaries of the Department of Health, Education, and Welfare (1971) issued regulations governing the use of human subjects in research funded by the National Institutes of Health. The rules require that, before research proceeds, an institutional review board functioning in accordance with specifications of the department must review and approve all studies. In 1981 two regulations were added. One excepted several categories of research from the review requirement. The other provided the option of an expedited review in instances where risks were presumed to be minimal (see Box 3–4).

Box 3–2   American Nurses' Association Human Rights Guidelines for Nurses in Clinical and Other Research

The guidelines in this table attempt to specify several important entities: (1) the type of activities that are involved, (2) the rights that are to be protected, (3) the persons to be safeguarded, and (4) the mechanisms necessary to ensure that protection is adequate.

Guideline I: Employment in Settings Where Research Is Conducted

Conditions of employment in settings in which clinical or other research is in progress need to be spelled out in detail for all potential workers. . . . Anyone employed in work that carries the potential of risk to others needs to be advised as to the types of risks involved, the ways of recognizing when risk is present, and the proper actions to take to counteract harmful effects and unnecessary danger.

Guideline 2: Nurses' Responsibilities for Vigilant Protection of Human Subjects' Rights

In all instances the prospective subject must be given all relevant information prior to participation in activities that go beyond established and accepted procedures necessary to meet his personal needs. . . . Nurses must be increasingly vigilant in their concern for subjects and patients who by reason of their situation and/or illness are not able to protect themselves effectively from externally imposed threat or injury. They must be sensitive to the tendency toward exploitation of "captive " populations such as students, patients, and inmates in institutions and prisons. All proposals to be used need to be discussed with the prospective subject and with any workers who are expected to participate as a subject or data collector or both. Special mechanisms must be developed to safeguard the confidentiality of information and protect human dignity.

Guideline 3: Scope of Application

The persons for whom these human rights guidelines apply include all individuals involved in research activities and include the following groups: patients, donors of organs and tissue, informants, normal volunteers including students, vulnerable populations that are "captive" audiences such as the mentally disordered, mentally retarded, and prisoners.

(Continued)

Box 3–2   American Nurses' Association Human Rights Guidelines for Nurses in Clinical and Other Research (Continued)

Guideline 4: Nurses' Responsibility To Support the Accrual of Knowledge

Just as nurses have an obligation to protect the human rights of patients, so do they also have an obligation to support the accrual of knowledge that broadens the scientific underpinnings of nursing practice and the delivery of nursing services.

Guideline 5: Informed Consent

To safeguard the basic rights of self-determination, consent to participate in research or unusual clinical activities must be obtained from the prospective subject or his legal representative. The subject needs to receive:

- A description of any benefit to the subject or to the development of new knowledge that might be expected

- An offer to discuss or answer any questions about the study

- A clear statement to the subject that he is free to discontinue participation at any time he wishes to do so

- Full freedom from direct or indirect coercion and deception

Guideline 6: Representation on Human Subjects Committees

There is increasing public support for systematic accountability to ensure that individual rights are not denied human subjects who participate in research studies. In most instances, the protective mechanism takes place through a committee judged competent to review studies and other investigative activities that involve human subjects. The profession of nursing has an obligation to publicly support the inclusion of nurses as regular members of Institutional Review Committees of this kind.

Source: Adapted and summarized with permission from the American Nurses' Association, *Human Rights Guidelines for Nurses in Clinical and Other Research* (ANA Publication No. D-46 5M 7/75), 1975. Also found in ANA, *Guidelines in Nursing Research*, Kansas City, Mo.: 1975.

Four Basic Rights

Balancing the obligation to conduct the most valuable study with the obligation to safeguard the rights of human subjects is not an easy task and embroils researchers and reviewers alike in stormy ethical issues. In all instances, however, from a moral point of view, the following list of four rights of research subjects must be protected.

The Right Not To Be Harmed The regulations of the Department of Health, Education, and Welfare (now the Department of Health and Human Services) defined **risk of harm** to a research subject as exposure to the possibility of injury going beyond everyday situations. They included physical, emotional, legal, financial, and social harm. Directly withholding treatment in order to study the course of a disease is clearly a physiological danger. But risks to human subjects in a nursing study may be more subtle. For example, subjects who are asked to complete a

---

Box 3–3   Articles of the Nuremberg Tribunal

1. The voluntary consent of the human subject is absolutely essential. . . .

2. The experiment should be such as to yield fruitful results for the good of society, unprocurable by other means of study, and not random and unnecessary in nature. . . .

3. The experiment should be so designed and based on the results of animal experimentation and knowledge of the natural history of the disease or other problems under study that the anticipated results will justify the performance of the experiment. . . .

4. The experiment should be conducted to avoid all unnecessary physical and mental suffering and injury. . . .

5. No experiment should be conducted where there is a prior reason to believe that death or disabling injury will occur. . . .

6. The degree of risk to be taken should never exceed that determined by the humanitarian importance of the problem to be solved by the experiment. . . .

7. Proper preparations should be made and adequate facilities provided to protect the subject against . . . injury, disability, or death.

8. The experiment should be conducted only by scientifically qualified persons. . . .

9. The human subject should be at liberty to bring the experiment to an end. . . .

10. During the experiment the scientist . . . if he has probable cause to believe that a continuation of the experiment is likely to result in injury, disability, or death to the experimental subject . . . will bring it to a close.

Source: From J. Katz, *Experimentation with Human Beings*, New York: Russell Sage Foundation, 1972, pp. 289–290.

questionnaire, ostensibly dealing with "health issues," after the death of a child in their family may experience undue anxiety and the awakening of guilt if the questionnaire includes sensitive items that could evoke disturbing feelings. This is particularly true if no **debriefing** (a process of disclosing to the subject all information that was previously withheld) is conducted afterward and no provision for referral to counseling is included in the study protocol. Merely agreeing to be confined for an extended period in a hospital for research purposes exposes a subject to an increased risk of hospital infections, boredom, and missed opportunities. The risk associated with participating in a randomized treatment study places the subject at a 50% risk of receiving care or treatment that may not be as effective as the standard or control treatment with which the experimental treatment is being compared. Simple procedures such as venipuncture performed for research purposes involve risks that range from a small bruise to death. Other risks include:

- Loss of confidentiality, which could occur if a nursing faculty member required that students enrolled in a course complete a questionnaire about personal experiences with recreational drugs.

- Loss of privacy by becoming a subject in multiple studies because of one's serious illness or condition (for example, a cancer patient who is terminally ill may be willing to agree to anything to sustain hope for recovery).

- Being subject to additional procedures and tests as a consequence of participating in clinical research and then being charged for them. Most institutions require that investigators assume costs for tests done for research purposes.

- Being duped into thinking that participating in a study will positively affect one's care or condition directly, when in fact the advancement of knowledge or the development of a new commercial product may be the only benefit.

- Exploitation by commercial sponsors who ask patients to donate extra blood or endure discomfort or inconvenience so that the firm can develop a new, marketable product.

In summarizing the risks associated with research procedures, Reynolds (1972) identified *five categories*:

1. No positive or negative effects expected on the research subjects. These studies include chart reviews and tissue studies, and formal consent procedures and forms may be waived by some review boards in such cases.

2. Temporary discomfort, anxiety, or physical pain. Here the discomfort is no more than would be encountered in day-to-day living and ceases with the termination of the experiment. Simple venipuncture for taking a blood sample would fit into this category.

3. Unusual levels of temporary discomfort that may last beyond the end of the study and that may require a debriefing interview or conference to return a

---

Box 3–4   Research Activities Eligible for Expedited Review Under United States Rules

1. Collection of hair and nail clippings, in a nondisfiguring manner; deciduous teeth; and permanent teeth if patient care indicates a need for extraction.

2. Collection of excreta and external secretions, including sweat, uncannulated saliva, placenta removed at delivery, and amniotic fluid at the time of rupture of the membrane prior to or during labor.

3. Recording of data from subjects 18 years of age or older using noninvasive procedures routinely employed in clinical practice. This includes the use of physical sensors that are applied either to the surface of the body or at a distance and do not involve input of matter or significant amounts of energy into the subject or an invasion of the subject's privacy. It also includes such procedures as weighing, testing sensory acuity, electro-

cardiography, electroencephalography, thermography, detection of naturally occurring radioactivity, diagnostic echography, and electroretinography. It does not include exposure to electromagnetic radiation outside the visible range (for example, x rays or microwaves).

4. Collection of blood samples by venipuncture, in amounts not exceeding 450 milliliters in an eight-week period and no more often than two times per week, from subjects 18 years of age or older and who are in good health and not pregnant.

5. Collection of both supra and subgingival dental plaque and calculus, provided the procedure is not more invasive than routine prophylactic scaling of the teeth and the process is accomplished in accordance with accepted prophylactic techniques.

6. Voice recordings made for research purposes such as investigations of speech defects.

7. Moderate exercise by healthy volunteers.

8. The study of existing data, documents, records, pathological specimens, or diagnostic specimens.

9. Research on individual or group behavior or characteristics of individuals, such as studies of perception, game theory, or test development, where the investigator does not manipulate subjects' behavior and the research will not involve stress to subjects.

10. Research on drugs or devices for which an investigational new drug exemption or an investigational device exemption is not required.

Source: Federal Regulations for Human Research.

---

subject's anxiety to normal. An interview or questionnaire that evokes strong feelings or upsets the subjects might fall into this category, as would research in which subjects are not told from the start the question really under investigation.

4. Risk of permanent damage, such as might result from the use of an experimental drug or device.

5. Certainty of permanent damage. In this fifth category are the abuses of human subjects cited earlier in this chapter—the Nazi war experiments, the Tuskegee syphilis study, and the like. In fact, some subjects of the Tuskegee study suffered no permanent damage. Apparently, tertiary syphilis is in some cases asymptomatic and essentially dormant. This is not to condone the study but points out that certainty of harm, like certainty of lack of harm, is elusive.

EXAMPLE: The Prayer Experiment

Study problem

Experimental design
Treatment or independent variable

Study purpose

In a study entitled "Positive Therapeutic Effect of Intercessary Prayer on an Intensive Care Population," the subjects were unknowingly to be assigned to one of two groups, experimental or control. If they were assigned to the first group, their bed number, diagnosis, and prognosis would be given to a group of Christians who would then pray for them for the entire time they were in the hospital. The purpose of the study was to "evaluate some of the various ways in which prayer helps critically ill patients."

Discussion of the Prayer Experiment

Risks

Risks

No consent procedure

Low benefit

Although the study seems simple and innocuous on the surface, the institutional review board of the university hospital found that it contained myriad problems and issues that needed to be unraveled. These problems were in the areas of protection of patients' autonomy and in the transmission of private information. The review board acknowledged that although many people would be happy to have someone praying for them, others might not feel so positively and might, in fact, hold serious objections. The criticism was felt by some members to raise the constitutional issue of freedom of religion, by others, the issue of privacy, and by still others, the simple risk of upsetting very ill patients. Upon reading the results, were they to be published in the lay press, some subjects might be quite angry to learn that they had unknowingly participated in such a study. The Belmont Report (U.S. National Commission 1978) identifies "respect for persons" as one key ethical principle of research. What if a subject were a deeply committed non-Judeo-Christian or an atheist? It is not consistent with this principle to treat the intensive-care patients as if they were uninvolved persons with no feelings about whether a group of Christians who had been given private information about them should be praying for them. Thus, there appeared to be no adequate semblance of informed consent. Finally, the board raised questions about the risk-benefit ratio in this study. It noted that benefit to society is often dependent upon the strength of the research design. In this study it is very difficult to determine if the power of prayer can ever be empirically "proved." The committee questioned how the investigator would control for confounding variables, such as someone else, in or out of the prayer group, also praying for the control group members. How would the research distinguish spiritual help from physical help?

The prayer experiment ultimately earned approval from the board once a simple consent form with full disclosure about the risks to human subjects became part of the protocol and the hospital chaplain (not the patient's primary nurse) was designated as the person to approach patients about participating in the study. Even then, its endorsement by the full committee was weak, illustrating that radiation, withdrawal of care, surgery, and chemotherapy in no way embrace the full range of risks to subjects.

Concern for protecting human research subjects has been extended beyond research that threatens bodily harm, such as drug toxicity or discomfort, to include research that threatens a subject's self-esteem, self-worth, values, composure, privacy, and even religious freedom. The risks of anxiety, embarrassment, or other stressors must be weighted against the benefits in any study, and the **risk-benefit ratio** must be clearly disclosed to all research subjects before they agree to participate. Consider this ratio in the example of the prayer experiment. The case illustrates the two key considerations in attempting to ensure the right not to be harmed: (1) Certain subjects are vulnerable and may not be able to evaluate risks involved in a study (for example, unconscious patients). (2) The risk-benefit ratio of a research project may not justify exposure of subjects to the risks.

In the first instance, children, fetuses, the mentally disabled, the elderly, captives, the dying, and the sedated or unconscious are vulnerable groups of subjects. In such cases a guardian or advocate should be identified to provide special consideration and protection. Even here, however, there seem to be no simple answers, only complicated ones. For example, can a mother who has volunteered for an abortion have the interest of the fetus in mind when evaluating the risks associated with an untested intrauterine fetal research procedure? The fundamental rule here is that the less able a subject is to give informed consent, the greater the burden on the investigator to protect the subject's rights.

The second issue in calculating the risk-benefit ratio requires that risks to research subjects be justified by potential benefit to them in the case of clinical research or to society in the knowledge produced. The benefits, in short, should exceed the risks. Even then, the risks to a cancer patient may not always be justified by advancing society's knowledge about cancer treatment. Among these risks are increased side effects from combining multiple chemotherapeutic agents with reported adverse effects, including susceptibility to infection, bleeding, increased fatigue, nausea, vomiting, kidney damage, hair loss, hearing loss, and abnormal liver function. This risk-benefit ratio continues as a primary objective standard by which we can judge the ethics of certain research procedures. The calculation of it involves naming the benefits and weighing them as well as considering the following two questions: (1) "How important is the research?" and (2) "How serious are the risks to human subjects?" Some critics, however, cite this standard as "typically American" in its pragmatism, in that it judges the morality of research practices by the results produced. Often the benefits of "basic" research (see Chapter 1) are difficult to identify. In any case, if harm, be it physiological or psychological, is involved, the investigator must explain how these risks will be minimized. The subjects must be fully aware of them, and the nature of the benefits expected from the study must be convincing. **Minimal risk** means that the risks of harm anticipated in the proposed research are not greater than those ordinarily encountered in daily life or during the performance of routine examinations or tests.

The Right to Full Disclosure Nurses who become involved in clinical research are in particularly tempting positions with respect to the ethical requirement for full disclosure of the purpose, procedures, and risks of an investigation. This is true because of the ease with which research data about patients can be collected as part of clinical nursing practice without patients' knowledge or consent. In such situations, a potential conflict also exists between the roles of clinician and investigator, arising from the inclination to adhere to the study plan against the best interests of the patient's care. Full disclosure involves informing subjects about the following aspects of any study:

- the nature, duration, and purposes of a study

- the methods, procedures, and processes by which data will be collected, expressed in straightforward lay terminology—for example, teaspoons or ounces of blood to be drawn, rather than milliliters—in short, what will happen to them

- the use to which findings will be put and any personal or societal benefits that could derive from the research

- any and all inconveniences, potential harms, or discomforts that might be expected, including becoming a target for inclusion in future studies, risking loss of privacy or confidentiality, and commitment of personal unreimbursed time.

- any results or side effects that might follow from participation in a study, including follow-up interviews or questionnaires

- alternatives to participating in the study that are available to the subject

- the right to refuse to participate or to withdraw at any time

- the identities of the investigators and how to contact them

Full disclosure means that deception, either by withholding information about a study in the interest of protecting its validity or by giving a subject false information about the study, is unethical. Researchers have taken undercover jobs in mental institutions as nursing aides or attendants while engaging in observational research. Patients have been told that a study was focusing on child development rather than on their own attitudes and behavior toward their battered children. The scientific rationale for deception is that knowing the point of the research would either influence the natural behavior of the subjects or their willingness to consent to participate, or both. Researchers may argue, for example, that informing staff nurses that they are studying the amount of time the nurses spend on paperwork as compared with patient care might alter usual behavior. Furthermore, they may contend that in even the most extreme examples some experimental subjects, when looking back on their experiences, will report that the deception imposed on them was justified by the scientific knowledge gained and that they do not perceive the lack of full disclosure as unethical.

EXAMPLE: The Obedience Experiment

One of the best-known studies in which deceit about the purpose of the research and the procedures involved resulted in upsetting the subjects was Milgram's famous 1963 research on obedience to authority. The study tried to determine how far subjects would go in obeying the commands of an authority figure, even when they knew they were harming another person. The study procedures required the research subjects to give what they understood to be increasingly strong electrical shocks to another person, who was acting the part of a victim. Of the 40 subjects, 65% continued to administer the shocks to the end of the required series, even though they were led to believe that they might be endangering the life of a powerless person. The investigators in the process urged them to go on despite instances of trembling, sweating, stuttering, and other indications of severe discomfort and outright anguish experienced by the subjects.

Study purpose

Methods involving deception

Risks

Discussion of the Obedience Experiment

Many experts say that it is preferable for researchers to tell subjects that they cannot let them know the exact nature of the research question until their participation is completed because of the likelihood that the data would be affected. This approach certainly seems less humiliating and embarrassing than lying to them. If you are afraid that full disclosure would make your potential subjects angry or cause them not to participate in your study, you should probably reconsider the design of the research. Under the right of full disclosure, subjects can refuse to participate, participate selectively, or withdraw from current participation without fear of endangering the quality of their care, even if their withdrawal is detrimental to your research. It is the nurse's responsibility to be sure that they are aware of this right. Anytime a subject withdraws from or declines participation in a research project, the investigator must be prepared to accept the decision graciously.

The Right of Self-Determination Research subjects who have the right of self-determination will feel free from constraint, coercion, or undue influence of any kind. This means that researchers will avoid coercive or seductive language in introduction letters and consent forms. Instead of referring to a study as the investigation of "a promising new relaxation technique for the pain experienced by cancer patients," for example, investigators will use a more neutral expression, such as "an experimental pain-control technique involving meditation." Similarly, any promises of getting special attention or of becoming famous by making a contribution to science or other masked inducements are strictly avoided.

A nursing study investigating the effects of injection rates on the intensity of first and second pain of intramuscular injection stated forthrightly that (1) there were no known additional risks from being in the study, other than that the injection a subject received might be more or less painful than an injection given by another method, and (2) that there were no personal benefits to the study subjects, because the purpose of the study was to learn about intramuscular injection pain.

If financial compensation is being offered to all or some subjects, the investigator will so state from the onset in matter-of-fact terms, including arrangements for prorated payments should subjects withdraw from the study before its completion. Financial compensation is intended to make up for inconvenience, not act as an inducement to participate in a study.

Many research subjects feel pressured to participate in studies if they are in powerless, dependent positions, such as being a patient in a nursing home, or if they feel they must please nurses who are responsible for their treatment and care. Repeated follow-up letters, phone calls, or home visits to prospective respondents who have not returned mailed consent forms may be experienced as "pressuring" subjects to participate in research when they would really prefer not to do so.

Dementia research in nursing homes abounds with ethical problems. The critical question raised by Abrams (1988) and others is whether subjects' involvement in research is genuinely voluntary when patients cannot "walk away" from the study. Creative efforts in designing clearer guidelines are required to advance knowledge of patients who cannot protect themselves.

The Right of Privacy, Anonymity, and Confidentiality   *Privacy* enables a person to behave and think without interference or the possibility that private behavior or thoughts may be used to embarrass or demean the person later. A study is considered truly **anonymous** if even the investigator cannot link a subject with information reported. **Confidentiality** means that any information that a subject divulges will not be made public or available to others. Even with the apparent clarity of such definitions, review boards debate issues such as whether biomedical research using normal postcircumcision foreskins of infants should be treated like research on hospital records in a university teaching hospital, for which permission is not required, or should require informed consent from the infants' parents or guardians. Different definitions of these concepts result in different outcomes. The use of instruments such as hidden tape recorders, cameras, or one-way mirrors without a subject's knowledge or permission is an invasion of privacy. Personal activities, opinions, attitudes, beliefs, letters, diaries, and records are generally private property and may not be used as sources of research data without a subject's permission. Even such records as school or health records are released only with a person's consent. Privacy is invaded when the subject is not aware of the information being elicited and the use to which it will be put.

If private information is to be collected, at a minimum the investigator will:

1. Maintain the anonymity of subjects by avoiding personally identifiable information on data-collection forms, substituting code numbers instead of names, and keeping a master list under lock and key in a separate place.

2. Preserve the confidentiality of data sources by limiting people other than the principal investigator from access to the raw data. If a loss of confidentiality is threatened, all records and links to identity will be destroyed.

The investigator informs research subjects of the measures that will be used to maintain confidentiality and anonymity and to protect their privacy. In a study of stress and role strain in RN baccalaureate nursing students, subjects were told: "There is no identifier attached to the questionnaire, and once the data are pooled, they cannot be used to identify respondents in any way except for school attended." When publishing your research, you should use pseudonyms or general descriptions or report aggregate data only. Remember, however, that agreeing not to mention participants by name also means not identifying them by a combination of characteristics. For example, reporting the personality inventory data of a female full professor under the age of 40 in the department of psychiatric nursing of a Northern California university school of nursing that offers a doctoral program is tantamount to naming the data source.

Ensuring That Research Is Ethical

Although it is the responsibility of investigators to examine their own projects with all the conscience and candor they can summon, federal regulations require that institutions, including universities, hospitals, nursing homes, and health agencies, establish review committees on human research subjects, often called institutional review boards, or IRBs.

The Institutional Review Board

The activities that fall under the jurisdiction of board review were succinctly set forth in the 1974 *Code of Federal Regulations*:

> . . . any research, development, or related activities which depart from the application of those established and accepted methods necessary to meet the subject's needs or which increase the risk of daily life.
>
> (*Federal Register*, May 30, 1974)

Thus, an established nursing procedure with therapeutic benefit to patients does not fall under board jurisdiction, because it is not research. Yet a federally funded evaluation study of teaching strategies in a nursing course in which students are randomly assigned to one of two types of teaching will require that the investigator obtain informed consent from the student subjects and undergo board review.

Review boards are formed in any institution that receives significant federal funding or that does a significant amount of drug or device research regulated by the Federal Drug Administration (FDA). Many smaller hospitals and institutions have no board per se but have a research advisory committee that serves similar purposes.

Most boards establish written guidelines for investigators. These guidelines include steps to be taken to receive approval, forms for a human-subjects protocol, guidelines for writing a standard consent form, and criteria for qualifying for an expedited rather than a full committee review. Each of these essential points for acquiring clearance for a proposed study is taken up in subsequent sections of this chapter.

Institutional review boards make final decisions on all federally funded research protocols involving human subjects. Their duty is to protect subjects from undue risk and deprivation of personal rights and dignity. This protection is achieved by reviewing the study's protocol to ensure that it meets the major requirements of ethical research, as summarized in Box 3–5.

Informed Consent

Most review boards use the *Code of Federal Regulations* (pp. 9–10) to define the meaning of **informed consent**:

> . . . the knowing consent of an individual or his/her legally authorized representative, under circumstances that provide the prospective subject or representative sufficient opportunity to consider whether or not to participate without undue inducement or any element of force, fraud, deceit, duress, or other forms of constraint or coercion.

Documentation that research meets the criterion of informed consent relies heavily on the board's review of a signed consent form for subjects to be involved in research. The wording of this form features prominently in most reviews, because the board must verify that it is suitable for promoting the free self-determination of potential subjects, and otherwise it is difficult to verify the consent process.

Vulnerable Subjects You can expect the board reviewing your protocol to exercise special care if your research involves subjects with *diminished capacity* to give free and informed consent. Prisoners, minors, fetuses, unconscious persons, psychiatric patients, the mentally retarded, students, fellows, and employees are all categories of **vulnerable subjects** whom many boards will not approve if the desired research data can be obtained from the study of other adult or normal subjects.

Box 3–5   **Federal Ethics Requirements for Research**

In order to approve research covered by these regulations the IRB shall determine that all of the following requirements are satisfied:

1. Risks to subjects are minimized: (i) By using procedures which are consistent with sound research design and which do not unnecessarily expose subjects to risk, and (ii) whenever appropriate, by using procedures already being performed on the subjects for diagnostic purposes.

2. Risks to subjects are reasonable in relation to anticipated benefits, if any, to subjects, and the importance of the knowledge that may reasonably be expected to result. In evaluating risks and benefits, the IRB should consider only those risks and benefits that may result from the research (as distinguished from risks and benefits of therapies subjects would receive even if not participating in research). The IRB should not consider possible long-range effects of applying knowledge gained in the research (for example, the possible effects of the research on public policy) as among those research risks that fall within the purview of its responsibility.

3. Selection of subjects is equitable. In making this assessment the IRB should take into account the purposes of the research and the setting in which the research will be conducted.

4. Informed consent will be sought from each prospective subject or the subject's legally authorized representative, in accordance with, and to the extent required by §46.116

5. Informed consent will be appropriately documented, in accordance with, and to the extent required by §46.117.

6. Where appropriate, the research plan makes adequate provision for monitoring the data collected to ensure the safety of subjects.

7. Where appropriate, there are adequate provisions to protect the privacy of subjects and to maintain the confidentiality of data.

8. Where some or all of the subjects are likely to be vulnerable to coercion or undue influence, such as persons with acute or severe physical or mental illness, or persons who are economically or educationally disadvantaged, appropriate additional safeguards have been included in the study to protect the rights and welfare of these subjects.

Source: Federal Regulations for Human Research.

Prisoners are vulnerable because (1) no prisoner is truly a free agent, (2) financial compensation that might seem modest may constitute an excessive inducement in prison, where earning opportunities are minimal, and (3) prisoners may believe that participation in an experiment will shorten their sentence. *Minors, unconscious pa-*

tients, *psychiatric patients*, and *the mentally retarded* may be unable to evaluate the risks involved, and you will therefore need to seek consent from parents, guardians, or close relatives. *Students* should preferably be recruited from classes other than an instructor's own. Their participation, or lack of it, must never influence their grades or future recommendations from the faculty member conducting research. Similarly, *fellows* and *employees* must be clear that their job, promotion, salary, and status are in no way dependent on serving as a research subject.

Some nurse scientists argue that review boards devised to protect the rights of human subjects in research can sometimes obstruct the efforts of nurse researchers who study certain populations. Robb (1983) believes that researchers who strictly adhere to board conditions for obtaining written informed consent from the elderly in institutional settings risk losing entire study populations, because many elderly people prefer being interviewed or observed to signing a consent form. As an illustration, she cites a proposed study to evaluate perspiration patches for estimating digoxin levels. The researchers failed to recruit a single participant despite the fact that 107 of 312 institutionalized elderly patients were taking digoxin. She urges researchers to find creative solutions to the burdens of written consent based on the urgent need for research into this population.

Box 3–6   Elements of Informed Consent

A. Basic elements of informed consent. . . .

1. A statement that the study involves research, an explanation of the purposes of the research and the expected duration of the subject's participation, a description of the procedures to be followed, and identification of any procedures which are experimental;

2. A description of any reasonably foreseeable risks or discomforts to the subject;

3. A description of any benefits to the subject or to others which may be reasonably expected from the research;

4. A disclosure of appropriate alternative procedures or courses of treatment, if any, that might be advantageous to the subject;

5. A statement describing the extent, if any, to which confidentiality of records identifying the subject will be maintained;

6. For research involving more than minimal risk, an explanation as to whether any compensation and an explanation as to whether any medical treatments are available if injury occurs and, if so,

(Continued)

Box 3–6   Elements of Informed Consent (continued)

what they consist of, or where further information may be obtained;

7. An explanation of whom to contact for answers to pertinent questions about the research and research subject's rights, and whom to contact in the event of a research-related injury to the subject; and

8. A statement that participation is voluntary, refusal to participate will involve no penalty or loss of benefits to which the subject is otherwise entitled, and the subject may discontinue participation at any time without penalty or loss of benefits to which the subject is otherwise entitled.

B. Additional elements of informed consent. When appropriate, one or more of the following elements

of information shall also be provided to each subject:

1. A statement that the particular treatment or procedure may involve risks to the subject (or to the embryo or fetus, if the subject is or may become pregnant) which are currently unforeseeable;

2. Anticipated circumstances under which the subject's participation may be terminated by the investigator without regard to the subject's consent;

3. Any additional costs to the subject that may result from participation in the research;

4. The consequences of a subject's decision to withdraw from the research and procedures for orderly termination of participation to the subject;

5. A statement that significant new developed during the course of the research may relate to the subject's willingness to continue participation will be provided to the subject; and

6. The approximate number of subjects involved in the study.

Source: From *Code of Federal Regulations*, Title 45, Part 46, Washington, D.C.: U.S. Government Printing Office, January 26, 1981.

Box 3–7   Sample Form: Experimental Subject's Bill of Rights

The rights below are the rights of every person who is asked to be in a research study.

As an experimental subject I have the following rights:

1. to be told what the study is trying to find out

2. to be told what will happen to me and whether the procedures, drugs, or devices are different from what would be used in standard practice

3. to be told about the frequent or important risks, side effects, or discomforts of the things that will happen to me for research purposes

4. to be told if I can expect any benefit from participating, and, if so, what the benefits might be

5. to be told the other choices I have and how they may be better or worse than being in the study

6. to be allowed to ask any questions concerning the study both before agreeing to be involved and during the course of the study

7. to be told what sort of treatment is available if any complications arise

8. to refuse to participate at all or to change my mind about participation after the study is started. This decision will not affect my right to receive the care I would receive if I were not in the study.

9. to receive a copy of the signed and dated consent form

10. to be free of pressure when considering whether I wish to agree to be in the study

If I have other questions, I should ask the researcher or the research assistant. In addition, I may contact the institutional review board, which is concerned with protection of volunteers in research projects. I may reach the board office by calling 123-4567 from 8:00 A.M. to 5:00 A.M., Monday to Friday, or by writing to the Committee on Human Research, State University.

Participation in research is voluntary. I have the right to refuse to participate and the right to withdraw later without any jeopardy to my nursing care [my grades, my employment].

Careful ethical reflectiveness requires that Robb's position be reconciled with the duty to protect the rights of vulnerable subjects. Consent should be conceived of as an agreement between two parties, investigator and subject, who have different degrees of power. Investigators are responsible for clarifying to a board what their approach to the patient was. The official consent form is only one way of putting the agreement into written form. Letters of agreement or verbal agreements made after reading an information sheet are alternative ways to document it (see Appendix A).

Elements of informed consent under federal guidelines are summarized in Box 3–6.

Writing a Standard Consent Form

Most investigators obtain consent through personal discussion. This process is recommended, because it allows questions to be answered on the spot. Consent documents, added to oral consent, may appear to be an unnecessary and quasi-legal burden. In addition to the legal requirements, however, there are two practical uses for a **consent form**: (1) It can aid the investigator by providing a checklist of discussion items. (2) It can aid the subject as a memory tool to be used at a later time; this suggests that a consent form should be readable and even engaging.

A consent form should tell a reasonable person from the proposed population the information he or she would wish to know in order to make an informed decision, in language that he or she is likely to understand. The suggested formats and language that follow are meant to replace previous, often stilted, language. (See Boxes 3–7, 3–8, and 3–9.) The organization is adaptable; it can be put in narrative, letter, or outline form as desired. Short paragraphs with wide margins are easy for most people to read. Investigators should consult with their review board in the cases of special populations (children, pregnant women, the mentally disabled).

Guidelines

1. The title should mention research in some way—for example, "Consent to Be a Research Subject."

2. The form should be consistent in person and verb tense.

3. The date of typing and page number should appear in the lower left corner.

4. Legal language should not be used. There is no reason to use *herewith* or *hereby*, for example. "I understand that . . ." also tends to place words that might not be true in the subject's mouth. A consent form is at most a piece of evidence, not a legal document.

5. The name and phone number of the investigator should be clearly visible.

Investigators not subject to a review board should consult the state law for the elements of informed consent required by their state. The easiest organization is as follows:

Organization

1. *Statement of Purpose and Introduction:* This section should answer the questions "What is being studied? why?" "Why me?" "Who are the investigators?" "What is going on that is different from normal?" This part should set the stage for the remainder of the form and provide a quick review.

A study is being done by F. Nightingale, RN, Ph.D., to learn more about the causes of [whatever the condition is]. She has asked me to be in the study.

A diet called XX is currently the standard treatment for my condition. It is known that a percentage of people do not respond to XX.

An experimental diet called YY is being tested in people who have not responded to XX. Because I have not responded to XX, I have been invited to be in the study.

Note: The word *new* connotes *better* to many people. *Experimental* is a more descriptive word for use in applications.

Box 3–8   Sample Form: Consent to be a Research Subject

Ms Nightingale is a nurse studying the way a certain blood component, called XYZ, works. To do the study, she needs blood from healthy people and from people with colds. If I agree to be in the study, a technician will draw a maximum of 100 milliliters (approximately 3 ounces) of blood from my arm vein. This will be done in her lab at 1842 Clinics. Drawing blood may be uncomfortable and could produce a bruise or, rarely, an infection. There will be no benefit to me, though the study may produce information of use to nurses in the future.

I have had the opportunity to talk with Ms Nightingale about the study. I may reach her at 123-4567 if I have questions later.

I will be paid $5.00 for this donation of blood. (If I am an employee, I agree not to participate during my work hours.)

I have received a copy of this form and the Experimental Subject's Bill of Rights to keep. I have the right to refuse to participate or to withdraw at any time without any jeopardy to my employment, my grades, or my care at this clinic.

_____   _____
Date   Subject's Signature

_____   _____
Date   Investigator's Signature

2. *Procedures:* Subjects need to know "What will happen to me if I participate that would not otherwise happen to me?" Standard or new procedures that would not ordinarily be done to these patients should be included. They should be described in terms of the subjects' experience (blood drawing) rather than laboratory terms (CBC). Procedures affecting the selection of care (random allocation) or others that a subject might wish to know about (for example, contacting a relative) are included. The form must be complete enough to allow a subject to make plans (baby-sitting, transportation).

If I agree, I will return to see the nurse practitioner in the clinic for ten additional monthly visits of one hour each. At each visit I will have the following tests that will not be for my diagnosis or treatment . . .

If I agree to participate, I will be interviewed for one hour. The questions will concern my background and how I feel about the treatment my family has received in the clinic. This will take place in my home or another place we agree on. If I agree, the interview will be tape-recorded.

In the study I would be randomly assigned to one of two groups. I would have a 50/50 chance of assignment to either group. Neither my nurse nor I would make the choice. The two groups are:

- Group A will have the standard treatment for 6 weeks instead of the usual 3 weeks.

- Group B will have the usual treatment time (3 weeks but at twice the usual amount).

---

3. *Risks and Discomforts:* Subjects should be able to gain a fair idea of the risks they will be taking and of the discomforts they might experience as a result of consenting. These include potential legal, economic, and psychological risks as well as physical risks. In some behavioral or social science studies, the term *disadvantages* might be more useful. A rule of thumb is that a side effect that is "relatively" frequent or that is "relatively" serious or permanent should be included. A side effect a reasonable person would wish to know about (sterility, scarring) should obviously be mentioned.

This drug may cause an allergic reaction such as skin rashes or hives. It can also cause a rare allergic reaction, similar to an allergic reaction to penicillin, which can be life threatening.

Taking blood from a vein may cause a bruise or, rarely, an infection.

I may be assigned to a group that is later shown to have had more side effects or less effective treatment. This information will not be known until the study data are analyzed.

As a result of answering this questionnaire, there is a possible loss of my privacy. The investigators will separate names from responses and will keep the names coded and locked so my confidentiality will be protected as much as possible under the law.

Participation in this study may involve the risk of arousing concerns about my family members or the oncology unit that are upsetting to me. Counseling references will be available to me.

The amount of radiation I will be exposed to is relatively small. Small doses may have potential harm, but the risk is difficult to measure with any precision. If I have many x-ray exams or if I am, or might be, pregnant, I should discuss this with the investigator.

Do not forget to include the statement on treatment and compensation for harm if there is any real or foreseeable risk of physical harm that exceeds what is considered "minimal." Each institution has its own particular compensation statement. Here is an example:

If I am physically injured as a result of being in this study, treatment will be available. The costs of such treatment may be covered by the university, depending upon a number of factors. For information I may call 123-4567.

---

4. *Benefits:* An unbiased statement should be included discussing personal and societal benefits. It should not be overstated or read like an advertisement.

I will derive no direct benefit from participating. The investigators hope to learn more about diets XX and YY, which may help care for patients like me more effectively in the future.

The additional tests I will have done are not needed for my diagnosis or care. The information will be put in my record and could be of interest to my primary nurse.

Box 3—9   Sample Form: Consent Letter

Dear X:

B. Smith, RN, and L. Jones, RN, are educational researchers who are interested in learning about how students choose their nursing career. They have completed an initial study of people who have no idea what they are going to do, and now they wish to compare this group with people who have a very definite idea about their goals. They have asked me to contact a few of my nursing students to see if they would be interested in responding.

If you agree to participate, please return the questionnaire I have enclosed to them at the address listed. There is identifying information on the form. If you would agree to a further interview, please fill that in at the same time. If you would not agree, then leave the information blank to help protect your own privacy.

You might be interested in further information from them before agreeing to participate. You may call them at 123-4567. Of course, no one must participate in any research if he or she does not wish to do so.

Sincerely,
Professor X, RN, PhD

Note: Most review boards do not consider money paid to subjects to be a benefit.

5. *Alternatives:* This section should describe the therapeutic or treatment options open in lieu of participation in this study. If the only alternative is simple refusal (for example, to throw away the questionnaire) this section may be omitted.

Instead of having my care chosen by the study, I may ask my own nurse to make the decision. The treatments available are diets XX and ZZ, but not YY.

---

6. *Questions:* Few subjects comprehend all details immediately or without some discussion. It is essential to offer a way to contact an investigator for a later discussion. If there is a possibility of emergency reactions, a 24-hour number should be used.

I have talked with Ms Nightingale and her assistant about this study and have had my questions answered. If I have other questions, I may call her at 123-4567.

7. *Bill of Rights:* The experimental subject's bill of rights (see Box 3–7) must be used when physically invasive procedures are involved. If a bill of rights is not used in a study, the researchers ought to include the final paragraph from the Bill of Rights on any consent form.

Participation in this research is voluntary. I have the right to refuse to participate and the right to withdraw later without any jeopardy to my nursing care [my grades, my employment].

8. *Payment:* Money is offered to pay for expenses, inconvenience, time, and trouble. It should not provide "undue influence" or reflect payment for acceptance of risk.

I will be paid $10.00 for each visit plus an added $5.00 whenever blood is drawn. This will total X.00 if I complete all the visits.

9. *Signatures:* The subject's signature should always be placed first. Other signatures may be requested. When children are involved, they should be asked to sign if they are old enough (over 7) to consider the questions, and their parents should generally be asked to give "permission" for their participation. The investigator's signature should also be included. A witness is not necessary for most studies but may be desired by the investigator or sponsor.

Sample consent forms can be found in Boxes 3–8 and 3–9.

The letter in Box 3–9 could be used in conjunction with a more formal consent form to be presented at the time of the interview. That consent form would apply to the interview and tape recording. It might disclose further advantages (such as receiving a copy of the published report) and disadvantages (such as loss of time and inconvenience) of participation.

Preparing a Protocol for a Review Board

An institutional review board, once having established that informed consent procedures are being followed, is also charged with disapproving any activity that falls under its jurisdiction if the risks of that activity are not outweighed by the sum of the benefit to subjects and the importance of the knowledge to be gained. Most committees have difficulty approving protocols entailing high personal risks to subjects if the benefit is purely social or if the research design raises questions about whether it is possible to gain any benefits at all. The committee will look for evidence that you have taken precautions to minimize the risks of your procedures and will examine the strength of the research design in the protocol you submit. Making this determination requires that you prepare a full "human subjects protocol" and submit it to the board along with your consent form. The accompanying example will guide you in this task.

Checklist for a Human Research Application

The following material is not an outline. Use it as a checklist against which to review your protocol. Does your submission include the following?

A. *Cover Sheet:* Fill this out completely each year.

B. *Protocol:* This usually should be a maximum of ten pages of text, and it should generally not be a copy of your grant application. Instead it covers:

1. background
   (a) context of work
   (b) competence of investigator—previous work done by others and self
   (c) justification for current study in humans

2. specific aims of the study
   (a) hypotheses, questions to be answered, data to be gathered or tested, description to be made
   (b) relevance to continuing work in this field

3. significance
   (a) benefits to individual subject or patient, if any
   (b) benefits to the class from which the subject is drawn
   (c) benefits to science, society, or humanity in general

4. methods
   (a) general study design
   (b) methods of data analysis
   (c) subjects
      (1) number and number per group (Why this number?)
      (2) source and access to subjects (If subjects are recruited from an agency other than that represented by the IRB, permission should be obtained from them.)
      (3) criteria for inclusion and exclusion
      (4) discussion of risks (physical, social, economic, other)
      (5) methods used to minimize the risks
      (6) consent process
      (7) vulnerable population? why? (see special regulations)
   (d) duration of the study

5. procedures
   (a) detailed explanation of what will be done to each subject and how that compares with what would be done were it not for the study
   (b) risks of each procedure (added time? physical? psychological?)
   (c) precautions to minimize risks (such as coding of records, debriefing of subjects, erasing of audiotapes)
   (d) frequency and duration of each procedure or test
   (e) location of studies

6. compensation of subjects
   (a) amount (Why that amount? Will all subjects receive the same?)
   (b) amount, if any, to be withheld until the end (Why?)

7. records: Where will they be stored? Where will consent forms be stored?

C. *Consent form(s):* This should be in lay language and in consistent person and tense.

1. background: What is this study about? What are the investigators hoping to show?

2. procedures: What will happen or change as a result of agreeing to participate?
   (a) extension of time, if any
   (b) return visits, if any
   (c) randomization or placebo

3. risk, discomforts, disadvantages: obvious and subtle points that the subject should be aware of before agreeing

4. benefits: a balanced presentation of benefits to self or others

5. alternatives, if any, including that of refusing to be in the study and having standard care

6. questions: assurance of investigator's readiness to answer questions and a phone number at which to contact the investigator

7. money: terms of payment where applicable

8. refusal or withdrawal: assurance of right to refuse or withdraw without jeopardy to whatever is applicable

9. receipt: notice that the consent form and Experimental Subject's Bill of Rights (for health care experiments) are to be given to the subject

EXAMPLE: Procedure for Submitting a Protocol to a Review Board

1. In most institutions, no federally funded study involving human subjects may begin until IRB approval is obtained.

2. Investigators should usually allow a minimum of 6 weeks for IRB review of any moderately complicated study, although some institutions require 6 months.

   The committee must usually receive multiple copies of the protocol (complete with all required information). These protocols are then circulated and are discussed during the meeting following their receipt or are considered without a full meeting of the committee.

   Each IRB has its own specific guidelines

3. IRB review usually proceeds in the following way:

   (a) The committee may decide that the proposal does *not* involve subjects at risk. For the purposes of DHHS, this committee action is equivalent to approval.

   (b) The committee may decide that the proposal does involve subjects at risk. If this is the case, the committee must review the proposal for the risk-benefit balance, the protection of rights of subjects, and the adequacy of informed consent. After doing so the committee may:

   - approve the protocol as submitted
   - approve the protocol contingent on minor revisions
   - request outside review of the protocol and then reconsider
   - require significant modification of the protocol before approval
   - request the investigator to discuss problems with the committee
   - reject the protocol

   Possible outcomes of an IRB's deliberations

4. Notice of the committee's decision will be sent to the principle investigator following the committee consideration. In the event of a rejected protocol the following applies:

   The decisions of the committee on human experimentation made on the basis of technical and ethical judgments are final and may not be appealed. However, it appears that occasionally during committee consideration of a proposed protocol the investigator feels the committee is showing bias, or that an inordinate amount of time is being taken in reaching a decision. Mechanisms usually exist within an institution to review complaints about bias or delay.

   Bias or extraordinary delay can be grounds for a complaint against an IRB

Source: Adapted from Federal Regulations for Human Research.

Nursing and the Ethics of Research

This chapter began with questions about how to make your own scientific research ethical and how to tell if someone else's studies are ethically sound. Advocates for research subjects, your own conscience, and review committees whose members have no particular investment in a particular study all safeguard the rights of human subjects. Nurses who are research investigators or who assist in the research projects of others are in a position to assert and maintain the protective values of the profession. A study design that deprived one group of patients of relaxation techniques for labor pain or preoperative teaching, for example, would be unethical unless provisions were made for alternatively effective care. Projective psychological tests like the Rorschach inkblot test may represent an invasion of privacy if patients do not know that such tests may measure traits that the patients wish to conceal. Furthermore, patients are vulnerable to requests to participate in research when the person approaching them with the request is the nurse whom the patient depends on for care.

As Walker (1983) points out, obtaining approval for clinical investigations can be time-consuming and cumbersome, making it difficult for some nurses to conduct research in hospitals. But it is difficult for *anyone* to conduct clinical research unless he or she has demonstrated scientific rigor, sophistication, political savvy, and concern for the ethics of research on human subjects.

Guidelines for Critique

- Does the research report contain a statement that the study was approved by an ethical review board or similar institutional committee?

- Were vulnerable subjects used?

- Were subjects deceived in any way?

- Were subjects fully informed of all the procedures involved in the study?

- Were careful measures taken to protect subjects from harm and invasion of privacy?

- Were subjects apprised of the risks, both obvious and subtle, of participating in the study?

- Did the benefits resulting from the study outweigh the risks?

- Was informed consent obtained from all subjects? In what form?

- Did subjects have the right of self-determination (were they coerced in any way)?

■ Were subjects debriefed?

■ Have data been kept anonymous and confidential?

■ Has the researcher been objective in reporting results, as evidenced by inclusion of data that are unsupportive as well as those that are supportive?

■ Has credit been given to others who contributed to the research?

■ Has the researcher disclosed any sources of financial support or sponsorship?

SUMMARY OF KEY IDEAS AND TERMS

✔ In the past, many researchers have abused the rights of human subjects in the interest of advancing knowledge.

✔ Nursing research, because it regularly involves human subjects, has a particular responsibility for conducting ethical yet scientifically sound studies.

✔ Characteristics that make a study ethical are scientific objectivity, cooperation with authorized review boards, integrity about the nature of a study, equitability in acknowledging the work of others, nobility in advocating the rights of human subjects, truthfulness, impeccable observance of the researcher's role, forthright honesty about a study's funding sources and sponsorship, illumination of the knowledge base of the discipline, and courage in correcting distortions.

✔ Contemporary codes of scientific ethics are derived from the Nuremberg Code and the Declaration of Helsinki.

✔ Four basic rights of human subjects are (1) the right not to be harmed, (2) the right to full disclosure, (3) the right of self-determination, and (4) the right to privacy, anonymity, and confidentiality.

✔ One way of increasing the likelihood that your research will be ethical is acquiring approval from an institutional review board.

✔ Review boards protect human subjects by providing an impartial third-party review of the issues and protections for human rights such as (1) ensuring that informed consent is obtained from subjects and (2) ensuring that an appropriate balance exists between the potential benefits of a study and the risks to human subjects.

✓   Board approval is required for federal and much other funding of research.

✓   Particular care must be exercised in gaining informed consent from vulnerable subjects, such as children, the mentally disabled, and prisoners.

✓   It is important to follow your institution's board guidelines when writing a study protocol and consent form.

References

Abrams R. Dementia research in the nursing home. *Hoop Community Psychiatry* 1988; 39:257–259.

American Nurses' Association. *Human Rights Guidelines for Nurses in Clinical and Other Research*. Kansas City, Mo.: American Nurses' Association, 1975.

American Sociological Society. Toward a code of ethics for sociologists, *Am Sociol*, July 1984:1–4.

Berkowitz SB. Informed consent and the elderly. *Gerontol* 1978; 18:237–243.

Code of Federal Regulations. Title 45, Part 46. Washington, D.C., January 26, 1981.

Honor in Science, 2nd ed. New Haven, Conn.: Sigma Xi, 1986.

Jones JH: *Bad Blood: The Tuskegee Syphilis Experiment*. New York: Free Press, 1981.

Katz J: *Experimentation with Human Beings: The Authority of the Investigator, Subject, Professions and State in the Human Experimentation Process*. New York: Russell Sage Foundation, 1972.

Reynolds PD: On the protection of human subjects and social science. *Int Soc Sci J* 1972; 24:694–695.

Robb SS: Beware of the informed consent. *Nurs Res* May/June 1983; 32:132.

U.S. Department of Health, Education, and Welfare. *The Institutional Guide to DHEW Policy on Protection of Human Subjects*. Washington, D.C.: US Government Printing Office, 1971.

U.S. National Commission for the Protection of Human Subjects of Biomedical and Behavioral Research. *The Belmont Report: Ethical Principles and Guidelines for the Protection of Human Subjects of Research*. DHEW Publication No. (05)78-0012. Washington, D.C.: US Government Printing Office, 1978.

Walker M: As I see it . . . Research with patients requires commitment, savvy. *Am Nurse* July/August 1983:5.

A Consumer's Guide
to Nursing Research

C H A P T E R

4

How To Read Research Articles

HOLLY SKODOL WILSON

Chapter Objectives

After reading this chapter, the student should be able to:

- Explain why typical research articles are often low on readability

- Recognize when long or impersonal words and sentences can be translated into plain, conversational language

- Describe the arrangement of headings and subheadings in a typical research journal article

- Interpret presentations of information in each section of a journal article

- Define the meaning of some commonly used research terms

- Critically analyze information usually disseminated in graphs and tables

- Overcome attitudinal obstacles to reading nursing research reports effectively

In This Chapter . . .

Have you ever felt the frustration of not being able to understand what the author of a scientific article means? Did you ever become bogged down in what seemed to be heavy, stale, cliché-ridden jargon that obscured possibly forceful ideas? Did the research report you read catch and hold your attention, or did you find yourself eager to move on to a more interesting popular piece of clinical writing in the *American Journal of Nursing, Nursing '89* or *RN*? Did you conclude that it's no wonder that practitioners of the past have avoided participating in and implementing nursing research in their professional role?

In this chapter you will learn step-by-step instructions to decipher technical writing and foster mental processes that will help you think about the research-oriented writing you read. In the framework of analytic reading, *you will come to terms with research terminology*. Naturally, the arts of reading and thinking can be learned only by constant practice. In this chapter, I encourage you to set up a training program for yourself so that reading even highly complex research literature will become second nature to you. Don't stop practicing till you reach that point.

Topics covered in this chapter include (1) understanding the format of a research journal article, (2) translating the language of science, and (3) learning strategies for interpreting tables and graphs. You don't have to be a career researcher to decipher nursing research, evaluate it, and use research findings in your clinical practice.

Readability

In most dictionaries, *readable* is defined as "easy" *or* "interesting" to read. Actually, to most people, readability means ease of reading *plus* interest. Most of us want to make as little effort as possible while we are reading and want something to carry us forward like an escalator. We want to be inspired or interested as well as informed. Flesch (1960) puts forth a formula for successful communication in 25 rules for effective writing listed in Box 4–1.

Flesch adds that for most of us, graph and chart reading is *not* one of the three Rs! *People need training to learn from visual presentations*. In view of the preceding points, it should come as no big surprise that nursing research reports, protocols, and methodology at first seem low in readability according to Flesch's conception of it.

The plain-talk style of writing that makes popular magazine articles easy to read is decidedly absent in most reports of scientific research. The problem of reading research literature effectively becomes partly a matter of language translation and partly a matter of context translation. We will consider both in the pages that follow.

Box 4–1   Twenty-five Rules for Effective Writing

1. Write about people, things, and facts.

2. Write the way you talk.

3. Use contractions.

4. Use the first person.

5. Quote what you said.

6. Quote what was written.

7. Put yourself in the reader's place.

8. Don't hurt the reader's feelings.

9. Forestall misunderstandings.

10. Don't be too brief.

11. Plan a beginning, middle, and end.

12. Go from the rule to the exception, from the familiar to the new.

13. Use short names and abbreviations.

14. Use pronouns rather than repeating nouns.

15. Use verbs rather than nouns.

16. Use the active voice and a personal subject.

17. Use small, round figures.

18. Specify! Use illustrations, cases, examples.

19. Start a new sentence for each new idea.

20. Keep your sentences short.

21. Keep your paragraphs short.

22. Use direct questions.

23. Underline for emphasis.

24. Use parentheses for casual mention.

25. Make your writing interesting to look at.

Source: Rudolph Flesch, *How to Write, Speak, and Think More Effectively*, New York: Harper & Row, 1960. Copyright 1946, 1949, 1951, 1958, 1960 by Rudolph Flesch. Copyright 1950, 1951 by Printers' Ink Publishing Corporation. Reprinted by permission of Harper & Row, Publishers, Inc.

In Pursuit of Translation

As you read research literature, you will undoubtedly encounter multisyllable words, jargon-ridden paragraphs, and technical terminology. Here are a couple of preliminary strategies for understanding them when you meet up with them:

1. Give yourself time to understand different and unfamiliar words and expressions.

2. Pause between reading difficult sentences.

3. Mentally fill in the spaces between ideas with your own reasoning about them.

4. Think of illustrations or personal rephrasings that help you reach a personal understanding of an author's ideas.

5. Try to translate them into your own mental, conversational talk.

Some Plain Talk about Research in Nursing

In 1976 the American Nurses' Association's Commission on Nursing Research, with the cooperation of a distinguished list of nurse researchers, published a document called *Research in Nursing: Toward a Science of Health Care*. In it, using conversational, popular language and a lot of photographs, the authors explain what research in nursing is and give some superb examples of clinical discoveries made through scientific inquiry. They describe research in nursing as

> investigating . . . the area of knowledge where the physical and behavioral sciences meet and influence one another, in an effort to study how health problems relate to human behavior and how behavior relates to health and illness. . . . Research in nursing addresses the human and behavioral questions that arise in the treatment of diseases and the prevention of illness and maintenance of health (p. 1).

This document introduces the reader to some selected projects conducted by nurses that represent important advances in health care knowledge and the study of people with health problems. The project descriptions are excellent examples of how technical writing styles and esoteric language can be translated into highly readable material. After reading a few of these illustrations (Examples 1–5 on pp. 108–110), use the strategies in the rest of this chapter to translate some published research reports into plain talk yourself.

EXAMPLE 1: Alleviating Pain

A series of relaxation exercises carried out once or twice a day may relieve the intensity of pain or relax patients so that they are better able to cope with pain according to results of tests by a nurse researcher. Working with three groups of patients—those having elective surgery such as gallbladder removal or hernia repairs, those having rheumatoid arthritis and cancer patients—the nurse researcher was able to validate that pain can be relieved by methods other than medication (p. 3).

EXAMPLE 2: Understanding Obesity

Although the cause of obesity is not known and its treatment is notably unsuccessful, a nurse researcher believes that the answer to treatment of the obesity problems lies in understanding more about the mechanisms which underlie feeding behavior and control appetite. Her research project, which is directed at understanding hunger and satiety, is exploring the role of many different hormones and substrates contained in the blood and their influence on appetite and regulation of body weight. These studies are being carried out on monkeys whose anatomy and physiology is similar to that of humans (p. 7).

EXAMPLE 3: Screening for Cystic Fibrosis

A nurse research project has provided a breakthrough in effectively screening victims and carriers of cystic fibrosis, a process that has been impeded by lack of an efficient test system that could be readily made available to clinical laboratories (p. 9).

EXAMPLE 4: Womb Simulation for Premature Infants

Premature babies given special treatment and conditions to simulate prenatal womb life achieve a greater degree of development than similar infants provided standard conditions according to information compiled by a nurse researcher. Normal, full-term infants can usually sleep for 60 minutes at a time, while a baby who normally would be in the womb for another eight weeks lacks the nervous system development that controls sleep behavior, which in turn affects weight gain and physical development. . . . The nurse and her research team simulated womb conditions by playing a tape-recording of a heart beat for 15 minutes every hour, and rocking the mattresses of the isolettes in which the babies were placed. Those infants living in the womb-simulated situations slept more quietly and gained more weight than a group of similar babies of the same age used in comparison studies. The nursing research team is continuing efforts to determine the best time in an infant's life to begin simulation, how loud a heart beat is advantageous, the intensity of rocking that is most productive and at what point visual stimulation might be used (pp. 10–11).

EXAMPLE 5: Coping with Home Dialysis

Patients using an artificial kidney machine at home have advantages over those who continue treatment in hospitals according to a nurse researcher studying the relationships in home dialysis triads and patient outcomes. The study, which investigates how cooperation among patient, spouse, and doctor makes a difference for the patient using home dialysis, indicated that home treatment resulted in better physical health, closer adherence to medical regimen, greater amounts of work and leisure time activities, fewer hospitalized days and fewer emergencies for the patient. . . . The study of families successfully coping with dialysis is yielding information about the ways they make adaptations which maximize the quality of life for the patient and minimize the disruption of other family members (p. 13).
Source: American Nurses' Association, Commission on Nursing Research, *Research in Nursing: Toward a Science of Health Care*, Kansas City, Mo.: 1976.

Speaking the Language of Science

Meaning and Context

Before you can evaluate the worth of a scientific article, you have to understand it. Learning what may be a new vocabulary is part of the solution. But vocabulary alone isn't all of it. We understand the meaning of even unfamiliar words when we first understand their context. What this means is that you can use terms such as *vitamin deficiency* or *wound infection* when teaching patients who may never have heard them if you put them in a context that helps the patients interpret what they mean. Likewise, you understand unfamiliar research terminology once you grasp its context in the research process. Unfortunately, building a research vocabulary isn't as easy as merely looking up words in a resource such as the glossary at the end of this book. Even the term *science* has somewhat different meanings under different conditions. If you look it up in a glossary, you will probably find a definition like this:

> *Science*: A branch of study . . . concerned with the observation and classification of facts, esp. with the establishment of verifiable general laws.

If, however, you ask a nurse theorist what he or she means by *nursing science*, the response might be more like this:

Science is an interconnected series of concepts and conceptual schemes that have developed as a result of empirical observation and guide future observations, descriptions, and prediction.

Clearly, these two definitions of science are different. The first emphasizes facts, and the second emphasizes concepts. Having advanced an argument for placing the meaning of scientific language in the appropriate context as one way of making it easier to understand, I will now consider the language of science *within the context* of the format of a typical scientific article.

Typical Format of a Research Journal Article

Almost all research journal articles are divided into sections with headings and subheadings. The arrangement of these headings usually follows a somewhat standardized format. If you are familiar with it, you can get the most out of the time you spend reading, because you understand the context that each section intends to establish. You will also have a better chance of getting your own articles published in scientific journals if you should decide to conduct your own research (see Chapter 18). Huck, Cormier, and Bounds (1974), in a handy little book called *Reading Statistics and Research*, outline the typical sections of a research article with the headings arranged as follows (pp. 3–4):

1. Abstract
2. Introduction
   - Review of the literature
   - Statement of purpose
3. Method
   - Subjects
   - Design
   - Materials (data collection)
   - Procedure (data analysis)
4. Results (conclusions)
5. Discussion
6. References

Let us examine each of these sections with a bit more care.

Abstract An **abstract** is located at the beginning of a research article. Its purpose is to summarize the entire piece as briefly as possible. An abstract usually provides the following information about the study:

1. its purpose, objectives, or hypotheses

2. a description of the participants or sample members

3. a brief explanation of data-collection and analysis procedures

4. a summary of important findings (Huck, Cormier, and Bounds 1974 p. 4)

The accompanying example is an illustration of an abstract. It offers you an overview of what you will find in the article that follows. Because it is *located at the beginning* of an article, you can read it in a minute or two and then decide whether

Sample Abstract

A national survey of a stratified random sample (n = 240) of accredited hospitals with critical care units (CCUs) was conducted in order to describe the current practice of restrictions imposed upon myocardial infarction (MI) patients. A cross-sectional correlation survey with a two-stage mailing was used.

The first-stage mailing at the institutional level was sent to the head nurses of the CCUs (n = 600). Nurses were requested to give: (a) importance and frequency ratings of selected coronary care nursing practices; (b) information about the use of discontinuance of two specific restrictions: ice water and rectal temperature measurements. Follow-ups by mail and/or telephone yielded response rates for about 87%.

The conceptual framework, "Diffusion of Innovations," was used to assess the diffusion of the results of studies published in clinical journals. Despite findings that cast doubt on the practices of restricting ice water and rectal temperature measurement, coronary precautions are commonly practiced.

Hours spent reading and the number of journals read correlate (p less than .001) with greater levels of awareness in nurses that such restrictions are in question. Levels of awareness are *not* related to the importance and frequency ratings for those restrictions. Differences among nurses do not explain differences in ratings. If research is to be used, nurse researchers and managers need to actively intervene in care. Passive diffusion of research results is inadequate, unsure, and slow.

Source: K. T. Kirchoff, "A Diffusion Survey of Coronary Precautions," *Nursing Research*, July/August 1982, vol. 31, p. 196. Reprinted with permission. Copyright © 1982 American Journal of Nursing Company.

to skim systematically or read the whole article analytically. Because it helps you use your reading time wisely, an abstract serves a very useful purpose. It may also be your first encounter with some unfamiliar words. If the study relates to your interest areas, you will have a chance to read about the subjects in more depth and get a fuller grasp of the meaning of terms as you continue reading the article.

Let's go back to the components of an abstract and figure out what we've just read. First, an abstract provides the purpose, objectives, or hypotheses of the study. In this example, the purpose is "to describe the current practice of restrictions imposed on myocardial infarction (MI) patients" in CCUs throughout the United States. We'd probably add, in view of the conclusions, that another descriptive purpose of the study was to determine if practicing these restrictions had any relationship with whether nurses had read the latest research on the subject in professional journals.

Second, the sample abstract tells us that the participants in the study were a sample of 600 randomly selected nurses and head nurses from a stratified random sample of 240 CCUs in accredited hospitals throughout the country. The selection of random sampling tells us (as do the large sizes of the samples) that the investigator wanted to increase the possibilities of generalizing her findings to the total population of accredited CCUs by obtaining a representative sample, and not just to a case study of one institution or even a particular region's practices.

As far as procedures are concerned, the researcher mailed some instruments to head nurses and randomly selected staff nurses in accredited settings who were willing to participate. She asked them to provide information about the awareness and use or nonuse of coronary precautions and their typical journal reading habits as well as some additional information. She used a statistical technique to correlate these categories of information that yielded a number, called a *p value*, that she compared with values in a statistical table.

Fourth, the abstract gives us a summary of important findings. Although the researcher found that nurses who spent more hours reading had greater levels of *awareness* that coronary restrictions were in question, being aware didn't seem to alter clinical practice. This finding led the author to argue for the importance of active programs to get research findings into practice.

Introduction   The introduction of a research article usually contains two parts, (1) a review of the literature and (2) a statement of the study's purpose. Most authors begin with a **literature review**—discussion of previous relevant studies that they or others have conducted. This background of information helps the reader figure out how the study being reported relates to previous knowledge in a field. It is important to ask yourself if the study at hand is so original that little or nothing of any importance has preceded it, or if the investigator just didn't bother to look up the prior research or theoretical literature on his or her topic. The discussion of previous research can be as short as one or two sentences or as long as several pages. The following three paragraphs constitute the literature review in our sample study report by Kirchoff.

Sample Literature Review

The term "coronary precautions" covers a list of restrictions imposed upon myocardial infarction patients, including restriction of: hot and cold beverages, rectal temperature measurement, stimulant beverages, and sometimes vigorous back rubs (Kirchoff 1981).

Several clinical and laboratory studies of cardiac changes following the ingestion of ice water have been conducted (Cohen, Alpert, Francis, Vieweg, and Hagan 1977; Fitzmaurice and Simon 1974; Houser, 1976; Pratte, Padilla, and Baker 1973). The general conclusions were that a normally consumed amount of hot or ice water (200 cc) was *not harmful* to a recent myocardial infarction patient, although Pratte, Padilla, and Baker (1973) found that ingestion of 600 cc of ice water by normal males in the supine position was related to changes in electrical activity in the heart.

Two studies of the cardiac changes following the measurement of rectal temperature were found (Gruber, 1974; McNeal, 1978). Measurement of rectal temperatures *did not* cause bradycardia or arrhythmias. No studies were found that discounted the restriction of stimulant beverages, none were found that mentioned vigorous back rubs. Except for the findings of Fitzmaurice and Simon, and Pratte and colleagues, the results of the studies were rarely available to critical care nurses [Kirchoff 1982 p. 196].

Having summarized the relevant literature leading up to a current study, the author usually states the specific goals or purposes of the study. In our sample article, Kirchoff says:

Sample Purpose

A survey of current practice was designed to assess the impact of the published studies on the practices of restricting ice water and the measurement of rectal temperature. Nurses who read these publications might have reduced the frequency of or even eliminated these practices, rendering further research meaningless [Kirchoff 1982 p. 196].

One can paraphrase the paragraph above as follows: "Because published studies have demonstrated that nurses don't need to restrict ice water and rectal temperature-taking with coronary patients, one would expect that nurses who read these studies would have abandoned these restrictions. I decided to do a survey to find out if in fact they have." When you look for the literature review and study purpose in a research report, be prepared to find them either under separate headings or grouped under the heading "Background" or "Introduction."

Method   In this section of a research article, the author explains in detail exactly how he or she conducted the study. The reason for going into such elaborate detail is so that a reader could replicate the study. According to Huck and his colleagues (1974 p. 6), the author addresses four main questions in the method section of a research article:

1. Who participated in the study?

2. What type of research design was used?

3. What materials (data) were needed?

4. What procedures were the participants required to do?

The reader needs a full description of the subjects who participated in the study and the process by which they were selected (sampling procedure) because the conclusions of most studies are valid only for people who are similar to the subjects in the study. In our sample article, the author does a good job of telling us the criteria for including nurses in the sample to receive survey instruments and of the number (n = 524) who actually completed the data collection forms. She also tells us how she selected the head and then staff nurses, using a random sampling procedure from a list provided by the head nurse of settings who met study criteria.

For any study purpose, several designs can be used. Chapter 5 is devoted to a discussion of these in detail. The design gives you an idea of the overall plan for organizing the study and some predictions about how data might be statistically treated. In our sample article, Kirchoff informs us that she used "a cross-sectional national descriptive/correlational survey of critical-care nurses employed in acute medical-surgical hospitals." We understand that instead of comparing two or more groups on some characteristic or another (an experimental design), Kirchoff mailed a survey to a national sample of critical-care nurses and then correlated certain responses with other responses.

Materials are the measurement devices used to collect data from the subjects. One might use a questionnaire, a thermometer, or an interview, but whatever the instrument, the researcher should tell you whether he or she used a new instrument constructed especially for this study or an older instrument developed by somebody else. The author should describe exactly how the measurements were done and particularly report on a self-developed instrument's **validity** and **reliability** (see Glossary). If the instrument comes from somewhere else but is modified for use in the study being reported, the author should explain how the original was modified. In our sample article, Kirchoff describes the instruments in this way:

Sample Description of Instruments

A one-page questionnaire, printed on two sides called the *Unit Form*, contained closed-ended items. The questions were designed to elicit information about the institution (hospital) and the unit (CCU). Face validity of the items was assumed on the basis of the demographic nature of the items and simplicity of the format. Pretesting of the instrument on a small national sample of hospitals ($n = 24$) revealed no omitted responses and no apparent inconsistencies in the data.

The *Staff Nurse Selection Sheet* consisted of a one-page grid, which required the head nurse to list full-time registered nurses working the day or evening shift. . . . No changes in this instrument were needed on the basis of pretesting during the pilot study.

The Nurse Form was designed to obtain a national picture of current coronary care practices and to provide data for the analysis of the diffusion of the results of published research relating to two specific practices; the restriction of ice water and the restriction of rectal temperature measurement. The form consisted of a five-page questionnaire, divided into three parts. The first page contained explicit directions and described the clinical situation of an uncomplicated MI patient. . . . All the forms and the method were pretested in the pilot study. After the completion of the pilot study and preliminary analysis, the revised instruments were submitted to a nationally recognized cardiovascular nurse clinician for review [Kirchoff 1982 pp. 197–198].

The procedure section describes how the study was conducted. Remember, it is supposed to include enough detail so that a reader could replicate the study. Here's an excerpt from our sample article to give you a sense of how detailed the procedure discussion was:

Sample Procedure

A letter addressed to the director of nursing was mailed to each of the randomly selected institutions. At the sample time, a cover letter, Unit Form, Staff Nurse Selection Sheet, and a return stamped envelope were sent to the "Head Nurse, CCU" at each of the selected hospitals. A second letter and an additional copy of the Unit Form and Staff Nurse Selection Sheet along with another return envelope were sent to all head nurses who had not responded within three weeks. After another three and a half weeks, a third similar follow-up was sent to those nurses. . . . Attempts were made to contact the remaining head nurses by phone. About two months after the beginning of the first-stage mailing, with a majority of the responses from the CCU's received, the second-stage mailing was initiated [Kirchoff 1982 p. 198].

You can either skim through the specifics of the write-up of a study's procedure quickly to move to the results, or you can use it as a step-by-step road map to critique or replicate a study.

Results   The results of a study tend to be reported in the text, summarized in tables, or presented visually in a graph or figure. It is absolutely critical that you be able to understand and evaluate the results of any study that you read. Sometimes researchers have used a statistical test incorrectly, sometimes they have drawn conclusions that go far beyond what can be justified by the sample and study design, and sometimes the tables are inconsistent with what the authors explain in the text. Kirchoff reported the results of our sample study in the text like this:

Sample Results

Avoiding the use of rectal thermometer and restricting ice water received moderate importance and frequency ratings but large standard deviations, indicating high variability among the sample of nurses. . . . The most common origin for practice of both these restrictions is unit policy. . . . The most important nurse variable in a multiple regression is the number of years since most recent graduation, but the total explained variance despite the inclusion of 10 significant variables was only 6%. . . . Reading the *American Journal of Nursing*, the number of journals read and the hours spent reading per week were significantly correlated with level of awareness that the coronary care precautions were being questioned. But the effect of awareness (reading) on persuasion (the importance ratings) and on adoption (the frequency ratings) showed no significant differences. . . . *Being aware did not affect how important the nurses thought the restrictions were or how frequently they reported practicing the restrictions* [Kirchoff 1982 p. 200].

Discussion   The preceding section on results presents a report of how the statistical analysis turned out. The discussion section explains what the results mean with regard to the study's purposes and relates them to a theoretical context. Many authors also use this part of a research article to tell us why they think their results turned out the way they did and to suggest new types of study for future research. Sometimes the discussion section is called "Conclusions." In our sample study, Kirchoff conveys the nontechnical interpretation of the study findings this way:

Sample Discussion

Coronary precautions are widely practiced. The awareness of published studies has not changed practice. Although the passive diffusion [of research results] process has some effect on awareness, it has little effect on persuasion or adoption. . . . Some studies require a translation process before they are put to use. . . . Passive diffusion of research results is inadequate, unsure, and slow. A process of active intervention on the part of those nurses qualified to evaluate completed studies is needed [Kirchoff 1982 p. 201].

Our sample study also presents some of the results in tables. The final section of this chapter is devoted to overcoming some of the obstacles to interpreting visual representations of study findings.

References A research article ends with a list of books and articles to which the author referred during the study report. This list can be a useful resource if you want to tackle a comparative reading of the major ideas associated with a topic. Reading the references cited at the end of a study report can also familiarize you with the findings and logic that led the author up to the study being reported. The reference list at the conclusion of our sample article includes articles and books on research utilization and communication of findings as well as on coronary care precautions.

Now that we have at least an initial idea of what the article is about and have decided that it is of interest to us, we are in a position to read it at an analytic level with a particular eye toward coming to terms with the research terminology in context.

Coming to Terms with Research Terminology

Concepts, Constructs, Conceptual Frameworks, and Theory

Concepts are abstractions that allow us to categorize observations based on certain commonalities and differences. For example, nurses study a diverse array of concepts including *infection, bonding, activity level, elimination, stress, coping, loss, pain, self-esteem, accountability, self-care, rhymicity, locus of control, limiting intrusion,* and *in-*

stitutionalization, among others. Some concepts are names for concrete observations that can be measured directly, and others rely on what are called "proxy measures," because they cannot be directly measured by counting pulse rate or respirations or some other directly observable phenomenon.

Certain more abstract concepts are called **constructs**, because they have been created (constructed) by scientists for a research purpose. Examples of constructs include *positive reinforcement* from learning theory, *learned helplessness* from psychology, *bureaucratization* and *social class* from sociology, and in the case of our example study, *diffusion of innovation*, probably from social psychology and communication theory. Science is concerned with explaining and refining the concepts that classify and make sense of the order in the world and with generalizing from the specific or particular to the abstract, that is, with generating and testing theories. In our example, concepts included in the study were not only the major one, *diffusion of innovation*, but also *coronary precautions*, and *communication channels*. We are introduced to these concepts and the process of mental relations (awareness, persuasion, decision, and confirmation of decision) in a section of the early part of the article headed "Conceptual Framework." Here we learn that others (Rogers and Shoemaker 1971) formulated relationships between and among the concepts and constructs in this study in a model that included a source (researchers), an innovation (the discontinuance of two coronary precaution restrictions), communication channels (research publications), and communication receivers (staff nurses in coronary care units).

Operationally Defining a Concept

Although many of us can function adequately with a highly personal or even vague idea of what a concept means in day-to-day practice, a researcher must translate the concepts in his or her study into variables that can validly represent the concept under investigation and reliably be measured. An **operational definition** of a concept specifies what a researcher does to make the concept measurable. It defines a concept so that someone else will measure it in the same way. When concepts have been operationalized, they are called **variables**—meaning something that varies and has different values that can be measured. For something to be called a variable, therefore, it must be able to have at least two values. *Sex* is a variable; *female* is not a variable, but rather a value for the variable *sex*. Many studies are criticized primarily on the approach the researcher has used to operationalize concepts that are being studied. It is the researcher's job to make his or her operational definitions plausible in the eyes of critical readers. In order to replicate someone's study, we have to know how the concepts and other terms were defined. They are usually defined according to their relationship to the problem being studied in a particular investigation. In our sample study the study *settings* were coronary care units, selected using a stratified random sampling procedure, in accredited hospitals that were willing to participate. The *individual nurses* were randomly selected staff nurses (every possible sample member had an equal chance of being selected) identified by head nurses as "registered nurses with at least one year of experience in the unit, at least 75% of time spent in patient care, full-time employment, and assignment to the day or evening shift." In addition, the head nurses from participating units were included in the mailing. If you want to use research results from this or any other study in your own work, you have to look to operational definitions that are closest to your own definitions of concepts and other terms.

Distinguishing Independent from Dependent Variables

Variables are often labeled as *dependent* or *independent*. The **dependent variable** (DV), also called the output or criterion variable, is the study variable under investigation. It's the one that the researcher determines *as a result* of conducting the study. In some cases it is the *effect* or *outcome* of an experimental procedure. The variability in the dependent variable presumably *depends* on the cause or conditions that may be manipulated by the researcher in the study. The dependent variables in our example study were the persuasion about and adoption of research findings about coronary precautions. In most studies, the dependent variables are the ones that the researcher is intending to understand, explain, or predict. The dependent variables in our example are measures of the outcome of innovation diffusion. They constitute what the researcher measures about the subjects *after* they have experienced or been exposed to the independent variable.

Independent variables (IVs), in contrast, are the causes or conditions that the investigator manipulates or identifies to determine the effects or outcomes. Their values are established independently by the investigator ahead of time. They constitute the *input* of an experiment and precede the measurement of the dependent variable.

It is usually not too hard to spot the difference between the independent variables and the dependent variable(s) in a research study. Sometimes they are alluded to in the study title: "A Diffusion Survey of Coronary Precautions" means that the study is about the impact of the diffusion of research knowledge about coronary precautions on the practice arena. The statement of study purpose sometimes reveals that an investigator has set out to establish the effects of something (IV) on something else (DV) (for example, the effects of preoperative teaching on postoperative recovery or of therapeutic touch on perception of pain). The same statement is sometimes made in reverse order: "This study was conducted to see whether a client's self-esteem [DV] was affected by changes in levels of physical exercise [IV]." In both cases, though, the investigator is doing the same thing: manipulating or selecting an IV or several of them to determine whether it (they) affects or changes measurements in the DV(s).

It is possible to have both multiple dependent variables and multiple independent variables, but all must be operationally defined. In our study example, the investigator correlated nurse variables that included *11* independent variable measures with two important coronary care restrictions—on ice water and on rectal temperature-taking (see Table 4–1). Together, these independent and dependent variables allowed her to reach conclusions about research knowledge diffusion, at least when it came to CCU nurses and patients and the practice of coronary precautions.

Uncontrolled, or Confounding, Variables

So far everything seems straightforward in our sample article's new vocabulary. The investigator has decided what the independent and dependent variables are to be and has operationally defined them. She has obtained a sufficiently large sample, using a stratified random sampling procedure of accredited hospitals that have CCUs and nurses doing patient care on them who meet certain criteria. She has collected data about them, using a series of survey forms that allow her to classify them along 11 "nurse variables" related to her study question about innovation diffusion. She

TABLE 4–1   *Correlation of Two Importance Ratings with Nurse Variables[a]*

| | | | Restrictions | |
| | | | Rectal Temperature Measurement | |
Nurse Variable		Ice Water (n)	(r)	(n)
Years since basic education	.13[d]	513	.04	518
Years since most recent education	.13[c]	512	.08[b]	517
Years of nursing experience	.12[c]	516	.06	521
Years of CCU experience	.07[b]	516	−.01	521
Years of experience in unit	.03	513	−.01	518
AACN membership	.00	515	−03	520
ANA membership	.06	515	.08[b]	520
Reads *AJN*	.00	519	.08[b]	513
Reads *Heart & Lung*	.00	519	−.11[c]	513
Number of journals read	.06	519	−.01	513
Hours week reading journals	.01	506	−.05	510

[a]Pearson Product-Moment Correlation
[b]p<.05
[c]p<.01
[d]p<.001

Source: K. T. Kirchoff, "A Diffusion Survey of Coronary Precautions," *Nursing Research*, July/August 1982, vol. 31, p. 199. Reprinted with permission. Copyright © 1982 American Journal of Nursing Company.

has obtained dependent variable data from her subjects by asking about awareness and persuasion ratings on two important coronary-care precautions, restrictions on ice water and rectal temperature measurement. Finally, based on our outline of the typical format for a scientific article, you would expect her to interpret her statistical results and draw conclusions. But it isn't always that simple. The researcher has to take into consideration other relevant variables that might have effects on the DV other than or in addition to the IVs. If these other variables are not taken into account, they can confuse the interpretation of a study's results, because they con-found the effects of the IV. Not surprisingly, they are therefore called **confounding variables**, which, if they are not controlled in the study design or procedure, may be called *uncontrolled variables*. **Extraneous variables** is yet another term that may be used to refer to these factors.

In our sample study report, Kirchoff concludes that the effect of awareness (reading) on persuasion (the importance ratings for both restrictions) and on adop-tion (the frequency ratings) as determined by a statistical test called analysis of variance (ANOVA) was not significant or meaningful. That is, reading or being aware of research that challenged the value of the coronary-care precautions did not affect how important the nurses thought the precautions were or how frequently they practiced them. The investigator decided to take a look at any possible confounding variables that might account for her study findings. In doing so, her statistical anal-ysis allowed her to add the following information about potential confounding vari-ables:

1. Larger medical centers in urban locations, with educational programs for nurses, had significant but weak relationships to lower ratings on the frequency and importance of the two questioned coronary-care precautions.

2. Federal and nonprofit institutions had lower importance and frequency ratings for the rectal temperature measurement.

3. Nurses employed in units that used special procedures for measuring cardiac output (thermodilution technique) had lower ratings for restriction of ice water.

Including both head nurses and staff nurses and reporting these additional findings about practices on the unit that were not among the independent variable measurement list was one way that this researcher attempted to "control" for po-tentially confounding variables.

Hypotheses

A **hypothesis** is the statement of relationships the researcher expects to find be-tween a study's independent and dependent variables. This statement might be in the form of a question, but more often the question is called the study problem, and the hypothesis is a declarative sentence. This statement may be designated by the symbol H, or H_0 if the researcher is going to test the reverse of his or her hypotheses. In the latter case, H_0 is called the **null hypothesis**. If there are several hypotheses in any single study, a number might follow the letter H (H_1, H_2, H_3). Some studies are designed to *generate rather than test* preconceived hypotheses and thus don't begin with any formally stated hunches, let alone hypotheses about expected relationships. In our sample study's survey design, formal hypotheses weren't stated from the outset. But one might assume that the researcher had an informal hunch that being aware of the research literature would indeed influence practice decisions about coronary precautions—a hunch that was *not* substantiated in the study data.

Data

Data are the information the investigator collects from the subjects or participants in the research study. The values for variables or concerns in a study constitute its data. The data on importance and frequency (and difference) for selected CCU nursing actions collected in the course of our example study are summarized in Table 4–2. (Note that when referring to *data*, because it is a plural noun, the proper verb is *are* or *were*, not *is* or *was*.)

Instruments

Instruments are the devices used to record the data obtained from subjects. Many instruments are used in nursing studies, including interview transcripts, question- naires, intelligence tests, rating scales, performance checklists, pencil and paper tests, and biological measurement devices. Among the most important questions to evaluate when sizing up the worth of any instruments used to measure variables in a nursing study are their **reliability** and **validity**. A reliable instrument will produce consistent results, or data, on repeated use, usually because the investigator has standardized the procedure for administering it. For instance, if blood pressure is measured several times under unchanged conditions and the same readings are obtained, the measure is reliable. A valid instrument is one that measures what it is supposed to measure. A paper and pencil test of a client's knowledge about his or her diabetic diet may measure reading skill rather than grasp of nutritional in- formation. Obviously this issue is a lot more complicated when you are measuring an abstract variable, such as professional commitment or social network, than when you are measuring a more direct and concrete one, such as weight, height, or tem- perature.

TABLE 4–2 *Importance and Frequency Ratings and Difference Scores for Selected CCU Nursing Actions (n = 524 Nurses)*

CCU Nursing Action	Importance (I) M	s	Frequency (F) M	s	Difference (I–F) M	s
Insure EKG monitoring	6.98	.14	6.92	.37	.06	.37
Assess chest pain quality	6.88	.41	6.55	.82	.33	.73
Relieve anxiety	6.75	.53	6.17	1.00	.58	.93
Maintain IV	6.74	.90	6.74	.91	−.01	.53
Provide quiet	6.43	.84	5.53	1.25	.90	1.23
Teach Valsalva avoidance	6.30	1.12	5.68	1.58	.60	1.30
Restrict coffee[a]	6.00	1.46	6.16	1.52	−.16	1.29
Restrict visiting time	5.89	1.24	5.32	1.38	.36	1.26
Check temperature/4 hours	5.62	1.46	6.09	1.35	−.47	1.16
Bathe the patient	5.46	1.64	5.75	1.48	−.28	1.23
Avoid rectal thermometer use[a]	5.37	1.85	5.96	1.91	−.09	1.63
Restrict cola[a]	5.32	1.72	5.13	2.06	.19	1.60
Provide sedative at night	5.28	1.24	5.09	1.16	.19	1.02
Restrict ice water only[a]	4.90	2.15	5.15	2.22	−.22	1.68
Restrict tea[a]	4.76	1.96	4.28	2.31	.47	1.74
Restrict fluid intake	4.63	1.83	4.30	1.80	.33	1.19
Restrict cold fluids[a]	4.35	2.04	4.32	2.15	.04	1.51
Avoid vigorous back rub[a]	4.08	2.07	4.26	1.97	−.18	1.67
Restrict hot fluids[a]	3.81	2.07	3.70	2.17	.12	1.51
Feed the patient	2.92	1.91	3.10	1.84	−.20	1.46
Give bedpan for defecation	2.78	1.87	3.32	1.84	−.55	1.54

[a]Coronary precaution item

Source: K. T. Kirchoff, "A Diffusion Survey of Coronary Precautions," *Nursing Research*, July/August 1982, vol. 31, p. 199. Reprinted with permission. Copyright © 1982 American Journal of Nursing Company.

Population and Sample

The **population** for a study (symbolized by a capital N) is the total possible membership of the group being studied. But because it is not always feasible to study everybody, a microcosm of the population, called a **sample** (designated by a lower case n) of participants or respondents is usually selected. In the sample study, the n was 600 staff nurses and 235 eligible hospitals. Of these, 524 nurses returned usable questionnaires after three mailings, yielding a *response rate* of 87.3%. Completed questionnaires were received from 202 head nurses, or 86%, of the eligible sample. When a sample is representative, the investigator is in a better position to conclude that the study results are generalizable to the entire population of nurses and settings that make up the universe applicable to the study.

Hawthorne and Halo Effects

The *Hawthorne* and the *halo effects* are two terms often used in reference to research studies. The **Hawthorne effect** is the change in people's observed behavior that occurs merely because they know they are being studied. (It was first observed in the Hawthorne plant of the Western Electric Company.) Subsequent studies have shown that productivity or job satisfaction can change temporarily when management makes a change of any kind, purportedly due to the extra attention workers believe they are receiving. The Hawthorne effect can occur in all kinds of study situations when data reflect the effects of the study itself.

The **halo effect** refers to an observer's tendency to rate certain subjects as consistently high or low on everything because of the overall impression that the subject gives the rater. Strategies to lessen the effects of inaccurate responses include the **double-blind** method of studying a particular care or treatment approach. In this procedure, neither the caregivers nor the patients know whether the experimental or control treatment procedure is being administered.

TABLE 4–3 *Type of Restriction by Reported Frequencies for Origins of Restrictions (n = 524 Nurses)*

| Origins of the Restrictions | Type of Restriction | |
	Ice Water	Rectal Temperature Measurement
Not ordered	117	180
Physician	34	20
Unit policy	312	252
Nurses	30	35
Combinations of above	15	16
Other	8	9
Missing data	8	12
Total	524	524

Source: K. T. Kirchoff, "A Diffusion Survey of Coronary Precautions," *Nursing Research*, July/August 1982, vol. 30, p. 199. Reprinted with permission. Copyright © 1982 American Journal of Nursing Company.

Interpreting Visual Presentations

You'll have to discover the sometimes obscure trend hidden in the tables or charts of a research study. Take, for example, Table 4–3 from our sample article and use the following guidelines to understand it and others like it:

■ Try to spot trends. You must see in this table that the most frequent *source* of both coronary care restrictions cited by nurses in the study sample was "unit policy."

■ Decide whether the author has picked the right measure of central tendency (see Chapter 14). There are three statistical averages: the **mean** (the sum total

TABLE 4–4   *Factor Loadings for Importance Ratings of Selected CCU Nursing Actions with Rotated Factor Matrix (n = 524)*

Nursing Action	Factor 1 Temperature	Factor 2 Caffeine	Factor 3 Rest	Factor 4 Psychological	Factor 5 Cardiac Stimulants
Restrict cold fluids[a]	.85	.21	.23	−.01	.09
Restrict ice water only[a]	.46	.18	.04	.12	.10
Restrict hot fluids[a]	.75	.20	.13	.01	.11
Restrict coffee[a]	.22	.63	.00	.15	.21
Restrict tea[a]	.20	.65	.12	.03	.05
Restrict cola[a]	.17	.84	.12	.06	.09
Feed the patient	.16	.11	.58	.01	.10
Give bedpan for defecation	−.01	.01	.61	.03	.05
Avoid vigorous back rub[a]	.31	.12	.33	.02	.25
Relieve anxiety	.00	.03	−.01	.60	.07
Provide quiet	.12	.09	.16	.64	.12
Avoid rectal thermometer use[a]	.22	.17	.11	.08	.50
Teach Valsalva avoidance	.08	.12	.13	.25	.45
Eigenvalue	4.46	1.80	1.51	1.15	1.10
% Total variance	21.3	8.60	7.2	5.5	5.2
Cumulative % total variance	21.3	29.8	37.0	42.5	47.7

[a]Coronary precaution item
Source: K. T. Kirchoff, "A Diffusion Survey of Coronary Precautions," *Nursing Reasearch*, July/August 1982, vol. 31, p. 198. Reprinted with permission. Copyright © 1982 American Journal of Nursing Company.

divided by the number of cases); the **median** (the midpoint between the upper and lower halves); and the **mode** (the case that is most common). It's important for you to evaluate which is the *best* way to describe the central tendency for any study question.

■ Pay attention to the range of numbers in charts or graphs. In reporting "importance" and "frequency" scores, the author of the sample article writes: "Avoiding the use of rectal temperatures and restricting ice water received moderate importance and frequency ratings but large standard deviations, indicating high variability among the sample nurses" (p. 200) (see Table 4–4).

■ Look for exceptions. In Table 4–3 we can see that the category "missing data" accounted for only 8 and 12 of the 524 sample members. Had the number of exceptions been large, we would evaluate the apparent trends differently.

■ Compare figures presented in the text with those in the charts and tables, keeping alert for contradictions or inconsistencies.

■ Read the captions that accompany tables and figures carefully and compare them with the results and discussion presented in the text. Together they will tell you a great deal about any study that you read.

■ Look up unfamiliar statistics to determine if they were used correctly. Chapters 14 and 15 in this text offer resources. A good basic statistics book is another source.

In the methodology corner of the July/August 1981 issue of *Nursing Research*, Dr. Barbara S. Jacobsen wrote a guest essay entitled "Know Thy Data." She commented that inferential and confirmatory data analyses were rapidly becoming more widespread in nursing studies, perhaps because nurse researchers have greater access to and skill in using computers to analyze their data. An unfortunate side effect, according to the author, is that "researchers know their F ratio and p values (statistics), but do not know their data. . . . Confirmatory design and analyses may be easier to teach and computerize, but all too often they are learned in a mechanistic way and performed as a ritual" (p. 254).

The consequence is that you may be forced to make false interpretations of statistics. Jacobsen reports an incident in which an excited researcher raved that the computer had isolated a "key variable" in her questionnaire that correlated with everything! (Correlation shows the extent to which values of one variable are related to values of another variable.) Often these correlations were difficult to explain. An illustration of the latter case was that "number of people living in the household correlated with a measure of depression." It took a scatter diagram printout that looked like Figure 4–1 to illuminate the mystery. The two *outliers* (subjects who were very different from the rest of the group) simply lived in large institutions and also happened coincidentally to be depressed. When their scores were removed, the positive correlations between numbers of people in the household and depression score changed to reveal the *absence* of any correlation. The visual diagram of score frequencies solved the mystery.

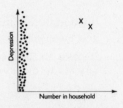

Figure 4–1   Scatter diagram

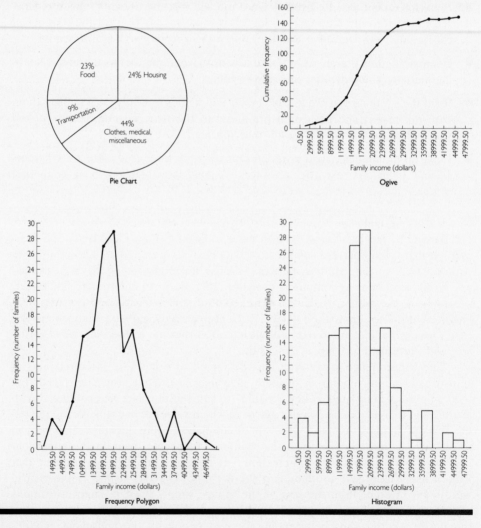

Figure 4–2   Types of graphs.

Extreme scores in a data set can likewise make it appear that no relationship exists between two variables. A single outlier (extreme score) can invalidate means, standard deviations, regression coefficients, and *t* tests. Jacobsen maintains that visual presentations (see Figure 4–2) can help a researcher know when to question the validity of statistical analyses. They can help you uncover patterns in the data that offer suggestions and cues for future research and enable you to better "know *their* data."

Guidelines for Critique

- What is the research report about? What type of report is it?

- What is the main theme ("little logic") of the report?

- What is the organization of this particular report? Does it follow the typical research journal article format, or does it differ in some way?

- What is the main question or problem the author set out to answer?

- Are there important and unfamiliar terms that you will need to "translate" in order to understand the report?

- What are the basic premises, propositions, or arguments in the report?

- What conclusions has the author reached? Are there other possible conclusions?

- What are the implications of the study's findings?

SUMMARY OF KEY IDEAS AND TERMS

✓ You can popularize a piece of scientific writing *for yourself* and make it more readable by *mentally* translating long or impersonal sentences and words into your own plain, conversational talk.

✓ The format for a typical research journal article usually follows these headings: (1) abstract, (2) introduction, (3) method, (4) results, (5) discussion, and (6) references. Each has a standard location and purpose that you can anticipate.

✓ Concepts, constructs, conceptual frameworks, and theories are abstractions that are used to classify observations of patterns in the world.

✓   An operational definition of a concept or construct specifies what a researcher does to measure it so as to be sure others will interpret its meaning in the same way.

✓   Independent variables (IVs) are the causes, conditions, and inputs that are established or manipulated before measuring the dependent variable(s).

✓   Dependent variables (DVs) are measures of outcome and consequences that depend on exposure to the independent variable.

✓   Confounding, extraneous, or uncontrolled variables are all those variables that might also affect the dependent variable and confuse your interpretation of the effects of a study's independent variable(s).

✓   Hypotheses are statements of relationship that the investigator expects to find between a study's independent and dependent variables.

✓   Data are the information collected from a study's subjects or participants.

✓   Instruments are the tools or devices used to collect data or information from study subjects.

✓   The population is the total possible membership of the group being studied.

✓   The sample is a microcosm of the population selected as actual participants or respondents.

✓   The Hawthorne effect refers to the tendency of people's behavior to change just because they know they are being studied.

✓   The halo effect refers to a person's inclination to respond to an entire set of items or questions in the same way or to an observer's tendency to rate subjects based on the overall impression that they have made.

✓   You can increase your ability to interpret visual presentations of data in tables and graphs by (1) trying to spot trends, (2) deciding whether the author has used the best measure of central tendency, (3) paying attention to the variability in a data set, (4) looking for exceptions and outliers in the data, (5) comparing figures presented in tables with those in the text, (6) reading captions for figures and tables, and (7) looking up unfamiliar statistics in a basic statistics book.

References

American Nurses' Association, Commission on Nursing Research: *Research in Nursing: Toward a Science of Health Care.* Kansas City, Mo.: 1976.

Campbell DT, Stanley JC: *Experimental and Quasi-Experimental Designs for Research.* Chicago: Rand McNally, 1966.

Flesch R: *How to Write, Speak, and Think More Effectively.* New York: Harper & Row, 1960.

Hays WL: *Statistics for the Social Sciences.* New York: Holt, Rinehart & Winston, 1973.

Huck S, Cormier W, Bounds W: *Reading Statistics and Research.* New York: Harper & Row, 1974.

Jacobsen B: Know thy data. *Nurs Res* July/August 1981; 30:254–255.

Kaplan A: *The Conduct of Inquiry: Methodology for Behavioral Sciences.* San Francisco: Chandler, 1964.

Kirchoff KT: A diffusion survey of coronary precautions. *Nurs Res* July/August 1982; 31:196–201.

Rogers EM, Shoemaker F: *Communication of Innovations*, 2nd ed. New York: Free Press, 1971.

5

Recognizing and Evaluating Study Designs

HOLLY SKODOL WILSON

Chapter Objectives

After reading this chapter, the student should be able to:

- Determine whether a study includes the six generic elements of a research design

- Evaluate the match between a study's overall purpose and the type of design employed

- Classify study designs according to whether their major emphasis is on discovery or on accuracy and control

- Differentiate between external and internal criticism in historical study designs

- Specify the major steps in each type of study design

- Compare the advantages and disadvantages of each major type of study design

- Recognize correctly the type of study design used in reports of nursing research

- Explain the three hallmarks of true experimental study designs

(Continued)

- Discuss the concepts of reliability and validity in relation to experimental study designs

- Formulate design remedies to counter potential threats to the internal and external validity of experimental designs

- Describe the major types of experimental design

- Compare and contrast quasi-experimental designs with experimental designs

- Account for the major disadvantages of ex post facto study designs

- Discuss the purpose of methodological research

In This Chapter . . .

Suppose you are responsible for providing nursing care to a 50-year-old woman during her postoperative recovery from gallbladder surgery. What do you do first? What do you avoid? How much of anything is going to be enough to prevent post-operative complications? What strategies will work? To help you answer these questions and accomplish the clinical goals set for this patient, you need to devise a *workable plan*. The plan is customarily called a *nursing care plan*. It offers you and the other clinicians working with this patient a blueprint, or organized design, for achieving certain specified objectives, such as the prevention of wound infection, pneumonia, thrombosis, and other complications that can follow such surgical procedures. The plan would take on quite different configurations if it were intended to accomplish an alternate purpose, such as decreasing a patient's anxiety or teaching someone about a diabetic diet.

Designs accomplish much the same thing for scientific research. They are the plans used to get answers to research questions that are valid and reliable according to scientific canons (see Glossary). The design is the overriding program, or protocol, for the research. It includes strategies for sample selection, data collection, and data analysis and a timetable. Strategies refer specifically to the methods and procedures that will be used to:

1. answer the research questions empirically as validly, objectively, accurately, and economically as possible

2. control the experimental, extraneous, and error variances that might be associated with the particular phenomena being studied.

Research designs suggest what observations or measurements to make, how to make them, and what to make *of* them. In effect, *research designs imply a set of instructions that tells an investigator how data should be collected and analyzed in order to answer a specified research problem.* There are almost as many designs as there are possible approaches for attempting to establish that something is or is not true. But as is the case with nursing care plans, certain designs are better suited to certain levels of inquiry, research purposes, and types of problem than are others. As Kerlinger (1973) observes:

> All man's disciplined creations have form. Architecture, poetry, music, painting, mathematics, scientific research—all have form. Man puts great stress on the content of his creations, often not realizing that without strong structure, no matter how rich and how significant the content, the creations may be weak and sterile. So it is with scientific research. Without content . . . good theory, good hypotheses, good problems—the design of research is empty. But without good form . . . adequately conceived and created . . . little of value can be accomplished. . . . Many of the failures of research have been failures of disciplined and imaginative form (p. 290).

Thus, researchers can choose from a wide variety of plans for addressing their study problems, but you as a reader must be prepared to evaluate critically not only the type of design that was used but also *the wisdom of selecting it*.

What follows in this chapter is an overview of the range and diversity of study designs. Specific sampling, data-collection, and data-analysis operations are discussed in detail in Part III. Here, we will consider the elements of a study design, the purposes for which research is done, and the design options best suited to each. We will compare and contrast nonexperimental, quasi-experimental, and true experimental designs and examine examples of nursing studies that have used various approaches. We will take a look at the advantages and disadvantages of each type of design within the framework of the key concepts of validity and reliability. After all, the scientific method is important to us insofar as it is really a process for knowing what is true (see Chapter 1), even though we believe that truth is less a static set of external laws than a representation of an episode in evolving history.

Elements of a Good Research Design

Some authorities on nursing research would have you believe that the more highly rigorous experimental and quasi-experimental study designs, in which phenomena of interest are isolated and controlled in laboratory settings, are by nature more elegant and therefore better than other designs. This view is associated with the logical positivist view of science (Silva and Rothhart 1984). Listening in on an institutional review board's meeting, a funding agency's grant proposal review, or even an editorial board's discussion of research manuscripts would undoubtedly reveal further supporters of such a position. After all, the nineteenth and twentieth centuries have witnessed the awesome achievements in the physical and biological sciences that the experimental approach to research questions generated. Furthermore, members of this camp suggest that researchers who use qualitative designs try too often to squirm out of describing the precise details of their methodology, expecting instead that their findings will be accepted on faith (Downs 1983).

Other authorities, representing an alternate point of view sometimes called *historicism* (Laudan 1977), caution us to reflect on the philosophical incongruence of nursing's commitment to belief in the whole person, individual uniqueness, personal autonomy, and experiential relativism and the scientific reductionism and instrumentalism that characterize experimental designs. Munhall (1982) points out that, in applying an experimental design and a logical positivist or empiricist philosophy, the scientist chooses an observable, measurable part of a person's human response or environmental context, becomes distant from the problem in order to be objective, places individuals into groups to eliminate the influence of confounding variables, and applies results to the mean, or average, of all cases stated. In her appraisal, the basic premises of the experimental design are that individuals are alike according to categories and that experience is all quantifiable and measurable. The result is a mechanistic, reductionist world view in which people's human responses are viewed as reactions to a predetermined stimulus selected to produce a desired outcome. Munhall asks, "[Are] nursing practice philosophy and nursing research philosophy in apposition or opposition?" She concludes by advocating the congruence of approaches outlined in this book's chapter on qualitative analysis and associated with a symbolic-interactionist intellectual tradition (see Chapters 12 and 13).

The position you take on the issue of *which* research design has the most potential for the advancement of nursing knowledge ultimately depends on *your* philosophy of science. Whatever stance you elect, it is important that you be able to recognize the type of design employed in any study you read or hear about and to evaluate its soundness on its own terms as well. The following list contains what Schantz and Lindeman (1982) isolated as the six generic elements of all research designs, whatever the type:

1. setting—where the research will take place

2. subjects—who will be the recipients of an experimental treatment or will be observed

3. sample—a reasonable number of subjects, so that the reseacher can make comparisons or describe a phenomenon, and the procedure for obtaining them

4. treatment—what the research intervention will be, in an experimental design, or conditions under which data will be collected, in a nonexperimental design

5. measurement, observation, or data-collection methods

6. plan for communication of results, including the way the data will be analyzed and interpreted

Spelling out each of these decisions in detail, so that the purpose of the research is served and the research question answered, increases the likelihood of creating a tight and logical study design. A correct experimental design, for instance, is intended to isolate variables of particular concern or interest so they can be examined under known conditions, to eliminate bias, and to reduce the margin of error, enabling the researcher to have confidence in the truth of his or her conclusions.

Matching Research Design and Research Purpose

Every study, of course, has its own specific substantive purpose. You might find, for instance, that a study is designed to find out whether structured preoperative teaching will significantly increase a postsurgical patient's ability to cough and deep breathe. Or a study might be designed to identify the mental health care needs of the deinstitutionalized elderly or to describe the influence of religion on nursing in Western civilization. Most investigators think of research purposes as falling into several main groups, or categories. Diers (1979) uses the following categories of research studies in nursing:

1. Factor-naming, or factor-searching, studies describe, name, or characterize a phenomenon, situation, or event in order to gain familiarity with it or achieve new insights. In more traditional sources this research is called exploratory and descriptive. It answers "what" questions and "who" questions.

2. Factor-relating, or relation-searching, studies are done to develop links among variables and describe the relationships that are found. These studies go on at the second level of inquiry after a phenomenon has been explored, named, and described. Many qualitative and grounded theory studies fall into this category. These studies address "how" questions.

3. Association-testing studies, also called explanatory or correlational studies, seek to determine what factors occur or vary together without either changing the natural situation (manipulating it) or attempting to reach conclusions about whether one causes another. They address "if-then" questions.

4. Causal hypothesis-testing studies test a causal relationship between variables and are also called true experiments, or explanatory studies, and attempt to answer "why" questions.

In the first two types of study, the major emphasis is on *discovery*, and the research design must be *flexible* enough to permit the investigator to use any strategy that might be helpful in obtaining rich and broad-ranging data on a phenomenon. In studies that are aimed at the third and fourth purposes, the prime issue is one of *control* and *accuracy*. Thus, the design must minimize bias, control variance, and enhance the reliability and validity of the evidence obtained. The fourth category of study seeks in addition to allow inferences to be made about cause and effect in the very particular scientific sense (see Glossary). When reading a report or proposal for a study, you may not always find its purposes as clear-cut as the preceding discussion might have led you to believe. In practice, a study may have some overlap of purpose. But the distinctions made by sorting studies into four types by purpose are helpful as we turn our attention to understanding the various types of study design.

Historical Study Designs

Most scholars agree that history is an activity engaged in for the purpose of learning the truth about the past. History is also a discipline of study that has established methods for collecting and evaluating evidence about the past. In fact, the clearest characteristic of the historical research method is that its data already exist. The purpose of historical research is to explain the present or to anticipate the future based on a systematic collection and critical evaluation of data pertaining to past occurrences. **Historical study** designs call for a prescribed approach to examining and interpreting data contained in historical sources such as diaries, letters, documents, and journals. Hockett (1955) emphasizes the importance of efforts to establish the validity and reliability of historical research:

> The aim of historical research is to ascertain facts, as they must be made the basis of all conclusions. . . . Statements are the raw materials with which the historian works and the first lesson he must learn is that they must not be mistaken for facts. They may be facts but that cannot be taken for granted. . . . In view of the possibilities for error, it becomes the duty of the historian to doubt every statement until it has been critically tested (p. 13).

Christy (1975) echoed this warning by reminding us that "the danger lies in the fact that we tend to believe anything in print, especially if it is found in an old document." Use of a historical design, therefore, requires that the researcher employ two separate processes to establish the validity and reliability of the data before using them to reach a conclusion: external criticism and internal criticism. These processes are hallmarks of sound historical research.

External Criticism

External criticism refers to examination of the historical data sources (maps, letters, books, documents, inscriptions, artifacts, and the like) for their validity, genuineness, or authenticity. Documents cannot be taken to reflect the truth unless they are really what they appear to be rather than forgeries or frauds. Techniques that historical researchers use to establish the authenticity of their data sources include consideration of the age of the paper, the kind of ink used, the appearance of watermarks, the match with other samples of handwriting, the congruity with other evidence of the author's or originator's ideas, or the use of a variety of laboratory procedures that determine characteristics (age, composition, and so on) of materials. In the case of book or article manuscripts, the historian must determine who the true author was. Questions that help establish authorship include:

- Is the manuscript an original or a copy?

- Is it dated?

- Could it have been written by anyone else?

- Might it be a forgery?

When evaluating data for their validity, the historian must consider the possibility that a previous historian misidentified a document, the chance of errors due to translations or even transcriptions from other languages, and the likelihood that documents have been altered or changed. Canons of historical research require that the historian get to original, primary sources in order to minimize the chance of distortion and error.

Internal Criticism

Once the validity of data sources is established, the historical researcher turns his or her attention to determining the *accuracy of the statements contained within the documents or historical material*. The process involved in making such a determination is called **internal criticism**. It requires the following steps:

- The researcher must be certain that he or she understands the information contained in the documents. As with all other designs discussed in this chapter, being aware of one's own biases and expectations is a basic requirement to avoid interpreting statements so that they provide false support for one's own hypotheses or pet notions.

- The investigator must be knowledgeable about the meaning of terms and statements in their historical and cultural context. Consultation with translators and linguists can sometimes help in this area. Munhall and Oiler (1985) remind us that words take on different meanings in different cultures, eras, and social settings. *Goodynurse*, for example, at the time of the Salem witch trials referred *not* to nurses but to married, middle-class women in the Puritan community.

- The researcher must subject the statements to a phase of negative criticism in which efforts are made to corroborate the truth reflected in them. Most authorities believe that the further an author moves from reporting an eyewitness account, the less reliable are the statements. Establishing the reliability of a rendition of what occurred usually requires *two independent primary sources that corroborate* each other. Comparing accounts of the same events and finding agreement increases confidence in the data. Evidence is considered "probable" when the researcher has information from *one primary source that passes the tests of authenticity* and *finds no substantial evidence to the contrary*. If neither of these routes to confidence in the truth of the data is available, the historian is dealing from the substantially weaker position of "possibility." Historical research requires the ability to find evidence, group it, evaluate it, interpret it, and communicate it in relation to important questions, themes, or hypotheses.

Steps in a Historical Research Design

The historical reseacher begins a study with a clearly stated research problem that has resulted from narrowing down a broader, more general area of interest. Christy (1969), a nurse historian, studied "the impact of the leadership of the Nursing Department at Teachers College, Columbia University, on changes and major events in American nursing during the first half of the twentieth century." Data in historical research such as Christy's study consist of evidence about events, people, and situations in the past. Instead of manipulating variables or designing data-collection tools, the historian must rely on documents from the past. Such documents are considered either **primary sources** (firsthand information) or **secondary sources** (second- or thirdhand accounts). Examples of primary sources include letters, eyewitness accounts, diaries, photographs, and legal or public documents. These are materials that existed at the time of the event. Secondary sources might be newspaper articles, reference books, and hearsay. These are the end products of studying primary data. Once the problems of data availability, data gaps, and evaluation of data validity and reliability are surmounted, the final step in a historical research design is synthesis, analysis, and articulation of the findings. During this last step, the historian must build into a related whole the facts that have been verified. Determining the meaning of facts, discovering relationships among them, and presenting them in a way that is interesting to the reader are among the challenges. Obviously, documentation in the form of footnotes and references is critical to verifying sources a historian uses to reach his or her conclusions. The steps implicit in the process of historical research described above are:

1. Formulate a researchable problem that is best approached with a historical research design.

2. Specify the data needed to address the research question.

3. Determine that sufficient data are available.

4. Collect known data, new data, and previously unknown data sources (primary and secondary).

5. Evaluate data sources through external and internal criticism.

6. Initiate the descriptive synthesis of findings in a written report while continuing to collect data.

7. Draw interpretive conclusions with respect to the original research question.

Advantages and Disadvantages of Historical Research

The value of historical research to nursing has only recently been recognized. Some of the archives established for the preservation of nursing's documents and other related material are listed in Box 5–1. Table 5–1 summarizes important general sources of information for the historian. The orientation to the past of historical research has as its major advantage the potential for illuminating a current question through the intensive study of carefully selected material that already exists.

Disadvantages of the historical research design include the following:

- The investigator must rely on finding data that already exist and cannot develop new data.

- The investigator cannot alter the form in which data appear but must attempt to understand them in their existing form.

TABLE 5–1   *General Sources of Information for Historical Research*

Reviews	Journals	Bibliographies	Newspapers and Journalism
American Historical Review	*Journal of American History*	*Historical Bibliographies*	*Journalism Quarterly*
Canadian Historical Review	*Journal of Modern History*	*A Guide to Historical Literature*	*American Journalism*
Catholic Historical Review	*Journal of the History of Medicine and Allied Sciences*	*A Bibliography of the Negro in Africa and America*	*Quill*
Economic History Review	*Journal of Southern History*	*Bibliographic Index*	*Columbia Journalism Review*
Book Review Digest	*Past and Present*	*Biography Index*	*New York Times Index*
Index to Book Reviews in the Humanities	*Social Sciences and Humanities Index*	*Guide to Periodical Literature*	*Journalism Educator*

Box 5–1   Archives of Historical Nursing Documents

- Archives of the Department of Nursing Education, Teachers College, Columbia University, New York

- Historical Book Collection, Sophia Palmer Library, American Journal of Nursing Company, New York

- Historical Collection, Reference Room, National League for Nursing, New York

- Lillian Wald Collection, Special Collections, Butler Library, Columbia University, New York

- Adelaide Nutting Historical Collection, Russell Library, Teachers College, Columbia University, New York

- Elizabeth Carnegie Nursing Archive, Schlesinger Library, Radcliffe College, Cambridge, Massachusetts

- Mary S. Gardner Papers, Women's Archive, Schlesinger Library, Radcliffe College, Cambridge, Massachusetts

- Maternity Center Association Archives, Maternity Center Association, New York

- Nursing Archive, Mugar Library, Boston University, Boston

- Nursing Historical Collection, Welch Memorial Library, Johns Hopkins University, Baltimore

- Nursing History Collection, National Library of Medicine, Bethesda, Maryland

- Nursing Museum, Pennsylvania Hospital, Philadelphia

- The investigator must analyze and interpret the meaning of data without the advantage of being able to ask clarifying questions.

- The data may be incomplete and have gaps in crucial areas.

- The investigator must be able to translate concepts, terms, and ideas in light of their historical period and context.

- The investigator must overcome obstacles of time, resources, freedom of movement, and language to search for and evaluate data resources.

■ The investigator cannot predict an accurate timetable for completion of a historical study. He or she must not only locate and evaluate data but also develop insights that tie together these masses of data.

EXAMPLES: Historical Designs in Nursing Research

The study question
Existing medical recording as a data source
The time period for the study was 10 years
Hospital records data source
The study question
The time period for the study was 26 years

In a study entitled "Social Characteristics of Death as a Recorded Hospital Event" Jeanne Benoliel (1977) attempted to discover these characteristics in teaching hospitals in the decade 1961–1971 through a retrospective analysis of 4380 patient medical records.

Helen Nakagawa and Oliver Osborne (1972) conducted a historical epidemiological investigation over a 26-year span of "presenting complaints" from records of first-admission state hospital patients in King County, Washington. Their purpose was to discover dominant trends in these complaints in the context of changing sociocultural, environmental, and treatment practices.

Two historical studies are noted in the accompanying example. Such studies can serve to interpret the past and supply perspective to contemporary problems and issues by suggesting parallels, differences, and trends. For example, the emergence of specific nursing leaders, the establishment of nursing education in hospitals or institutions of higher learning, and the proliferation of nursing functions are all studied against a background of social needs, economic constraints, and the political climates of given periods.

Case Study Designs

Case studies provide an in-depth analysis of a subject for investigation such as an individual patient, a family, a hospital ward, a health care agency, a professional organization, or a group such as Recovery Incorporated or Alcoholics Anonymous. A case study is customarily done under natural conditions. It examines only a single subject or a small number of subjects with respect to a number of variables pertaining to history, current characteristics, and interactions. The case study design is useful in accomplishing the following purposes:

■ gaining insight into little-known problems

■ providing background data for the planning of broader studies

- developing explanations of social-psychological and social-structural processes

- offering rich descriptive anecdotes or examples to illustrate generalized statistical findings

Steps in a Case Study Design

Case studies, by definition, are both more flexible and more vulnerable to bias than many other designs, in that the investigator must make judgments about sources, amounts, and credibility of data without many rules or guidelines. In general, however, the steps involved in a sound case study design are as follows:

1. Determine the purpose of conducting a case study.

2. Identify the unit of analysis (individual, family, group, aggregate, organization, community).

3. Determine how data sources will be selected.

4. Specify the data-collection plan and methods.

5. Collect, analyze, and interpret data.

6. Write a report of findings.

7. Suggest directions for further research on the basis of these findings.

Advantages and Disadvantages of the Case Study

Nurse scientists working in a relatively unstudied area of investigation, where there are few prior studies on which to base design decisions, have often acknowledged the value of intensive study of selected case examples to stimulate insight and suggest hypotheses or even directions for future research. Case studies have been the first step toward many discoveries in anthropology and medicine. Psychoanalytic theory is based for the most part on Sigmund Freud's carefully documented case studies of psychiatric patients. Case studies can often provide information that is rich and otherwise difficult to come by. They are also well suited for studying a process over time. Some believe that case study designs are virtually synonymous with descriptive research.

Descriptive single-subject research has indeed made valuable contributions to knowledge in psychopharmacology, psychotherapy, and medicine. Holm (1983) cites behavior modification studies in the areas of weight control and childhood eating disorders as bringing research and practice closer together. Other descriptive case studies report how particular patients respond to specific situations or nursing approaches.

Holm argues that experimental approaches can also be used in case studies by modifying experimental design principles so that a subject's baseline data are compared with his or her data after an experimental intervention. A **single-subject experimental design** can also include what is called a *reversal phase*, during which the intervention must be withheld while measures of the dependent variable continue. Holm uses a hypothetical study designed to determine if the 2g sodium diet results in a significant decrease in blood pressure in a 25- to 35-year-old newly diagnosed hypertensive who is otherwise normal as an example of a single-subject experimental design. Other topics that might lend themselves to this design are study of the effectiveness of a program of breathing exercises as measured by tidal volume, vital capacity, and respiratory rate; skin care interventions as measured by pre- and postintervention decubitus ulcer size and stage; or a stress-reduction program as measured by blood pressure, pulse rate, weight, and sense of well-being. Replication of such studies should be encouraged, because they can generate confidence in findings and foster generalizability and are practical and realistic research approaches in most clinical studies. After all, if a process or effect is documented in one person, it might reasonably recur in others.

The major disadvantages of the case study design are still its problems with generalizability. It is difficult to argue with certainty that what is learned from a single case is representative of patterns or trends in the entire population. Furthermore, the methods for compiling case study data are not as rigorously prescribed as those for data collection under alternate study designs, resulting in what critics consider outright ambiguity. This very ambiguity, however, may provide the flexibility necessary to bring inventive approaches to gathering a rich array of data and arriving at insightful interpretations of them. The other disadvantages of a case study design are those associated with its flexibility and lack of rigor and control. To elaborate:

- Investigators have no guidelines to help them decide how many data are enough.

- Because most of the data collected in case studies are based on interviews and observations obtained by the investigator and the circumstance is often one of a relatively long-term and close association between the investigator and the subject or subjects, the possibility of researcher bias influencing the findings and conclusions is always present.

- The cost effectiveness of case studies is open to criticism, because some authorities believe that the expenditure of money and time is high relative to the value of the information obtained.

- A case study design is not adequate for testing causal hypotheses and definitely unsuited for trying to establish scientific cause and effect.

EXAMPLE: A Case Study Design in Nursing Research

A research monograph entitled *Deinstitutionalized Residential Care for the Mentally Disordered: The Soteria House Approach* (Wilson 1982) used the case study design. It is a story of a community-based, residential care facility for severely mentally disordered, young diagnosed schizophrenics that professed a nonmedical approach. The book portrays a scene, a time in history, and a way of being in intimate detail: a locale is sketched, analyzed, and conceptualized. It is described in the foreword as "documentation of a true social experiment told in the words of the participants" (Wilson 1982 p. xi). It stands alongside an array of descriptive and conceptual case studies published by nurses and social scientists on topics related to delivery of health care.

A case study of one health care setting

Institutions as well as people can be subjects for a case study
Involved generating a description and a grounded theory

Survey Research Designs

Survey research designs are nonexperimental designs that involve studying populations or universes based on the data gathered from a sample drawn from them. The data are often gathered using self-report methods, such as a questionnaire completed by the study subjects. Survey research generally serves the purpose of *describing characteristics, opinions, attitudes, or behaviors as they currently exist in a population*, although other purposes are possible. The word **survey** means the collection of information from a variety of subjects who resemble the total population on the characteristic(s) of interest to the researcher. For example, a nurse working in the field of psychogerontology might conduct a national survey of factors that affect access to health care resources among elderly women with Alzheimer's disease. When a survey studies a sample of the total possible population, it is technically called a *sample survey*. If the entire population is studied—for example, all doctorally prepared nurses in the United States—the survey may be called a *census*.

Types of Survey

Survey designs can be classified by the subjects from whom data are collected (*sample survey* versus *census* or *group survey* versus *mass survey*); by the methods used to collect the data (*mailed questionnaire survey, face-to-face interview survey*, or *telephone survey*); by the study's time orientation (*retrospective survey, cross-sectional survey*, or *longitudinal survey*); or by the study's purpose or objective (*descriptive, comparative, correlational, developmental*, or *evaluative*.) A quick review of issues published in the last several years by *Nursing Research* reveals the kinds of problem investigated using

STUDENT SURVEY

ID (1-5) 1. Code Number: /____/____/____/____/____/ (to be assigned)

2. Name (print): /_____ /_____ /_____/
                             First   *Mid. Init.*   *Last*

MOEDUC (7) 3. Mother's level of education (Check one):

      _____ Elementary school or less

      _____ Some high school

      _____ High school graduate

      _____ Some college

      _____ College graduate

      _____ Post-graduate degree

      _____ Other: _____

DEGHOPE (8) 4. What is the highest degree you expect to receive in your educational career? (Check one):

      _____ Master's in nursing

      _____ Master's in another field

      _____ Doctorate in nursing

      _____ Doctorate in another field

      _____ Other (Identify) _____

      _____ Don't know

5. What are the sources of financial support for your education this year? (Check all that apply).

SUPSELF (9)	_____ Self-support	SUPSCSHP (13)	_____ Scholarship	
SUPSAVNG (10)	_____ Savings	SUPGRANT (14)	_____ Grant	0 = No
SUPPARNT (11)	_____ Parents or relatives	SUPTRSHP (15)	_____ Traineeship	1 = Yes
SUPSPOUS (12)	_____ Spouse	SUPOTHER (16)	_____ Other	

EMPSTATS (17) 6. Which of the following describes your employment status while in school? (Check one):

      _____ Full-time employment

      _____ Part-time employment

EMPHOURS
(18-19)

      _____ Hours per week, if part time

      _____ Armed Forces, reserve or active

      _____ Traineeship

      _____ Fellowship

      _____ Research Assistantship

      _____ Other: _____

      _____ More than one check

EMPHOURS

#	Frequency
0	13
8	2
11	1
12	1
16	5
20	5
24	6
26	1
27	1
32	1

Figure 5–1 Student survey for program research and development in a nursing school

different types of survey. Although types of surveys may overlap and interact, let's consider each of them separately.

Mass Survey Mass surveys involve collecting a relatively limited amount of superficial information from a large population or universe. The survey of all nursing education programs in the United States conducted every ten years by the National League for Nursing is one example. The kind of information collected in this instance is often demographic (age, sex, occupation, income, social class, educational level). Although identifying characteristics of the entire population or universe may be the study objective, a survey can be based on information collected from a sample carefully drawn from that population using a systematic sampling procedure.

Group Survey In a group survey the sample size may be smaller than in a mass survey but usually the information elicited is of greater depth and scope. First, almost all surveys of this type ask respondents some identifying or descriptive information about their personal background and current situation. These preliminary questions often include age, sex, ethnicity, marital status, education, religious affiliation, political preference, income, parents' educational level, number of people living in the household, siblings, and occupation. See Figure 5–1 for an example of typical survey questions coded for computer processing. The value of collecting these data along with data that bear on the actual research question is that knowing the characteristics of the sample allows an investigator to feel more confident about generalizing findings from the sample to a population. Occasionally, even a sample selected using random sampling procedures turns out by chance not to represent the population from which it was drawn.

A second category of data often elicited in group surveys involves the subject's social context, be it home or work environment. A study of stress experienced by nurses who work in intensive care or critical care units may include questions about the noise level, the frequency with which people die on the unit, the staff-patient ratio, the provisions for avoiding burnout, and so on.

Yet a third category of questions addresses behaviors. A survey of kidney transplant recipients,* for example, might include questions such as:

1. What two foods that are high in salt do you avoid?

2. What two things do you do every morning at home to monitor your kidney function?

3. What do you do to decrease fluid retention in your tissues caused by the prednisone you take?

4. What do you do to prevent muscle weakness that can be related to taking prednisone?

---

*Source: Questions related to kidney transplants taken with permission from Wirth P, Barton C: Barton-Wirth kidney transplant knowledge questionnaire (Draft of unpublished instrument.) Kidney Transplant Unit, Moffitt Hospital, University of California, San Francisco, 1983.

5. What do you do when you miss a dose of prednisone?

6. What have you done when you notice you are having undesirable effects from your prednisone?

A fourth category of questions addressed in group surveys determines how much information about a topic the sample members have. The same survey of kidney transplant patients might also contain the following items.

Sample

1. Circle the five things in the following list of symptoms that might indicate a rejection:
   a. pain over my kidney   f. decreased urine output
   b. yellowish skin or eyes   g. nausea
   c. smelly urine   h. elevated temperature
   d. weight increase   i. increased urine
   e. flulike feeling
2. If you were to wake up at home at 2:00 A.M. with pain over your kidney, what should you do? (Circle two answers.)
   a. Go to the hospital immediately.
   b. Call the transplant unit.
   c. Go back to sleep and see how you feel in the morning.
   d. Take your temperature and weigh yourself.

Yet another category of questions includes those that deal with psychological variables—subjects, opinions, feelings, attitudes, and values. A study designed to answer the question "What are the attitudes of adolescent diabetics who fail to comply with their diet regimen?" for example, would contain such psychological items or scales.

Face-to-Face Interview   In-person surveys can be used to address any of the possible content areas mentioned above, as can telephone interviews or mailed questionnaires. Certain topics, however, are best studied when trained interviewers meet with subjects in person and use a structured or semistructured interview schedule to collect data from them. Consider a study dedicated to answering a highly personal and sensitive question, such as "What are the personal, physical, cognitive, and psychological needs of young paraplegic men in the first six months after diagnosis?" This study would be difficult to conduct through an impersonal mailed questionnaire. Sensitive subjects and sensitive questions usually should be studied through interviews. So should questions whose answers may need clarification or elaboration. But interviews, especially face-to-face ones, are very costly. They require planning, interviewer training, travel, and so on. They obviously have the distinct advantages of allowing for clarification and elaboration of a topic and high subject participation.

Telephone Interview   Surveys over the telephone are less costly than face-to-face interviews, but they are also potentially less effective as a data-collection approach. They may be perceived as intrusive or annoying by respondents, and they certainly don't allow for the development of rapport needed to explore highly personal or sensitive topics. Interviewers must be trained for telephone interviews, an interview schedule must be developed, and telephone bills must be paid. The costs associated with travel, however, are avoided, and thus telephone interview surveys may be a necessary compromise when face-to-face interviews are too costly. They may also be preferable to relying exclusively on mailed questionnaires.

Mailed Questionnaire   Mailed surveys require that the subject be able to read, understand, and respond to the questionnaire and be sufficiently motivated to return it to the investigator. Although the response rate for mailed questionnaires is generally considerably lower (sometimes as low as 15% or 20%, even if stamped, self-addressed envelope and engaging cover letter are included), they are often the only option available to a researcher who wants to collect data from a population spread over a great distance—for example, a multinational sample of executives in schools of nursing throughout the world.

Cross-Sectional Survey   In most of the examples discussed thus far, the researcher sees a single snapshot of certain variables in a sample, that is, data are collected at a single point in time. If, however, a research question is about change or development (or stability) over time, the investigator usually uses either a cross-sectional survey or a longitudinal survey. The **cross-sectional survey** involves subjects who are at different points in the process of moving through an experience; they are surveyed at the same time and assumed to represent data collected from different times. For example, oncology patients who have recently begun radiation treatments and chemotherapy might be asked to respond to a set of interview questions or questionnaire items at the same time that other patients who have experienced at least one remission and exacerbation are asked to do so. The two groups are assumed to reflect different stages of the same process. One of the major limitations of this kind of time sampling is that the researcher is always really talking about *different* people in the different phases, and a lot of intervening and confounding variables can affect the findings. Yet collecting data about change with this approach eliminates the possibility that respondents become "test-wise," and it is economical.

Longitudinal Survey   As opposed to the cross-sectional survey, the **longitudinal survey** collects data from the *same* people at different times. At several major American university hospitals, large studies on normal aging have been conducted. Researchers have followed adults for more than 20 years to uncover heretofore unknown aspects of the aging process. The primary strength of the longitudinal design is that the researcher does not have to assume that different groups are sufficiently comparable to designate them as representing different points of the same process. Its disadvantages are the amount of time it takes to complete even a short-term longitudinal study (less than five years) and the influence of studying subjects who become test-wise from repeated completion of similar data-collection instruments. Unless some dramatic shift has taken place in the study setting (a change of institutional mission, composition, or policy), most authorities agree that the cross-sectional design functions reasonably well as an approximation to at least a short-term longitudinal study.

Descriptive Survey   Descriptive surveys are conducted for the purpose of accurately portraying a population that has been targeted because of some specific characteristics. Such surveys are often used to determine the extent or direction of attitudes or behaviors. In a survey sponsored by the University of Miami, interview and questionnaire data were collected from 50 midwestern couples who were in their 70s or older and had been married for 50 years or more. The purpose was to describe the quality of a long-lasting marriage (Secrets of making marriages last, 1984). According to the study findings, these couples spent time together and shared household chores.

Comparative Survey   Comparative surveys are used to compare or contrast representative samples from two or more groups of subjects in relation to certain designated variables. A national survey of attitudes toward "professionalism" or "leadership aspirations" among graduates of baccalaureate and associate degree nursing programs is an example of a comparative design. Sampling procedures must be carefully followed so that the groups to be compared will be as similar as possible on all variables that are not the focus of the study and to ensure that the sample is as representative as possible of the population from which it is drawn.

Correlational Survey   Surveys designed to discover the direction and magnitude of relationships among variables in a particular population of subjects are called correlational surveys. Another way of saying this is that in correlational study designs the investigator studies the extent to which changes in one characteristic or phenomenon correspond with changes in another. One might investigate, for example, whether adaptive functioning in the year before the onset of an illness is related to coping with the stresses of illness and hospitalization. A correlational survey might show a relationship among factors that are of interest to nursing practice and health care. If so, the correlational survey might be the basis of a more precisely controlled experiment that addresses cause and effect.

Evaluative Survey   Surveys conducted for the specific purpose of making judgments of worth or value are called evaluative surveys. More precisely, evaluation surveys allow the investigator to delineate, obtain, and provide information that is useful for judging decision alternatives when conducting a program or service. Evaluation studies can focus on **formative** (process) or **summative** (outcome) questions. In the former, the purpose is to *provide ongoing feedback* to people who are responsible for carrying out a plan or programs. In the latter case, the study is designed to focus on the *effectiveness of the outcome of the plan or program*. An evaluation study can serve these purposes:

1. identifying goals or objectives to be evaluated

2. discovering how well objectives are met

3. determining the reasons for specific successes and failures

4. analyzing the problems with which a program must cope

5. ascertaining how long the effects of a program last

6. studying the success of alternative techniques

7. redefining the objectives or the means for attaining them

8. interpreting the meaning of changes found

9. identifying unexpected outcomes of a program

The survey format is viewed by evaluators as a relatively effective and efficient way to gather information about achievement of a program's goals or objectives. Some authorities argue that unanticipated consequences should also be examined, and they advocate what are called **goal-free evaluation** plans. A survey should establish the variables to be measured, the sample population and sampling plan, the availability of existing scales or the need to develop them, and in the case of evaluation based on program goals, the yardsticks used to make judgments about the meaning of data that are collected.

A good evaluation survey design includes the following (Wilson 1976):

■ consideration of why one is evaluating and how the results will be used

■ decisions and choices about what the objectives of data collection are or what questions require answers

■ decisions about the nature of the sampling plan—from whom information will be needed and at what times

■ formulation of a system for recording and storing data

■ plans for checking out the objectivity, reliability, comprehensiveness, validity, and relevance of data

■ plans for comparing groups, if possible

■ strategies for summarizing and reporting findings so that they can be used for decision making and program improvement

■ task assignments and time schedules

A poorly designed survey can produce masses of irrelevant information that make drawing conclusions difficult, and, in the case of mailed survey instruments, the problem of low return rate must be expected.

Criteria for judging the merit of evaluation study designs include familiar ones: internal and external validity, reliability, objectivity, relevance, significance, scope, credibility, timeliness, pervasiveness, and efficiency.

EXAMPLE: A Context Evaluation Study

Context evaluation

Steele and associates (1978) conducted three surveys to determine the need for a program to prepare clinical nurse specialists in child health nursing in a northeastern state. They considered their work to be an example of context evaluation, which looks outside a program or procedure to gather evidence that will be helpful in the planning process. In their first survey they attempted to determine whether graduates of the proposed master's program in child health nursing would have opportunities for employment. Some authors would equate this type of evaluation with *needs assessment research*. In their second survey, they focused on the functions and tasks performed by clinical specialists in child health nursing. And the third survey was a modified *focus Delphi* technique, a special type of survey used for forecasting. This final survey was designed to identify the events that a large number of people felt would influence the field of child health nursing in the future. Data compiled from this survey were later used in determining content in the curriculum. The authors concluded retrospectively about their initial effort: "The survey attempted to elicit too much information and fell victim to one of the ills of survey research—loss of a great deal of data" (p. 8).

Needs assessment research

Authors' self-critique

Steps in Survey Research

There is clearly overlapping in the types of survey we have just considered. They are not mutually exclusive. An evaluation survey can also be a mailed questionnaire and longitudinal survey. In general, all survey designs require that these steps be addressed:

1. State the research question.

2. Ascertain that the research question can be addressed with a survey design.

3. Decide on the type of survey to be used.

4. Translate the objectives of the survey into categories of question or item.

5. Identify the population of respondents or settings.

6. Use sampling procedures to identify a representative sample.

7. Design data-collection procedures.

8. Plan for analysis of data.

9. Pilot test the data-collection and analysis approach.

10. Modify as indicated.

11. Collect and analyze data.

12. Write descriptive, comparative, or evaluative findings and draw conclusions.

EXAMPLE: A Survey Design in Nursing Research

Maria O'Rourke (1981) conducted a cross-sectional correlational survey of 633 healthy women between the ages of 21 and 44 to address the study question of *whether women's subjective appraisal of their psychological well-being differed in relation to the presence of menstrual and nonmenstrual symptoms.* Her study data were collected using a structured mailed questionnaire that included the General Well-Being Schedule and the Moss Menstrual Distress Questionnaire. Her results after statistical analysis indicated that although women experienced specific menstrual symptoms that were distressful, symptoms did not negatively affect their assessment of their psychological well-being. She viewed the implications of her findings as important in clarifying misconceptions about the effect of menstrual cycle symptoms on women's mental health.

Cross-sectional correlation survey

Study question

Mailed questionnaires used to collect data

Study findings

Conclusions

Advantages and Disadvantages of Surveys

It is probably obvious in light of the diversity of types of survey that the strength of the survey design lies in its ability to combine flexibility of content and purpose with elements of precision and control. It can be used to gather information from a large number of subjects with comparatively minimal expenditure of time and money. Its methodology can be explicitly stated, making it easier to evaluate and to replicate in comparison with alternative designs that are high in flexibility. It can take advantage of existing standardized scales and questionnaires and can be structured so that data analysis can be accomplished by computer.

Limitations of survey designs include:

1. the possibility of a low return rate due to the impersonal approach that often characterizes survey research

2. the possibility that preconceived questions are irrelevant or confusing to the respondents and therefore yield meaningless data

3. the necessity of developing a system for storing and keeping track of a vast amount of data

4. the tendency of data obtained to be relatively superficial

5. the fact that survey data do not allow an investigator to answer cause-and-effect questions about related variables

Experimental Study Designs

The term *experiment* is sometimes used interchangeably in everyday conversation with *study* or *research project*. In the language of science, however, an *experiment* or experimentally designed study has a very specific meaning. In this kind of study, the researcher *manipulates* and thus controls one or more independent variables and observes the dependent variable or variables for the consequences, change, outcome, or effect. Furthermore, in a true experiment, the investigator has the *power to assign subjects to either an experimental or control group* and ideally has the *power to use random sampling procedures to select them* in the first place. Experimental designs allow for the greatest control over confounding and intervening variables and thus are used to examine questions of cause and effect. Summarizing, then, true experiments are characterized by the following features:

1. control over at least one dependent variable and manipulation of at least one independent variable by the investigator

2. random selection of sample members

3. random assignment of sample members to experimental and control groups

In the opinion of many philosophers of science, the true experiment is the ideal study design, because it measures relationships among variables with the most precision, rigor, and control. The control accomplished with an experimental design is best understood in terms of the idea of control over **variance**. The experimental study design can:

1. maximize systematically introduced experimental variance

2. control extraneous variance

3. minimize error variance

Let's look at each of these notions in more detail, because they are the strengths of a true experimental design.

Strengths of Experimental Designs

Maximizing Experimental Variance   A typical experiment begins with a hypothesis about the existence of a relationship between an independent variable and a dependent variable. The hypothesis, for example, may be that holding a newborn at time of delivery (IV) is related to postpartum bonding behaviors in first-time fathers during the first three days after a baby's birth (DV) (Toney 1983). The investigator then randomly selects a sample of first-time fathers who meet specific inclusion criteria—for example, married, aged 20 to 32, father of a baby without deformities, delivery uncomplicated, and the like. At delivery, the fathers who meet the sample criteria are randomly assigned to two groups by the investigator. The fathers in the experimental group are offered their newborn infant to hold for ten minutes during the first hour after delivery. The fathers in the control group don't hold their babies until 8 to 12 hours after delivery. The null hypothesis tested in the study is H_0. There will be no significant difference in the frequencies of father-infant bonding behaviors between fathers who have early contact and those who do not. An experimental study design is selected because it can most accurately determine how much variance in the dependent variable (father-infant bonding behavior) can presumably be due to manipulation of the independent variable (holding or not holding an infant at birth). An experimental design is set up to show most fully how great a variance in the dependent variable is due to the independent variable. This is accomplished by separating this experimental variance from the total variance in the dependent variable, which can be due to a lot of things, including chance. The way to maximize the experimental variance is by operating according to a precept of *planning and conducting the research so that the experimental and control conditions are as different as possible*. In the case of our example study, holding the newborn for 10 full minutes was contrasted to not holding the infant at all. Every effort was made to avoid introducing the ambiguity of holding for a few seconds or even touching for a moment.

Controlling Extraneous Variables   Controlling extraneous variables means nullifying or eliminating that variance in the dependent variable that might be due to something other than the influence of the independent variable. This goal is accomplished in an experimental design in five ways:

1. A reseacher can eliminate extraneous variables altogether. For example, if the researcher studying bonding had suspected that fathers' years of college education might have an effect on the dependent variable of father-infant bonding, she might have selected sample members for both her experimental and control groups who had zero years of college. In short, to eliminate the variance that might be due to some extraneous factor, the investigator can select sample members so that they are homogeneous for that particular factor or variable.

2. The investigator can control the influence of extraneous variance through random selection of sample members and random assignment of subjects to the

experimental and control groups. Proper randomization allows the investigator to assume that the experimental and control-group members are statistically equal on all possible extraneous variables.

3. The researcher can build an extraneous variable into the design of the experiment as yet another independent variable and collect data about its effect on the dependent variable (and its interaction with other independent variables).

4. The experimenter can match subjects in the control and experimental groups on the variable in question.

5. Finally, certain statistical methods can isolate and quantify the amount of variance due to extraneous variance (see Chapters 14 and 15).

Minimizing Error Variance Error variance can be associated with individual differences among subjects and measurement errors, such as those due to test fatigue, lapse of memory, fleeting feelings, and other unpredictable phenomena. The primary precept in experimental designs to reduce error variance is that *to increase the reliability of measures is to reduce error variance*. This means that the less scores or values fluctuate randomly on subsequent administrations of an instrument, the more reliable and free of error variance they are. The visual representation of the meaning of measurement is:

$$M = \text{Actual Value} \pm (+ \text{ or } -) \text{ Error}$$

Because the more reliable and accurate the measures are, the easier it is to identify systematic variance in the dependent variable, systematically controlled testing circumstances and procedures are also a requisite in an experimental design. In our sample study the researcher's trained observers observed both the experimental and control-group fathers for the same amount of time (10 minutes), while the father changed the infant's shirt and diaper. They assessed the father-infant bonding using an instrument for interaction assessment that had been tested in a number of prior studies.

Internal and External Validity in an Experiment

The ability of the researcher to control variance through the experimental design contributes to internal validity. **Internal validity** is a measure of whether or not the manipulation of the independent variable really makes a significant difference on the dependent variable. In the study we have used as an illustration, Toney found no statistically significant differences in bonding behaviors between fathers who had contact for 10 minutes with their newborn infants in the first hour after delivery and those who did not. The author explained this finding by reflecting on the possibility that certain demographic and situational factors that were not controlled in her design may have detracted from the study's internal validity.

External validity refers to the representativeness or generalizability of a study's results. In our study, the author acknowledged that, without cross-cultural replication, her study findings were limited to predominantly middle-class Caucasian fathers who are married and have some college education. She acknowledged that cross-cultural sampling would be indicated to increase her study's external validity, because different subcultures have different beliefs and methods of expressing affection and attachment. Toney structured the variables as well as the basic experimental study design with control and experimental groups and pre- and posttests (often called a 2 × 2 design) to increase the experiment's internal and external validity.

Campbell and Stanley (1966), in their classic resource on experimental and quasi-experimental designs, list seven classes of extraneous variable that can threaten the internal validity of an experiment. These are presented in Table 5–2.

The seven extraneous variables are not the only ones that can occur in the conduct of an experimental design, but most authorities agree with Waltz and Bausell (1981) that they are the most common. Many of the strategies used in true experimental designs are intended to control or prevent their influence or the influence of yet another set of factors that act as threats to *external* validity. Most researchers deal with the threats to internal validity first because they are easier to control by altering features of experimental designs than are many of the threats to external validity.

External validity, as you recall, is defined as the extent to which the results of an experiment can be generalized to different subjects, populations, settings, treatments, and dependent variables. The primary threats to external validity derive from (1) population validity problems, (2) ecological validity problems, and (3) pretest sensitization.

Population Validity **Population validity** means that the researcher can reasonably generalize from his or her actual sample to all possible sample members and likewise to the total population of interest to the investigator. For example, a nurse researcher conducting an experimental study to determine the effects of touch as a means of communication with profoundly retarded children would want to be sure that:

- the responses obtained from sample members would be representative of potential responses from the target population

- results for subsets in the sample (for example, different sexes or age groups) would occur similarly in the population

Two strategies to minimize problems with population validity are to (1) define the accessible population as broadly as possible and then randomly sample as many subjects as is feasible and (2) use sampling procedures to increase the likelihood that the sample has the same constituencies (or characteristics) as the target population. If a researcher designs an experiment without employing these two sam-

TABLE 5–2 *Extraneous Variables That Can Threaten Internal Validity*

Classes of Extraneous Variables	Remedy and Rationale
1. *history*, which is defined as the influence of events that occur during the course of the experiment that might affect the dependent variable	1. Randomly assign subjects to experimental and control groups, because both groups could be assumed to have had exposure to the events that occur
2. *maturation*, which refers to processes that go on within the respondents themselves as a function of the passage of time	2. Complete the experiment in as short a time as possible to minimize developmental changes. Random assignment to control groups for the same reason as #1
3. *testing*, which is defined as the effect of having taken the test on retest scores	3. Don't test the same subjects. Build in a second control group that is tested the same number of times as the experimental group so as to be able to account for amount of change due to subjects becoming test-wise
4. *instrumentation*, which refers to lack of reliability or consistency in the way scores are assigned to a dependent variable	4. Keep scorers "blind" to which subjects are experimental-group and control-group members. Use standardized procedures and protocols for rating or scoring, to avoid biases. Give scorers as much practice as possible before they work with actual research data
5. *statistical regression*, which means that there is a tendency for subjects who score at extremes of a distribution to have less extreme scores when they are retested	5. This is only a factor when subjects are chosen for a study *because* of their extreme scores and can be taken care of through random assignment to control and experimental groups
6. *selection*, which refers to a tendency for certain types of subject to be alike if they are not randomly assigned to experimental and control groups	6. Avoid volunteers, and randomly assign to treatment groups to try to make groups as much alike as possible
7. *differential loss of subjects* from treatment groups during the course of an experiment	7. Little can be done about this factor except to document it as a potential limitation of the study when it occurs and try to prevent it by making every ethical effort to enable willing subjects to continue participating in the study.

Source: D. T. Campbell and J. C. Stanley, *Experimental and Quasi-Experimental Designs for Research*. Copyright © 1963 by Houghton Mifflin Company. Adapted with permission from Houghton Mifflin Company and American Educational Research Association.

pling strategies and instead simply grabs subjects in a single setting as they become available, it is likely that the sample will be systematically biased or different from the population to whom he or she hopes to generalize the findings, and the study's external validity is compromised.

Ecological Validity A study has **ecological validity** if the experimental environment in which it is conducted is sufficiently explicit, clear, and consistent that it could be replicated by another investigator. In practical terms, avoiding problems with ecological validity requires that the researcher operationalize both the independent and dependent variables in detail and prevent the occurrence of the Hawthorne effect. Replication is said to be the final arbiter of all external validity questions (Waltz and Bausell 1981). In the study of touch with profoundly retarded children, the investigator would need to spell out in detail the nature of the touching (IV) and the indicators of responsiveness (DV), so that another researcher could replicate the study with different subjects or under different circumstances. Furthermore, effects that might be due just to knowing about participating in a study (the Hawthorne effect) would need to be counteracted by keeping caregivers blind as to the exact indicators being recorded (without, of course, violating ethical research conduct).

Pretest Sensitization **Pretest sensitization** occurs when subjects are pretested (for example, on an attitude scale) and the taking of the pretest itself sensitizes the subjects to the experimental intervention that follows. If, for example, nurse practitioners were being studied for their attitudes toward caring for homosexuals before and after a series of workshops designed to clear up misconceptions and decrease prejudice, the test taken before the workshops could tip the subjects off about the researcher's interests or even the desired responses. The design strategy used to counter this tendency is to include a second control group that does not attend the workshops but receives only the posttest. Comparing this second control group's posttest scores with the posttest scores of the first control group—which was both pre- and posttested but also didn't attend the workshops—should allow the researcher to estimate how much change in the dependent variable (attitudes) could be attributed to the pretesting itself. See Figure 5–2. Subtracting for the pretest influence allows the researcher to compare the posttest scores of the control and experimental groups and assume that any difference found is due to the workshops (IV).

Types of Experimental Design

The most common true experimental designs reflect four strategies. These typical experimental design strategies are:

	Pretest	Workshop	Post test
Control group 1	Score = 50	No	Score = 60
Control group 2	No	No	Score = 55
Experimental group	Score = 50	Yes	Score = 65

Figure 5–2   A design to control for pretest sensitization.

1.   manipulation of the IV(s)

2.   an experimental group, which is exposed to the IV, and at least one control group that is not exposed to the IV

3.   random selection of sample members and random assignment of them to control or experimental groups

4.   measurement of the effects of the IV(s) on the DV(s) by measuring the DV before and after manipulation of the IV.

The logic of experimental designs is to structure the situation so that you have a sound basis for determining how much of the effect on a dependent variable is related to the independent variable and how much is due to chance.

After-Only Experimental Design   The *after-only*, or **posttest-only**, design is the simplest experimental design. In it the investigator assigns subjects to an experimental group and control group but *collects data only at the end of the treatment or exposure to the independent variable.* The soundness of the design relies on the soundness of the assumption that the two groups are comparable. Its weakness is that one must make this assumption at the beginning of the study without testing for it. From what we've seen earlier in this chapter, random sampling and random assignment to the two groups help the investigator to have confidence in this assumption.

An example of an after-only experimental design is Toney's 1983 study of the effects of holding the newborn on paternal bonding. She randomly assigned 37 married, first-time fathers attending uncomplicated deliveries of normal infants to experimental and control groups (those who held and did not hold their infants at delivery). From 12 to 36 hours after the babies were born, bonding behavior frequencies were recorded during 10 minutes of father-infant interaction. Her findings suggest that early contact (IV) did not appear to enhance bonding behaviors (DV). Her study necessitated, by virtue of the nature of her question, an after-only design (see Figure 5–3).

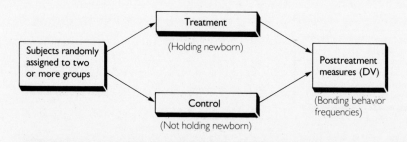

Figure 5–3 An after-only study design.

Before-After Design In the **before-after design**, subjects are measured before the experimental treatment on the same variables as after the treatment. The following example (Figure 5–4), published in *Nursing Research*, illustrates the most familiar and classic version of an experimental design called by some "the true experiment," "the pretest-posttest control group design," or "the 2 × 2 design."

Randomized Block Posttest Design A variation on the after-only design is the *randomized block posttest* design, which involves assigning subjects to experimental and control groups *after they have been ranked* with respect to some variable that is important to the dependent variable. For example, in a study of preoperative teaching methods and their respective effect on patient recovery rates, subjects might be matched according to the extensiveness of their surgical procedure before being assigned, one to the experimental group and one to the control group, by the flip of a coin (see Figure 5–5).

Factorial Design When two or more different variables are studied in the same experiment, factorial designs are used. **Factorial designs** allow you to examine the effects of two or more IVs as well as the interaction of the IVs. Factorial designs

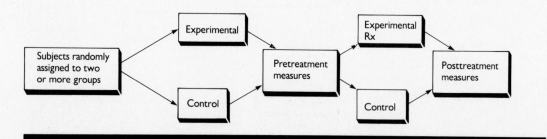

Figure 5–4 A before-after study design.

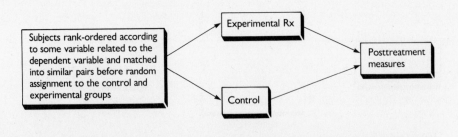

Figure 5–5 A randomized block posttest design.

can be constructed using three or four variables, which results in increased numbers of cells and the need for larger samples. The basic 2 × 2 factorial posttest design appears in Figure 5–6. A 2 × 2 factorial design produces a study with four cells. This design is used to study multiple causality.

The types of experimental design we have examined generally reflect a comparison of the experimental treatment or intervention with *no* treatment or intervention. Sometimes, control groups receive an alternative treatment or intervention (for example, "standard practice"), because receiving no treatment or a placebo would not be ethical. In this case, what is typically called the control group may be called the comparative group. As long as two groups are randomly assigned to experiences that differ from each other in an important way, the conditions for an experimental design have been met. This is true even when a second independent

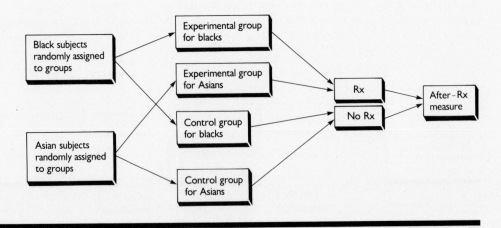

Figure 5–6 A 2 × 2 factorial design.

variable such as race or sex is not randomly assigned to subjects, as occurs in a factorial design. Any experimental design can be expanded to a multivariate design that uses complex statistics (see Chapter 15) to study complex relationships among variables.

Study designs with posttest only and no control group have neither pretesting nor the potential for comparison and as such are considered weak, or **preexperimental**, designs. The design with pretest, posttest, and no control group is considered the second weakest. It has a few advantages over the former model in that changes in the DV can be identified, but without a control or comparative group, of course, it's impossible to determine which of all the possible extraneous or error variances they might be due to. This design is also called preexperimental by some authorities (Waltz and Bausell 1981).

Steps in Experimental Designs

Students wishing to study varieties of experimental design in more depth are encouraged to consult the most widely used classic resource on the subject, Campbell and Stanley's book *Experimental and Quasi-Experimental Designs for Research* (1966). In general terms, however, the array of experimental designs introduced in this chapter involve these steps:

1. State the research problem.

2. Determine that an experimental design is well matched to the problem.

3. Operationalize the independent and dependent variables.

4. Formulate the hypotheses to be tested.

5. Identify measures for the dependent variable.

6. Specify the full range of potential intervening variables and decide which should be controlled, which can be permitted to vary, and which can be ignored.

7. Design the experiment to test the hypotheses, including selecting the sample.

8. Collect data on "before" measures.

9. Implement experimental and control conditions.

10. Collect data on "after" measures.

11. Analyze data.

12. Present findings in relationship to hypotheses being tested.

13. Prepare discussion of conclusions, limitations, and implications for further study.

EXAMPLE: An Experimental Design in Nursing Research

Hypotheses tested

Slavinsky and Krauss (1982) tested the hypotheses that chronically ill psychiatric outpatients who received nursing services explicitly designed to meet patient needs for both support and growth in regard to both dependency and social competence over a two-year period would

1. show a lower rehospitalization rate

2. spend more days outside of the hospital annually

3. have less treatment dropout

4. show a greater average decrease in symptom ratings

5. have fewer medication increases

6. show a greater average increase in socialization ratings

7. have a greater average increase in satisfaction with life situation ratings

8. have a greater average increase in satisfaction with care

9. show a better overall clinical adjustment in the group

Control group—
experimental group,
before-after study
design

Interviews were the
data collection
method
Sample inclusion
criteria

Study procedures

These nurse researchers used a before-after design with an experimental group and a control group. Forty-seven medication-maintained patients were assigned to the treatment condition by starting randomly and then alternating assignment to the groups. Measures of the dependent variables were obtained, using home interviews, at three points: before treatment, after one year of treatment, and after two years of treatment. The sample was drawn from a population of long-term outpatients who spoke English and were stabilized on maintenance dosages of psychotropic medication. The experimental and control-group patients were not different on age, sex, race, social class, number of previous hospitalizations, years of illness, psychopathology ratings, and other indices. The 25 patients assigned to the nursing group received "nursing services designed to meet needs for growth and support in regard to social competence." Services included group therapy, on-call crisis intervention, and medication maintenance. Control-group patients ($n = 22$) attended medication clinics that did not use group or individual therapy. Both groups had similar care insofar as they had the same number of contacts each month and were assigned to one "therapist." Data were collected by trained raters, and the validity and reliability of the ratings were demonstrated. Analysis of variance (ANOVA) was used where possible to explore the interrelationship of baseline ratings, demographic data, and outcomes.

Findings

Ratings after one year of treatment were of limited value as predictors of final (two-year) outcome. And finally, to the surprise of the nurse researchers, their findings reflected that the individually oriented medical clinic model of care appeared more effective than the nurse-run clinic aimed at improving social adjustment. Flaws in the study design were cited as a possible explanation for findings that failed to support their initial hypotheses, but the

Study limitations

investigators questioned whether it was reasonable to find that all three independent raters could have consistently introduced a systematic bias against
the research hypotheses. In fact, the more likely bias would probably have
been in support of the experimental intervention's outcomes. They did acknowledge, however, that "when an intervention is complex, demanding,
tedious, extended in time, involving multiple participants, and so on, there
can be serious problems in maintaining treatment integrity." All of these characterized their independent variable, and thus their findings may have been
influenced by problems of internal and external validity. Figure 5–4 depicts
a classic pretest-posttest experimental design.

Source: A. Slavinsky and J. B. Krauss, "Two Approaches to the Management of Long-
Term Psychiatric Outpatients in the Community," *Nursing Research*, September/October
1982, vol. 31, pp. 284–289. Reprinted with permission. Copyright © 1982 American
Journal of Nursing Company.

EXAMPLE: An Experimental Design in Nursing Research

Levin (1982) sampled 138 preoperative adult patients and randomly assigned   **Random assignment**
them to choice (experimental) and no-choice (control) conditions to answer
the question of whether the choice of site for an injection and locus of control   **Study question**
affect the perception of pain. Her experimental study tested four hypotheses:

Hypotheses

1. Individuals given a choice in determining their injection site report less
   pain from an injection than individuals not given a choice.

2. There is no relationship between locus of control (as measured by Rotter's
   Internal versus External Control Scale) and perception of momentary pain
   from injection when no choice in site is given.

3. When choice in site is given, persons with internal locus of control report
   less pain from injection than persons with external locus of control.

4. The addition of "locus of control" to "choice" accounts for more of the
   variance in perception of momentary pain than "choice" alone.

Levin's sample consisted of 54 male and 84 female preoperative patients   **Sample size**
who met specified criteria for inclusion, including being between the ages of   **Inclusion criteria**
21 and 65, awaiting elective surgery, and having no history of neurologic
dysfunction, chronic pain, drug addiction, or psychiatric history. Furthermore,
all participants were able to read and speak English.

Pretreatment measures were obtained from both experimental and con-   **Pretesting**
trol patients when they were asked to rate the amount of injection discomfort
from previous intramuscular injections (using graphic rating and visual analog   **Data collection tools**
scales). Participants were then randomly assigned to choice and no-choice
groups. Those in the choice group were asked *where* (hip or thigh) they would
prefer to receive their preoperative medications. Participants in the no-choice

Study procedures

Posttesting

Statistical analysis done with a computer program

Findings are related to hypotheses; additional unanticipated findings are reported

group were given their preoperative medicines without asking them to decide upon the site. Injection procedures were standardized, and nurses administering them were blind as to which group a patient was in, because the investigator told the nurse which site to use before she entered the patient's room. After receiving the preoperative injections, patients rated on pain scales the degree of pain they felt from the injection. Data were analyzed using the SPSS program for statistical analysis (see Chapter 14). Hypotheses 1, 3, and 4 were not supported. Hypothesis 2, which predicted no relationship between locus of control and perception of pain, was the only one supported. Unanticipated findings were that the pain of injection was apparently more closely related to the background and experience of the nurse who gave the injection and, among the female patients, their age. Younger women experienced injections as more painful than did older women.

Advantages and Disadvantages of Experimental Designs

The rigor, precision, and control properties of experimental designs enable them to be the most powerful way for scientists to establish **cause-and-effect** relationships, or test causal hypotheses. Causal relationships are important to science because they allow us to predict and explain. For example, an experimental design could tell us if using a dry-abraded skin preparation caused poor quality EKG signals. Or it could tell us if using sterile saline solution and K-Y jelly caused an increase in the number of pathogens at the meatal introitus of male patients with an indwelling urinary catheter. *Causation* in the scientific sense requires three criteria:

1. *A cause must precede an effect in time.*

2. *There must be evidence that the causal variable (IV) and the dependent variable are associated.*

3. *There must be evidence ruling out other factors as possible determining conditions for the dependent variable.*

The scientific notion of causality acknowledges that in most cases it is a multiplicity of determining conditions that together make up the necessary and sufficient conditions for an event. A **necessary condition** is one that must occur if an effect is to occur. For example, trying drugs is necessary for drug addiction to occur (except, of course, with newborns). A **sufficient condition** is one that is always followed by the effect. For example, destruction of the optic nerve is a sufficient condition for blindness. Some phenomena are both necessary and sufficient, but these are rare (Sellitz et al 1976). The experimental design's strategies of (1) manipulation, (2) comparison, and (3) randomization help the investigator to rule out alternative causal explanations for changes in dependent variables.

Disadvantages of experimental designs also exist:

- Some variables are not feasible or ethical to manipulate. For example, assigning pregnant women to take a new drug found to be dangerous to fetal development in animal studies would not be ethically possible.

- Randomization and otherwise equal treatment of control and experimental groups can occur in a laboratory, but these conditions do not resemble what goes on under real-world conditions, and experimental findings can therefore be based on rather artificial circumstances.

- Experimental designs attempt to reduce variables to measurable terms. Many of the phenomena that are of importance to science in nursing are complex, multidimensional, and holistic and defy the reductionism that has worked reasonably well in the physical or natural sciences.

Despite these limitations, however, the evolution of nursing's research and theory base will probably yield increasing numbers of studies that employ experimental designs in the years to come.

Quasi-Experimental Designs

When it is not feasible for a researcher to implement all of the characteristics of an experimental design—for example, random assignment to control and experimental groups—alternative designs, usually called **quasi-experimental designs**, are selected. We will now take up several of the most familiar quasi-experimental options.

The Nonequivalent Pretest-Posttest Control Group Design

The most basic quasi-experimental design uses **nonequivalent pretest and posttest** and a control group. Huckaby (1978) used it in her study of cognitive and affective consequences of formative evaluation in graduate nursing students. One group of nursing students was taught the first quarter of the graduate program using formative evaluation as a mastery strategy. The students enrolled in the second quarter of the program were taught using conventional lecture and discussion. Pretreatment and posttreatment measures were compared for the groups. (They found that the innovative teaching strategy was associated with more positive affective behavior.) This type of quasi-experimental design is useful when a researcher cannot randomly assign subjects to different treatments but must rely instead on comparative groups. Collection of the pretreatment data allows the investigator to determine how similar the groups are on the variable of interest even though one cannot assume that the experimental and comparison groups are equal.

The Time Series Design

The **time series design** is used when the investigator can study only one group but uses "before" measures to establish a baseline against which to compare the posttreatment measure of the dependent variable. If, for example, a psychiatric inpatient unit policy shifted to include a system for implementing Joint Commission on Accrediting Hospitals (JCAH) standard compliance treatment plans, the nurse executive could design a study to compare observations associated with the quality of patient care in the setting before and after the treatment planning system. The time series design can be used either when a comparable group is not available or when it is not feasible to do other than use experimental subjects as "their own control" because of limited resources. Even though some authors include the time series design as a quasi-experimental design, Campbell and Stanley (1966) consider it to be preexperimental, because it fails to control so many confounding or extraneous variables. Expanding the design to include a more extended time series and multiple data collection points both before and after introduction of the independent variable is one possible adaptation. Campbell and Stanley say this expansion changes the design from preexperimental to a quasi-experimental design with considerable integrity, because of the researcher's greater ability to attribute change in the dependent variable to the experimental treatment or manipulation.

EXAMPLE: A Quasi-Experimental Design

Study question

Sample size

Study procedures

Findings

Pamela Mitchell and her colleagues (1981) employed a quasi-experimental design to determine intracranial pressure (ICP) as measured by ventricular fluid pressure (VFP) with eight selected nursing-care activities in each of 20 patients. VFP was measured before and after turning the body to four positions, after passive range of motion (arm extension and hip flexion), and after rotation of the head to the right and to the left. Mean ICP increased for at least 5 minutes in all patients after one of the four turns and in 88% after half of the turns. Large increases in ICP occurred in the five patients for whom head rotation was done, but there was minimal change in ICP for passive range of motion procedures. A cumulative increase in ICP occurred with activities spaced 15 minutes apart regardless of what the activity was. No cumulative increase in ICP was found if procedures were spaced at least 1 hour apart.

Advantages and Disadvantages of Quasi-Experimental Designs

From the point of view of controls for internal validity, quasi-experimental designs are thought to be superior to the preexperimental designs. Their disadvantages, however, include:

- They cannot test causal hypotheses.

- They do little to ensure external generalizability.

- They are more susceptible to the effects of both testing and experimental settings because of the frequent testing schedules.

These disadvantages can be mitigated by adding a nonequivalent comparative group, thus combining the features of the two major types of quasi-experiment presented earlier.

Ex Post Facto Study Designs

In an **ex post facto study**, the researcher attempts to study something after the fact. Instead of introducing or manipulating an independent variable, the investigator selects subjects who have undergone some life experience. He or she then attempts to describe or explain it and, often, its possible relationships to some variable. Such correlations might be the presumed causes, but these cannot be confirmed, only tentatively suggested. Without the control that is possible in an experiment, the investigator must take things as they have already occurred and try to untangle them. Many nursing studies use ex post facto study designs. Andreoli (1981) attempted to determine if there were differences among diagnosed hypertensives who were compliant versus those who were not compliant on their prescribed therapy, at least with respect to measures of self-concept and health beliefs. Other investigators might wish to study the health habits of people who have early heart attacks, or drug use after the birth of a deformed baby, or cigarette-smoking patterns of men who develop lung cancer. In ex post facto studies the researcher selects and studies preexisting groups that have not been randomly selected but, in Kerlinger's (1973) terms, have been "self-selected" in that they have a common experience or characteristic.

The major disadvantage of ex post facto studies is that the investigator cannot establish cause-and-effect relationships, only correlational ones. This disadvantage is due to three weaknesses in the ex post facto design: (1) the researcher cannot actively manipulate the independent variable, (2) the researcher cannot randomly assign subjects to experimental treatments, and (3) the possibility for misinterpretation of study results is keen. Suggesting the plausibility of cause-and-effect links when strong correlations are found can be very tempting when an investigator discusses conclusions in an ex post facto study. It takes a sharp and critical reader to recognize that a researcher has gone beyond the data when writing up a study's interpretations.

Methodological Studies

One of the most difficult and challenging aspects of nursing research is the development of tools or instruments that are suited to answering nursing questions. Almost all published nursing studies use existing tools, modify existing tools, or require that the investigators develop their own data-collection instruments. For the most part, nursing research has tended to rely on psychometrics, biological measures, and sociometrics. Many authorities believe that nursing science needs to develop measurements that are specific to the interests of nursing research. Generally speaking, **methodological studies** are those that are designed to develop, validate, or evaluate research tools or techniques. Hurley, at New York University, is pioneering the use of the Psychological Stress Evaluator (PSE), a machine that translates the inaudible microtremors of focal muscles from a recording onto a paper tape in patterns that resemble electrocardiograms. Hurley has used the PSE in a study of communication between marriage partners and in a study of a family whose child had cancer. Winstead-Fry, also of NYU, is developing a statistical technique called multidimensional scaling to study intergenerational patterns in family systems. Ketefian has developed a scale called Judgments about Nursing Decisions (JAND) to study the moral behavior of nurses. Kreuger developed the Subjective Experience of Therapeutic Touch measure as part of a study on touching during childbirth. Other examples of attempts to address methodological problems in nursing studies include a Nurse Practitioner Rating Form (Prescott et al 1981), an adaptation of the Organizational Climate Description Questionnaire so that it could be used to study neonatal intensive care units (Duxbury et al 1982), and Hinshaw and Atwood's work (1982), originally devised to develop strategies for evaluating the impact of change in staffing patterns on both nursing staff and clients.

Of particular interest to nurse researchers engaged in methodological studies has been the effort devoted to constructing approaches to measuring the *quality of nursing care*. Some have focused on structural variables, that is, the organization of the patient-care system; others have emphasized the actual process of giving care; and yet others have examined outcome as reflected in patient welfare. Some of the instruments developed for this purpose are the Slater Nursing Competencies Rating Scale (Wandelt and Steward 1975), which measures the competencies displayed by a nurse; the Quality Patient Care Scale (QUALPAC) (Wandelt and Ager 1974) for measuring the quality of nursing care received by a patient while care is being given; and the Nursing Audit (Phaneuf 1972) for measuring the quality of nursing care received by a patient after a cycle of care has been completed and the patient has been discharged.

The contemporary trends toward prospective payment for hospital care and consumer requirements for accountability from health professionals add to the importance of advancing the methodology and instrumentation of nursing science. Until nursing science moves from a preparadigmatic to a paradigmatic state in its evolution, both its legitimate problems and the corresponding methods for studying them are still in the state of becoming. "Acquiring a paradigm and the subsequent research it permits are signs of maturity in any scientific discipline . . . maturity not yet characteristic of nursing science. Students conducting research within existing paradigms learn the basis of their fields from similar models and usually agree about the fundamentals of methodology or acceptable evidence" (Meleis et al 1980 p. 119).

Nursing science—its philosophy, theories, and methods—is in transition. The informed clinician can become a highly valued and integral part of the development and testing of nursing theory by critically evaluating whether or to what degree the varieties of nursing study described in this chapter contribute to the actual solution of patient-care problems. In the opinion of many, herein will lie the criteria for assessing nursing's scientific progress as a professional discipline.

Designs Fit Study Problems

Earlier chapters in this text considered questions such as "What do nurses study?" and "Why are such topics important?" The emphasis in this chapter has been on "*How are nursing research questions studied?*" If you as a research consumer or as a participant in research expect to have confidence in the credibility of research findings, you must be convinced that the plan or blueprint for conducting the study effectively fits the question being asked. The design must not only suit the study purposes and answer the question but also control for unwanted variance. As you may surmise, research designs can be simple or quite complex. By now, however, you should have a good sense of the range, diversity, advantages, and disadvantages of the ones that are used most frequently in nursing research.

Guidelines for Critique

- What type of design has been used in the study?
- Is the design carefully described in the methods section?

- Has the researcher examined the strengths and weaknesses of this particular design approach?

- Is the design well suited to the research problem? To the purpose of the study?

- If the design is a case study, what procedures has the researcher used to impose order on the data collection?

- If the design is historical, have rules for external and internal criticism been met?

- If the design is a survey, were survey questions relevant to the research problem? Was the return rate sufficient to draw meaningful conclusions?

- If the design is experimental, what methods were used to control for extraneous variables? What attempts were made to keep research conditions the same for all subjects? Does the design demonstrate internal validity? External validity?

- If the design is quasi-experimental, why was this approach chosen? What steps were taken to mitigate the disadvantages of this type of design?

- If the design is ex post facto, has the researcher gone beyond the data in drawing conclusions from the study?

SUMMARY OF KEY IDEAS AND TERMS

✔   *Study designs* are the overall plans, or blueprints, for collecting and analyzing data to answer research questions as validly and reliably as possible and control for unwanted variance.

✔   An intelligent reader of research findings should be able to recognize the design used in a study report and evaluate its suitability for addressing a study's purpose.

✔   Designs for *factor-naming* and *factor-relating studies* emphasize flexibility and discovery; designs for *association-testing* (explanatory) and *causal hypothesis-testing studies* rely on control and accuracy.

✔   Researchers using *historical study designs* explain the past and its implications for the present and future by systematically collecting, evaluating, and interpreting evidence—such as letters, maps, books, artifacts, diaries, and public documents—that already exists.

✔   Processes of external criticism—to establish the authenticity of data sources—and internal criticism—to establish the accuracy of the statements or information contained within the data sources—are the critical hallmarks of sound historical research.

✓ Establishing the reliability of accounts of what occurred usually requires two primary (firsthand) sources that corroborate each other. Secondary sources (products of studying primary data or secondhand accounts) must be carefully verified before a historian can base conclusions on them.

✓ *Case study designs* provide in-depth analyses of a single subject of investigation—such as an individual patient, a family, a hospital ward, a professional organization, or the like—to gain insight, provide background information for broader studies, develop explanations of human processes, and provide rich, descriptive anecdotes.

✓ Despite notable contributions made by single-subject studies in a number of disciplines, many critics believe they are limited in their generalizability.

✓ Surveys are also called *nonexperimental designs* by some authorities, because they lack the control associated with true experiments. Researchers can survey large or small groups, using mailed or distributed questionnaires or interviews, for descriptive, comparative, correlational, developmental, and evaluative purposes. In general, surveys involve collecting information from a variety of sample subjects and generalizing the findings to the population of interest to the investigator.

✓ Survey items are well suited to the study of demographic information, social characteristics, behavioral patterns, and information bases. They have been used in a variety of nursing research studies.

✓ A *cross-sectional survey* samples subjects who are at different points in moving through an experience. The investigator assumes that data collected from them represent different points in time. In a *longitudinal survey* data are collected from the same people at different points. In the latter, the investigator doesn't have to assume that the two groups are sufficiently comparable to designate them as representing different points in the same process or experience.

✓ *Evaluative surveys* are used to judge the value or effectiveness of a program or strategy by providing formative (in-process) or summative (outcome) data and measuring them against specified criteria (for example, the program's goals). Context evaluation is called needs assessment research by some authorities.

pendent variable, (2) random selection of sample members, and (3) random assignment of sample members to control and experimental groups.

✓   The strengths of an experimental design are that it can (1) maximize systematically introduced experimental variance, (2) control extraneous variance, and (3) minimize error variance.

✓   The ability of an experimental design to control variance contributes to its internal validity, that is, whether or not manipulation of the IV really made a difference on the DV. External validity refers to the representativeness, or generalizability, of a study's results. The experimental study design's use of randomization, control groups, and experimental groups; manipulation of the IV; and pre- and posttests, or measures of the DV, are all remedies to ward off threats to internal and external validity.

✓   Experimental designs are the only ones that can establish scientific causality. Causality requires three criteria: (1) A cause must precede an effect in time. (2) Evidence must indicate that the IV and DV are associated. (3) Evidence must as far as possible rule out other factors as determining conditions for the DV.

✓   *Quasi-experimental designs* are used when the investigator cannot randomly assign subjects to control and experimental groups but instead uses some form of comparative group.

✓   *Ex post facto designs* study something after the fact. Instead of introducing or manipulating an IV, the researcher selects subjects who have undergone some life experience and attempts to relate it to other variables. Such correlations, when they are found, should not be interpreted as cause and effect.

✓   *Methodological studies* aim to develop tools, instruments, or methods appropriate for answering nursing research questions. Of particular interest are instruments that measure quality of nursing care in terms of patient outcomes.

References

Andreoli KG: Self-concept and health beliefs in compliant and noncompliant hypertensive patients. *Nurs Res* November/December 1981; 30:323–328.

Benoliel JQ: Social characteristics of death as a recorded hospital event. In *Communicating Nursing Research*. Vol 10. Boulder, Colo.: WICHE, 1977.

Campbell DT, Stanley JC: *Experimental and Quasi-Experimental Designs for Research.* Chicago: Rand McNally, 1966.

Christy TE: *Cornerstone for Nursing Education.* New York: Teachers' College Press, Columbia University, 1969.

Christy TE: The methodology of historical research. *Nurs Res* May/June 1975; 24:189–192.

Diers D: *Research in Nursing Practice.* Philadelphia: Lippincott, 1979.

Downs F: One dark and stormy night. *Nurs Res* September/October 1983; 32:259.

Duxbury ML et al: Measurement of the nurse organizational climate of neonatal intensive care units. *Nurs Res* March/April 1982; 31:83–88.

Hinshaw AS, Atwood JR: A patient satisfaction instrument: Precision by replication. *Nurs Res* May/June 1982; 31:170–175.

Hockett HC: *Critical Method in Historical Research and Writing.* New York: Macmillan, 1955.

Holm K: Single subject research. *Nurs Res* July/August 1983; 32:253–255.

Huckaby LM: Cognitive and affective consequences of formative evaluation in graduate nursing students. *Nurs Res* 1978; 27:190.

Kerlinger FN: *Foundations of Behavioral Research.* New York: Holt, Rinehart & Winston, 1973.

Laudan L: *Progress and Its Problems: Toward a Theory of Scientific Growth.* Berkeley: University of California Press, 1977.

Levin RF: Choice of injection site, locus of control, and the perception of momentary pain. *Image* February/March 1982; 14:26–32.

Meleis AI et al: Toward scholarliness in doctoral dissertations: An analytical model. *Res Nurs Health* 1980; 3:115–124.

Mitchell P et al: Moving the patient in bed: Effects on intracranial pressure. *Nurs Res* July/August 1981; 30:212–218.

Munhall PL: Nursing philosophy and nursing research: In apposition or opposition? *Nurs Res* May/June 1982; 31.

Munhall P, Oiler C: *Nursing Research: A Qualitative Perspective.* Reston, Va.: Reston Publishing Co., 1985.

Nakagawa H, Osborne, O: An epidemiological study of psychiatric symptom pattern change: Pilot study findings. *Communicating Nursing Research.* Vol 5. Boulder, Colo.: WICHE, 1972.

O'Rourke M: Psychological well-being and menstrual symptoms. *Communicating Nursing Research.* Vol 14, Boulder, Colo.: WICHE, 1981, p. 34.

Phaneuf MC: *The Nursing Audit: Profile for Excellence.* New York: Appleton-Century-Crofts, 1972.

Prescott P et al: The Nurse Practitioner Rating Form. *Nurs Res* July/August 1981; 30:223.

Schantz D, Lindeman CA: Reading a research article. *J Nurs Adm* March 1982; 30–33.

Secrets of making marriages last. *San Francisco Chronicle* February 3, 1984; 28–30.

Sellitz C et al: *Research Method in Social Relations.* New York: Holt, Rinehart & Winston, 1976.

Silva MC, Rothhart D: An analysis of changing trends and philosophies of science on nursing theory development and testing. *Advances in Nursing Science* January 1984; 6:2–13.

Slavinsky A, Krauss JB: Two approaches to the management of long-term psychiatric outpatients in the community. *Nurs Res* September/October 1982; 31:284–289.

Steele S et al: *Educational Evaluation in Nursing.* Thorofare, N.J.: Charles B Slack, 1978.

Toney L: The effects of holding the newborn at delivery on paternal bonding. *Nurs Res* January/February 1983; 32:16–19.

Waltz C, Bausell, RB: *Nursing Research: Design, Statistics, and Computer Analysis.* Philadelphia: FA Davis, 1981.

Wandelt MA, Ager JW: *Quality Patient Care Scale.* New York: Appleton-Century-Crofts, 1974.

Wandelt MA, Steward DS: *The Slater Nursing Competencies Rating Scale.* New York: Appleton-Century-Crofts, 1975.

Wilson HS: Curriculum evaluation research. In: *The Second Step.* Searight MW (editor). Philadelphia: FA Davis, 1976.

Wilson HS: *Deinstitutionalized Residential Care for the Mentally Disordered: The Soteria House Approach.* New York: Grune & Stratton, 1982.

Wirth P, Barton C: Barton-Wirth kidney transplant knowledge questionnaire. (Draft of unpublished instrument.) Kidney Transplant Unit, Moffitt Hospital, University of California, San Francisco, 1983.

6

Preparing a Formal Critique of Research

HOLLY SKODOL WILSON

Chapter Objectives

After reading this chapter, the student should be able to:

- Recognize the value of critiquing skills to nurses as research consumers

- Distinguish between a research critique and a review

- Formulate strategies that contribute to making a critique constructive rather than destructive

- Comprehend seven basic criteria for critiquing and operationalize them in a framework of questions that the reader should raise

- Comprehend the rationale for asking the framework of critiquing questions and interpreting responses to them

- Discuss three major sources of error in research studies

- Explain 14 hallmarks of well-presented tables

- Analyze issues critical to the theoretical and logical basis of inquiry that underpin a thoughtful critique

(Continued)

- Apply the critiquing process to research proposals and reports of findings

- Appreciate the importance of preparing critiques that are concise, readable, rational, sensitive, accurate, and impartial

In This Chapter . . .

Criticism, in everyday parlance, is full of negative connotations. To criticize is "to censure, to blame, to reprove, to flay, to nitpick, to find fault, and to pan." But in particular literary, artistic, and scientific terms, criticism takes on an entirely different meaning—one associated with analyzing, reviewing, carefully dissecting, evaluating, or judging the merit of a piece of work. In this case, criticism refers to a finely sharpened skill for ascertaining an author or creator's meaning through an unbiased endeavor to examine the characteristics and qualities of his or her contribution to art or science. In fact, criticism as it was first introduced by Aristotle was meant to be a standard for "judging well."

Leaders in nursing all seem to agree that all nurses, regardless of their educational level, should be prepared with the skills that are essential to functioning in the role of research consumer (ANA 1976, Flemming 1980, Kramer et al 1981, Krampitz and Pavlovich 1981, Mallick 1983, Wilson 1982):

> In this role practitioners read research reports of others, determine the scientific merit and clinical utility of the studies and apply findings where appropriate (Horsley and Crane 1982).

The ability to do all this depends ultimately on the nurse's skill in conducting a critique of the scientific merit of research proposals and reports. Unfortunately, the majority of resources available to students do not provide sufficient opportunities to learn to become an intelligent "consumer" of research literature. Mallick (1983) and Krampitz and Pavlovich (1981) reviewed articles in nursing journals and existing textbooks to determine (1) whether the issue of teaching skills of criticism was addressed and (2) what methods were used to present the process of critical appraisal. The consensus was that little has been written on the development of these critical evaluation skills.

This chapter culminates Part II of this text, which has been devoted expressly to the skills of research consumership. In it, critiquing scientific proposals or reports is both described and illustrated in detail sufficient to allow students and practitioners to replicate the process themselves with confidence and credibility. A thoughtful critique of a research report requires more than merely knowing about a list of pertinent questions to ask, such as "Is the study question clearly stated?" or "Is the review of the literature sufficiently comprehensive?" Readers need standards against which to make such judgments, and perhaps equally important is a comprehension of the rationale for both asking and attempting to answer such questions when conducting a scientific critique. This chapter presents a framework of fundamental questions and principles that underpin the process of critiquing a research proposal or report. Then it takes the reader through a sample critiquing experience, focused on all aspects of a simulated proposal using the criteria, questions, and logic of scientific criticism.

What Is a Research Critique?

According to Leininger (1968), a research critique should be distinguished from a research review. A **critique** is "a critical estimate of a piece of research which has been carefully and systematically studied by a critic who has used specific criteria to appraise . . . the general features. . . . A research **review**, by contrast, merely identifies and summarizes the major features and characteristics of a study" (p. 51). A research critique encompasses a descriptive account of what is in the study, but unlike a book report that merely summarizes the plot, the emphasis is on *making a judgment about the proposal or report's scientific merits and ultimate worth*. As must be evident from reading other chapters in this text, the scientific way of knowing is often far from flawless. Even the most conscientious researcher may have to compromise great ideas and inquiry strategies because of pragmatic and ethical considerations. The critic's challenge is to determine what the researcher has tried to do and to evaluate the strategies selected, given the overall constraints of the study. A critique presents both the criteria and the evidence for the judgments that are made. These must be sufficient to allow another reader to form an opinion based on the critique. The art of scientific criticism can be demonstrated verbally or in a formal written document, but according to Leininger's classic article, "The most distinctive behavior of a research critic is to act in a judiciously critical but kind manner as he (or she) analyzes another person's work" (p. 53).

What Is the Purpose of a Research Critique?

The purpose of a research critique is to help an investigator refine and improve his or her program of inquiry and to help research consumers decide how to use findings from a study, based on a judicious appraisal of its strengths and limitations. Consider the example on page 179.

Responding to such health-related questions is a regular part of a clinical nurse's role. Responding correctly requires that the nurse be skillful in critiquing studies like the one in this example.

Whether the research critique is undertaken so that scholarly colleagues can exchange information or perspectives that will advance a particular line of inquiry, or whether it is done for the purpose of better informing health care consumers or other clinicians, a competent critique ought to represent a contribution to knowledge and be helpful.

Yet the critic must not confuse helpfulness with a lack of objectivity or be so earnest in his or her wish not to discourage or offend the investigator as to suppress or drastically disguise the critical points. Nurses who have practice in exercising their critical sensibilities on the day-to-day problems of clinical practice can most certainly learn to bring the same inquiring, honest, benevolent mind to bear on the problems of research quality. Inculcating an involvement with the research enterprise in the role of research critic can foster identification and a sense of communality with the scientific community in nursing. Furthermore, it can integrate a research perspective into the evolving tapestry of each nurse's clinical interests. When critiques of research proposals and reports are objective, comprehensive, correct, respectful, and humane, the nurse scientist, the nurse clinician, and the patients they serve all benefit.

EXAMPLE: Beer Therapy

Mr. H., a 65-year-old retired attorney with a history of hypertension and coronary heart disease, appeared for his regular blood pressure check and presented the nurse practitioner with an article he had clipped from his local newspaper. The headline read: "Beer or Jogging: A Hearty Choice." The article reported on a study, published in the *Journal of the American Medical Association* and conducted in Houston, which concluded that "drinking three beers a day is about as good as jogging when it comes to producing an effect that may decrease the risk of coronary heart disease." The researchers had found that volunteer runners and joggers registered about the same high-density lipoprotein (HDL), a type of cholesterol associated with heart disease, as did volunteer sedentary men who drank three cans of beer each day for the three-week period of the study. The rationale was that moderate drinking causes the liver to respond by producing the same or similar enzymes it produces in response to exercise. Mr. H.'s question to the nurse, of course, was whether he could now substitute three beers a day for the daily walking that he'd been encouraged to do, in view of these new scientific findings.

Clients seek health information from nurses

Partial reports of health research appear regularly in the popular press

Findings

Are the client's conclusions from the findings warranted?

Achieving these mutual goals requires that a critic and an investigator be able to differentiate between *constructive* and *destructive criticism*.

Constructive criticism is evident when the critic offers thoughtful comments which are given in such a way that they stimulate the researcher to use suggestions and motivate him (or her) to continue work on the study. In contrast, destructive criticism tends to thwart the researcher's interest in his (or her) work (Leininger 1968, p. 55).

TABLE 6–1 *Do's and Don'ts for Sensitive Critiques*

Do	Don't
1. Try to convey a sincere interest in the study you are critiquing	1. Avoid excessive nitpicking and fault finding on trivial details
2. Be sure to emphasize the points of excellence that you discover	2. Never ridicule or demean an investigator personally
3. Choose clear, concise statements to communicate your observations rather than ambiguous ones	3. Don't try to include flattery that is designed merely to boost a researcher's self-esteem
4. When pointing out a study's weaknesses, include explanations that justify your comments about them	4. Don't base your summary and recommendations about the study on some loose and perhaps biased attitude toward the state of all science in a particular discipline or on a particular topic
5. Include supportive and encouraging statements where they are warranted	
6. Be aware of your own negative attitudes toward a particular approach to science or any personal hostilities that could distort your ability to judge a study on its own merits	5. Don't write your critique in condescending, patronizing, or condemning language
7. Offer practical suggestions that are not overly esoteric or unrealistic	6. Don't forget that your purpose is to adivse the researcher and to improve the work
8. Remember that empathy for the researcher is often crucial to being an effective critic	

The careful choice of words in a critique is often cited as one of the most important features of artful and sensitive criticism. When the critic's words are well chosen, the researcher being criticized is more likely to use the criticism to benefit rather than become defensive about it. A few helpful do's and don'ts in dealing with the interpersonal aspects of critiquing research are summarized in Table 6–1. Critics who bear in mind their real purpose and attend to the potentially delicate social psychology of the researcher-critic relationship can provide valuable opportunities for scholarly and intellectual exchanges that can advance both the science and the professional practice of nursing.

What Are the Criteria for Good Research?

Recognizing the importance of upgrading standards of reporting clinical research, Field (1983) and Fleming and Hayter (1974) suggest that a combination of the following criteria be used to evaluate reports of nursing studies:

1. clarity and relevance

2. researchability of the problem

3. adequacy and relevance of the literature review

4. match between the purpose, design, and methods

5. suitability of the sampling procedure and the sample

6. correctness of the analytical procedures

7. clarity of the findings

Clarity and Relevance of the Study

All researchers should specifically state the aims of the study. The author should clearly explain the reasons for doing the study and indicate why it is of importance. Finally, the reader should be convinced that conducting the study is indeed worthwhile. A judgment about the potential value of a nursing study is easier to make if you ask three questions about it:

1. Will the study solve a problem relevant to nursing?

2. Will the facts collected be useful to nursing?

3. Will the study contribute to nursing knowledge?

Many authorities believe that in order to be classified as *nursing research*, studies have to make a first-order contribution to testing clinical nursing interventions or patient responses to them (Field 1983). Others argue that contributions to nursing education and nursing administration, although termed *research in nursing*, are equally justifiable. The key point is to be sure that your critique does not condemn a researcher for failing to accomplish something that was not part of his or her purpose in the first place.

Researchability of the Study Problem

Chapter 7 details how to state a researchable study problem. A well-stated study problem should at least be able:

1. to be answered through measuring empirical evidence or data

2. to be stated as a question that involves the existence of a relationship between two or more variables

Having established that a study problem meets the two most fundamental criteria, the reader can consider other questions relevant to critiquing the quality of a study problem:

3. Is the statement of the problem clearly and specifically articulated *early* in the proposal or report?

4. Have the investigators placed the study problem within the context of existing knowledge and prior work on the topic?

5. Are the hypotheses, or research questions, explicitly stated?

6. Are the concepts or variables operationally defined so that the methods for measuring them could be replicated?

7. Are the limitations and assumptions of the study included, and are they logically justifiable?

8. Does the problem statement accurately reflect the title of the study?

9. Are the study questions, or hypotheses, clear, specific, testable, and consistent with the study title, purpose, and subsequent literature review?

Adequacy and Relevance of the Literature Review

Whether it is called a "review of related literature" or "a theoretical framework" for the study, evidence that the researcher has a mastery of current knowledge on his or her topic of inquiry and has placed the proposed or reported study within its context is a third criterion for judging the scientific merit of research. Not only should you the critic find such a section in the material and the references listed at the end of the document, but you must also be convinced that:

1. the investigator has selected references that logically pertain to the subject being studied and the methodology being used

2. the investigator has not merely presented a laundry list of sources but instead has integrated them into a background synthesis that suggests how the present study resolves controversies, fills gaps in knowledge, extends or refutes what is already known, and so on

3. the literature review section is logically organized

4. the review does not omit classic or landmark sources (You may need to consult an expert in the substantive field of the investigation on this point if you are not familiar with the body of literature on a certain topic.)

5. the investigator has been open-minded enough to include references to prior work that may not be supportive

6. the literature review or theoretical framework makes sense as a rationale for framing the specific hypotheses or research questions being examined

7. the review provides justification for operational definitions of concepts or variables that have been advanced

8. the review supports the choices of data-collection tools and instruments in the present study

Agreement of Purpose, Design, and Methods

As you recall, the study design is the overall blueprint selected to answer the research question and enhance the study's validity and reliability, and the methodology is a description of the procedures for data collection and analysis to be used in a study. As a critic you should ask:

1. Does the investigator name and describe the study design, including its strengths and weaknesses for the problem under scrutiny?

2. Is the study design well matched to the task of answering the specified study questions and controlling extraneous variables that could detract from the value of study findings? (See Box 6–1 for sources of error in research studies.)

3. Does the investigator provide evidence from pilot tests or published literature that the data-collection procedures are reliable and valid?

4. Does the investigator include a copy of the data-gathering instrument or other evidence that it is free from ambiguity, bias, or significant omissions?

5. Are the sources for and adaptations of nonoriginal data-collection tools provided?

6. If the data-collection tools are self-developed, are the processes for developing them and reports for establishing their validity and reliability included?

7. Are the techniques for data collection logical and practical ways of acquiring empirical evidence on study variables?

8. Does the researcher include checks to guard against possible errors in collecting, recording, and tabulating data?

9. If the design was experimental, do you find evidence of control of extraneous variables, manipulation of independent variables, randomization in both sample selection and assignment of sample members to treatment groups, and replicability?

10. What attempts were made to keep research conditions the same for all sample members?

11. Did the investigator try to keep subjects and researchers who were recording outcomes "blind" with regard to which intervention was being administered to whom?

Box 6–1   Potential Causes of Research Error

Data Characteristics

1. Inadequate sampling
2. Inaccurate measurement
3. Unrepresentative data
4. Careless observation
5. Intentionally distorted data

Analytical Characteristics

1. Mathematical errors
2. Incorrect choice of formulas
3. Comparison of nonanalogous data
4. Generalization based on insufficient data
5. Failure to acknowledge significant factors
6. Confusion of correlation with causation
7. Interpretation manipulated to support prejudice or preconception
8. Elimination of contrary evidence

Suitability of the Sampling Procedure and the Sample

Because it is usually not feasible to obtain data from every member or element in an entire population, the researcher should explain his or her approach to deciding which of all those possible study elements are to be used as sample members and data sources. When critiquing the study sample, you should be able to determine:

1. Did the investigator choose to use a probability or nonprobability sample? Why one or the other?

2. What strategies were incorporated to avoid collecting a biased sample about which one could not generalize to the target population?

3. Is the sample representative of the population to which findings are to be generalized?

4. Is the sample size large enough to meet the assumptions of any statistical test that may be used in data analysis? (See Chapters 14 and 15.)

5. Is the sample size large enough to reduce the standard error?

6. What are the descriptive characteristics of the sample, particularly with respect to any variables that might influence study findings, such as age, education, sex, or physical or psychological condition?

7. What criteria were used to enter eligible sample members into a study?

8. How was informed consent obtained, and how were the rights of the human research subjects protected? For example, did each subject get a complete and honest explanation of the purpose of the research? Were they told what was going to happen to them and how the findings would be used?

9. Finally, were subject losses due to lack of follow-up or to dropping out detailed?

Correctness of Analytical Procedures

Data-analysis methods, including both statistical procedures and qualitative methods and appropriate references to them, should be clearly presented. Presentations of summary data should be clear enough to allow the reader to determine whether the statistical methods were the appropriate ones. Mention of the *power* of the test (**power analysis**) should be made, so that you and other readers can decide whether the study was conducted on a viable number of subjects and whether an increase or decrease in number of subjects could have affected the results and to what extent. Assumptions related to the use of statistics should all be made clear. In the case of qualitative analysis methods, sufficient detail about the analytic approach should be included so that another investigator could replicate the analytic operations (see Chapter 13). Specific questions that you, in the role of research critic, should ask include:

1. Does the author specifically name the statistical tests applied, along with the probability associated with significant values?

2. Does the author explain and provide references for analytic strategies for non-numerical data?

3. Are the statistical tests used appropriate to the level of measurement (nominal, ordinal, interval, or ratio) represented by the data?

4. Is the statistical procedure the right one to answer the specific research question?

Clarity of Findings

The results section of a research report normally contains a technical report of how the statistical or qualitative analyses turned out with respect to study questions or hypotheses to be tested. The discussion of results is usually devoted to a non-technical interpretation of them. In addition to telling us what the results mean, some researchers use the discussion section to explain why they think the results turned out the way they did. Some authors use the discussion section to suggest ideas for further research. Results themselves usually appear in the text of the article, in one or more tables, or in graphs (technically called figures). As a research consumer, you must be able to read, understand, and critically evaluate the results in a research report to avoid uncritical acceptance of findings just because they appear in print. You don't have to be a whiz in math to get the drift of a results section in a scientific article. Becoming familiar with research terminology and the principles of scientific evidence that follow in this chapter will enable you to become much more comfortable with this task. In your role of research critic of reports and discussions of findings, you should ask the following questions:

1. Are interpretations of results clearly based on the data obtained?

2. Are reasons given for tabulating or presenting data in particular ways?

3. Can you detect error in any computations?

4. Are there any discrepancies between results presented in graphic form and results presented in the text of the report?

5. Do all the tables and graphs have titles?

6. Are the relationships of the variables in tables clear and easy to figure out? (See Box 6–2 for additional characteristics of good tables, and see Chapter 18.)

7. Has the researcher distinguished between actual findings, on the one hand, and interpretations made by the researcher, on the other?

8. Are the findings explicit enough for you, the critic, to decide if the interpretations are justified? (For example, some authorities believe that conclusions of any kind cannot be drawn from data returns of less than 51% of the sample.)

9. Are minor or secondary findings overemphasized in the report and major or primary findings underplayed?

10. Are the findings clearly and logically organized?

11. Is the presentation of findings impartial and unbiased?

12. Do generalizations or conclusions go beyond the data collected or the population represented by the sample?

13. Are recommendations for further research offered?

14. Does the researcher include unsuccessful efforts and negative outcomes?

15. Are limitations that might have influenced the results noted?

Box 6–2   Hallmarks of Well-Presented Tables

1. *Every table should have a title.* The title should be a succinct description of the contents of the table and should help make it intelligible without reference to the text. The title should be clear, concise, and adequate and should answer the questions *what? where?* and *when?* The title should always be placed above the body of the table.

2. Every table should be identified by a number to facilitate easy reference. *The number is in arabic numerals,* and it can be centered above the title or placed on the first line of the title.

3. The captions, or column headings, and the stubs, or row readings, of the table should be clear and brief.

4. Any explanatory footnotes concerning the table itself are placed directly beneath the table.

5. If the data in a series of tables have been obtained from different sources, it is ordinarily advisable to indicate the specific sources in an inconspicuous place just below the table.

6. To emphasize the relative importance of certain categories, different type, spacing, and indentation can be used.

7. It is important that all column figures be properly aligned. Decimal points and plus and minus signs also should be in perfect alignment.

8. Sometimes the columns are numbered to facilitate reference.

9. Miscellaneous and exceptional items are generally placed in the last row of the table.

10. Since it may be confusing to read a long table when all the rows or lines are single spaced,

it is a common practice to group the stubs or sideheads. Generally, grouping of stubs by fives or fours is very satisfactory.

11. Abbreviations should be avoided whenever possible, and ditto marks should not be used in a statistical table.

12. The arrangement of the major classes in the table depends on the facts and relationships that are to be emphasized. However, a statistical table should be as logical, clear, accurate, and simple as possible.

13. Columns and rows that are to be compared with one another should be brought close together.

14. Totals can be placed either at the top or at the bottom of the table. *The most conspicuous part of the table is the upper left corner.*

What Are the Standards of Scientific Merit?

Good-quality research can reflect a variety of study designs (including descriptive and fieldwork techniques in which the investigator does not attempt to manipulate an independent variable). A sound research project can be based on numerical or nonnumerical data. Research settings can be laboratories or natural conditions. The study can be based on a large number of subjects or a single case. A research project can be a one-shot study or an integral part of a continuing series of replicated studies. No one design or method is "best," and no one approach is scientifically most powerful. This attitude of flexibility and diversity also applies to techniques of analysis. *The critical point is that researchers should always employ the study design and analytic procedure that answer the particular questions being studied.* Openness to experience can be seen as being fully as important a characteristic of the scientist as is the understanding of a research design. And the whole enterprise of science can be seen as but one portion of a larger field of knowledge in which truth is pursued in many equally meaningful ways, science being one.

Understanding the principles behind the framework of specific criteria and questions that are useful in the process of scientific criticism is as important to becoming a skilled research consumer as is knowing which questions to ask. A clinician conducting a mental status examination of an 83-year-old woman in a psychiatric outpatient department knows to include interview questions about distant and recent memory. The clinician also knows that answers that indicate, for example, that the patient remembers the name of her high school principal but not the name of the current president of the United States or mayor of her city constitute evidence of memory impairment. But the most critical point is that this kind of memory impairment along with other specific evidence of diminished intellectual functioning signify the presence of dementia. In other words, the nurse must not only know what questions to ask, in which areas to ask them, and what the answers may signify but must also comprehend why knowing all this is relevant in the first place. This idea is also true for the research critic and skillful research consumer. The rationale for asking the elaborate array of precise questions and considering the preceding seven specific criteria when appraising a research proposal or report of findings rests on principles or conventions associated with the logic of scientific work and the logic of inquiry.

Considering some of the more theoretical aspects of research critiques seems justified, if not essential, because these assumptions tend to be neglected in most books and articles on the subject of critiquing research in favor of a "cookbook" approach. We devoted the first half of the chapter to pragmatic strategies for undertaking a critique of scientific research. We now turn our attention briefly to examining them in their relationship to broader logical and theoretical considerations about science. The goal here is to help the research consumer transcend a technician's role and attain the knowledge base appropriate for a true professional engaged in the application of scientific findings. Mere technical virtuosity without attention to rationale is unfortunately likely to lead to sterile results.

The Theoretical and Logical Bases of Inquiry

Certain theoretical assumptions about the nature of reality and the logic of scientific inquiry guide researchers in their choices of topics and their research procedures. They also offer a basis for evaluating or critiquing the research enterprise as reflected in study proposals and reports of findings. The principles set forth in this section, though not necessarily exhaustive, include those that strongly influence a critic's thinking when preparing a research critique. Sjoberg and Nett (1968), among others, believe that such principles influence the rules, procedures, and methods for conducting "good" science. Certain choices or actions are thereby judged as preferable to others in aiding the scientist's search for truth or empirically grounded knowledge. These rules have become the bases for the norms of science and the conventions on which scientists and scientific critics have reached some points of consensus. Even with agreement on conventions that reject the explanatory value of hunches, guesswork, or casual observation, methodological scrupulousness does not yield unquestionable, universal, or unalterable truths about reality. These principles should be used as keys to evaluating the merits of nursing research studies, not as methods for unlocking the doors to incontrovertible scientific laws. In Kaplan's words (1964 p. 5), "Standards governing the conduct of inquiry in any of its phases emerge from inquiry and are themselves subject to further inquiry." Because nurse executives and clinicians base the decisions that affect nurses' future on findings from nursing studies, however, we ought to be as well-informed as possible. Research consumers apply their skills and understanding of scientific criticism to help make that happen.

The Nature of Reality

A long-standing debate about whether reality is stable or fluid and whether humans respond to or create their environment underlies nursing studies. Scientists who argue that a fixed, stable order characterizes social as well as physical reality subscribe to canons of science directed toward accurately and precisely uncovering "what actually exists." Others, while conceding that there is a degree of order in the world, stress its ever-changing and complex nature and posit scientific methods that allow them to study this fluidity. Additionally, those who think of the environment as fluid tend to conceive of humans as interpreting and shaping their reality, whereas those who are committed to a conception of a fixed set of relations in the objective world tend to conceive of humans as responding, adapting, or coping with physical and social forces. Studies with the former orientation emphasize the value of the flexibility of field methods, and those with the latter assumptions require reliability and validity of measurement instruments that reflect the "actual value" of an operationally defined variable at a static point in time.

The Observer's Relationship to Observed Phenomena

Every nursing study indicates some assumption about the scientific observer vis-à-vis the variables being observed. The most marked divergence is between those associated with the *logical positivist* perspective, who assume that observers should be able to distance themselves and make unbiased observations, and the adherents of the *verstehen* approach, who contend that the observer always influences and is influenced by the reality under investigation. Obviously, the logical positivist values strategies or instruments designed to eliminate observer bias, and the *verstehen* scientist emphasizes the value of being aware of and reporting on the subjective, interpretive nature of the observer-observed interaction and his or her *attempts* to approach the ideal of objectivity (which many philosophers of science believe the logical positivist takes for granted but rarely achieves).

The Relationship between Theory and Data

As Sjoberg and Nett (1968) point out, theory as a system of concepts or ideas is not unique to science but is basic to all systems of philosophy and religious thought. The essential difference lies in the use of empirical observation as the method of discovery or validation. Although scientists seem to agree that both theory and data are essential features of the scientific method, they disagree, as have philosophers since Kant and Hume, about the relationship between the two. Some nursing scientists define theory in rigorous terms that are applicable only to systems that involve sets of postulates from which testable hypotheses (**propositions**) can be derived. In the opinion of others, any logically related statements that explain an investigator's observations or make them meaningful can be considered as scientific theory in a broad sense. Nurse scientists and scholars sometimes disagree about whether theory or data have priority in the research process. The split between those researchers who stress theory and those who emphasize observation (data) in effect reflects the difference between adhering to a **deductive** theory-testing approach in science and more **inductive** inquiry that is oriented toward discovery. Clearly, evaluation criteria that address the quality of hypotheses, identification of independent and dependent variables, and the like are much more appropriate when the study under examination is in the deductive tradition.

The Value of Natural or Artificial Language

Natural language, on the one hand, is ordinary language. It may be vague, convey shades of emotion, and be somewhat ambiguous when used by different people. Artificial, or scientific, language systems, on the other hand, primarily try to free the scientific discourse from the perceived inadequacies of ordinary language. The ultimate artificial language is, of course, a mathematical formula. Many nursing studies should be judged on their adherence to a traditional "axiomatic" system of logic. That is, (1) a system of hypotheses is derived from previous research, (2) definition of key terms is advanced in "scientific" language, and (3) the hypotheses are subjected to test through empirical observation. Other studies reflect research procedures based on the notion that science is and should be inductive, in that it extracts out of nature (data) an order (a conceptual but "natural" explanation) to produce truth. A critic can't hope to resolve the controversy about the proper language and logical systems in nursing research, but he or she can be sensitive to the view about induction or inference that shapes the study problem and mode of analysis reflected in a particular study and resist evaluating it according to inappropriate criteria. Study designs and research procedures selected to maximize discovery and flexibility necessarily require somewhat different yardsticks for measuring their quality and effectiveness than studies that emphasize accuracy, precision, exactness, and control (see Chapter 13).

Selection of Units of Analysis and Sources of Data

The way a nurse scientist elects to choose sample members and the kinds of data collected say a lot about his or her conception of the scientific method. Many of the technical procedures, particularly those involved in choosing a random sample, depart considerably from commonsense thinking. Before the investigator selects the sample members from whom data will be collected, he or she must have a clear conception of the ultimate range of generalizations from the study. Regardless of the type of sampling procedure (probability or nonprobability), most authorities alert us to the error of drawing generalizations from data that cannot be demonstrated to be typical, random, or representative in any sense. Even when one is studying the extremes of human action, where probability sampling would not be appropriate, one can expect to see careful, purposeful sampling and plans to discover whether the patterns that are discovered can be replicated with different groups.

The Nature and Adequacy of Proof

The nature and adequacy of proof engage the critic in the questions related to when data are considered adequate to support a given analytic scheme or set of hypotheses. The controversies surrounding this topic involve at least three related issues:

1. the necessity of quantifying data and the relative merits of tests of statistical significance versus multivariate analyses

2. the question of whether prediction or understanding is the key criterion for judging the adequacy of one's data relative to one's theory or hypotheses

3. the most meaningful techniques for establishing the reliability and validity of evidence

The quantification of independent, dependent, and extraneous variables in any research situation is a function of the researcher's broader conception of the reality being studied. Many nurse researchers find it difficult to isolate and measure these variables precisely when they are investigating human problems that are amorphous and complex without imposing an artificiality or fictional nature on the problem. On one side of the debate are nurse scientists advocating the rigid adoption of measurement and statistical rules used so productively in many of the physical sciences. Others argue that to apply measurement and statistical rules and procedures to complex, interactional human systems, investigators must conduct much more methodological research before all the issues associated with the use of such rules and procedures can be resolved. Proponents of the latter view point out that many of the proxy indicators used to "measure" nonunitary and abstract concepts or variables in nursing studies are often controversial, crude, or even meaningless. The problem is compounded when nurse researchers apply powerful statistical procedures to nominal and ordinal scale measures. To manipulate nominal or ordinal data through the use of inappropriate statistics is viewed as imposing an artificial order on the nature of social reality.

Similarly, there is no firm consensus among nurse scientists about the criteria for judging the adequacy of an explanation or theory. Nurses who align themselves with the positivist scientific tradition contend that prediction is the key requirement. In this view, nursing theory must ultimately be evaluated for its predictive power. From the symbolic-interactionist perspective, however, the function of nursing theory should be to promote understanding, thus rejecting the notion that human action can be predicted in mechanistic terms. Among advocates of this philosophy of science, understanding is the goal of inquiry, and coherence is the basis for judging truth. If the analysis or theory makes sense of the data under study in a coherent and internally consistent way, the explanation meets the criterion of adequacy.

Yet another point bearing on the nature and adequacy of proof is the matter of determining the reliability and validity of data. You will recall that reliability refers to the consistency among observers (or data-collection tools), and validity refers to the accuracy or adequacy of the data in view of the study question being asked. The test-retest and split-half techniques are procedures regularly used to determine whether data collected are consistent over time or across raters or observers. And the prediction or some variant thereof is basic to the means of validating measurement techniques. Critics of the standard techniques for establishing reliability charge that they tend to lead nurse researchers to sacrifice generality for specificity and reductionism. Critics of validity techniques based on predictability protest that nurse researchers require a fuller grasp of the conditions in which prediction can and cannot be effectively employed.

The preceding paragraphs merely highlight some of the issues related to an extremely complex matter. Blalock (1964) probably summarizes them best:

> We would suggest flexibility as the guiding theme. In our haste to become "scientific" we have perhaps overrigidly followed the few rules . . . which have been rigorously set forth (p. 185).

Norms That Govern the Dissemination of Research Findings

Advancement of nursing science must be built on prior achievements, and thus a body of nursing knowledge and theory depends on rapid and widespread communication of research findings. When judging the effectiveness of dissemination of findings, a critic must consider evidence that the author has attended to:

- the nature of the audience or reference group (readership)

- the style employed in research reporting (see Chapter 18)

- the ethical norms that govern what should and should not be published (see Chapter 3)

The critic's task is to spot potentially significant contributions to knowledge in an expanding sea of research publications of variable quality. Conventions of form may dominate the questions a critic raises about a report of research, but true scientific advancement depends on creative ideas for both controversy and inspiration.

Critiquing a Sample Proposal

You will now have an opportunity to practice applying the critiquing criteria presented earlier in this chapter to a hypothetical sample research proposal (see Box 6–3). Doing so will help you extrapolate the knowledge and skills of critiquing research to other studies you encounter.

Once you've read the study proposal, you are in a position to apply the criteria for a research critique, raise the set of questions related to each of them, and think through the important considerations concerning the logic of inquiry.

Clarity and Relevance of the Study Purpose   Reducing postoperative distress is indeed relevant and useful to nursing. Knowing if a specific training program can achieve it would contribute to nursing knowledge and perhaps even alter and make more effective the nature of "standard" preoperative preparation. Thus, our sample study is both clear and relevant insofar as its purpose and value for nursing are concerned.

Researchability of the Study Problem   The investigator has met many of the standards for a researchable study problem. The problem can be answered by collecting or measuring empirical data. The investigator has explicitly asked the question: "Can training in cognitive coping skills reduce postsurgical distress in adult patients?" Coping-skills training has been identified as the independent variable and been given an operational definition. Postsurgical distress has been identified as the dependent variable and provided with an operational definition. A specific hypothesis to be tested in the study has been stated: that the training will reduce postsurgical distress. And the study question is accurate and consistent with the title, purpose, and literature review.

Box 6–3   Sample Study Proposal

Title:

Training in Cognitive Coping Skills and the Reduction of Postsurgical Distress

Purpose:

Nursing's major goal after a patient experiences surgery is his or her uncomplicated recovery. Most patients who are admitted to a hospital for surgery experience anxiety and feel helpless. They are surrounded by unfamiliar machinery and subjected to invasive procedures. Yet ample literature supports the conclusion that the events themselves rarely cause patient anxiety but rather the patients' views and information about the events. This study will demonstrate that training in cognitive coping skills can reduce patient anxiety and contribute to a less distressing postsurgical recovery. Implications of this study are that nurses will have empirical support for their role as a health educator, and patients will experience surgery as less traumatic because they feel more independent and in control of their experience. In sum, the specific question for this research is whether cognitive-coping skills training can reduce postsurgical distress in adult patients.

Hypothesis:

The specific hypothesis to be tested in this study is: Patients who are trained in the use of cognitive coping skills before surgery experience less postoperative distress than similar patients who do not receive such training.

Review of Related Literature and Conceptual Framework:

The conceptual framework for this study is drawn from related literature in the fields of nursing and psychology. Meichenbaum, Golfried, Mahoney and colleagues have demonstrated that an individual's internal dialogue and images influence not only feelings related to a situation but also a person's behavior. Langer and associates (1975) trained surgical patients to use cognitive coping skills, including reappraisal and rehearsing positive aspects of a surgical experience, and found that in their sample there was a significant reduction in postsurgical distress. Further clinical evidence of the value of using cognitive coping skills was present in studies by Meichenbaum and Wine (1970). In their research, students after receiving training in coping skills began to label physiological arousal like sweating, increased heart and respiratory rate, and the like as coping rather than debilitating. Other studies have likewise reported reductions in test and speech anxiety following similar training (Wine 1971, Sarason 1973, Norman 1974). Based on the literature cited above, it seems reasonable to assume that surgical patients' internal dialogue and images related to their surgical procedures may influence their

(Continued)

Box 6–3   *(continued)*

postsurgical distress. This study addresses the question of whether a surgical patient's postsurgical distress can be reduced by altering his or her views about the surgical experience through coping-skills training.

Definition of Terms:

Cognitive-coping-skills training: a process by which a nurse teaches patients to change distress-provoking thoughts and styles of thinking in order to produce thoughts that decrease distress.

Postsurgical Distress: constitutes the dependent variable in this study and will be measured operationally using the following indicators:

1. length of stay in the recovery room
2. frequency of pain medication requested
3. time required before eating again by mouth
4. length of hospital stay
5. time required to attain normal routine at home
6. self-report of experience after discharge
7. incidence and severity of postoperative complications

The cognitive-coping-skills training program constitutes the independent variable in this study and will be carried out for all sample members according to the following procedure:

I. Educational Phase:

The purpose of the first phase is to convey the idea that there is no 1:1 correlation between a situation and a feeling; rather, it is the individual's style of thinking and images that are the major influencing factors in distress.

This section will incorporate didactic and experiential examples of the idea above. Discussion involving members will be encouraged. Charts and diagrams will be used to aid in understanding the relationship between events and thoughts. Patients will be told that they probably have not been aware of the influence of thoughts on behavior because they were taught to believe that there is a correlation between the two. They will be told that thinking and thinking styles have become routine and automatic, and thus we are not aware of them. Demonstration of this concept of automatic thinking will be carried out.

(Continued)

Box 6–3 *(continued)*

There will be a homework assignment given to members to bring back the following day. The patients will be asked to visualize the situation of their upcoming surgery and to record their thoughts, images, and feelings concerning the surgery.

II. Rehearsal Phase:

The next day, we will work with the data provided by each member in the following way:

Cognitive Reappraisal   1. Identify with the patients their distressful thoughts (for example, "I am going to die").

2. Teach the patients to identify their assumptions and distinguish them from facts. (Assumptions are neither true nor false but are only probabilities.)

3. Teach the patients to counter their assumptions, using thoughts and images that are incompatible with the original distress-producing thoughts.

A homework assignment will be given to reinforce what the patients have learned.

III. Calming Self-Talk:

Patients will be taught how a stress situation occurs and how to prepare themselves. Examples will be given.

Stress comes about in stages:

Stages	*Examples of Calming Self-Talk*
1. what we say to ourselves when preparing for surgery	1. "I can develop a plan to deal with this situation."
2. the actual situation (the surgery)	2. "One step at a time. I can handle this situation."
3. coping with being overwhelmed	3. "When fear comes, just pause."
4. reinforcing self-statements	4. "I can be pleased with my progress."

IV. Cognitive Control through Selective Attention:

Patients will be shown that selection of a particular focus (regular breathing, repeating a statement) is incompatible with negative thoughts that produce distress.

(Continued)

Box 6–3 *(continued)*

Data Collection Procedures and Methodology:

Settings for this study will be four private and public hospitals in a West Coast urban area. Patients of either sex who are in the age range 30–55, have had no previous surgery, have no clinically documented illness, are scheduled for a cholecystectomy without common duct exploration, are willing to give informed consent, and have their physician's referral will be admitted to the study *sample* until a total *n* of 100 patients is achieved. Patients will be assigned alternately to Group A or Group B. Group A will receive cognitive-coping-skill training, and Group B, the control group, will receive no special preoperative preparation other than standard care.

The training will be done by the same nurse with special skills in this method and take 1 hour for each of four days before admission to the hospital for surgery. Patient data will be obtained from the following data sources:

1. the recovery room chart
2. the ward patient chart
3. telephone interviews to obtain self-reports
4. one follow-up home visit conducted one month after discharge

Limitations in the form of uncontrolled *extraneous variables* that are acknowledged consist of the following:

1. Patients at the younger end of the age range may recover more quickly than patients at the older end.

2. Self-report data may be influenced by sample members' attempting to please the interviewer.

3. No comparable preoperative intervention for the control group leaves unanswered the questions of whether any differences are due to the training per se or just any form of special attention.

Data Analysis

The following mock tables reflect the data analysis plan. Scores will be constructed for frequencies of behaviors, summarized in Table I, and frequency of negative and positive comments reported in postoperative phone and home-visit interviews, reflected in Table II. Statistical-analysis procedures will include descriptive data summaries that characterize the study sample and specific techniques appropriate for comparing frequencies for significant differences. Expectations are that the hypothesis will be supported and

(Continued)

Box 6–3 *(continued)*

that both statistically and clinically significant differences will be found between Group A and Group B on the dependent variable of postoperative distress.

Table I: Frequency of Postoperative Distress Behaviors

Distress Behavior	Total Frequency *Group A*	Total Frequency *Group B*
1. Length of stay in recovery room (hours)		
2. Number of pain-medication requests		
3. Time required to begin eating by mouth (hours)		
4. Length of hospital stay (hours)		
5. Time required to attain normal routines at home (hours)		
6. Numbers of postoperative complications		

Table II: Self-Report on Postoperative Distress

Number of Negative Comments		Number of Positive Comments	
Group A	*Group B*	*Group A*	*Group B*
Total	*Total*	*Total*	*Total*

Source: Adapted from a research proposal of B. E. U. Stroud. Rohnert Park, Calif.: Sonoma State University, 1977.

The investigator includes some of the study's limitations. But—and this is a rather big *but—justification* for accepting the study with those limitations is not included. The influence of age could be controlled for, either through sampling techniques that matched comparative groups by age or through using statistical means to account for any differences in findings that could be attributed to age differences rather than to the independent variable. Similarly, strategies to minimize the Hawthorne effect—the likelihood that any significant differences between groups A and B are due to the fact that group A got some kind of "special attention" for four extra hours plus homework activities and group support—could have been incorporated into the study design. Four hours of other individual or group interaction could have been provided to the control group (for example, a general discussion group with the nurse in which the coping skills were *not* taught). Finally, the possibility of biased self-report data could have been decreased by using a mailed, objective self-report form rather than a face-to-face or even telephone conversation with the nurse (particularly if the nurse doing the follow-up interviews was the same one who did the training program).

Adequacy and Relevance of the Literature Review   Again the investigator has met a number of the standards for an acceptable literature review. The references are pertinent to the subject under investigation, are integrated and logically organized, and provide a rationale for the present study. We can also note the following deficiencies, however:

1. The references are dated (not current).

2. We are left unsure about how this particular study will extend prior work.

3. One of the dates is omitted from the references.

4. The literature review does not provide us with the investigator's rationale for measuring the dependent variable of postsurgical distress in the manner chosen.

5. We really don't get much insight into the researcher's awareness of the range of opinion and extent of research findings in the problem area. For example, we don't know if this is a well-studied area or whether the references incorporated represent the totality of the work previously done on this topic.

Agreement of Purpose, Design, and Methods   Although the study has been designed to answer the research question, a number of omissions make it difficult to conclude that efforts to increase its validity and reliability will be successful. For example, the investigator does not ever actually discuss the choice of a study design and therefore does not comment on its strengths and weaknesses. Because sample members are not randomly selected or assigned, we can surmise that this is a quasi-experimental design with a comparative group. But we are not assured that the two groups are actually comparable once they have been constructed, because analysis of demographic data is not included in the analysis plan. We have commented earlier on the way in which the procedures fail to control for some of the extraneous variables that could affect the study findings. We also have no results of pilot studies or power analyses on which to base any decisions about the reliability and validity of data-collection operations and adequacy of sample size. For example, is it correct to assume that the number of requests for pain medication is necessarily an indicator of postoperative distress? Might cultural or personal preferences about taking medication be a factor here? The investigator also does not provide us with copies of the data-collection and data-recording tools, making it hard to assess exactly how self-report data, in particular, will be obtained and making it impossible to replicate the study. Not knowing what tools or instruments will be used makes it impossible for us to know the sources of them, their tested validity and reliability, or how they were developed—if they were. Finally, although conditions were apparently to be the same for all members of group A, who experienced the experimental treatment, conditions for group B were not comparable to those for group A, and we have no reason to believe that the rater or interviewer was blind when collecting the postoperative data on the dependent variable.

Suitability of the Sampling Procedure   The investigator does tell us the size of the intended sample, the fact that it will be collected from four different hospital settings, and the criteria used to enter eligible sample members into the study. What we find missing is the rationale for these choices. Why not a random sample and assignment to groups? On what basis was the decision for a sample size of 100 made? Addition of more of the sampling logic and reporting on the characteristics of the two groups in the final report are two areas for improvement.

Correctness of Analytical Procedures   The logic of analysis of data in the study is underdeveloped and incomplete. Why focus exclusively on absolute frequencies? Are they all of equal weight or importance? What specific statistical techniques will be used to answer the study question and test the hypothesis for significant differences between the two groups? The analysis section is perhaps the single weakest aspect of the study proposal. We are unable to answer any of the questions appropriate for conducting a critique of a study's analytic procedures, even though sample tables are incorporated. For instance, we don't know the name of the statistical tests to be applied or the probability associated with significant values. Further, we don't know how any extra qualitative data might be analyzed or if they will be, whether the intended statistical tests are appropriate to the level of measurement and study question, and what the researcher intends to do about clinically significant findings that may not be "statistically" significant.

Clarity of Findings   Because this is a study proposal rather than a study report, there are, of course, no research findings. Instead, review the questions under this criterion and apply them to a report of findings in a current nursing research journal. And remember that it is neither just nor reasonable to criticize a piece of work such as the simulated proposal we have just dissected for failing to be or do something that the author never intended for it. Our sample proposal could, however, be improved by a less abrupt conclusion that would serve as an abstract or summary of the entire study.

Critiquing Research—Some Final Tips

The preceding criteria, questions, principles, and illustrations are all intended to serve as guidelines in critiquing research proposals or reports of study findings. It is never justifiable to apply them without giving sufficient rationale for your opinion that they are appropriate and your conclusions in relation to them. Try to keep in mind the audience for whom the research was intended, and think about the work as a whole even as you scrutinize it for details like the ones suggested in the questions associated with each of the seven criteria. Remember to avoid nitpicking about trivial details and thereby sacrificing the good in favor of the perfect. How you evaluate a piece of research may influence the decisions of others to replicate it or base their practice on it. Try to consult experts and other resource persons on technical aspects that you may feel uncertain about to ensure the accuracy and precision of your interpretation. Be considerate in your language. *Science* magazine advises its reviewers: "If you find you have to devote the last paragraphs of your critique to correcting a false impression [about the quality of the research], reconsider your criticisms of it." This doesn't mean that you should withhold criticism, but the merits of the work (or the lack of them) should emerge as the overriding theme of your critique. Be concise, readable, rational, sensitive, accurate, and impartial. Offer explanation and examples. And practice.

Guidelines for Critique

- Have you written a critique or a review of a study proposal or report of findings?

- Have you attempted to be constructive in your criticism?

- Have you considered the basic critiquing questions?

- Did you evaluate all possible sources of error?

- Are research tables well-presented?

- Are research procedures consistent with underlying assumptions?

- Can you apply the critique process to study proposals as well as to reports of findings?

Summary of Key Ideas and Terms

✓   To fulfill the role of research consumer, which is expected of all nurses regardless of their educational preparation, you must acquire skills of critiquing research.

✓   Conducting a good critique of a study proposal or report of findings requires not just a list of pertinent questions to ask but criteria or standards against which to evaluate answers to the questions and a comprehension of the rationale for asking and answering them in the first place.

✓   A *research critique* is a critical estimate of a piece of research that has been carefully and systematically studied by a critic who has used specific criteria to appraise its general features.

✓   A *research review* identifies and summarizes the major features or characteristics of a study.

✓   The critic's challenges are to determine what a researcher has tried to do, to evaluate the strategies used in light of the realistic constraints of the study, and to present both criteria and evidence for making judgments about the quality of the research.

✓   A competent critique ought to represent a contribution to knowledge and scholarly exchange and be helpful to the author of the research.

✓   A helpful critic uses strategies to differentiate his or her criticism from destructive criticism and trivial nitpicking.

✓   Seven conventional criteria can be used as a basis for conducting a critique of a research proposal or report of study findings. These are: (1) clarity and relevance of the study purpose, (2) researchability of the study problem, (3) adequacy and relevance of the literature review, (4) agreement of purpose, design, and methods, (5) suitability of the sampling procedure and sample size, (6) correctness of the analytic procedure, and (7) clarity of findings.

✓   Well-presented tables ought to conform to a set of characteristic hallmarks.

✓ To avoid a "cookbook" approach to critiquing research, the reader should attempt to comprehend scientific issues that underpin the theoretical and logical basis of inquiry.

✓ A high-quality critique can be influential in that others may use it to make decisions to replicate studies or base practice decisions on it. The critic should strive to be concise, readable, rational, sensitive, accurate, and impartial, and he or she should offer explanations for judgments made.

References

American Nurses' Association: *Preparation of Nurses for Participation in Research*. Kansas City, Mo.: American Nurses' Association, 1976.

Blalock HM Jr: *Causal Inferences in Nonexperimental Research*. Chapel Hill: University of North Carolina Press, 1964.

Field WE: Clinical nursing research: A proposal of standards. *Nurs Leadership* December 1983; 6:117–120.

Fleming JW, Hayter J: Reading research reports critically. *Nurs Outlook* March 1974; 22:172–175.

Flemming J: Teaching nursing research content. *Nurse Educator* 1980; 5:24–26.

Horsley J, Crane J: *Using Research to Improve Nursing Practice: A Guide*. New York: Grune & Stratton, 1982.

Kaplan A: *The Conduct of Inquiry*. San Francisco, Chandler, 1964.

Kramer M et al: The teaching of nursing research. Parts 2, 3. *Nurse Educator* 1981; 6:30–37.

Krampitz SD, Pavlovich N (editors): *Readings for Nursing Research*. St. Louis: Mosby, 1981.

Leininger MM: The research critique: Nature, function and art. Pages 20–32 in: *Communication Nursing Research: The Research Critique*. Boulder, Colo.: WICHE, 1968.

Mallick MJ: A constant comparative method for teaching research critiquing to baccalaureate nursing students. *Image* Fall 1983; 15:120–122.

Sjoberg G, Nett R: *A Methodology for Social Research*. New York: Harper & Row, 1968.

Wilson HS: Teaching research in nursing: Issues and strategies. *West J Nurs Res* 1982; 4:365–377.

Conducting Research
in Nursing

C H A P T E R

7

Discovering Research Problems in Clinical Practice

HOLLY SKODOL WILSON

Chapter Objectives

After reading this chapter, the student should be able to:

- Recognize sources of research problems

- Distinguish between researchable and nonresearchable clinical questions

- Describe why "value" questions and "yes or no" questions are not amenable to answering with the scientific method

- Compare and contrast types of research problems, including factor-isolating, factor-relating, situation-describing, and situation-predicting questions

- Formulate a researchable problem from a general topic area of interest

- Evaluate problem statements in published research reports according to the criteria of significance, researchability, and feasibility

- Appreciate problem identification as an investigative role for all nurses regardless of their level of preparation

In This Chapter...

To build a scientific basis for their practice, nurses need a wide variety of investigative skills. One of the most important ones is being able to ask sensitive, astute, and potentially *researchable* questions in practice situations. Clinicians are in the best possible position to converse with colleagues and patients and learn about how they interpret their experiences. A nurse who sees research as inquiry, not just technical instrumentation, watches and listens for the underlying reality of the practice world. A nurse with an inquiring mind develops skills in observing and analyzing that help him or her discover important questions and problems in the course of giving nursing care. Each dressing change, catheterization, and bed bath becomes an opportunity, not only to care for other human beings, but also to learn about topics that demand research-based explanations. Theoretical and clinical sensitivity begin with your ability to raise the important and meaningful questions in your nursing practice. In fact, the American Nurses' Association Commission on Nursing Research agreed that (1) demonstrating awareness of the value and relevance of research in nursing, (2) assisting in identifying problem areas in nursing practice, and (3) assisting in collecting data within a structured format, have become investigative functions that *all nurses*, including those prepared in diploma and associate degree programs, should be able to perform (ANA 1981a). In the language of the commission:

> Building a scientific base for clinical practice is the priority for nursing research in the 1980's. To maximize the benefits of developing a scientific base for use in practice, mechanisms are required that ensure that scientific knowledge contributes to practice and in turn that the problems encountered in practice have an impact on the focus of the knowledge generated. Nurses performing different roles in nursing contribute to the interplay between practice and research (ANA 1981b).

This chapter gives you strategies for thinking about sources of research questions and ways to differentiate between clinical problems that can be researched and those that cannot. It discusses kinds of research problem, an approach to writing them, and criteria for evaluating those that served as the basis for studies that you read or hear about.

Finding Research Problems

Research begins with a study question, or what is called a **researchable problem**. This problem may concern nursing education, nursing administration, history, ethics, or a social or natural science question related to health that interests a nurse researcher. But if it is to address the priorities cited by leaders in the profession and meet the strictest definition of nursing research, the problem will most likely stem from nursing practice or patient care. Patient-care problems have generally been defined as difficulties or concerns experienced by patients or the nurses caring for them. Often, there is a *discrepancy* between what is actually practiced and what is desirable.

Even though every clinical situation is replete with possible study questions, deciding on a specific one can be difficult for a beginning investigator. It is sometimes hard to settle on one problem when so many seem to demand attention. In other cases, we are so accustomed to explaining things automatically to ourselves based on common sense or conventional wisdom that we fail to see the possible light that scientific inquiry could shed. Sometimes the stress, hectic schedule, and even boring routine of our work suppress our tendency to be curious about connections, trends, patterns, and ideas. At other times, low morale, rapid turnover, fatigue, and habit obstruct our ability to bring curiosity, imagination, and critical sensibilities to bear on our practice. But once, as Diers (1979 p. 12) says, "you are in the right frame of mind, researchable problems in nursing will probably find you!"

Sources of Research Problems

Valid sources of research problems in nursing include your own experience, patterns or trends, somebody else's completed research, and your intellectual and scientific interests.

Your Own Experience   The best source of clinical research topics is probably your own experience. All of the personal reactions listed in Table 7–1 can be used to generate researchable questions.

TABLE 7–1 *Experience As a Source of Research Problems*

Type of Reaction	Illustration
Wishes and desires	"I wish these children wouldn't get so upset when I come in to change the dressings on their burns."
Gripes	"There's never enough time for discharge planning with these postmastectomy patients."
Questions	"I wonder if it's feasible to start a cardiac rehab program for post-MI patients here?"

Patterns or Trends   A second major source of research problems can be tapped when a practitioner makes the imaginative leap that transforms an undifferentiated accumulation of individual cases into a reasoned pattern. It takes an inventive mind to notice the way a particular phenomenon occurs and to become involved in asking why. Such a nurse becomes an observer and interpreter of reality. One curious nurse working with patients in a nursing home noted certain incidents over a three-month period (see example).

EXAMPLE: Trends in Using Psychotropic Medication among Elderly Clients

Hazel S. came to the nursing home when her husband Sam of over 60 years was admitted because of pneumonia. Since no one else was available to look after her, she was admitted with him. Her anxiety and confusion over Sam's illness resulted in a prescription for regular Mellaril. She subsequently became stuporous and combative. She lost control of bowel and bladder function and was confined to bed. Weeks later when her husband took her home and she was no longer oversedated, her orientation returned completely to normal.

Mary M., an 80-year-old woman with dementia, was admitted to a nursing home screaming. Thorazine was prescribed to "quiet her down." A week later we discovered that she had a fractured femur.

Jerry C., a 74-year-old man, became confused and agitated following loss of consciousness after a fall. He was given Thorazine but became more disruptive, so Haldol and Mellaril were added. He finally developed a severe parkinsonian syndrome that led to discontinuation of his drug therapy. From then on, his mental status improved dramatically.

This nurse's list of anecdotes and case studies extended beyond the few examples described above. She eventually began to wonder whether nursing home staff members tended to adhere to a *pattern* of using psychotropic agents continuously to ease their burden rather than episodically to ease the temporary distress of the elderly patients. Her observations of a pattern resulted in a national survey that addressed questions of misuse of psychotropic drugs in nursing homes with elderly patients. Her findings had a direct impact on changing patient care for the better.

Somebody Else's Completed Research   Research problems that don't develop from your own first-hand experience are often suggested by literature that reports the work of others. Sometimes specific recommendations that a study be replicated with another group of patients or in another setting prompt research. At other times, an author's suggestions for further research in the discussion section of his or her report of findings can be a source of a study question. Most often, however, study questions suggest themselves when you read about contradictory results or controversial nursing issues that have limited or no empirical findings on which to base a conclusion or decision. For example, recent research on the relationship between holding and touching newborns in the delivery room and subsequent parental bonding has yielded mixed results.

Similarly, questions about the advisability of a 25-pound weight gain during pregnancy, seven-day-a-week jogging, and the growing array of diets arise from contradictory "hospital studies." A review of others' published research can not only help you formulate a researchable question but also guide you in deciding whether replicating the work of others is useful or unnecessary. You need not confine your reading to the formal research reports of others. Case studies and clinical descriptions often yield valuable nuggets of what Diers (1979 p. 25) calls "clinical nursing wisdom." In using this kind of literature you can build up a rich accumulation of common events and experiences and compare them with your own to discover themes and patterns that lead to research questions.

Your Intellectual and Scientific Interests The major difference between research topics that grow out of real-world practical concerns and those that are primarily dictated by scientific interest is that the latter are less likely to involve study of a particular clinical situation for the sake of knowledge that can be used in *that situation*. Research topics generated from scientific interests usually concern themselves with more general and abstract explanations of phenomena. Questions that derive from this source are directed toward developing an organized accounting of the universe by discovering systematic relatedness in seemingly unconnected statements and descriptions of facts and events.

Despite continuous polemics about nursing's focus, mission, responsibilities, and scope of practice, much of nursing science remains a grab bag collection of data, unverified assumptions, ritualized practices, and vague hunches. Some research questions are expressly directed toward developing a grand theory of nursing that would fit together nursing concepts into logical and systematic relationships. The example below illustrates such a study.

Gill and Atwood's question illustrates research intended to test the applicability of a nursing theory under real-world conditions.

EXAMPLE: An Experiment in Healing

Nurse researchers Barbara Gill and Jan Atwood published a report in *Nursing Research* (March/April, 1981) entitled "Reciprocy and Helicy Used to Relate mE6F and Wound Healing." The concepts *reciprocy* and *helicy* are drawn from the homeodynamics principles of Martha Rogers's theory of nursing. They deal with "the integration between human and environmental fields, and the unindirectionality of their curvilinear progression along the space-time dimension" (p. 68). These researchers asked if these two concepts adequately organize and explain the healing and/or reepithelialization of a small epidermal wound made on the back of a young Yorkshire-mix pig.

A grand theory of nursing

Test of Rogers' theory in a clinical situation

Identifying Research Questions

Identifying a research question is one of the earliest steps in the research process (see Chapter 1), and the subsequent procedures depend on its being clear and explicit. There are, unfortunately, no foolproof rules to guide a researcher in formulating truly significant questions about a topic. He or she can only try to create the conditions that some experts believe are conducive to formulating important questions. These conditions are:

- systematic immersion in the subject by firsthand observation

- study of existing literature and discussion with people who have accumulated practical experience in the field

- maintaining a critical, curious, and imaginative frame of mind in order to be alert to the new and unexpected

Whenever you find yourself surprised, frustrated, or puzzled, or whenever you express a complaint, a wish, a question, or a hope, you have the basis for a research question that can be refined under the conditions above.

Nonresearchable Questions   By this time you must be convinced that a constant parade of research questions is passing before your eyes each day in your clinical work. But all questions that are personally interesting to you or even clinically relevant are not necessarily researchable. If you are going to participate in research yourself or evaluate the usefulness of research that you read, you must be able to make the distinction. A *researchable question is one that can be investigated using the process of scientific inquiry set out in Chapter 1.* Two major types of nonresearchable questions need to be differentiated from questions that can direct scientific inquiry. These are (1) "value" questions and (2) "yes or no" questions. Let's look briefly at each to see why they don't qualify as sound researchable questions.

Questions of value are "should" questions. They seek information that reflects the values that people have or the policies that institutions have. You can recognize them because they either start with the word *should* or include it in the question. For example:

- Should all mothers be encouraged to breastfeed their babies?

- Should all fathers participate in the experience of labor?

- Should nurses on pediatric units wear white uniforms?

- Should hospital shifts be 8 hours or 12 hours in length?

- What should be the nurse's role in the AIDS epidemic?

- What should be the educational level for entry to professional practice?

None of these questions qualifies as truly researchable. These are questions of value. Questions that are designed to discover what values people hold can be researchable, but these are not the same as questions about what values people *should* hold. To be researchable questions about values held, they would have to read something like this:

■ What percentage of newly employed staff nurses in postpartum-care settings believe that all new mothers should be encouraged to breast-feed their babies?

■ What is the extent of agreement among first-time fathers that they should participate in the experience of labor and delivery?

■ What are the opinions of pediatric nurses about the advisability of wearing white uniforms?

■ What is the preferred shift length among hospital nurses?

■ What definitions of the role of nurses in the AIDS epidemic are advanced by nursing leaders?

■ What do members of the ANA believe is the basic educational preparation for entry into professional nursing practice?

Transforming the first list of value questions into researchable questions has meant editing out the *should*s. The revised list deals with statements of fact, of *what is* or of *how things compare*. In summary, as long as a proposed research question is really a matter of opinion or philosophy, it can't be answered by conventional research methods without transforming it. Research can provide a basis of facts addressing the consequences or outcomes of holding one value or policy position or another, but "should" questions are better answered by logic or persuasion than by empirical investigation.

The second category of question that does not meet the requirements of researchability comprises those that can be answered with a simple yes or no (or even maybe). Such questions may prompt collection of facts or data, but they don't really link up to a broader theoretical problem and offer explanations or predictions. What makes research, research is its obligation to go beyond data collection to influence theory. Examples of static "yes or no" questions are:

■ Do most nurses in city hospitals have a baccalaureate degree?

■ Are patients kept waiting for pain medication after they request it?

■ Do patients rest well in ICUs?

■ Do most prostate surgery patients become confused after surgery?

To qualify as researchable, these questions must be transformed so as to suggest a reason for bothering to collect the information needed to answer them. For example:

- What is the relationship between educational preparation of nurses and quality of care at city hospitals?

- What are the consequences of keeping patients waiting for pain medication after they request it?

- What conditions in ICUs contribute to diminished rest patterns for patients?

- What behavioral cues can nurses use to predict that a patient will become confused after prostate surgery?

These changes involved asking a question about the relationship of two variables associated with the topic of interest.

Researchable Questions   Questions of value, opinion, or policy and accumulations of data can be immensely valuable in clinical problem solving. But it takes questions that produce generalizable information for guiding practice under other conditions to make a nursing problem a nursing *research question*. Good research questions reduce a complex area of interest or topic to a set of simple questions that demand answers, answers that can be found by taking some action. The question "Should mothers bathe newborns daily?" must be transformed into "What is the relationship between daily baths for newborns, maternal bonding, and infant infections?"

Asking a clear, significant, researchable question becomes a key to subsequent decisions about research design, data collection, and data analysis. An overly complex, fuzzy, or nonresearchable question bogs a study down in confusion and inconsistency. Table 7–2 summarizes some sample types of researchable questions and offers an illustration of each.

As you search for your own researchable questions or advise others about doing so, remember that many of the conventional routines ingrained as "standard nursing practice" have never been scientifically studied.

Asking Research Questions

Basic Question Forms

Research questions or problems ultimately involve the use of terms that can be measured. The basic stem words are:

- *Who?*
- *What?*
- *When?*
- *Where?*
- *Why?*

TABLE 7–2 *Types of Researchable Question*

Type	Illustration
Why are things this way?	Why do some settings use primary nursing?
	Why do AIDS patients without hope participate in painful drug experiments?
What would happen if . . . ?	What would happen if third-party payers were reimbursed specifically for nursing care?
	What would happen if all nurses were doctorally prepared?
	What would happen if sex education were taught in all the schools?
Which approach would work better?	Is group or individual counseling more effective with clients who abuse alcohol?
	Does a back rub with conversation or a back rub without conversation result in greater relaxation?
Who might benefit from this?	Would laboring mothers benefit from being encouraged to choose their own position in the delivery room?
	Would hospitalized children have faster recoveries if parents were taught to participate in their care?
	Would infant mortality rates in developing countries be influenced by a prenatal teaching program?

When there is a change in the stem question attached to a substantive topic, the entire direction of the study changes. "Who" questions require that you describe and categorize such information about populations as ethnicity, sex, age, social class, race, health status, sexual behavior, and so on. "What" questions are either specific descriptive questions or more complex "what if" questions, in which you must describe relationships. "When" and "where" questions again include specific descriptive answers, including a time frame and a location. "Why" questions seek an explanation, as do "how" questions. I began my own doctoral dissertation many years ago by asking, "How is social order possible under conditions of espoused freedom in an antipsychiatric community?" My master's thesis several years earlier asked a "what" question—"What is the meaning of current dance forms to adolescent girls?"

Some researchers have sorted these kinds of question into what are called *levels*, suggesting that different questions are appropriate when our level of existing knowledge is at a lower or higher level. For example, if we already know a great deal about a certain topic, asking lower-level "what" or "who" questions is not appropriate. Likewise, if we don't even know the exploratory and descriptive "whats," "whos," and "wheres," asking "how" or "why" questions is premature (see Chapter 8).

Types of Research Questions

One system for distinguishing among the major types of research questions (and the types of answer they yield) has been advanced by nurse researchers and philosophers originally associated with the school of nursing at Yale University. According to Dickoff et al (1968a,b), these types are:

1. factor-isolating
2. factor-relating
3. situation-relating
4. situation-producing

Factor-isolating questions ask, "What is this?" They are sometimes called factor-naming questions. They isolate, describe, categorize, or name factors or situations and provide descriptive definitions. In such studies, the researcher doesn't attempt to introduce a change or to test hypotheses about theory. Instead, factor-isolating questions require that the investigator characterize as fully as possible a particular phenomenon. Sample factor- or situation-isolating questions are:

- What are the properties of parental bonding?
- What are the stages of the grieving process?
- What features characterize hospitals that have low turnover and high morale and function as magnets in recruiting nurses?
- What are the phenomena of concern for psychiatric nursing practice?

Factor-relating questions can be raised after factor-isolating studies have provided at least names for the important factors operating in a situation. Factor-relating questions ask, "What is happening here?" The goal is to determine the relationship among the factors that have been identified. In some cases, a factor-relating study question is not preceded by formal factor-isolating studies. Instead, the researcher draws on his or her own experiential knowledge or published literature to determine what the relevant factors in a given situation might be. A question such as "What is the relationship of parents' own childhood experiences to engaging in subsequent child abuse or neglect?" is a factor-relating question. Studies of drug interaction or correlates of uncomplicated postsurgical recovery are examples of others.

Situation-relating questions ask, "What will happen if . . .?" These questions usually yield hypothesis-testing or experimental study designs in which the investigator manipulates variables to see what will happen. Two examples are "Will reinforcement in the form of a token economy program decrease phobic behavior in a particular group of psychiatric patients?" and "Will biofeedback training decrease suffering among patients with chronic pain?" These questions require answers that allow the researcher to make situation-relating and explanatory state-ments that specify both the direction and strength of relationships.

Situation-producing questions ask, "How can I make it happen?" These questions establish explicit goals for nursing actions, develop plans or prescriptions to achieve the goals, and specify the conditions under which the goals will be accomplished. Most researchers agree that situation-producing questions are the most complicated ones to answer. Example questions might include:

■ How can I intervene to prevent postoperative vomiting?

■ How can I best prepare a woman for labor and delivery?

■ How can nursing services be organized to promote job satisfaction and quality of care?

Many experts believe that situation-producing research questions occur at the highest level of inquiry and must be based on the other three types of study. Situation-producing, or prescribing, questions are used eventually in studies that will guide activity in the empirical environment of the practice setting. They are goal based and concerned with more than what is. They ask, "What must be done in order to achieve what is desired?" Situation-producing questions are based on what Johnson (1968) terms "knowledge of control." This is knowledge of action that can change a sequence of events toward specified desirable outcomes. The task is to discover the sequence of steps that will produce the goal state from the initial state.

Writing Research Problems

A Four-Step Approach

Writing a research problem can begin with any of the sources of questions discussed earlier in this chapter. Let's take the nurse's *wish* that the burned children she took care of wouldn't get so upset when she came in to change their dressings. To trans-form her wish into a researchable problem, all she need do to begin is to turn that wish around and ask, "Why can't I get my wish?" In other words, step 1 is to *state the discrepancy clearly*. Step 2 is simply to identify the *constraints that contribute to the discrepancy between what is going on now and what ideally should occur.* This involves thoughtful periods of brainstorming and consultation with others that might yield the following list of constraints:

1. fear

2. prior experience of pain

3. lack of familiarity with the nurse

4. lack of trust in the nurse

5. fatigue

6. separation from parents

7. lack of information about what to expect

8. being caught off guard

9. low pain threshold

10. emotionally expressive personal style*

Constructing a list like this one is, in effect, specifying the possible variables that might be studied. Once the list of constraints has been completed, a researchable problem can be formulated in step 3 by *focusing on the most likely explanation*. Step 4 involves *rephrasing the problem in conceptual terms* to determine the impact of different approaches on burned children's levels of "being upset." So the hope that began as "I wish they wouldn't get so upset when I come in to change their dressings" becomes the researchable problem:

> Will prior introduction of the nurse and explanation of the dressing change procedure result in a less upset response by burned children who are anticipating a dressing change when compared with children who have not had a prebriefing meeting with the nurse?

The steps involved in refining a general concern or area of clinical interest into a research problem, then, are:

1. Clearly state the discrepancy.

2. Brainstorm all the plausible obstacles or constraints or explanations.

3. Narrow the focus by selecting a few specific high-priority variables.

4. Rephrase the problem in conceptual terms.

This is only one of a long list of possible study questions that range from altering nurse activities to looking for a relationship between personality variables, developmental level, or cultural background and children's reactions to anticipated trauma. Researchers must choose from all of them the ones that will be most fruitful, eliminating those that are trivial or difficult to study, and then refine them into a question that can direct a study design.

---

*Adapted with permission from Cogen Television Cassettes, University of Nevada, Reno, 1975.

A Two-Stage Approach

If you decide to conduct your own research or to participate with a research team, you will probably have a central role in specifying the details of the research question. Lindeman and Schantz (1982) offer an alternative system for moving from interest in several broad topics to a narrowed, formal problem statement or question that will guide the conduct of the study: Stage 1 is formulating the question, and stage 2 is refining the question.

Stage 1: Formulating the question   Most authors agree that research questions have two components, a stem and a topic. Stems can be simple or complex. For example, you might ask, "What are the effects of several types of oral hygiene on the dental health of leukemic patients?" (This is a simple stem that asks "what.") Or you might ask, "What causes postoperative infections, and when do they occur?" (This question asks about causes and occurrence; that is, it is a complex question that asks both "what" and "when.") The way you ask a question influences the way you will answer it, and so it is important to choose the stem of your research question carefully. Reread the section of this chapter that tells you what kinds of answer different kinds of stem question will produce.

   The *topic* is the other part of a research question. In nursing it may be attitudes, behaviors, feelings, beliefs, people, families, communities, health care problems, and so on. The important point about your topic is that you will need to specify how you intend to measure it through working, or operational, definitions. Some of the phenomena of interest to nursing are easier to measure than others. The greater the correlation between the topic and some observable indicator of it, the easier it is to define operationally. It's a good idea to write out all the topics that interest you in one column on a piece of paper and all the significant stem questions in another and then ask yourself: "Which of these questions is the one I really want to ask about the topic?" and "Which of the aspects of the topic best expresses what I really want to know about?" See the example in Table 7–3.

   Once you have narrowed your focus to a specific stem and a topic of interest, *write an unedited statement of the question.* Free yourself from the self-imposed tyranny of correct grammar for the moment and think about satisfying only two criteria:

1.   Your question is answerable by empirical evidence or data.

2.   Your question involves a relationship between two or more variables.

Questions that meet both criteria include: "Does imaging affect patients' ability to cope with health crises?" "Does nursing monitoring increase compliance with a diabetic diet?" and "What is the relationship between massage therapy and pain relief?" In contrast, "Is imaging any good?" and "Should nurses use massage therapy?" are questions of value rather than questions that can be answered through empirical observation.

TABLE 7-3 *Aid to Writing a Research Question*

Stem Question	Topic
What?	Swallowing problems
What kinds?	Aspiration precautions in poststroke patients
How many?	
How often?	
How intense are . . . ?	
When do . . . ?	
Where do . . . ?	
Why do . . . ?	
How do . . . ?	

Having written a rough statement of your question, it is useful to *set up a simple three-column table of variables.* In the first column, write the variable that is being manipulated or examined (the IV). In the last column, write the variable you intend to measure to evaluate the effect of the first variable (the DV). In the middle column, write the variables other than the ones you wish to test that could influence the one you intend to measure. These are called extraneous variables, and a list of them can become fairly long. So our sample question, "Does imaging affect patients' ability to cope with health crises?" might be written up like this:

Independent Variable(s)	Other Factors	Dependent Variable(s)
Imaging	Type of crisis	Coping with health crises
	Support system of patient	
	Relationships with therapist	
	Past life experiences	
	Psychological traits	
	Cultural background	

Once your three-column table is complete, you may want to request critiques from peers to determine whether you should add variables to any column, modify any variable, or delete variables from any column. The edited table is a rough conceptualization of your research problem and is ready for refinement in stage 2.

Stage 2: Refining the Question   The second stage of writing a good research question, according to Lindeman and Schantz (1982), is refining it. In the refinement stage you must build a bridge between the current research-based knowledge related to your topic and the step you intend to undertake. Lindeman and Schantz suggest using a matrix, or building-block, approach to sort through related studies that you have discovered in the course of reviewing the literature. On the *y*-axis of the matrix, put types of study, and on the *x*-axis, put categories of variables related to your study question. Table 7–4 shows a hypothetical matrix for our proposed question about the use of imaging to help patients cope with health crises.

Organizing existing literature and integrating it helps you decide whether to formulate your research question as an experiment or as a nonexperimental study. This process can also help you to make decisions about instruments and about methods for controlling extraneous variables.

Evaluating Research Problems

Deciding which research studies are worth trying to carry out at an individual or institutional level in practice requires that you evaluate the adequacy of the research question or questions on which the study was based. Some studies that you read clearly look as if they were done as exercises in methodology for a course or program requirement. They give the impression that the investigator chose the question

TABLE 7–4   *Literature Review Matrix*

Type of Literature	Effects of Imaging	Timing	Patient Characteristics/ Nurse Characteristics
Theory			
Replication			
Experimental			Doe, 1985
Exploratory	Smith, 1983		
Descriptive			
Survey		Jones, 1984	

because he or she thought it would make for an *easy* study. The topic may be trivial, the instruments self-made or imported, and the sample a one-shot captive population of "volunteers" in a single setting. Study questions sometimes grow out of a researcher's idiosyncratic interests but may make little or no conceivable contribution to either practical problems or nursing theory. Finally, keep an eye open for study questions that are so ambiguous, vague, or difficult to define that variables can't be measured. To evaluate the potential usefulness of any particular study question, consider using the following criteria:

- significance
- researchability
- feasibility

Significance

Kaplan (1964) recalls an anecdote involving a drunkard searching under a street lamp for his house key, which he dropped some distance away. Asked why he isn't looking for it where he dropped it, he replies, "It's lighter here." Much research, according to Kaplan, is conducted in much the same way as the drunkard's search. Really important problems are not always those that are most interesting to the researcher or easiest to study.

The problem studied should advance knowledge of phenomena that are objects of inquiry in the field. Even though a question may reflect an individual researcher's thoughts and imagination, it must be articulated in a conceptual system that is understandable to others in the scientific community. Significant research problems make contributions to the science or the discipline of nursing in a meaningful way. Insignificant study questions are trivial, obvious, or expedient.

Researchability

Researchability demands that a study problem admit the possibility of empirical testing. This means not only that a question about the possibility of a relationship between variables is asked but also that the variables under scrutiny must somehow be measurable. As we saw earlier in this chapter, certain questions of value or policy may be important to philosophers and administrators but cannot be studied using empirical testing procedures.

Within nursing, according to Donaldson and Crowley (1978), there is a need to know and to work from descriptive theories as well as prescriptive ones. As Gortner and Nahm (1977) have also pointed out, some studies are basic, in that they are applicable to a general understanding of human behavior or responses to illness, and other studies are applied. Both are needed and significant in a professional discipline, because each discipline has a principal aim that influences the perspective of that field, the way it conceptualizes the relevant world, and the questions it poses for investigation. Because of the uniqueness of each discipline's perspective, it is not possible to simply borrow theory or knowledge from other disciplines. Viewing phenomena from the perspective of healthy functioning of individuals in interaction with their environments will generate distinctive research at all levels and a defined, structured body of knowledge. Studies that raise significant clinical questions are emphasized in this text and reflect contemporary priorities in nursing. However, *the need persists for philosophical, historical, and other types of inquiry within the discipline of nursing*, not only to build the knowledge base but also to refine the social relevance and value orientations of the discipline itself. Important research questions are those raised in the context of theoretical considerations that have meaning to the discipline *and* the practice of nursing.

A researchable problem is stated clearly and unambiguously as either a question or a statement. For example, an investigator can ask, "What are the effects of group meetings on locus of control among psychiatric inpatients?" Other ideas can be best stated in a declarative sentence: "The problem in this research is to identify nursing functions that help patients achieve behaviors necessary for control of their hypertension" or "The study problem is to determine the effect of episodic apnea on sleeping patterns among patients with chronic respiratory problems." Questions have the advantage of putting study problems in a simple and direct way. For that reason, I recommend asking a question. A problem put in statement form is also easier to confuse with the statement of a study's purpose, and the two are not the same.

A researchable problem or question follows logically and consistently from a review of what is already known about a topic. It is the next logical question to pursue given what has been learned in the past [Lindeman and Schantz 1982).

Feasibility

Polit and Hungler (1987) remind us that a good study problem should also be feasible in terms of:

- Time. The problem should be sufficiently restricted that enough time will be available to study it.

- Availability of subjects. There must be enough participants with the desired characteristics who will be willing to cooperate.

- Cooperation of others. The problem must be one that host settings and approval boards (see Chapter 3) are likely to endorse.

- Facilities and equipment. Research problems must be framed in such a way as to be possible given the space, office equipment, transportation, consultation, and computer facilities available.

- Money. Study questions must not only be proposed in the context of sufficient budget but must also be sufficiently worthwhile to justify the anticipated cost of studying them.

- Experience of the researcher. The problem "should be chosen from a field about which the investigator has some prior knowledge or experience." Furthermore, the investigator should either possess the requisite skills to collect and analyze data or have access to those who do.

- Ethical considerations. A research problem may not be feasible if unfair or unethical demands are made on potential subjects (see Chapter 3).

Having considered the significance, researchability, and feasibility of a study problem in general, you can then use the following set of questions to evaluate the problem in a piece of research, whether your own or a colleague's.

1. Have you stated the problem clearly early in the report?

2. Have the investigators placed the study problem within the context of existing knowledge and prior work on the topic?

3. Are the concepts or variables that are included in the study problem measurable?

4. Is the problem significant to the development of knowledge about the discipline or the practice of nursing?

5. Can a feasible study design be developed to address the question?

To sum up, knowledge of the characteristics of a good research question helps researchers formulate valid problem statements for their own research and helps research consumers select study findings of scientific merit to put into practice.

Your Role

Whether you are evaluating the research of others to decide whether to use their findings in your clinical practice or are engaging in your own research enterprise, you need to know what characterizes a good question, where to find one, and how to articulate your question to others in proposals, presentations, or reports of findings. This chapter has presented some tools and strategies useful in accomplishing all three. No matter how technically correct a research question is, however, nothing can substitute for being genuinely interested in and curious about the topic or area you elect to study. You may be spending a long time on it, and your future career may be shaped by your research interests, so choose a research topic that really matters to you and to the goals of the profession.

Guidelines for Critique

■ Have you stated the problem clearly?

■ Have you placed the study problem within the context of existing knowledge and prior work on the topic?

■ Are the concepts or variables that are included in your study problem measurable?

■ Is the problem significant to the development of knowledge about the discipline or the practice of nursing?

■ Can you conduct a feasible study to address the question?

SUMMARY OF KEY IDEAS AND TERMS

✓   All nurses, regardless of their educational preparation, share the investigatory role of discovering and evaluating research problems.

✓   Most clinical research problems reflect a discrepancy between what is desirable and what is actual in nursing practice.

✓   Important sources of research problems include (1) your own experience, (2) patterns or trends, (3) somebody else's completed research, and (4) your intellectual and scientific interests.

✓   A researchable problem can be differentiated from a "value" question or a "yes or no" question by its ability to be solved using the process of scientific inquiry.

✓   Most research questions in nursing fall into the categories of factor-isolating questions, factor-relating questions, situation-relating questions, and situation-producing questions.

✓   The following steps will help you move from a topic of interest to a research question:

■ Step 1 State a discrepancy between what exists and what is ideal or desired.

✔   In a true *experimental design* one finds the following hallmarks: (1) control over at least one independent variable and/or manipulation of at least one inde-

■   Step 2 Identify the constraints that contribute to a discrepancy between what goes on and what should occur.

■   Step 3 Focus on the most likely explanation.

■   Step 4 Rephrase it to interpret the problem in conceptual terms.

✔   A well-stated research question should:

■   be answerable by empirical evidence

■   involve a relationship between two or more variables

✔   A table of variables and literature review matrix are additional tools useful in formulating and refining research questions.

✔   The criteria for evaluating your own or somebody else's research problem are significance, researchability, and feasibility.

References

American Nurses' Association, Commission on Nursing Research: *Guidelines for the Investigative Function of Nurses*. Kansas City, Mo.: American Nurses' Association, 1981(a).

American Nurses' Association, Commission on Nursing Research: *Research Priorities for the 1980's*. Kansas City, Mo.: American Nurses' Association, 1981(b).

Cogen Television Cassettes, Reno: University of Nevada, 1975.

Dickoff J, et al: Theory in a practice discipline part I: Practice oriented theory. *Nurs Res* September/October 1968(a); 17:415–435.

Dickoff J, et al: Theory in a practice discipline part II: Practice oriented research. *Nurs Res* November/December 1968(b); 17:545–554.

Diers D: *Research in Nursing Practice*. Philadelphia: Lippincott, 1979.

Donaldson SK, Crowley DM: The discipline of nursing. *Nurs Outlook* February 1978; pp. 113–120.

Gill B, Atwood J: Reciprocy and helicy used to relate mE6F and wound healing. *Nurs Res* March/April 1981; 30:68–72.

Gortner SR, Nahm H: An overview of nursing research in the United States. *Nurs Res* January/February 1977; 26:10–33.

Johnson D: Theory in nursing: Borrowed and unique. *Nurs Res* November/December 1968; 17:545–554.

Kaplan A: *The Conduct of Inquiry*. San Francisco: Chandler, 1964.

Lindeman CA, Schantz D: The research question. *J Nurs Admin* January 1982; 6–10.

Polit D, Hungler BP: *Nursing Research*, 3rd ed. Philadelphia: Lippincott, 1987.

8

Getting Started on a Study

SALLY A. HUTCHINSON

Chapter Objectives

After reading this chapter, the student should be able to:

- Formulate a research question
- Differentiate between levels of inquiry
- Specify the steps in a literature review
- Specify the scope of a literature review
- Specify the rationale for a literature review
- Formulate a statement of purpose
- Formulate hypotheses, if appropriate
- Recognize criteria for and types of hypothesis
- Identify variables
- Formulate operational definitions
- Choose an appropriate design for the study purpose
- Classify sampling methods according to probability and nonprobability methods

(Continued)

- Discuss the relevant issues related to sample size
- Discuss sampling with special population groups
- Discuss the relationship of sampling to external validity

In This Chapter . . .

Florence Nightingale, known as the first nurse statistician, can also be credited with advocating that nursing research focus on nursing practice. In 1975, Notter, former editor of *Nursing Research*, echoed Nightingale, and in 1979, Hodgeman predicted such a move in the practice setting, with the actual research to be done by practicing nurses. If nursing is to be based on scientific knowledge, it is vital that practicing nurses identify relevant, researchable problems and participate in the research process. It is toward this end that this chapter moves.

As a practicing nurse or a nursing student in a diploma, A.D., B.S.N., or graduate program, you may find yourself in a number of situations that force or encourage you to get started doing research. For instance, a physician or a faculty member involved in research may ask you to collaborate. If you are working on your B.S.N. degree you may be required to do a research project as part of your senior practicum. You may be a student in a master's program and choose to do the thesis option that earns you an M.S.N. degree. Perhaps the director of nursing of the hospital where you work is making resources available for nurses involved in clinical practice to do scientific studies. Furthermore, you recognize that promotions and merit increases for nurses in the future are going to reflect this new emphasis on research productivity. Finally, research can be exciting, intellectually stimulating, and rewarding.

Although you may not be initially aware of it, you have many research ideas. Each nurse has observed some aspect of patient behavior or patient treatment that is perplexing or annoying. These observations can lead you to formulate a general research question, which after a literature review can be refined into a research purpose. The research purpose is the objective of your study.

After choosing a research design that is appropriate for your purpose, you select a sample. It is soon time to collect data. By now you are more than halfway through the research process and are on your way toward making a much-needed contribution to nursing knowledge.

"Science becomes the creative search to understand better, and it uses whatever approaches are responsive to particular questions and subject matters addressed" (Polkinghorn 1983 p. 3). It is up to the researcher to make decisions at each step of the research process. This chapter was written to help you make them. It deals with the questions "How do I formulate a research question?" "What literature do I review, and what do I do with it after I review it?" "How do I state my research purpose?" "How big should my sample be?" "Do I need hypotheses?" "What type of research design is appropriate for my study?" Chapter 13 covers qualitative research in detail. This chapter, focusing most directly on quantitative studies, covers the research process from choosing a question to sampling. Other chapters in this book cover the rest of the research process, from data collection to data analysis and discussion. Reading and reflecting on this chapter and on the illustrations from nursing studies that it contains will help you get started as a nurse researcher.

The Research Question

Planting the Seed

Imagine that you are a cardiac rehabilitation nurse and notice that many cardiac bypass patients do not comply with the suggested regimen of diet, exercises, and no smoking. You wonder what sort of nursing intervention would increase their compliance, giving them the opportunity to reap the benefits of their surgery and to live a more comfortable life.

Or assume that you are new to the medical unit of a small community hospital. You notice that hospital procedure requires the application of ice to the injection sites of patients who are receiving heparin, for 15 minutes before the injection and 15 minutes after the injection. You are told by coworkers that the ice is used to decrease bruising from the heparin. You recently worked in a hospital in the nearest large city, and ice was also applied to the heparin site there. You wonder if the ice really does what it is supposed to do.

Or perhaps you work in the labor and delivery units of an urban hospital. You notice that the fathers who go through Lamaze training classes are participating in the labor and delivery process. Men who do not go through the training are excluded from the delivery room. You wonder if the two groups of fathers differ in their

TABLE 8–1   *A Comparison of Two Schema of Levels of Inquiry*

Level of Inquiry	Brink and Wood (1983)	Diers (1979)
1	What is . . . ?	What is this?
2	What is the relationship between . . . and . . . ?	What's happening here?
3	Why does . . . affect . . . ?	What will happen if . . . ?
4		How can I make . . . happen?

feelings about their partner's birth experience or their new baby.

Or imagine that you read in a nursing journal that young male schizophrenics who have female counselors are more likely to keep follow-up appointments and call for help than those who have male counselors. You wonder if this is an accurate picture of the mental health clinic in which you work.

These situations are examples of research problems in the early phase of development. The seed of an idea appears, and you must cultivate and nurture it until it becomes a full-grown research project. Research problems can come from your experiences, observations, and reading of articles, books, or study reports. Nursing theory or theories from other disciplines, if they are relevant to nursing practice, are excellent sources of research problems. See Chapter 9.

Determining Your Level of Inquiry

Once you recognize the seed of a worthwhile idea, you are faced with the task of refining the idea into a researchable question and designing the procedures for answering it. Different nurse experts present different levels of research questions. Table 8–1 compares a schema by Pamela Brink and Marilyn Wood to one by Donna Diers.

Level 1 Inquiry   Level 1 questions are used when little knowledge is available about a topic. (You can determine this through your literature review.) Level 1 questions begin with "What" (see Box 8–1). These questions are used in **exploratory** and **descriptive studies** whose goal is to describe an unknown phenomenon, for example, patients' responses to organ transplants. Qualitative studies are examples of level 1 studies. Diers (1979) also calls these studies factor-isolating research.

Nurses often become concerned when they find little in the literature review of direct relevance to their research question. The references are often only indi-

---

Box 8–1   Level 1 Research Questions

Stem	Topic
1. What . . .	are the experiences of fathers who are in the delivery room with their wives?
2. What . . .	are nurses' attitudes toward obese patients?
3. What . . .	do insulin-dependent diabetic patients want to know about their disease?

rectly related to their specific interest. Nursing is a new and evolving science, and nurses have been actively engaged in research for a mere 20 to 30 years. For this reason, a dearth of information is not uncommon.

Writing a level 1 question is the perfect solution to the problem of minimal information. If very little information exists, you can design a study to explore and describe your subject, and your findings can be the basis for subsequent higher-level studies. In this way scientists build knowledge and develop theory. Each level of inquiry contributes to the maturation of the science.

After you formulate your specific research question, Brink and Wood (1988) suggest, you should check it to be sure that it has (1) one variable or topic and (2) a reference to the population in which the variable or topic will be found (p. 13). The variables and populations in the three questions in Box 8–1 are summarized in Table 8–2.

Level 2 Inquiry   Level 2 questions are used to look for the *relationship between variables*, and they begin with "What is the relationship?" or, "What is happening here?" Qualitative studies and quantitative studies that are exploratory and descriptive are examples of level 2 inquiry. In these studies, which Diers (1979) calls factor-relating studies, investigators look for relationships between things that have already been named and described.

Your literature review helps you determine if the research question should be a level 2 question. If the variables you are interested in are discussed in the literature, you must then think of a theoretical rationale for the relationship implied in the question. If you ask, "What is the relationship between the public's political beliefs (liberalism versus conservatism) and their image of nurses?" your literature review should support the idea that the variable *public's political beliefs* is related to the variable *public's image of nurses*. The literature will not specify the precise nature of the relationship between the variables, but it will give you enough information to make a conceptual leap in assuming that the relationship might logically exist.

TABLE 8–2   *Variables and Populations for Three Level 1 Research Questions*

Question	Variable	Population
Question 1:	Experiences	Fathers in the delivery rooms
Question 2:	Attitudes	Nurses
Question 3:	Desire for Knowledge	Insulin-dependent diabetic patients

---

Box 8–2   Level 2 Research Questions

Stem	Topic
1. What is the relationship . . .	of patient education to patient compliance in a cardiac rehabilitation program?
2. What is the relationship . . .	of continuing in-service education in their specialty to the turnover rate of cardiac care unit (CCU) nurses?

For example, the literature may report that people who have conservative political views tend to prefer that women remain in traditional roles. Those with liberal political views are better able to see women in a variety of roles. A researcher can assume, then, that conservative people may view nurses (97% women) in the traditional role of dependent handmaiden to the physician. In contrast, those with liberal views may more readily see the nurse as being more autonomous, creative, and professional. Other examples of level 2 research questions are summarized in Box 8–2.

Level 2 questions make reference to two variables. (Remember, level 1 questions have only one variable and identify the population in which the variable is of interest.) A **variable** is any factor that varies, so be sure that any variables you choose to examine do, in fact, vary and vary in the population of interest. In the variables listed in Table 8–3—patient education, patient compliance, in-service education, and turnover rate—every factor can vary. There may be a patient education program or the absence of such a program—thus, the variability. Patients may or may not comply, or they may comply in part. There may be continuing specific in-service education, no education, or just general education. The turnover rate can be stated as a percentage of nurses leaving over a certain period of time.

If you asked, "What is the relationship of the discussion method of in-service education to the nurse turnover rate?" you would soon recognize that the factor of "discussion method of in-service education" does not vary as stated. Consequently, you would need to change the "variable" to the more general category of "method of in-service education," which would allow you to examine the discussion method versus the lecture method versus videotape, demonstrating the variability of methods.

Level 3 Inquiry   Level 3 inquiry, also called situation-relating research by Diers (1979), assumes a relationship, either causal or influential, between two variables and asks "Why?" or "What will happen if?" These studies test causal hypotheses. Your literature review will reveal theory (or other findings) that predict the nature

---

TABLE 8–3   *Variables and Populations for Two Level 2 Questions*

Question	Variables	Population
Question 1:	(a) Patient education (b) Patient compliance	Cardiac rehab patients
Question 2:	(a) In-service education (b) Turnover rate	CCU nurses

---

of the relationship. For example: "Why does a behavior modification program decrease the acting out of adolescent patients on a psychiatric unit?" Learning theory (classical conditioning) is used to predict how rewards (for not "acting out," for "good" behavior) elicit the desired response of "good" behavior (Wilson and Kneisl 1988 pp. 81–82). Two other examples of level 3 questions appear in Box 8–3. You can see how the questions in Box 8–3 imply cause and effect—that self-care behaviors do have an effect in patients with chronic illness and that attending AA meetings affects the drinking behaviors of alcoholics.

Box 8–3   Level 3 Research Questions

Stem	Topic
1. Why. . .	do self-care behaviors increase the feelings of well-being in patients with chronic illness?
2. Why. . .	does attending Alcoholics Anonymous meetings decrease the drinking behavior of alcoholics?
3. What will happen if . . .	self-care behaviors are taught to patients with chronic illness?
4. What will happen if . . .	alcoholics attend Alcoholics Anonymous meetings?

Level 3 studies lend themselves to replication under different conditions. Nursing studies suffer from a lack of replication, which is necessary to support research findings. Master's theses are ideal for replication research. Researchers duplicate the sampling strategy and experimental procedures, or they may, based on a critical analysis of the first study, alter these slightly. Then the data are interpreted and linked to the first study. In this way, knowledge is built.

Level 4 Inquiry Diers (1979) views her fourth level of inquiry (How can I make . . . happen?) as an extension of the other levels and as a goal for the future, when we have enough knowledge to prescribe a treatment or behavior to bring about a certain situation. The idea here is to use theory to improve practice, to change the way we give patient care.

Determining the Correct Level Depending on your literature review, questions may be written at different levels. For example, you may initially write a level 2 question: "What is the relationship of patient education to patient compliance in a cardiac rehabilitation program?" As you search the literature, you find theory to support the notion that a patient education model using lecture and discussion is more effective in changing behavior than one using videotapes. Therefore, the original question could be rewritten as a level 3 question: "Why does a lecture and discussion form of education increase patient compliance in a cardiac rehabilitation program?" *If there is theory to predict the nature of the relationship between the variables, then use a level 3 or level 4 question.*

One mark of a good research study is that the research question is written at the appropriate level. As you refine your research question, be sure you meet the criteria for the level at which you are writing it. Aim for clarity and conciseness.

Some complex studies may lend themselves to both hypotheses-testing research (level 3) and research about relationships (level 2). That is, theory may predict the nature of a relationship between two variables but perhaps ony suggests a relationship between two other variables. In this case, both hypotheses and research questions are appropriate.

Review of the Literature

After you have written your question, the next step is to return to the literature and conduct a systematic search to find out more precisely what is known about your topic. As we have seen, the level of your question may change after you do an extensive review of the literature. One nurse wrote a level 1 exploratory question, "What are the experiences of young women with cancer?" His literature review revealed hundreds of articles dealing with psychological and physiological effects of cancer, but none of them focused on young women. The nurse could have written a level 2 question and examined any number of variables to test for a relationship, and he could have found a theory (perhaps crisis theory) and tested the relationship of selected variables. But because his interest was in *young* women, he elected to formulate a level 1 question. This example demonstrates that questions can often be written at different levels of inquiry, but as you refine what you specifically want to know about your topic, the question level will become apparent.

Steps in Conducting a Literature Review

Find the Sources   A literature review helps support and clarify why you are doing your particular study. As you read, you will make decisions about your problem, purpose, relevant variables, design, sample, and instrument(s) to use for measurement.

You may begin your literature review by examining relevant specialty journals (such as the *Journal of Critical Care Nursing*, *Oncology Nursing*, or *Neonatal Network*), the *Cumulative Index to Nursing and Allied Health Literature* (CINAHL), other indexes (such as *Nursing Abstracts* or abstracts from other disciplines), *Dissertation Abstracts International* or *Masters Theses Index*. Alternatively, you may do a computerized search. Often, skimming through the last five years of nursing research journals, the specialty journals, and CINAHL will give you a notion of what research has been done in your area of interest. If you find one or two good articles, the reference lists at the end are often very useful in suggesting other sources.

If you do a computerized search, first, select a few key words from your question, and discuss with a reference librarian the appropriate terms to put into the computer. Librarians can suggest which data bases are the most useful for your research problem. The review should include all variables (key terms) relevant to your study. For example, if you are interested in the question "Why do self-care behaviors increase the feelings of well-being in patients with chronic illness?" you might look up Orem's theory of self-care (1980), articles on self-care behaviors in patients with chronic illness, and articles on patients' feelings of well-being. Reference librarians are helpful in selecting key words that elicit relevant printouts of references.

You may find few directly relevant research articles. However, don't be too easily discouraged. Do an exhaustive search, using the suggested multiple sources, that covers at least the last five years. This way, you will really find out how much is known about your topic. The aim of the search is to place your question in the context of existing knowledge.

Take Notes   Take notes on the major points of the article, such as the journal name, the authors' names, the research question or hypothesis, the method, and the findings (see Figure 8–1). These notes help you keep a record of what research has been done in your area. You will use them to write the literature review. Note significant points, such as an especially small sample size, an interesting instrument, or the use of a unique theoretical framework.

As you read, take notes on cards. Five-by-eight cards are particularly useful, because they can hold a good deal of information. Although note taking may seem like a lot of work at the time, it is very necessary and will prevent you from the fate of one nurse, who did a review of the literature, reading approximately 100 articles. Because she felt none were particularly relevant to her study of fathers' perceptions of their pregnant wives, she took no notes. At the end of weeks of work she had nothing recorded. After reexamining the research purpose and re-thinking the level of the study, she recognized that her readings were indirectly related to the topic and thus supported the need for a level 1 exploratory study. Consequently, she had to start all over again.

Even if an article is only peripherally related to your study, jot it down. Especially when little is known about your topic, you may be doing a level 1 study, and you ought to review studies that are indirectly related to clarify the gap your study is designed to fill.

On your note cards write the bibliography and a few major headings (see Figure 8–1).

Authors: Mishel, Merle & Murdaugh, Carolyn

Title: Family Adjustment to Heart Transplantation: Redesigning the Dream

Source: Nursing Research, 1987, 36:332–338

Research Question or Hypothesis:
What are the processes used by the family members to manage the unpredictability elicited by the need for and receipt of heart transplantation?

Method: Field study (grounded theory): Twenty family members were sampled. They attended support groups conducted by the investigators. The groups focused on any topic of concern to the family members and met for 12 weeks for 1 1/2 hours. The aim was to generate substantive theory.

Findings: The integrative theme, Redesigning the Dream, described how family members gradually modify their beliefs about organ transplantation and develop attitudes and beliefs to meet the challenge of living with continual unpredictability. Three concepts central to the theory are immersion, passage, and negotiation; these parallel the stages of waiting for a donor, hospitalization, and recovery.

Figure 8–1   Sample research note card   Source: Mishel, M and Murdaugh, C. "Family Adjustment to Heart Transplantation: Redesigning the Dream" *Nursing Research* 1987, 36:332–338. Reprinted with permission. Copyright 1987 by American Journal of Nursing Company.

Scope of a Literature Review

Your review should include six major types of literature:

1. Relevant nursing research.

2. Theoretical literature. This part of the literature review is addressed in Chapter 9.

3. General and specialty nursing literature. If research studies are minimal, and you see yourself heading for a level 1 study, search the general nursing literature—*American Journal of Nursing, Heart and Lung, Maternal Child Nursing,* and the like—and other specialty journals not expressly dedicated to research. Reading these journals will give you a notion of how closely your colleagues have approached your topic. In the study on the experiences of young women with cancer, the researcher found no scientific articles relating to experiences but several anecdotal articles in the general nursing literature describing a nurse's experience as a patient with breast cancer.

When you do level 2 and 3 studies, general nursing literature may be interesting, but you need to find research that can support (level 2) or predict (level 3) the relationship between two variables.

4. Methodological literature. If you notice that all the studies on your subject use a certain method of analysis, you may want to say something about the method. For example: "All previous studies of patients' psychological responses to myocardial infarctions (MIs) have used specific psychological instruments to determine degrees of anxiety." You may want to read something on instruments dealing with anxiety to give you new ideas or sources for criticisms of the instruments. If all the studies deal with psychological instruments, perhaps you want to build a case for using an instrument that measures social or cultural responses. Or maybe you don't want to use an instrument at all but instead to explore (level 1) the patients' experiences with a myocardial infarction with in-depth semistructured interviews.

5. Research literature from other disciplines. Most nursing research can benefit from research done in related disciplines—sociology, psychology, anthropology, political science, physiology, or economics, depending on the nature of your question. Do not limit yourself to nursing research, because multidisciplinary literature can offer useful information about theory and methods. Nursing can be viewed as an applied science, so literature in social and natural science may be relevant. Society's pressing problems today are both political and economic, so literature from these disciplines may offer a broad yet relevant perspective on certain nursing research questions. If you are unsure of yourself in these areas, find an expert—an economist, an anthropologist, a psychologist, a physiologist—and ask for help (see the heading "Using Other Resources," later in this section).

6. Popular literature. Popular literature includes books like *First You Cry*, *Anatomy of an Illness*, *In the Company of Others*, and *Heartsounds*. These are written by patients or family members and in journalistic fashion describe a hospitalization or illness through the eyes of the involved participants or subjects. Often newspaper (professional and popular) and magazine articles deal with health issues. Such reports are not appropriate for a level 2 or 3 study but may be helpful for a level 1 study. The American Medical Association newsletter and the Associated Press reported on a California case in which two physicians were tried for murder for discontinuing a patient's life-support systems. Articles such as these would be relevant for a level 1 study focused on the experiences of intensive care unit nurses caring for nonviable patients. These studies add context and history and emphasize the rich descriptive nature of the problems. They also help in identifying particularly relevant variables, such as the legal aspects, ethical aspects, and physicians' perceptions versus nurses' perceptions of discontinuing life support, for example. The value of reviewing popular literature is not supported by the nurse researchers who conduct level 2 and 3 studies, but a new trend among selected researchers in several disciplines is to view such literature as a useful source of information.

As you prepare your literature review, you will read many articles that you won't mention in the written literature review. In your reference section, list only those articles that you use for the written review.

How to Review

As you review the six types of relevant literature, do not merely read for content but analyze and compare.

A literature review requires not just the reading of large amounts of information but also a criticism of each piece. Critique the research articles for their credibility and soundness (see Chapter 6). If the sample size is five, yet the researchers make generalizations to a larger population, be skeptical of the study. You may want to critique the research articles on separate index cards, recording any problems. When you compose the literature review, mention the serious flaws that may affect your rationale for doing your particular study. For example, if a researcher used five subjects to understand the problems of feeding children with cerebral palsy, you might want to replicate the study using a larger sample. Or if a researcher used an inappropriate method of data analysis or did not sample the appropriate population, a replication study might be in order.

If the popular books written by patients focus mainly on changing body image after a mastectomy, note this narrow thematic focus in your literature review. If an instrument for measuring ethical judgment is used to measure nursing students' levels of decision making but has been used before only with male prisoners, mention this fact.

As with most steps of the research process, no rigid rules exist for all studies. At each stage, the researcher makes many decisions, presumably based on logical consideration of the factors discussed above. As you critically analyze the books and articles, you will be making decisions about what information is vital and relevant to include in your literature review.

Comparative reading relates all of the studies and reports to one another and to your research question. As your sources increase, you may want to categorize your reference cards based on a scheme that makes sense to you and fits your study question or decision. Perhaps you need to categorize research literature according to which studies had experimental designs and which were observational. Popular literature could be categorized according to biographical and autobiographical reports. Use any scheme that helps you compare your references to obtain an overview.

Why Review?

You may wonder why reviewing other literature is important. Why can't you just formulate your question, conduct your study, and report the findings? Remember that the purpose of science is to build theory and that research is the tool of science. Although many studies do not directly contribute to theory—for reasons that will become clear in the next chapter—they need to have contextual links. That is, a study in isolation cannot be clearly evaluated for significance and meaning, whereas a study that links up with previous research or theory provides a sense of context and a sense of history. We can analyze and understand the extent of existing knowledge and can determine where we should go in the future. The relevant books and articles that you read are the references that form the foundation and rationale for your own research.

Rationale for Your Research

Your observations and experiences often give rise to an initial research question. This question is a general idea that sends you to the literature and other sources. If you derived your question from experience or observations and not exclusively from a literature review, you need to describe the experience to the reader as an integral part of the background literature review. This personal account is usually placed at the beginning or end of the review in a research proposal or report. It can be placed anywhere in the literature review, however, as long as it is integrated in a logical fashion. For example, in her study, May (1982) writes:

> In spite of increased interest in expectant fatherhood and father involvement, we know very little about men's experiences of pregnancy prior to the last trimester or how they come to be with their partners in birth classes or the delivery room.

Use such an account to lead into the literature review, or use it at the end of the literature review to add a human, experiential element to the existing scientific reports.

Using Other Resources

As you begin the phase of starting your research, take advantage of all the resources available, not just the literature. Sometimes this means tracking them down and waiting long periods. If you are doing physiological research and you don't know a physiologist, find one or two or three. Talk with them, share your problems and dilemmas, and ask for suggestions. Ask them for the names of people who might be interested or helpful.

"Networking" in person, by phone, or by mail has many positive payoffs. Don't be intimidated by an author of a research article or by a national leader who does research in your specialty. Rather, view these people as resources, and use them as consultants or as sources of information. Most people who do research are excited about their work and enjoy sharing their expertise with others. Talking with one key person can sometimes be more useful than reading 50 articles, so in the interest of efficiency view people as vital resources in addition to the literature.

Networking occasionally results in several people doing collaborative research. The investigators may represent different disciplines or may be nurses sharing a similar interest. Being part of a joint effort can be exhilarating and can produce a study with more breadth and depth than a project by a single researcher. Collaborative research, sometimes called programmatic research, also enables investigators to pool such resources as statistical, computer, and editorial assistance.

A New Way of Seeing

Coming up with a research question and doing a literature review are challenging tasks that require much thinking and many rewrites. The process is not always totally efficient. You may read a lot of articles that ultimately are not relevant; you may have several ideas that appeal to you but are not feasible, researchable, or significant; and your final question may evolve to be far different from the original one.

Nurses are often task-oriented, and because of this tendency they may need to learn a new way of seeing and thinking to do research. Recognizing this need from the start should make the task somewhat easier. Try to avoid viewing the research enterprise as linear (step by step) and always efficient. Instead, think of getting started as a time for intellectual exploration; a time for musing and changing your mind; a time for checking things out before making a decision and a commitment. All of these considerations take time, but the early phase will solidify a definitive research question that is:

- substantiated by literature and rationale

- feasible (the possibility or practicality of conducting the study)

- significant

- researchable (the problem is a *research* problem and does not invite a yes or no answer, values, or opinions)

Statement of the Problem

The statement of the problem reflects a synthesis of the broad, often abstract issues that underlie the more specific research purpose. The problem introduces the study by providing a context and a rationale. Sometimes the statement of the problem is identified as such (typically in theses and dissertations); at other times (typically in journals), the problem is under the heading "Literature Review."

Statement of Purpose

The statement of purpose answers the question "Why do the study?" Researchers hold different views about stating a purpose for the research. Some believe that a question or hypothesis is sufficient and that including a statement of purpose is redundant. Others believe that both a statement of purpose and a research question or hypothesis are necessary. Brink and Wood (1988) suggest that the purpose be written as a *statement* for a level 1 study, as a *question* for a level 2 study, and as a *hypothesis* (or hypotheses) for a level 3 study. Box 8–4 illustrates this approach.

Planning your research begins with formulating a research question, moves through a review of the related literature and your rationale (often synthesized in a problem statement), and culminates with a concise statement of purpose.

Writing Hypotheses

A **hypothesis** (used with level 3 and 4 questions) is the statement of a predicted relationship between two or more variables (see Glossary). In the level 3 example in Box 8–4, the variables are teaching versus nonteaching and feelings of well-being. The hypothesis suggests that there is a relationship between teaching self-care techniques and patients' feelings of well-being. The hypothesis predicts that

---

Box 8–4   Levels of Inquiry and Their Statements of Purpose

Level 1   In a study that asks the question "What are the eating habits of bulimics?" the purpose can be expressed in the statement: *The purpose of this research is to explore and describe the eating habits of bulimics.*

Level 2   In a study that asks the question "What is the relationship between smoking and prematurity in primiparous mothers?" the purpose is written as: *The purpose of the study is to answer the question "Is there a significant relationship between smoking and prematurity in primiparous mothers?"*

Level 3   In a study that asks the question "Why does the teaching of self-care strategies increase the feeling of well-being in chronically ill patients?" the purpose is written as: *The purpose of this study is to test this hypothesis: Chronically ill patients who are taught self-care techniques will have higher scores on feelings of well-being than those who do not receive the teaching.*

---

those receiving the teaching will have higher scores on a measure of feelings of well-being.

Criteria for a Hypothesis

As you write your hypothesis, think about the following criteria, suggested by Polit and Hungler (1987), that are required if a statement is to be considered a hypothesis:

Testable: To be testable, a hypothesis must predict a relationship between variables, an independent variable and one or more dependent variables. Consider this hypothesis: "Nursing schools with flexible curricula will retain and graduate more students." Here, there is only one dependent variable (retention and graduation of students) and no independent variable, making the hypothesis untestable because there is nothing to compare. Rewritten as "Nursing schools with flexible curricula will retain and graduate more students than nursing schools without flexible curricula," the hypothesis is testable. You can measure the retention and graduation rates of schools with both curricula—flexible and inflexible (the type of curriculum is the independent variable)—and compare them.

A hypothesis can be tested only if the variables can be observed or measured. Operational definitions make the variables observable or measurable. For example, you may wonder what a "flexible curriculum" is. A flexible curriculum can be operationally defined as a curriculum that allows the students to (1) take a test to demonstrate knowledge of lower-level courses, (2) challenge upper-level courses, and (3) meet at a variety of times and places for classes. An inflexible curriculum refers to programs that do not meet these three criteria. Because of this clear definition, the variables *flexible curriculum* and *inflexible curriculum* can be measured.

Justifiable: A hypothesis must be justifiable, meaning that you have derived your hypothesis from theory. For example, if you read that behavior modification is more effective in encouraging obese people to lose weight than lectures on nutrition and dieting are, you can write a hypothesis to that effect. For example, obese people who participate in behavior modification training lose more weight than obese people attending lectures on nutrition and dieting. This hypothesis clearly is derived from behavioral theory.

However, suppose you have an idea that meditation might help people lose weight, and you propose to investigate the relationship between meditation and weight loss in two groups (one that attends meditation classes and one that does not). Your hypothesis does not meet the criterion of being justifiable, because it was not deduced from a theoretical framework. Rather, the idea was merely a personal hunch. It is a good practice to list all possible hypotheses and to follow your hunches to the hypothesis stage, but they must always have some theoretical support. If they do not, a research question is more appropriate.

Components of a Hypothesis

Hypotheses must be written clearly and concisely. Each word should add meaning to the hypotheses and have a purpose. Brink and Wood (1988) identify the three essential components of a well-written hypothesis: (1) the experimental group; (2) the expected result, and (3) the comparison group (p. 78). Table 8–4 shows the different parts of hypotheses in studies published in *Nursing Research*.

Types of Hypothesis

Hypotheses can be:

- simple
- complex
- directional
- nondirectional
- research hypotheses
- statistical hypotheses

A *simple* hypothesis predicts the relationship between one independent variable (IV) and one dependent variable (DV), whereas a *complex* hypothesis predicts the rela-

TABLE 8–4 *Required Parts of Hypotheses**

Hypothesis	Experimental Group	Expected Result	Comparison Group
1. Use of operating room (OR) restrictive shoes or shoe covers results in less bacterial transfer to clean areas than use of unprotected street shoes. (Copp, Slezak, Dudley, and Mailhot 1987)	Operating room nurses and orderlies who wore OR restricted shoes or shoe covers.	Will result in less bacterial transfer to clean areas.	OR staff who wear unprotected street shoes.
2. Women who experience cesarean birth will differ from those who deliver vaginally in the frequency over time a particular part of the body is used to initially handle their infants (Tulman 1986).	Women who experience cesarean birth.	Will differ in the frequency over time a particular part of the body is initially used to handle the infants.	Women who experience vaginal birth.
3. The incidence and degree of severity of subject discomfort will be less following administration of the 2-track intramuscular injection technique than following administration of the standard intramuscular injection technique (Keen 1986).	Subjects who are administered injections by the 2-track technique.	Will have less discomfort.	Subjects who are administered injections by the standard technique.

*According to the usual criteria for experimental groups, the subjects in examples 2 and 4 are not truly an "experimental" group because they were not randomly assigned to treatment. Rather, they already have had a cesarean birth or tachypnea. However, for purposes of explaining the required parts of a hypothesis, they can be considered the experimental group.

TABLE 8—4   *Required Parts of Hypotheses* (continued)*

Hypothesis	Experimental Group	Expected Result	Comparison Group
4. Tachypneic subjects will show a greater rectal/oral temperature difference than those who breathe normally (Durham, Swanson, and Paulford 1986).	Subjects with tachypnea.	Will show a greater rectal/oral temperature difference.	Subjects who breathe normally.

tionship between two (or more) independent variables and two (or more) dependent variables. Note the examples in Table 8–5.

As you might guess, a simple hypothesis is easier to test, measure, and analyze than a complex hypothesis. Because nursing research deals with human beings, who are complex, however, many hypotheses in nursing research are complex. The most important considerations for you as a researcher to think about are: (1) What type of hypothesis is best for your study? and (2) Is the study you are planning feasible? That is, if a complex hypothesis is appropriate for your study but you cannot collect the data to test it, then by all means write a simple hypothesis.

A **directional hypothesis** specifies the direction of the relationship between variables, whereas a *nondirectional* hypothesis only predicts that there is a relationship. Note the difference:

- *Directional Hypothesis*: Patients who receive reconditioning have less bladder dysfunction after indwelling catheter removal than patients who receive no conditioning (Williamson 1982).

- *Nondirectional Hypothesis*: There is a difference in bladder dysfunction after indwelling catheter removal in patients who receive reconditioning and patients who receive no conditioning.

Because theory always suggests the direction of the relationship, hypotheses should be directional. But you will read many examples of nondirectional hypotheses. Such hypotheses were not derived from theory but generally from hunches or a literature review. In such situations, a research question should be written.

As with much of research, there is controversy over the use of directional and nondirectional hypotheses. Some researchers believe that if you can't write a di-

TABLE 8–5 *Simple and Complex Hypotheses and Their Variables*

	Independent Variables	**Dependent Variables**
Simple Hypotheses		
1. Scrubsuits worn outside the OR without protection from covergowns show an increased level of bacterial contamination compared with scrubsuits worn solely inside the operating suite (Copp et al 1986).	Where scrubsuits are worn	Level of bacterial contamination
2. Husband's condition has a direct negative effect on anxiety (Bramwell and Whall 1986).	Husband's condition	Anxiety
Complex Hypotheses		
1. Mother's anxiety and perception are related to changes in infant satiety, anxiety, and feeding behavior (Blank 1986).	Infant satiety, anxiety, feeding behavior	Mother's anxiety and perception
2. Newborns fed either formula or sterile water at 1, 2, and 3 hours of life (HOL) produce stool earlier, have lower serum levels of indirect bilirubin at 48 HOL, have less observed jaundice at 48 HOL, and have a lower percentage of weight loss at 48 HOL than infants initially fed sterile water at 4 HOL and formula at 8 HOL.	Time and type of feeding	Time of first stool, serum level of indirect bilirubin, presence or absence of observed jaundice, percentage of weight loss

Source: Boyer, D. and Vidyasagar, D. "Serum Indirect Bilirubin Levels and Meconium Passage in Early Fed Normal Newborns," *Nursing Research* 1987, 36:174–78. Reprinted with permission. Copyright 1987 by American Journal of Nursing Company.

rectional hypothesis, then you should not design your study to test hypotheses but should instead ask a level 1 or 2 question—"What is . . ." or "What is the relationship between . . ." Other authorities believe that you can use directional or nondirectional hypotheses depending on your level of knowledge about a topic. They suggest that if there is not enough knowledge to predict the relationship, you should use a nondirectional hypothesis. For your research, I suggest writing directional hypotheses, because they are clearer and more logical and because hypotheses should be derived from theory that is sufficiently evolved to deduce them.

A *research hypothesis* states the anticipated relationship between variables; all the examples to this point have been research hypotheses. A *null*, or *statistical*, *hypothesis* is written in the form that predicts no relationship between the independent and dependent variables: "There is no relationship between modes of intervention and weight loss in obese people" is an example of a null hypothesis. Principles of statistical inference require that all research hypotheses be tested in the null form. For clarity in research studies, however, hypotheses should be stated in the research form, which clearly indicates the thinking of the investigator.

Defining Variables

Now that you have completed the literature review and defined your research purpose as a statement, question, or hypothesis, you are ready to define your study's variables operationally so that you can move on to collecting data. In level 1, or factor-searching, studies, the variables are unknown and thus are not defined. In the other three levels of studies, it is impossible to collect data until you have made your variables clear and until you have decided how to study them.

A variable is, as the name suggests, any factor that varies. See Table 8–6 for examples of hypotheses and their variables. For example, age, weight, height, temperature, PCO^2 values, stress, political beliefs, and attitudes are all variables, because all vary to some degree. Sex varies from male to female and is an example of a **dichotomous variable**, that is, a variable with only two categories. **Polychotomous variables**, such as race, have more than two categories, for example, Caucasian, Asian, and Hispanic. Dichotomous and polychotomous variables are examples of **categorical variables** that represent unordered categories, groups, or classes. Age, weight, height, and PCO^2 have a range of variability and are examples of **continuous variables** (see Glossary). It is important to know the types of variable you are working with because this determines the types of data analysis technique you will use.

Nurse researchers are interested in studying variables, particularly how they vary in relation to one another. For example, how does alcoholism vary with different types of treatment methods? How does surgical patients' anxiety vary with different types of anesthesia? An independent variable can stand alone, whereas a *dependent variable* depends on another (see Chapter 4). In some studies, independent variables are thought to influence dependent variables in a cause-and-effect fashion; for example, exposure to the sun over time may cause skin cancer. Independent variables are those that the researcher manipulates. For example, you, through the sampling process, can study people with much sun exposure and people with little sun exposure, thus manipulating the independent variable. Or, the researcher can introduce a cardiac rehabilitation education program (independent variable) and study patients' understanding (dependent variable) of their illness.

If you are testing hypotheses (levels 3 and 4), you will have an independent and a dependent variable. Since level 1 studies are exploratory, the relevant variables are not all known at the outset. All variables are assumed to be independent until there is sufficient knowledge to predict the nature of the variables. In level 2 studies, in which the researcher asks if there is a significant relationship between variables—for example, "Is there a significant relationship between women's age and sleep patterns?"—there is the underlying assumption or hunch that women's age (independent variable) does affect sleep patterns (dependent variable). But until

TABLE 8–6   *Hypotheses and Their Variables*

Hypothesis	Variables	Type of Variation
1. Scrubsuits worn outside the OR without protection from covergowns show an increased level of bacterial contamination compared with scrubsuits worn solely inside the operating suite (Copp et al 1986).	Where the scrubsuit is worn Bacterial contamination	The scrubsuit is worn outside OR or inside OR. The bacterial contamination is of different levels.
2. Tachypneic subjects will show a greater rectal/oral temperature difference than those who breathe normally (Durham, Swanson, and Paulford 1986).	Rectal/oral temperature Type of breathing	Temperature is greater or lesser Breathing is normal or tachypneic.
3. The incidence and degree of severity of subject discomfort will be less following administration of the 2-track intramuscular injection technique than following administration of the standard intramuscular injection (Keen 1986).	Subject discomfort Intramuscular injection technique	Incidence and degree of severity of subject discomfort The intramuscular injection technique is 2-track or standard.
4. The further women have progressed through the menopause transition (menopausal stage), the more positive their perceived health status will be (Engel 1987).	Menopause transition (menopausal stage) Perceived health status	Premenopause, perimenopause, or postmenopause Scores on a perceived health status questionnaire

the research is completed, one cannot justifiably predict a cause-and-effect pattern.

Once your research statement, question, or hypothesis is written clearly, with the appropriate delineation of variables, you need to write *operational definitions* for them. You will have already defined your variables conceptually in your literature review. A conceptual definition, derived from existing theories or even a dictionary, defines the concept under study in abstract terms. Operationally defining your variables requires that you clearly specify them and say how you are measuring them. The operational definition is closely linked to the conceptual definition. For example, if a researcher plans to study the response of women to tubal ligations and she or he believes that the women's feelings about their femininity are relevant, the concept of femininity should be described in the literature review and operationally defined along with any other variables being used in the study. The researcher will need to acquire or generate a reliable and valid instrument that measures femininity.

If your variable is age, how will you collect data on the subjects' age? Ask them? Have them write it on a questionnaire? Here, for example, is an operational

---

Box 8-5   Operationalizing Variables: Examples from Nursing Research

Purpose/Question/Hypothesis	Operational Definition
Newborns fed either formula or sterile water at 1, 2, and 3 hours of life (HOL) produce stool earlier, have lower serum levels of indirect bilirubin at 48 HOL, have less observed jaundice at 48 HOL, and have a lower percentage of weight loss at 48 HOL than infants initially fed sterile water at 4 HOL and formula at 8 HOL.	Time of stool: documented as time of initial meconium passage. Serum indirect bilirubin level: drawn at 48 hours. Observed jaundice: at 48 HOL get consensus of the subjective evaluation of presence or absence of jaundice by three experienced neonatal nurses. Weight loss: Weight change at 48 HOL as a percentage of birth weight (to standardize loss when birth weights are variable).

Source: D. Boyer and D. Vidyasagar, "Serum Indirect Bilirubin Levels and Meconium Passage In Early Fed Normal Newborns," *Nursing Research*, 1987, vol. 36, pp. 174–178.

The purpose of this study was to identify predictors of both a predominantly physiological outcome of care (blood pressure control) and a psychosocial outcome of care (adjustment of chronic illness) in hypertensive patients.	Physiological outcome of care: This was evaluated by physician judgment of the control status of the patient at the time of interview. Psychosocial outcome of care: Adjustment to chronic illness was assessed by the Psychosocial Adjustment to Illness Scale (PAIS) (Derogatis 1977).

Source: Boyer, D. and Vidyasagar, D. "Serum Indirect Bilirubin Levels and Meconium Passage in Early Fed Normal Newborns," *Nursing Research* 1987, 36:174–78. Reprinted with permission. Copyright 1987 by American Journal of Nursing Company.

---

definition of age: "The age of the subject will be asked during the interview session and will be recorded in number of years and months." An operational definition of sleep pattern is: "Sleeping electroencephalograms will be recorded over one eight-hour period, and the pattern will be assessed according to the Bannon Sleep Pattern Instrument." In both examples, you can see clearly what variable is being studied and how it will be measured. The operational definition permits you to go from the abstract idea of variables to a concrete definition of how to measure the specific variables. (See Box 8–5 for examples from published nursing research.)

Variables can be concrete (sex, age, height) or more abstract (stress, depression, political beliefs, spiritual beliefs). Abstract variables can be measured with many different instruments (see Chapters 10, 11, and 12). Stress and depression can be measured psychologically or physiologically; depression can be studied by projective techniques, self-report, or observation. Political beliefs and spiritual beliefs can be assessed by in-depth interviews or questionnaires. Because of all the possibilities, too numerous to list here, you must carefully specify your own approach to measuring your study's variables.

A word of caution about measuring variables is necessary. Some people think that writing a few questions for a questionnaire is an acceptable but quick and easy way to measure variables. In most cases, investigator-developed instruments must be tested for reliability and validity before use. Previously used instruments need to be examined initially for reliability and validity. To ignore this important step invites justified criticism: "How do you know this instrument really measures what you say it does?" (validity) and "How consistently does this instrument measure this variable in repeated trials?" (reliability). Measuring variables is a complex process.

Choosing a Design

In Chapter 5 you learned that a design is a blueprint, or plan, for conducting your research, and you learned about the different types of design. The question that faces all researchers is "What is the best design for my study?" A good design follows logically from the study's purpose and level of inquiry. Suppose the purpose is to explore and define unstudied variables, such as experiences of ICU nurses caring for nonviable patients. If the purpose is to explore and define variables, the study can also be called a factor-naming study. Certain designs lend themselves to studies intended to search for factors and to explore and define a given problem. See Table 8–7 for Dier's conceptualization of the relationship of level of inquiry to study designs and answers.

Historical and Case Study Designs

A historical design, as you saw in Chapter 5, aims to synthesize facts, thereby extending knowledge. Analyzing the creation and consequences of "the central dilemma of American nursing—the order to care in a society that refuses to value caring"—is an example of a historical research purpose (Reverby 1987).

TABLE 8–7   *Questions, Study Designs, Answers*

Level of Inquiry	Kind of Question	Study Design	Kind of Answer (Theory)	Other Names for Study Design
1	What is this?	Factor-searching	Factor-isolating (naming)	Exploratory Formulative Descriptive Situational control
2	What's happening here?	Relation-searching	Factor-relating (situation-depicting, situation-describing)	Exploratory Descriptive
3	What will happen if . . . ?	Association-testing	Situation-relating (predictive)	Correlational Survey design Nonexperimental Natural
		Causal hypothesis-testing		Experimental Explanatory Predictive
4	How can I make . . . happen?	Prescription-testing	Situation-producing (prescriptive)	

Source: D. Diers, *Research in Nursing Practice*. Philadelphia: Lippincott, 1979, p. 54.

The descriptive case study design, using in-depth analysis, is an appropriate exploratory (level 1) approach to a new problem. A case study design would have been appropriate to study the "bubble boy" (who had the rare immunological disease called severe combined immunodeficiency), because he was the first child to spend his entire existence, except for his last 15 days, in sterile plastic chambers (Begley and Shapiro 1984). An exploration and description of his relationships with staff or family members would have made a significant contribution to knowledge. Case study designs are not used much in nursing, perhaps because they require much analytic rigor and much time. However, Meier and Pugh (1983) advocate the case study as a viable approach to clinical research.

Case study designs that use experimental (level 3) approaches (discussed in more detail in Chapter 5) are useful if you want to use an intervention with one patient and measure a selected dependent variable before, during, and after the intervention. Some nurse researchers are beginning to see the value of this type of case study design, especially in selected situations (Barnard 1983, Holm 1983).

Survey Designs

Survey designs can have the purpose of describing characteristics, opinions, attitudes, or behaviors as they currently exist in a population (Chapter 5). If you want to explore and describe (level 1 inquiry) the attitudes of nurses with associate degrees, bachelor's degrees, and master's degrees toward "no-codes," you can do a comparative survey. You are comparing samples from three groups (A.D., B.S.N., and M.S.N. nurses) in relation to specific variables (attitudes toward no-codes). If you study patients' opinions about being treated by nurse practitioners, you can use a descriptive survey design that will portray types of feelings or attitudes about the designated group (nurse practitioners).

A cross-sectional survey design can answer such questions as "What are the experiences of parents who have two children with a fatal disease (muscular dystrophy, cystic fibrosis) when each child dies?" Remember that in the cross-sectional survey design subjects are at different points of an experience but are measured one time. So, parents who have lost their first child are surveyed, as are parents who have lost their second. In a longitudinal survey, these same parents would be interviewed over time, and their experiences would be assessed at predetermined stages.

If the purpose of your research is to answer the question "What is the relationship between x variable and y variable?" (level 2 inquiry) you are doing a factor-relating, or association, study. A correlational survey design is appropriate if you want to discover the magnitude of variables and the direction of the relationship between them. For example, if you have theoretical reasons to believe that socioeconomic status may be related to how the public views nurses, you can do a survey to assess that relationship. Or if you wonder how the new, untested method of indirect calorimetry correlates with the accepted Harris Benedict Equation (these are two methods for measuring nutritional needs of patients with chronic obstructive pulmonary disease), you can investigate the magnitude of the relationship with a correlational survey design. If the new method has a high correlation with the traditional method, then perhaps either method could be used, depending on cost, the ease of using each, and other relevant factors.

When you do correlation research, you look for relationships between variables and try to find whether one or more variables can predict another. For this reason representativeness is very important (see the section "Sampling," in this chapter). If you wonder whether undergraduate grade-point average or score on the Graduate Record Examination can predict success in graduate school, you need a representative sample, or your study will show little about how these predict success.

Evaluation surveys are used to make judgments and to evaluate a program, policy, or method. Such surveys embody research questions that ask about the relationship between a program and another variable or variables—for example, "What is the relationship between parent education and child abuse?" An evaluation survey is one way of eliciting the desired information.

Any design that has the purpose of answering a question about the relationship between or among variables is used only after the area of interest has been explored and defined. Factor-relating studies (level 2) are conducted before there is enough information to design a level 3 hypothesis-testing study.

Experimental Designs

Level 3 or 4 or causal hypothesis-testing studies require a design that maximizes control of variance. Consequently, experimental designs are the best choice, because they demand random selection of the sample, random assignment to groups, and control and manipulation of the independent variable.

Use an experimental design if (1) your hypothesis is derived from the literature, (2) your variables are operationally defined, (3) you can randomly assign subjects to control and experimental groups and impose a treatment or intervention, and (4) you can control intervening variables.

The study "Patient Management of Pain Medication after Cardiac Surgery" (King et al 1987) is an example of an experimental design. The authors investigated the effects of self-administered versus nurse-administered pain medication (independent variable) after cardiac surgery. A volunteer sample of 64 adults who had coronary artery bypass or valve replacement surgery were randomly assigned to treatment groups. The experimental group self-administered their pain medication, and the control group received the traditional nurse-administered pain medication. Both groups were assessed for their desire for control, their perception of pain intensity, disruption in daily activities, emotional responses, and use of pain medication over time (dependent variables). Few significant differences were found between the groups.

Because random assignment and controlling variables in nursing research are so difficult, experimental designs are rare. You should sensitize yourself to your everyday nursing practice, however, and be alert for research questions that may lend themselves to experimental design. The 1987 study by Shelly et al that examines the aggressiveness of nursing care for older patients and those with do-not-resuscitate (DNR) orders is another good example of experimental research. In this study simulation measurement was used to manipulate the two independent variables, DNR orders and age (see also Shelley 1984).

Quasi-Experimental Designs

Quasi-experimental research is similar to experimental research in that different groups or subjects are exposed to different treatments, but the groups are preexisting. Differences between groups in identified dependent variables are measured. Quasi-experimental designs (level 3 or 4 inquiry) are useful if the researcher cannot randomly assign subjects to control and experimental groups. The varieties of quasi-experimental designs are described in Chapter 5. Boyer and Vidyasagar's 1987 study entitled "Serum Indirect Bilirubin Levels and Meconium Passage in Early Fed Normal Newborns" is an example of a quasi-experimental design. Thirty normal newborns were sequentially (not randomly, as in experimental research) assigned to the control group (given routine hospital feeding) and two experimental groups (a water-fed group and a formula-fed group). Time and type of feeding are independent variables. The groups were then measured on several dependent variables—time of initial meconium passage, serum indirect bilirubin levels at 48 hours of life (HOL), observed jaundice at 48 HOL, and percentage of weight change at 48 HOL. The authors found the following:

1. The time of initial meconium passage was significantly earlier in both groups of early fed infants than in the control group.

2. The mean time of passage was earlier in formula-fed infants.

3. Serum indirect bilirubin levels at 48 HOL did not differ significantly, but the mean for the formula-fed group was lower.

4. Nine infants in the control group were jaundiced, and six infants in each experimental group were jaundiced. This was statistically significant.

5. Although the finding is not statistically significant, all infants in the control group lost weight, and two water-fed and one formula-fed infant gained weight.

6. Infants in the early-fed groups had stools significantly earlier than infants in the control group; however, a significant relation between earlier meconium passage and lower serum bilirubin levels at 48 HOL was not demonstrated (Boyer and Vidyasagar 1987).

The authors recommend that the study be replicated with larger numbers of infants. In addition, randomizing the infants to groups, that is, making the study truly experimental, would increase generalizability.

Quasi-experimental designs are the next best thing to experimental designs. Think about experiences that patients face during diagnosis and treatment and imagine how you could design a quasi-experimental study that measures patients on some variables before and after a treatment or compared with another group undergoing a similar experience.

Preexperimental Designs

Although similar to experimental designs, preexperimental designs use a single group of subjects that experience a treatment manipulation over time. Thus, one group of subjects is assessed for change over time. Each subject acts as his or her own control on the independent variable, which is manipulated. The dependent variable is measured and reveals if the treatment is effective. In the study "Controlled Supplemental Oxygenation during Tracheobronchial Hygiene," Walsh et al (1987) examined the effect of controlled supplemental oxygenation without bag ventilation (independent variable) on transcutaneous partial pressure of oxygen measurements (dependent variable) during tracheobronchial hygiene. Each of 16 premature infants experienced two procedures—procedure A, no supplemental oxygenation; and procedure B, controlled supplemental oxygenation—in random order. Findings indicated that in most infants, controlled supplemental oxygenation without manual bag ventilation (1) prevented hypoxia during tracheobronchial hygiene and (2) shortened recovery time from hypoxemia resulting from the bronchopulmonary hygiene procedure (Walsh et al 1987).

Ex Post Facto Designs

Ex post facto designs are common in nursing research, because they study an event or experience after the fact. Many patients are perfect subjects because they have had to undergo a certain experience (brain surgery, bone marrow transplant, lumbar puncture) that warrants close scientific examination. Kosko and Flaskerud (1987) compared the health beliefs of Mexican Americans concerning the specific symptom of chest pain to the beliefs of two groups in the predominant culture—a nurse practitioners group and a lay group. The authors hypothesized that Mexican Americans would have different beliefs about the etiology and treatment of chest pain than the nurse practitioner and the lay group and that nurse practitioners would have different beliefs than the Mexican Americans or controls. They felt that understanding these different belief systems was important for nurse practitioners in giving culturally specific nursing care.

As you look around your work environment and notice patients who are different in any way or who have experienced something—a specific nursing intervention, a diagnostic procedure, a crisis of any type—think about how theory could be used to suggest a hypothesis for study.

When you cannot manipulate an independent variable and randomly assign subjects to control and experimental groups, an ex post facto study is appropriate and worthwhile. Just remember that because of the design you are not studying cause and effect but rather correlations among variables. Thus, your conclusions and interpretation need reflect this fact clearly.

Methodological Designs

Methodological designs are vital to nursing research. Such studies develop or validate research instruments that are specifically designed to answer nursing questions. In "A Social Support Measure: PRQ 85," (Weinert 1987) describes the history of the development and the psychometric evaluation of the Personal Resource Questionnaire, a tool to measure situational and perceived social support.

Methodological research requires long-term study and is often the source of a dissertation. The investigator then follows up testing and validating the instrument in the period after the dissertation. In fact, the development of a valid and reliable instrument to measure some aspect of nursing inquiry could be a life's work and would represent a valuable contribution to nursing theory and practice.

If you decide to develop an instrument, you include in the literature review the same types of literature you would in other studies but you focus on methodological literature—the "how to's" of instrument construction and measurement. Additional examples of methodological studies are given in Chapter 5.

You have now had a glimpse of the design possibilities that may be appropriate for your research purpose. Issues of reliability and validity are vital to any design, and Chapter 5 offers an in-depth discussion of study designs and concerns of reliability and validity. The related issue of bias in sampling is discussed in the next section. Your design is a good one if it allows you to pursue your research purpose with accuracy and with control of variables (internal and external validity).

Sampling

Assume that you have just been selected to be a taster for the nutrition department of your small community hospital. Your job is to taste 30 low-calorie desserts and rate them according to specific criteria. Eating the entire 30 desserts is unnecessary and probably impossible. Rather, you take a small bite, a sample, of each, which you assume to be representative of the entire dessert.

In your research you also will be sampling. Sampling is a vital part of the research process, and the strategies for choosing your sample will influence your results and your interpretation of them. Now that you have formulated your purpose and chosen a design, you need to decide who or what you will study. Your research purpose should lead you to *relevant* subjects. If you plan to study disgruntled patients or patients who are unhappy with their nursing care, be sure to select patients who are, in fact, disgruntled.

Sampling for level 1 studies is described in Chapter 13 because it is quite different from sampling in level 2, 3, and 4 studies. A *sample*, a subset of the population, is a group (of people, records, organizations) drawn from the *population*. The population is the total group that meets your criteria, and it is often referred to as the *universe* or the *target population*. If you plan to study quadriplegic patients with decubitus ulcers, all such patients are your target population. Because you cannot find and contact all of these people, you choose a sample of quadriplegics with decubitus ulcers. Your sample comes from the *accessible population*, the population that is feasible to study. Perhaps you have access to two large rehabilitation hospitals, to five general hospitals, or to a home health service, all of which care for quadriplegic patients with ulcers. Any patients you can use as subjects compose your accessible population.

All researchers use sampling, because it is a feasible and logical way of generalizing from a smaller group to a larger one. Investigators can make inferences from the sample to the population if the sample selection process is a systematic one. The method of selecting a sample is thus crucial to the research design. You

TABLE 8–8 *Types of Sampling*

Probability Sampling	**Nonprobability Sampling**
Simple Random Sampling	Accidental or Convenience Sampling
Systematic Sampling	Snowball Sampling
Stratified Random Sampling	Purposive or Judgment Sampling
Cluster Sampling	Expert Sampling
	Quota Sampling

must be concerned with how you can get the most *representative* sample possible. You wonder if a certain treatment method decreases the incidence of decubitus ulcers in quadriplegic patients, compared with another treatment method. To say with assurance that one method is better than the other, you must be sure that your sample represents the characteristics of the population.

The next obvious question is "How do you make your sample representative?" Probability and nonprobability sampling are the two major approaches to sampling (see Table 8–8). **Probability sampling** is the more rigorous. It requires that every element in the population have an equal chance, that is, a *random* chance, of being selected for inclusion in the sample. **Nonprobability sampling**, in contrast, provides no way of estimating the probability that each element will be included in the sample. With the nonprobability approach the results are representative of your sample only and cannot be generalized to the accessible population.

Types of Probability Sampling

Simple random sampling   The best-known probability sampling approach is simple **random sampling**. Each individual in the **sampling frame** (all subjects in the population) has an equal chance of being chosen. If you plan to study patients with acquired immune deficiency syndrome, for example, you will need a list of all of these patients who make up the population. To select the sample:

1. Assign a number to each member of the population, and go to a table of random numbers (see Table 8–9).

2. Close your eyes and with a pencil point to a number on the table.

3. Move in a systematic way—up, down, or diagonally—choosing your sample by picking those subjects whose numbers correspond to the table of random numbers.

4. Ignore numbers that do not appear on your frame (for example, 100 if your frame goes only to 99).

5. Once a number is selected and becomes part of the sample, ignore it if it appears again in the table of random numbers.

6. Stop when your sample size is obtained. (Sample size is discussed later in the chapter.)

Other methods of random selection may be used as long as they ensure that each subject has an equal chance of selection. Such methods include putting well-mixed names in a hat or shuffling name cards thoroughly and then selecting the required number from a deck. Some people confuse random sampling with random assignment to treatment groups (as is possible in a convenience sample). Random assignment to groups does not turn a nonprobability sample into a probability sample. Another caution about random sampling concerns the fact that if some people (e.g., 25%) in the proposed random sample refuse to participate or cannot be located, the sample then is not a random sample, but rather a *convenience sample* or a *volunteer sample*.

Systematic Sampling **Systematic sampling** involves drawing every n^{th} element from a population. If you wanted to do a survey of nurses who subscribe to the *American Journal of Nursing*, you could select a systematic sample of 1000. You start, as with the random sample, by closing your eyes and pointing to a number and then choosing every n^{th} number that follows. For example, if you start at number 11, you may decide to pick every tenth number (this interval is arbitrary). You then

---

TABLE 8–9 *Listing of Random Numbers*

09 18 82 00 97	32 82 53 95 27	04 22 08 63 04	83 38 98 73 74	64 27 85 80 44
90 04 58 54 97	51 98 15 06 54	94 93 88 19 97	91 87 07 61 50	68 47 66 46 59
73 18 95 02 07	47 67 72 62 69	62 29 06 44 64	27 12 46 70 18	41 36 18 27 60
75 76 87 64 90	20 97 18 17 49	90 42 91 22 72	95 37 50 58 71	93 82 34 31 78
54 01 64 40 56	66 28 13 10 03	00 68 22 73 98	20 71 45 32 95	07 70 61 78 13
08 35 86 99 10	78 54 24 27 85	13 66 15 88 73	04 61 89 75 53	31 22 30 84 20
28 30 60 32 64	81 33 31 05 91	40 51 00 78 93	32 60 46 04 75	94 11 90 18 40
53 84 08 62 33	81 59 41 36 28	51 21 59 02 90	28 46 66 87 95	77 76 22 07 91
91 75 75 37 41	61 61 36 22 69	50 26 39 02 12	55 78 17 65 14	83 48 34 70 55
89 41 59 26 94	00 39 75 83 91	12 60 71 76 46	48 94 97 23 06	94 54 13 74 08
77 51 30 38 20	86 83 42 99 01	68 41 48 27 74	51 90 81 39 80	72 89 35 55 07
19 50 23 71 74	69 97 92 02 88	55 21 02 97 73	74 28 77 52 51	65 34 46 74 15
21 81 85 93 13	93 27 88 17 57	05 68 67 31 56	07 08 28 50 46	31 85 33 84 52
51 47 46 64 99	68 10 72 36 21	94 04 99 13 45	42 83 60 91 91	08 00 74 54 49
99 55 96 83 31	62 53 52 41 70	69 77 71 28 30	74 81 97 81 42	43 86 07 28 34

pick number 21, 31, 41, 51, and so on until all subjects are obtained. Systematic sampling results in a representative sample if the sampling frame doesn't have any built-in bias. For example, bias would result if the journal's nurse subscribers were listed by state or year of beginning subscription. Instead of getting a sample representative of subscribers, you might be getting a sample that included only nurses in the Northeast or only nurses who had subscribed for 10 years or more. If you decide to do systematic sampling, be sure to study the list carefully for potential systematic bias.

Stratified Random Sampling   A *stratum* is a subpopulation, and *strata* are two or more homogeneous subpopulations. Examples of strata of interest to nursing include patients who have certain diseases, patients who live in specified areas, or patients who require certain treatments. Major political polls use **stratified random sampling**, assessing different strata of the population. To use this method:

1. Select a population and determine the relevant strata.

2. Sample a number of people in each stratum. The number in a sample should reflect the proportion of the group in the total population. For example, if your population is patients with collagen diseases and your strata are patients with lupus, (3% of the population), patients with arthritis (95% of the population), and patients with scleroderma (2% of the population), you will use the same proportions in your sample—3% lupus patients, 95% arthritis patients, and 2% scleroderma patients.

3. After you decide on the strata and proportions, choose the subjects within each of the categories according to random sampling methods. Remember, randomly does not mean haphazardly.

When you decide to do a stratified random sample, think carefully about your population and the concept of relevancy. If you know your population composition and its relation to a specific characteristic, *and* if the factors are relevant based on logic and the literature review, stratify your sample. If you do not know your population composition or if the factors are not relevant (for example, the hair color of new mothers who elect rooming in on obstetric units), then do not stratify your sample.

Cluster Sampling   **Cluster sampling** requires that the population be divided into groups, or clusters. If you are studying associate degree nursing students, you may not have the time, money, or ability to get all the individuals' names, but:

1. You have a list of the associate degree schools in the area.

2. You randomly derive your sample from this list of clusters (schools).

3. You sample all students in each chosen cluster, or you sample only randomly selected students from each cluster.

You are randomly sampling both schools and subjects. Depending on your research problem, you move in stages from the most complex to the most simple unit, which is why cluster sampling is also called *multistage sampling*.

Most large-scale surveys use cluster sampling, because simple or stratified random sampling involves too few subjects from too few places, resulting in much wasted time, money, and energy.

A Critique of Probability Sampling   Probability sampling is based on probability theory, which focuses on the possibility that events will occur by chance (Kerlinger 1973, Winer 1962). Probability sampling is less likely to result in a biased sample that is not representative of the population, because each element in the population must have an equal chance of being selected. The ability to obtain representative samples makes probability sampling superior to nonprobability sampling. Ensuring a representative sample avoids bias, making it possible to generalize research results to the accessible population.

Sampling error can be estimated with probability sampling. Sampling error refers to the differences between sample values and population values. Some amount of sampling error is inevitable in any research study, but probability sampling does allow estimates of the degree of expected error. (For more about this see Cohen 1977 and Chapter 14.)

Probability sampling with small populations (for example, patients with liver transplants) may be efficient and effective. If the group is homogeneous, however, then sophisticated sampling is not necessary. In nursing, because we deal with human beings and thus many variables, it is unlikely that our population is ever homogeneous. Most people are different psychologically, culturally, or socioeconomically, bringing homogeneity into question.

In life, it is said, death and taxes are the only certainties. In sampling, there is no certainty that a probability sample ensures everyone's participation. If a group is underrepresented or refuses to participate for whatever reasons, a biased sample may result.

Types of Nonprobability Sampling

Nonprobability sampling is nonrandom sampling of subjects. Therefore, there is less chance of obtaining a representative sample than with probability sampling. Most nursing research involves nonprobability sampling.

Accidental, or convenience, sampling   **Accidental**, or **convenience**, **sampling** allows the use of any available group of research subjects. For example, to study children in well-baby clinics, you might pick a public clinic because of its geographical proximity and ready access. These children are relevant subjects, and they are available. Because of a lack of randomization in sampling, however, they may not be typical of well babies but may be atypical in some unidentified ways. The investigator has no control over the sampling process—the sample, the sampling representativeness, or the possible biases.

Snowball sampling is a kind of accidental sampling. It involves subjects' suggesting other subjects to the researcher, so that the sampling process gains momentum, like a snowball rolling down a hill. A nurse was studying women prisoners with an in-depth interview technique. Because only certain women were willing to be involved, the researcher asked each prisoner after the interview to suggest one or two other prisoners who might be interested in participating. This was a convenient and effective way of soliciting subjects. Of course, sampling bias is likely to be present, because women who agree to participate may be different from those who don't.

Snowball sampling is used if subjects are difficult to identify because they are hidden in the population (transsexuals, faith healers, women who have had abortions), but they may be part of an informal network. Brink and Wood (1988) use the term **network sampling** and say it is useful in finding "socially devalued urban populations such as addicts, alcoholics, child abusers, and criminals," because these people are usually hidden from outsiders (p. 128).

Purposive, or Judgment, Sampling   In **purposive sampling**, the researcher selects a particular group or groups based on certain criteria. In this subjective sampling method, the researcher uses his or her judgment to decide who is representative of the population. Because objectivity is lacking, this method is not recommended except in certain circumstances. For example, if you wanted to test an instrument to measure stress in patients who have just been admitted to the hospital, you could use a purposive sample of patients from surgical units, CCU units, labor and delivery units, medical units, and outpatient units. A pretest with such heterogeneous groups might offer interesting information. Or if you wanted to validate an instrument measuring self-concept or locus of control, you might give it to normal adults, normal teenagers, depressed adults, and depressed teenagers. You would expect group differences to be evidenced in the test scores. If there were no group differences, you would question the validity of the instrument.

Expert sampling is a type of purposive sampling that involves choosing experts in a given area because of their access to the information of relevance to your study. The Delphi technique uses expert sampling. Several rounds of questionnaires focusing on a specific topic are sent to experts, with the aim of eliciting their opinions. After data analysis, the questions are reformulated and sent out again. The aim is for fairly rapid group consensus. For example, a study at the Univerity of Florida preceded planning for a master's degree in nursing administration. When curriculum planning began, the program director questioned hospital administrators and nursing administrators, using the Delphi technique.

A conscious bias that cannot be measured exists in purposive sampling. Therefore, you should use it only if there are no other sampling alternatives, and you must be very wary in interpreting the data.

Quota Sampling   **Quota sampling** is different from stratified sampling in two ways. Quota sampling is not random and may or may not sample proportions representative of the population. (Remember, in stratified sampling the proportions are representative.) In quota sampling, the researcher makes a decision, based on judgment, about the best type of sample for the study. For example, if you are studying nurses' attitudes toward nurses who have problems with chemical abuse, you may want to get a representative quota of male and female nurses from different age groups and with different educational preparation.

The researcher decides what the strata are, depending on the variables that might affect the dependent variable being investigated. The sex and age of nurses probably affect their attitudes toward nurses with chemical abuse problems (dependent variable). Their educational preparation might also be a meaningful stratum. Since 3% of nurses are male and 97% are female, similar percentages can be drawn for the study. Since W% of nurses are between the ages of 20 and 30, X% between 30 and 40, Y% between 40 and 50, and Z% over 50, the sample can reflect these same proportions.

If you study chemically dependent nurses' responses to different treatment programs, you may want to study equal numbers of male and female nurses, and an equal number of nurses from different age groups. In this case, the sample is not representative of or drawn proportionately from the population.

Using quota sampling you can sample *matched pairs*. This means you select your sample on predetermined important characteristics. For example, if you wonder how preoperative education affects the behavior of cardiac bypass patients postoperatively compared to the behavior of angioplasty patients, you might match the patients according to risk factors—age, weight, exercise, smoking.

Quota sampling is used when an investigator cannot select a random sample but aims for more control than is possible with accidental, or convenience, sampling. Subjects are selected if they fit the criteria for each stratum as set by the researcher. The aim is to reduce bias or sampling error.

A Critique of Nonprobability Sampling   In most nursing studies we settle for nonprobability sampling, because the population is too unknown to obtain a random sample or because the expense in time and money of a random sample is too great. Also, informed consent is vital in research, and this requirement decreases the possibility of a random sample. Instead, our subjects are willing, informed participants who have the freedom to withdraw from a study at any time.

Because nursing research studies regularly use nonprobability samples, we need to be knowledgeable about the strengths and limitations of each type and attempt to make the sample as representative as possible. Caution in generalizing findings beyond what is warranted in studies with nonprobability samples is important.

Sample Size

Of vital importance in every researcher's mind is "How many subjects do I need?" As is true of much of the research process, there are no hard and fast rules for sample size. Rather, you must consider the research purpose, the design, the size of the population and the requirements of statistical tests. Depending on circumcumstances, a large or small number of subjects may be appropriate. Actually, however, with the exception of case studies, the larger the sample, the more valid and accurate the study, because a larger sample is more likely to be representative of the population. The following general guidelines may be helpful in determining sample size (n):

- If the population is homogeneous, you can use a smaller sample than if it is heterogeneous. On the one hand, a study examining the experiences of breast-feeding mothers will involve much variability, because mothers of all ages, of all socioeconomic groups, and of all ethnic groups breast-feed their babies. A study of the health habits of eighth-grade girls in a private school on the other hand, will have less variability. The girls are approximately the same age and come from the same socioeconomic group, so a smaller sample will be more likely to yield "typical" subjects. The review of the literature and your nursing experience will help you estimate the population variability.

- If you use a research design that requires numerous treatment groups (experimental design), then you must determine the number of subjects needed for the smaller groups (called cells) and not just for the larger group heading. For example, if you study the use by chronically ill geriatric patients of Orem's self-care model, do not base decisions about sample size exclusively on the larger group of geriatric patients needed. Perhaps your design requires you to compare patients in a private hospital with patients in a Veterans Administration hospital or cardiac patients with cancer patients and kidney patients. Because of all the subgroups, you will need more subjects than if you merely looked at a single group of chronically ill patients. You should decide the cell size for each sub-sample or treatment group and then add these together to get your total n. If the cell size is too small (often 10 or fewer), the treatment mean, a frequency calculation, is more likely to be skewed by one atypical number. A cell size of 20 or more generally yields more accurate results and allows more options when it comes to statistical analyses.

- Survey designs frequently use many more subjects than observational or experimental designs, because telephoning or mailing questionnaires to a large number of people is feasible, whereas observing large numbers of people may not be. One must also plan ahead for the possibility of less than a 100% return rate and of subject attrition over time. However, in experimental research it is not feasible to do experiments with many human subjects. In nursing, because of all the variables we must control, getting a cell size of ten is often very difficult and, at times, impossible. Case studies and case histories require even fewer subjects, usually between one and ten.

- A thorough review of the literature will give you ideas about what size sample is typical for certain types of research questions and designs used in nursing research (see Table 8–10). However, be aware that in many studies the sample size is too small and, therefore, should be viewed with a critical eye.

- The statistical analyses you choose to use may impose certain requirements regarding sample size. Be sure you know at the proposal stage of your research what statistical analyses you will use. If you leave this choice until later, your

TABLE 8–10   *Sample Sizes Used in Selected Nursing Studies**

Abstract	Design	Sample Size
1. The processes family members of heart transplant recipients use to manage the unpredictability evoked by the need for and receipt of heart transplantation were explored. Twenty family members were theoretically sampled using the grounded theory approach. Three separate family support groups, each of 12 weeks duration, provided data for constant comparative analysis. Redesigning the dream was identified as the integrative theme in the substantive theory that described how family members gradually modify their beliefs about organ transplantation and develop attitudes and beliefs to meet the challenge of living with continual unpredictability. The theory consists of three concepts—immersion, passage, and negotiation—which parallel the stages of waiting for a donor, hospitalization, and recovery.	Exploratory/ descriptive	20

Source: M. Mishel and C. Murdaugh, "Family Adjustment to Heart Transplantation: Redesigning the Dream," *Nursing Research*, 1987, vol. 36, pp. 332–338.

2. The question of whether personality hardiness moderates the impact of job stressors on burnout was studied in 107 registered staff nurses from an urban, community hospital who responded to a self-administered questionnaire. Consistent with previous research, burnout was significantly associated with higher levels of perceived job stress and lower levels of personality hardiness. Hierarchical multiple regression analyses further indicated that work stressors (particularly stress due to workload) and hardiness were significant additive rather than interactive predictors of burnout. That is, hardiness had beneficial main effects in reducing burnout, but did not appear to prevent high levels of job stress from leading to high levels of burnout.	Descriptive survey	107

Source: E. McCranie et al., "Work Stress, Hardiness, and Burnout Among Hospital Staff Nurses," *Nursing Research*, 1987, vol. 36, pp. 374–378.

3. Fourteen nursing research findings that meet the Conduct and Utilization of Research in Nursing (CURN) Project (1982) criteria for clinical use were identified from research journals and CURN publications. Data collected from 216 practicing nurses in small, medium, and large hospitals were analyzed to determine their awareness of, persuasion about, and use of the findings. The majority of nurses were aware of the average innovation, were persuaded about it, and used the average innovation at least sometimes. Use of the innovations had no relationship to hospital policies or procedures concerning the nursing research findings.	Descriptive survey	216

Source: J. Luckenbill Brett, "Use of Nursing Practice Research Findings," *Nursing Research*, 1987, vol. 36, pp. 344–349.

4. This study compared the health beliefs of Mexican Americans concerning the specific symptom of chest pain to beliefs of a group of predominant culture nurse practitioners and a lay predominant culture control group. Two hypotheses were examined: (a) The health beliefs of groups differ significantly with culture and	Correlational survey	90

TABLE 8–10 *Sample Sizes Used in Selected Nursing Studies (Continued)*

Abstract	Design	Sample Size

(b) the health beliefs of groups differ significantly with professional education. A 43-item structured questionnaire was developed, based on literature review and unstructured interviews with Mexican American respondents. The questionnaire was administered to three nonprobability samples of 30 subjects each: Mexican Americans, nurse practitioners, and lay controls. Significant differences were found between Mexican Americans and the predominant culture groups of nurse practitioners and lay controls on folk beliefs regarding chest pain. On some items significant differences between nurse practitioners and the lay groups of Mexican Americans and predominant culture controls were based on professional education.

Source: D. Kosko and J. Flaskerud, "Mexican American, Nurse Practioner, and Lay Control Group Beliefs about Cause and Treatment of Chest Pain," *Nursing Research*, 1987, vol. 36, pp. 226–230.

5. *The impact of menopausal stage, current life change, and attitude toward traditional women's role on perceived health status was studied in 249 women 40 to 55 years of age. Instruments included the Life Experiences Survey (LES), Index of Sex Role Orientation (ISRO), and the Perceived Health Status (PHS). The relationship between menopausal stage and PHS was inverse and significant, though small. That between the LES score and PHS was inverse and significant. No direct, significant relationship between the ISRO score and PHS was observed. Multiple regression analysis accounted for 15% of variance in PHS.* — Correlational survey — 249

Source: N. Engel, "Menopausal Stage, Current Life Change, Attitude Toward Women's Roles, and Perceived Health Status," *Nursing Research*, 1987, vol. 36, pp. 353–357.

6. *The purpose of this study was to investigate the effects of a personal control intervention in the form of self-administered versus nurse-administered pain medication after cardiac surgery, and its interaction with patients' desire for control, patients' perception of pain intensity, disruption in daily activities, emotional responses, and use of pain medication over time. Subjects were 64 adults undergoing coronary artery bypass or valve replacement surgery. Instruments included the Krantz Health Opinion Survey; a 7-point measure of discomfort scale to assess pain intensity, disruption in daily activities due to pain, and emotional upset due to pain; a shortened form of the Sickness Impact Profile; and the Bi-polar Profile of Mood States. No main effects were found between experimental and control groups on any of the dependent measures nor were interaction effects found between individuals' measured desire for control and the personal control intervention. A time by group interaction was found in reports of pain intensity, $p < .05$, with subjects in the experimental group reporting higher levels of pain intensity than subjects in the control group in the early postoperative period.* — Experimental — 64

Source: K. King, L. Norsen, R. Robertson, and G. Hicks, "Patient Management of Pain Medication after Cardiac Surgery," *Nursing Research*, 1987, vol. 36, pp. 145–150.

TABLE 8–10 *Sample Sizes Used in Selected Nursing Studies (Continued)*

Abstract	Design	Sample Size
7. *The purpose of this study was to investigate the effect of early feeding of the normal newborn with formula and sterile water on: time of initial meconium passage, serum indirect bilirubin levels at 48 hours of life (HOL), observed jaundice at 48 HOL, and percentage of weight change at 48 HOL. Thirty normal, term newborns were sequentially assigned to one of three treatment groups: a control group given the routine hospital feeding of up to 30 ml of sterile water at 4 HOL and up to 30 ml of formula at 8 HOL; a water-fed group given up to 30 ml of sterile water at each feeding at 1, 2, and 3 HOL; and a third group fed formula at the same times and in the same amounts as the water-fed group. The time of initial meconium passage was significantly earlier in both groups of early fed infants than in the control group, F = 4.202, p = .026. The difference between the water-fed and the formula-fed groups was not statistically significant, but the mean time of passage was earlier in formula-fed infants. Serum indirect bilirubin levels at 48 HOL did not differ significantly, F = 0.412, p = .666, although the mean for the formula-fed group was lower. The correlation between the time of initial meconium passage and serum indirect bilirubin levels at 48 HOL was r = .3271, p = .083. Nine infants in the control group were jaundiced, compared to six in the water-fed group and six in the formula-fed group, a difference that was statistically significant, x^2 = 6.79, p = .034. There was no significant difference in percentage of weight loss at 48 HOL, although all infants in the control group lost weight, and two water-fed infants and one formula-fed infant gained. Infants in the early fed groups had stools significantly earlier than infants in the control group in this study, but a significant relation between earlier meconium passage and lower serum bilirubin levels at 48 HOL was not demonstrated.*	Quasi-experimental	30

Source: S. Boyer and D. Vidyasagar, "Serum Indirect Bilirubin Levels and Meconium Passage in Early Fed Normal Newborns." *Nursing Research*, 1987, vol. 36, pp. 174–178.

8. *The effect of controlled supplemental oxygenation without bag ventilation on transcutaneous partial pressure of oxygen ($TcPO_2$) measurements during tracheobronchial hygiene was evaluated. Procedure A, no supplemental oxygenation, was compared to Procedure B, in which controlled supplemental oxygenation was used. For controlled supplemental oxygenation, the FiO_2 was increased until $TcPO_2$ measurements rose to levels between 90 and 100 torr. Sixteen premature infants who required mechanical ventilation were studied in the neonatal center. Both procedures were performed on each patient in random order. In both procedures, a precipitous decrease in $TcPO_2$ was observed during chest vibration, and further decrease in $TcPO_2$ was noted with endotracheal suctioning. Except for baseline readings, throughout the tracheobronchial hygiene $TcPO_2$ measurements were significantly higher and more subjects maintained $TcPO_2$ valves greater than 40 torr in Procedure B. In Procedure A corresponding $TcPO_2$ measurements were 40 torr or less. Mean recovery time was shorter in Procedure B, 2.1 ± 2.3 minutes, than in Procedure A, 4.9 ± 2.8 minutes, p < .003.*	Preexperimental	16

TABLE 8–10   *Sample Sizes Used in Selected Nursing Studies (continued)*

Abstract	Design	Sample Size
Thus in most patients, controlled supplemental oxygenation without manual bag ventilation seems sufficient to prevent hypoxia during tracheobronchial hygiene; it also shortens recovery time from hypoxemia as a result of the bronchopulmonary hygiene procedure.		

Source: C. Walsh et al., "Controlled Supplemental Oxygenation during Tracheobronchial Hygiene," *Nursing Research*, 1987, vol. 36, pp. 211–215.

*All abstracts used by permission. Copyright 1987 American Journal of Nursing Company.

sample size may be too small, prohibiting you from conducting the planned statistical analysis.

- **Power analysis** is vitally important when you are making decisions about sample size. Power refers to the probability that an inferential statistical test (see Chapter 14) will reject the null hypothesis when it is false and allow you to declare that the research hypothesis is supported when, indeed, it should be.

Determining sample size is one way of increasing power; this is in part because a larger sample size decreases error variance and increases the degrees of freedom for the test (see Chapter 14). Also, decreasing variance by increasing homogeneity of subjects or by increasing your controls aims to ensure an increase of power. A third method of increasing power is increasing the effect size. Increasing the *effect size* merely means that you, in any way possible, increase the intensity or frequency of your treatment in an experimental design. For example, if you are applying ice after heparin injections to decrease bruising, you might leave it on longer than the original 5 minutes to be sure of its effect. Perhaps ice will prevent bruising if it is left on for 15 minutes instead of 5 minutes. Treatment, however, should not be intensified unless there is theoretical justification for the supposition that increased frequency or duration will increase the effect size. These three methods—(1) increasing sample size, (2) decreasing variance, and (3) increasing effect size—all increase power.

Cohen (1977) writes authoritatively and extensively about power analysis, but a statistical consultant can be helpful in determining your required sample size with a power analysis. The computational procedures for conducting power analyses are, however, beyond the scope of either this chapter or Chapters 14 and 15. Tables in many statistics books help you estimate the probability of a type 2 (beta) error (incorrectly labeling a difference as due to chance when it's actually a real difference) for commonly used statistical procedures. Such tables can be used to estimate the needed sample size before research begins. If you know in advance that the sample size is necessarily small—say 20 patients—and you need a larger sample to avoid type 2 errors, you may choose to redesign or even abandon the project rather than doing research that, from a statistical point of view, is not worth doing.

The major focus in sampling should be on design. You should do everything possible to ensure representativeness of the sample to the population. The unnecessary use of small or nonrandom samples is a wasted effort. However, a large sample size cannot correct a poor design (Polit and Hungler 1987 p. 427).

Sampling from Special Population Groups

Special population groups present practical and ethical problems to researchers. Access to certain patient groups may be difficult or require extra effort by the researcher. According to Sexton (1983 pp. 378–380), some problems confronting researchers who study the chronically ill (COPD patients) include:

- identification of subjects and their reluctance to participate in studies—a problem of sufficient sample size

- implementation of certain designs (a panel study, longitudinal, experimental, or correlational) due to the exacerbations, remissions, and mortality of the illness—a problem of limited study designs

- consideration of the feasibility of the energy and the abilities required of the patient for each type of data collection—a problem of data collection

Nurses should not be reluctant to pursue research with chronically ill patients but must focus energy on working toward the best and most feasible approach, taking into account the typical problems these patients present.

Children, the mentally ill, the mentally retarded, and the elderly also require special consideration by the nurse researcher. Although informed consent (see Chapter 3) aims to protect patients' rights, it sometimes is less than effective. Most informed consent procedures have three conditions:

- The individual subject must volunteer to participate.

- The individual must be mentally competent.

- The individual must be informed of the risks, benefits, discomforts, and compensation.

Mitchell (1984) discusses the questions of when children are capable of informed consent, the difference between assent and informed consent, and parental permission versus consent. Nurses historically have been advocates of children and are now (because of new 1983 regulations from the Department of Health and Human Services) legally accountable for protecting children's rights.

Watson (1982) writes on informed consent of special subjects, including captive groups (prisoners), the acutely ill and dying patients, and the mentally ill and legally incompetent, including children. She raises the question, "What is voluntary consent and who can give it?" (p. 43). Can a subject who is impaired or vulnerable physically or psychologically really give informed consent? Hayter (1979 p. 125) says that general agreement seems to exist on two points:

1. Persons who are unable to give their own informed consent should not be research subjects if other subjects can be used.

2. The less able a person is to protect himself or herself, the more vigilant the investigator must be in protecting that person.

Mann and Whall's (1984) research on informed consent and the deinstitutionalized patient suggests that extra time and additional written explanations about research are useful to this special group. Reminding patients of their right to avoid participation or stop participation at any time also may help make consent truly informed.

Robb (1983), however, cautions us to beware the "informed consent," and expresses her fear that in our willingness to comply with legal and ethical restrictions we may be "protecting" the elderly to death by avoiding using them as research subjects. She urges "creative solutions" to "the burdens of written consent." Informed consent issues are clearly related to practical considerations of obtaining an adequate sample.

Sampling and External Validity

Your research purpose and design affect how important representativeness, yielding external validity, is. Different types of research question require, to a greater or lesser degree, representative samples. If you are doing descriptive research, which aims to describe behaviors or attitudes of a group, representativeness is very important, because you are aiming for descriptive accuracy (external validity). If your sample is biased or not representative, your description will be inaccurate and invalid.

In methodological studies you will need to be concerned with all types of reliability and internal validity—content-, construct-, and/or criterion-based validity (see Chapter 10). In case studies or case histories, you may be more concerned with illustrating or generating theory, and the issue of representativeness is not critical. In contrast, representativeness and external validity are of great significance in experimental studies. Because obtaining representative samples in experimental nursing studies is sometimes impossible, however, replication studies are useful in establishing external validity.

Sampling is a complex but essential stage in the research process. Some authors have devoted entire books to the various sampling procedures. For more information, review the References at the end of the chapter.

Box 8–6   Steps in Getting Started

1. Write a research question based on your experience, observations, or literature.

2. Review the literature—nursing research literature, general nursing literature, research from other disciplines, methodological literature, popular literature, theoretical literature.

3. Network—interview resource people.

4. Refine your specific study question.

5. Write your purpose—as a statement, question or hypothesis—depending on the level of inquiry of your question.

6. For Level 2 and 3 studies, operationally define your variables.

7. Choose an appropriate research design.

8. Select a sample.

As you get started on a research project, constantly evaluate where you are and where you are going. Think of the consistency and the logic of the entire process. (Note the summary of steps in Box 8–6.) Your initial question leads to a relevant literature review, which results in a purpose. Whether you focus on a statement, a question, or a hypothesis, clarify your variables and operationalize them so that they can be measured. Based on the purpose, you choose an appropriate design, which almost always suggests a sample. After you ascertain the feasibility of obtaining subjects and carrying out your study, and you get approval from the institutional review board (IRB), you are ready to collect and analyze data. Once you have reached this point conceptually, you are ready to put all your planning into action.

Guidelines for Critique

- From where have the research questions/hypotheses been derived?
- Is the literature review comprehensive, covering the required types of literature?
- Is the level of inquiry appropriate to the nature of existing knowledge?
- If there are hypotheses, are they written correctly?

- Are the variables operationally defined?

- Is the design appropriate to the study purpose?

- Are the sampling methods appropriate to the research purpose and design?

SUMMARY OF KEY IDEAS AND TERMS

✓   A *research question* can be derived from observations, experiences, or the literature.

✓   Classifying research questions into one of three levels of inquiry helps in the choice of a research purpose and design that are appropriate for your question.

✓   An extensive literature review provides contextual relevance for the research question, suggesting the correct level of inquiry.

✓   *Level 1 inquiry* is used for exploratory, descriptive studies in which there is little available literature on the research question.

✓   *Level 2 inquiry* looks for the relationship between variables. The literature suggests the relationship between variables but does not specify the nature of the relationship.

✓   *Level 3 inquiry* assumes a significant relationship between variables. A literature review reveals theory that predicts the nature of the relationship.

✓   A thorough literature review covers the last five years and includes nursing research literature, theoretical literature, general and specialty nursing literature, methodological literature, research literature from other disciplines, and popular literature.

✓   Writing a research question and doing a literature review are challenging and time-consuming tasks. Allowing time for intellectual exploration is useful. Such exploration involves networking with appropriate experts and thinking about the feasibility, significance, and researchability of the problem.

✓ The statement of the research purpose derives from the level of inquiry. The purpose of a level 1 question is written as: "The purpose of this research is to explore and describe . . ." The purpose of a level 2 question is written as: "The purpose of the study is to answer the question . . ." The purpose of a level 3 study is written as: "The purpose of this study is to test the hypothesis . . ."

✓ A *theoretical framework* that predicts the nature of the relationship between variables is necessary for a level 3 hypothesis-testing study.

✓ For a hypothesis to be testable, the variables must be observable and measured. The *dependent variable* must be observed under at least two different conditions. Variables, to be measurable, require operational definitions.

✓ A hypothesis must have three components (Brink and Wood 1988): an *experimental group*, the *experimental result*, and a *comparison group*.

✓ Hypotheses can be simple or complex, directional or nondirectional, and stated as research or statistical hypotheses.

✓ In level 1 studies (exploratory) all variables are assumed to be independent until research is done that indicates the nature of the variables. In level 2, 3, and 4 studies, independent and dependent variables need to be clearly identified.

✓ After the identification of the variables, operational definitions are written that specify how the variables will be measured.

✓ A good research design follows logically from the study's purpose. Historical and case study designs are appropriate for level 1 studies. Survey designs, depending on the type, are used in level 1 or 2 studies. Experimental and quasi-experimental designs and ex post facto designs are used in level 3 studies. Methodological study designs are used to develop and validate an instrument.

✓ The *research purpose* should lead an investigator to appropriate subjects for the sample. The sampling process, whereby a researcher studies a subset of the population, is a feasible and logical way of generalizing statements about a smaller group to a larger group. For such inferences to be valid, a sample should be as representative of the total population as possible.

✓   *Probability sampling*, the most rigorous sampling approach, requires that every element in the population have an equal (random) chance of being included in the study. With *nonprobability sampling* the results are representative of the sample only and cannot be generalized to a larger population.

✓   Most nursing studies use nonprobability sampling, because the population is too unknown to obtain a random sample or the expense of time and money of a random sample is too great.

✓   *Sample size* is very important and is dependent upon the research purpose, the design, and the size of the population. Generally, the larger the sample, the more valid and accurate the study.

References

Barnard K: The case study method: A research tool. *Am J Matern Child Nurs* 1983; 8:327.

Begley S, Shapiro D: The death of the 'bubble boy.' *Newsweek* March 5, 1984:71.

Blank D: Relating mothers' anxiety and perception to infant satiety, anxiety, and feeding behavior. *Nurs Res* 1986; 35:347–351.

Boyer D, Vidyasagar D: Serum indirect bilirubin levels and meconium passage in early fed normal newborns. *Nurs Res* 1987; 36:174–178.

Bramwell L, Whall A: Effect of role clarity and empathy on support role performance and anxiety. *Nurs Res* 1986; 35:282–287.

Brink P, Wood M: *Basic Steps in Planning Nursing Research, from Question to Proposal*. Boston, MA: Jones & Bartlett, 1988.

Cohen J: *Statistical Power Analysis for the Behavioral Sciences*. New York: Academic Press, 1977.

Copp G, Mailhot C, Zalar M, Slezak L, Copp A: Covergowns and the control of operating room contamination. *Nurs Res* 1986; 35:263–267.

Copp G, Slezak L, Dudley N, Mailhot C: Footwear practices and operating room contamination. *Nurs Res* 1987; 36:366–369.

Diers D: *Research in Nursing Practice*. Philadelphia: Lippincott, 1979.

Durham M, Swanson B, Paulford N: Effect of tachypnea on oral temperature estimation: A replication. *Nurs Res* 1986; 35:211–214.

Engel N: Menopausal stage, current life change, attitude toward women's roles, and perceived health status. *Nurs Res* 1987; 36:353–357.

Hayter J: Issues related to human subjects in *Issues in Nursing Research*. Downs F, Fleming J (editors). New York: Appleton-Century-Crofts, 1979.

Hodgeman E: Closing the gap between research and practice; changing the answers to the "who," the "where," and the "how" of nursing research. *Int J Nurs Stud* 1979; 16:105–110.

Holm K: Single subject research. *Nurs Res* 1983; 32:253–255.

Keen MF: Comparison of intramuscular injection techniques to reduce site discomfort and lesions. *Nurs Res* 1986; 35:207–210.

Kerlinger F: *Foundations of Behavioral Research*. New York: Holt, Rinehart & Winston, 1973.

King K, Norsen L, Robertson R, Hicks G: Patient management of pain medication after cardiac surgery. *Nurs Res* 1987; 36:145–150.

Kosko D, Flaskerud J: Mexican American, nurse practitioner, and lay control group beliefs about cause and treatment of chest pain. *Nurs Res* 1987; 36:226–230.

Luckenbill Brett J: Use of nursing practice research findings. *Nurs Res* 1987; 36:344–349.

Mann L, Whall A: Informed consent and the deinstitutionalized patient. *J Psychosoc Nurs* 1984; 22:22–27.

May K. Three phases of father involvement in pregnancy. *Nurs Res* 1982; 31:337–342.

McCranie E, Lambert V, Lambert C: Work stress, hardiness, and burnout among hospital staff nurses. *Nurs Res* 1987; 36:374–378.

Meier P, Pugh E: *The Case Study: A Viable Approach to Clinical Research*, Unpublished paper, 1983.

Mishel M, Murdaugh C: Family adjustment to heart transplantation: Redesigning the dream. *Nurs Res* 1987; 36:332–338.

Mitchell K: Protecting children's rights during research. *Ped Nurs* January/February 1984; 9–10.

Notter L: The case for nursing research. *Nurs Outlook* 1975; 23:760–763.

Orem D: *Nursing: Concepts of Practice*. New York: McGraw-Hill, 1980.

Polit D, Hungler B: *Nursing Research*, 3rd ed. Philadelphia: Lippincott, 1987.

Polkinghorne D: *Methodology for the Human Sciences*. Albany, N.Y.: State University of New York Press, 1983.

Powers M, Jalowiec A: Profile of the well-controlled, well-adjusted hypertensive patient. *Nurs Res* 1987; 36:106–110.

Reverby S: A caring dilemma: Womanhood and nursing in historical perspective. *Nurs Res* 1987; 36:5–11.

Robb S: Beware the "Informed consent." (Editorial.) *Nurs Res* 1983; 32:132.

Sexton D: Some methodological issues in chronic illness research, *Nurs Res* 1983; 32:378–380.

Shelley S: *Research Methods in Nursing and Health*. Boston: Little, Brown, 1984.

Shelley S, Zahorchak R, Gambrill C: Aggressiveness of nursing care for older patients and those with do-not-resuscitate orders. *Nurs Res* 1987; 36:157–162.

Tulman L: Initial handling of newborn infants by vaginally and cesarean-delivered mothers. *Nurs Res* 1986; 35:296–300.

Walsh C, Bada H, Korones S, Carter M, Wang S, Arheart K: Controlled supplemental oxygenation during tracheobronchial hygiene. *Nurs Res* 1987; 36:211–215.

Watson A: Informed consent of special subjects. *Nurs Res* 1982; 31:43–47.

Weinert C: A social support measure: PRQ 85. *Nurs Res* 1987; 36:273–277.

Williamson M: Reducing post-catheterization bladder dysfunction by reconditioning. *Nurs Res* 1982, 31:28–30.

Wilson H, Kneisl C: *Psychiatric Nursing*, 2nd ed. Menlo Park, CA: Addison-Wesley, 1988.

Winer BJ: *Statistical Principles in Experimental Design*. New York: McGraw-Hill, 1962.

Winer BJ: *Statistical Principles in Experimental Design*. New York: McGraw-Hill, 1962.

9

Relating Your Study to a Theoretical Context

LINDA E. MOODY ■ SALLY A. HUTCHINSON

Chapter Objectives

After reading this chapter, the student should be able to:

■ Explain the terms *concept, construct, proposition, theory, model, framework, paradigm,* and *metaparadigm*

■ Differentiate between conceptual and theoretical frameworks on at least four points

■ Interpret Kaplan's empirical-theoretical framework and its relevance for nursing theory development

■ Explain the purpose of a conceptual map

■ Discuss various types of theory

■ Describe four purposes of theory in a discipline

■ Analyze the relationship of theory and research

■ Describe the meaning of paradigmatic, preparadigmatic, and paradigm-transcending research and discuss the place of nursing as a science in this typology

■ Discuss questions raised in recent literature concerning nursing theories

(Continued)

- Define *metatheory*

- Analyze and evaluate nursing theories by applying the basic questions in metatheory

- Discuss the difference between internal and external criticism of a theory

- Describe and interpret ten criteria for theory evaluation

- List concepts that customarily serve as a focus for a nursing theory

- Understand the intellectual contributions of historically important nurse theorists

- Discuss the use of nursing and nonnursing paradigms in research

- Explain approaches for linking the theory and the research process

In This Chapter...

The words *theory*, *concept*, *construct*, *theoretical framework*, and *nursing model* have become common in contemporary nursing literature. This chapter aims to make these terms, which frequently evoke anxiety, confusion, and dismay, understandable and relevant to the nursing student and practicing nurse who are interested in research.

Theories play a big role in our conceptions of events and people in our everyday life. If you work in a hospital or health care agency, you are probably familiar with systems theory. Understanding why a private psychiatric hospital did not survive, for example, was made possible in part through a systems analysis. This process involved analyzing the subsystems of organizational structure, technology, economics, and symbolic systems (Hutchinson 1984b). Perhaps you are attempting to analyze why a nurse colleague appears to have a fear of success. Psychoanalytic theory offers a possible explanation, as does feminist theory, if your colleague is a female. Shopping at the grocery store and being forced to pay higher prices for certain items may cause you to reflect on the economic theory of supply and demand. If you have ever cared for young children, the development theories of Piaget (1958) or Erickson (1963) can be helpful in understanding their behaviors at various ages. If you are in a patient-care situation, the theory of gravity helps you understand why patients with dependent edema due to venous insufficiency are placed in various positions.

Theories from other disciplines, such as those mentioned above, often provide the framework for nursing research. One goal of research is to extend the scope of our knowledge. To do this successfully, a research study must be placed in a theoretical context or be designed to develop one. When a study is placed in a theoretical context, the theory guides the research process from the research questions through the design, analysis, interpretation, and conclusions. This chapter discusses the use of theories (nursing and nonnursing) in the research process.

You may wonder what qualifies as a theory. Does a nursing theory differ from any other theory? Are there different levels and types of theories? How are theories developed, and how are they used in the research process? How can you tell a good theory from a bad theory? These questions constitute the focus of this chapter, and examples drawn from nursing research serve as illustrations.

The Purpose of Theories

The word *theory* derives from the Greek *theoria*, which means *vision*. **Theories** are conceptual inventions of reality that are used to describe, explain, predict, or understand phenomena of concern. A "good" theory, then, provides a useful vision or perspective of reality. Theorizing is not just an academic exercise, because useful theories are tied to reality. Further, good theories expand our vision and guide our thinking, our practice, and our research. Theories also serve as heuristic devices by which we can discover new knowledge or revise old ways of thinking. Kaplan (1964), in his classic book *The Conduct of Inquiry*, makes another very important point:

> Theories are not just means to other ends, and certainly not just to ends outside the scientific enterprise, but they may also serve as ends in themselves—to provide understanding, which may be prized for its own sake [p. 310].

How is theory related to the research process? A theory, conceptual model (paradigm), theoretical framework, or model serves to provide parameters for the study, guides data collection, and provides a perspective for interpreting the data, enabling the scientist to structure the facts into an orderly system. Through this process, the potential for theory building or theory generation is enhanced. Analogous to the DNA molecular structure, Fawcett (1978a) views research and theory as a double helix, as two intertwining parts that are inextricably linked (see Figure 9–1).

> Theory is one helix, spiraling from the conception of an idea through modifications and extensions to eventual confirmation or refutation. Research is the second helix, spiraling from identification of research questions through data collection and analysis to interpretation of findings and recommendations for further study. The core of the double helix is the pairing of theory development with the research process. In the core, theory directs research and research findings shape the development of theory [1978a p. 50].

The current issues in theory development for nursing are in these major areas:

■ a deficient theoretical base to guide practice

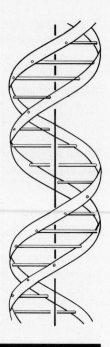

Figure 9–1   The helix is illustrated by the structure of DNA, which has a double helix.

- an excess of isolated studies that are not tied to an integrating theoretical framework or placed in a theoretical context
- a premature focus on experimental research

These are a few of the issues we explore in this chapter. But first, we provide an introduction to the special language of theory.

The Language of Theory

As you read about theories and their relationship to nursing research, you will immediately become aware of the frequent use of some new and esoteric language. An understanding of this vocabulary is essential for you to appreciate and apply the ideas in your reading and in your practice and research.

We begin by defining the most basic components of a theory, then follow with a discussion of the more complex terms that you need to know to appreciate the process of theory development.

Concept

Concepts are linguistic labels that we assign to objects or events. Concepts are the building blocks of theories and vary in level of abstraction. Examples of highly abstract concepts are *stress*, *pain*, *grief*, and *wellness*. Less abstract or more concrete concepts are *blood loss*, *temperature elevation*, *weight*, and *height*. Several classification schemes exist for categorizing concepts.

Concepts may have a *theoretical* or *operational* definition. In a *theoretical* definition, the concept is defined in relation to other concepts. The *operational* definition links the concept to the real world and identifies empirical referents (indicators) of the concept that permit observation and measurement. Regardless of level of abstraction, the researcher needs to provide both theoretical and operational definitions of the concepts to link the theoretical perspective with the research aims. Fawcett and Downs expand on this point: "Operational definitions are necessary regardless of the type of research. This is true whether the operational definition identifies the paper and pencil questionnaire used in a survey or the domain of the researcher-informant experience of an ethnography" (1986 p. 22). Thus, concepts may vary from the empirical, that is, observable *(blood loss)* to the theoretical, that is, abstract *(grief)*; constructs tend to be more symbolic *(social loss)*; and theoretical terms are generally derived from specific theories *(ego, id, superego, individuation, reinforcement)*. Recognition of this continuum from the empirical to theoretical should help when you read theories and attempt to understand how they are linked

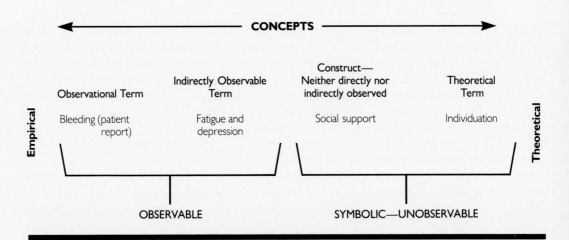

Figure 9–2 An empirical-theoretical continuum   Source: Adapted from A. Kaplan, *The Conduct of Inquiry*, San Francisco: Chandler, 1964, pp. 57–60. Reprinted with permission.

up with observable reality. If you are generating a theory in your own research, you need to be aware of where your terms are located on the continuum as you aim for a fit between the empirical and theoretical worlds (Figure 9–2).

Construct

When you read about concepts and theories, you may also read about *constructs*. **Constructs** are a group of concepts that are directly or indirectly observable (Jacox 1974 p. 6). They are derived from a combination of academic and clinical knowledge and contribute theoretical meaning and scope to a theory (Glaser and Strauss 1967 p. 70). Familiar examples of constructs are *society*, *socioeconomic status*, and *health status*. **Theoretical constructs**, which are terms specific to a given theory, are not observable. Examples of theoretical terms are *superego* and *Oedipal complex*, from psychoanalytic theory (Jacox 1974 p. 6). *Creating meaning*, from a theory about how nurses survive the horror of some of their work (Hutchinson 1984a), and *limiting intrusion*, from a theory about the social processes in a nontraditional treatment setting for psychiatric patients (Wilson 1982), are examples of theoretical constructs discovered by nurses in their qualitative research.

Proposition

Theories require **propositions**, and propositions describe the relationship of two or more concepts. As you can see from the definitions, theory development begins with the identification and description of concepts and constructs and proceeds to formulate propositions that describe the nature of the relationships between these concepts. Nursing studies on empathy (Forsyth 1980), privacy (Rawnsley 1980), restlessness (Norris 1975), and humor (Hutchinson 1976) offer a beginning look at these concepts and their relevance to nursing. Conceptual analysis has as its goal the examination of parts, of operations, and of the interrelated whole of a thing (Chinn and Jacobs 1987). Theoretical and operational definitions are derived from this knowledge. Before nursing can claim to have its own unique theories, it first must have concepts, constructs, and propositions.

Conceptual Model or Paradigm

A **conceptual model** refers to concepts that provide a structure or pattern for organizing phenomena of interest in practice or research. Kuhn (1970), a philosopher of science, popularized the term **paradigm** and used it to mean a model or world view about the major phenomena of concern to a discipline. Fawcett (1984), Parse (1987), and others in nursing use the terms *conceptual model* or *paradigm* to mean the same thing. Although not empirically testable, conceptual models or paradigms serve as heuristic devices or springboards for developing theories.

Theory

What qualifies as a theory? Theories are viewpoints or ways of perceiving reality. Kerlinger (1973) provides a formal definition of **theory**: "A *theory* is a set of inter-related constructs (concepts), definitions, and propositions that present a systematic view of phenomena by specifying relations among variables, with the purpose of explaining and predicting the phenomena" (p. 9). Henkel points out that "theories refer to a hypothetical universe—hypothetical in the sense that it encompasses all past, present, and future cases to which the theory applies, wherever they may occur" (1976 p. 84). Examples of theories you have probably heard about and per-haps even used in your practice are psychoanalytic theory, the theory of relativity, the theory of evolution, the theory of gravity, learning theory, systems theory, and the theory of homeostasis.

Stevens (1984 p. 1) provides a less restrictive definition of theory: " . . . a statement that purports to account for or characterized some phenomenon." Thus, Stevens's definition permits classification of nursing paradigms, models, or frame-works as theories, in the broad sense of the term. As you will note from the lit-erature, theories vary in scope, purpose, significance, level, and type. The term *theory* is used liberally and often in a generic sense to refer to any statement that attempts to describe, explain, predict, or shed light on some puzzle, problem, or phenomenon of interest. Later in this chapter, we discuss types and levels of theory and present examples of nursing theories developed through a variety of research methods, from causal modeling to grounded theory, such as Mercer's (1985) theory of maternal role attainment, Cox and Roghmann's (1984) model of client health behavior, and Hutchinson's (1987) theory of self-integration in nurses who experi-enced chemical dependence.

Theoretical Framework, Model, or Theory?

A theoretical framework is derived from one or more theories or paradigms through the processes of induction and deduction. A theoretical framework postulates re-lationships among concepts and permits empirical testing. Differences between con-ceptual and theoretical models are shown in Table 9–1.

Fawcett points out that although there is a difference between conceptual and theoretical models, *theoretical model* and *theory* are frequently used interchangeably. In fact, a *theoretical model* "refers to a group of interrelated theories which provide rationale for the hypotheses, policies and curricula of a science, whereas a theory encompasses fewer phenomena" (1978b p. 19).

Model or Paradigm   *Model* and *paradigm* are terms you will encounter in your education and practice. There are curricular models, administrative models, teach-ing models, and practice models or paradigms. Bush (1979) writes, "A model rep-resents some aspect of reality, concrete or abstract, by means of a likeness which may be structural, pictorial, diagrammatic or mathematical" (p. 16). A model or

---

TABLE 9–1   *Differences between Conceptual and Theoretical Models*

Conceptual Models or Paradigms	Theoretical Models or Frameworks
1. They are pretheoretic bases from which substantive theories may be derived.	1. They propose frameworks derived from theories.
2. They are highly abstract.	2. They are less abstract than conceptual models.
3. Concepts are related and multidimensional.	3. Concepts are narrowly bounded, specific, and explicitly interrelated.
4. They provide a perspective for a science.	4. They postulate relationships. They are descriptive, explanatory, or predictive (Reilly 1975). In applied science they are prescriptive.
5. They are derived from unsystematic empirical observations and intuition.	5. They are constructed from available theories and findings of empirical research (Reilly 1975).
6. They are developed through the process of induction.	6. They are developed through the processes of induction and deduction.
7. They must be evaluated on logical grounds and cannot be empirically tested.	7. They permit empirical tests (Torgerson 1958).

Source: Adapted from J. Fawcett, "The 'What' of Theory Development," in *Theory Development: What? Why? How?*, New York: National League for Nursing, 1978, pp. 18–19.

paradigm, unlike a theory, does not focus on the relationships among phenomena but rather on their structure or function. A model is essentially an analogy, a symbolic representation of an idea. You will probably remember the model of the heart or the eye that you used in anatomy class. The structure of the organs was accurate and complete, but the model did not tell you how or why the parts were interrelated.

Perhaps in your psychiatric nursing experience you have read Hildegard Peplau's *Interpersonal Relations in Nursing* (1952) and learned how to interact with patients based on her model. Fitzpatrick and her associates (1982), in their book *Nursing Models and Their Psychiatric Mental Health Applications*, examine a number of therapy models (individual, family, crisis) and discuss their relationship to selected nursing models (Rogers, King, Orem, Roy). All of these models or paradigms essentially offer a system for understanding and analyzing phenomena.

Nurses borrow models from other fields, just as they borrow theories, if these models can explain nursing phenomena. For example, one nursing student analyzed nurse-physician relationships by using a model of exchange from economic theory. Rhythm models, from many disciplines, are useful in examining healthy and unhealthy human functioning such as menstrual and sleep cycles and, as such, have implications for nursing (Floyd 1982). Because these borrowed models often don't fit nursing phenomena exactly, nurse scientists work on adapting them to nursing's perspective, using what works and altering or discarding what doesn't.

Models, Paradigms, and Theories   You may now wonder about the relationship between models, paradigms, and theories. Bush (1979) identifies three types of relationship between models and paradigms on the one hand and theories on the other:

1. Models or paradigms may be constructed for theories. For example, Figure 9–3 demonstrates an example of the Orem self-care model. This visual, symbolic model essentially simplifies Orem's theory, making it visible in the same way a model of the eye demonstrates its structure.

2. Models or paradigms may serve to stimulate theoretical explanations. For example, a biochemical model of how certain cancer cells are believed to behave offers scientists a perspective that encourages theoretical thinking. A proposed nursing model can function in the same way.

3. Mathematical models exist at a higher level of abstraction, based on theory, yet are functional in suggesting theories in any discipline. Here is a typical mathematical model (Estes 1963):

$$gn = (1 - \frac{1}{N})\,(1 - C)n$$

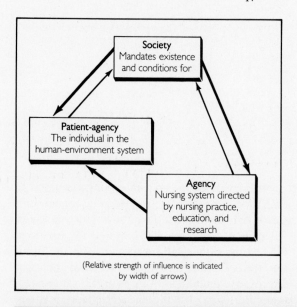

(Relative strength of influence is indicated by width of arrows)

Figure 9–3   A model of Orem's self-care theory   Source: Based on J. Fitzpatrick et al., *Nursing Models and Their Psychiatric Mental Health Applications*, Bowie, Md.: Robert J. Brady Co., 1982, p. 59. Reprinted with permission.

These models transcend the subject matter by proposing a more or less universal structure.

When you are doing research, you can conceptualize your thoughts by building a model (diagrammatically, physically, mathematically, or symbolically, depending on what you are studying). Such models simplify and clarify theory or stimulate theoretical explanations.

Artinian's (1982) article "Conceptual Mapping" deals with the value of such maps (which are theoretical models) for understanding the relationship among variables in a study. In experimental and correlational studies, mapping or model making helps in conceptualization of the research problem. If you are doing a qualitative research study with the aim of theory generation, mapping helps you see your theory, and this visualization of the interrelationships of the variables is surprisingly helpful in encouraging further conceptualization. Figure 9–4 is an example of a conceptual map for the study of chronic dyspnea.

Conceptual maps can be useful to you at all stages of the research process, from your proposal to the final writing of your report of findings. The conceptualization required for map making results in a logical and organized model, accurately depicting your research.

Paradigms (Models) and Research   The process of research, according to Bush (1979), can be conceptualized by a model. Chinn and Jacobs (1987) offer a paradigm of the scope of the research process for nursing. They view the research process as having four steps:

1. evaluation and analysis of concepts

2. formulation and testing of relational statements

3. theory construction

4. practical application of theory

You can relate this model in part to the levels of research questions discussed in Chapter 8. The first step in developing theory is to explore and describe the relevant variables or concepts in nursing practice. The second step is to test which variables are related to each other and to what degree. Once the variables and the nature of the relationships have been identified, propositions can be written, and the interrelated system of propositions forms the structure of a theory. Once a theory is proposed, it must be tested and, if necessary, modified until it is useful for nursing. Chinn and Jacob's model demonstrates the unity that the research-theory relationship should have. You can see from this paradigm how different types and levels of research are all necessary to contribute to nursing knowledge. This supports the idea of pluralism of nursing research.

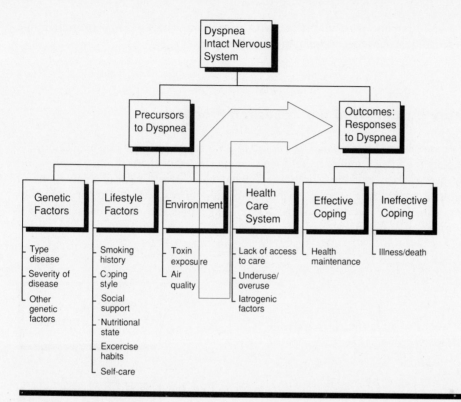

Figure 9–4   A conceptual map for the study of chronic dyspnea (Moody 1988)

Metaparadigm

The term *metaparadigm* is derived from Kuhn's (1970) original work on paradigms. The **metaparadigm** defines the domain of interest, establishes the questions to be addressed, and identifies appropriate theories, methods, and instruments to be used in research. The metaparadigm is therefore *the most global perspective* of a discipline and serves as an encapsulating unit or framework within which the more defined models, theories, or paradigms develop. Several authors have noted that there is general agreement regarding the central concepts of the metaparadigm of nursing: the nature of nursing, the individual who receives care, society-environment, and health (Donaldson and Crowley 1978, Flaskerud and Holleran 1980, Yura and Torres 1975).

There appears to be consensus among nurse scholars about the central concepts of the metaparadigm of nursing, often referred to as the domain concepts: nursing or nursing action, person, client (individual, family or community), health (health states or illness-wellness continuum), and environment. A *nursing metaparadigm* provides the discipline with the most global world view (*Weltanschauung*) or cognitive map to guide knowledge development in nursing.

Theory Building and the Research Process

There are several ways to view the issue of a metaparadigm for nursing. Figure 9–5 depicts the more commonly held view, suggesting that there is one global, world view accepted by nursing. From that global view derive multiple paradigms or models to guide practice and serve as heuristics for research and theory development. Paradigms, theories, models, frameworks, concepts, constructs, and propositions are all abstractions of reality.

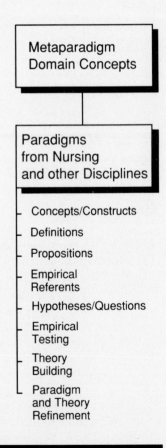

Figure 9–5 Theory building and the research process

Most scientists believe that there is a reality "out there" and that it is worthwhile to obtain knowledge about it. Figure 9–5 demonstrates that theory building begins with a few concepts or constructs that are usually derived from within the metaparadigm and paradigm structure of a discipline. **Paradigm-transcending research** or theorizing occurs when concepts are derived outside the metaparadigm. These concepts or constructs are then further refined and related in propositions or statements that can be submitted to empirical testing. The process is not necessarily linear; it may be iterative or retroductive, combining induction and deduction. Theory building and paradigm refinement are accomplished through empirical testing, regardless of whether the research approach is qualitative or quantitative.

A Typology of Theories

At one time or another, most of us have been theoreticians, if only in a primitive sense. Perhaps we announced our theory as to why a certain patient did not respond as expected to treatment or we noted what needed to be done. With these formulations, we placed the problem in a theoretical context to better understand it. In the broadest sense, then, theory can be defined as a systematic abstraction of reality that serves a goal or purpose. Thus, the theoretical is utilitarian, but only if it serves some goal or purpose.

Broadly speaking, we assess the value or utility of a theory by how well it provides us with a perspective of reality or truth. We revise theories according to our perspectives of reality. Our perceptions of reality change in reference to time and context. An important point is that *theories are not discovered by scientists; rather, they are invented* to describe, explain, or understand phenomena of concern or to solve nagging problems.

Similarly, Dickoff and James define theories as intellectual inventions designed to describe, explain, predict or prescribe. They note four types of theory, each building on the other, and point out that, as a practice discipline, nursing needs to develop prescriptive theories (1968 p. 202):

1. *factor-isolating theories:* observing, describing, and naming concepts

2. *factor-relating theories:* relating named concepts to one another

3. *situation-relating theories:* interrelationships among concepts or propositions

4. *situation-producing theories:* prescribing activities necessary to reach defined goals (also known as prescriptive theories)

Diers (1979) expands the ideas of Dickoff and James by identifying the interrelationship of the process of theory building and research for a practice discipline:

1. *Factor-naming or factor-searching research* describes, names, or characterizes a phenomenon, situation, or event to familiarize or yield new insights (descriptive or exploratory research).

2. *Factor-relating or relation-searching research* develops links among variables and describes the relationships that are discovered after a phenomenon has been explored, described, and named. Many qualitative and grounded-theory studies fit into this category.

3. *Explanatory/correlational research* aims to determine factors that occur or vary together. No attempt is made to control or manipulate the environment or to test interventions. An explanation of phenomena is sought.

4. *Causal hypothesis-testing research* addresses causal relationships between variables in an attempt to predict what will happen if *x* occurs.

The causal hypothesis-testing research (level 4) has been given high priority in nursing research in the hope that it will yield prescriptive or middle-range theories that can be applied to nursing practice.

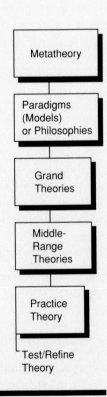

Figure 9–6 Levels of theory

Levels of Theory   Theories have not only been defined according to their purpose (that is, teleologically) but also classified according to their scope or breadth. One of the most helpful classification systems for viewing levels of theory is shown in Figure 9–6. The greater the scope of the theory, the nearer it is to the upper end of the continuum. Some conceptual models in nursing are *macro* or **grand theories** that address phenomena of concern. As such, these grand theories are not testable but are viewed as theory-generating models or models from which hypotheses can be derived and submitted for testing.

Much has been written about the need for practice disciplines, such as nursing, to develop **middle-range theories**, a term proposed by Merton (1968) a sociologist and the founder of sociology of science. Many nursing scholars who studied sociology in the 1960s and 1970s were profoundly influenced by Merton and other sociologists. Merton describes middle-range theories as those that examine a portion of reality and identify a few key variables. In middle-range theories, propositions are clear, and testable hypotheses can be derived. The scope of the problem is limited, and this restriction encourages in-depth exploration and analysis. To develop middle-range theories, the researcher links the study closely to the empirical world in which the phenomena occur. Although the approach may be inductive, deductive, or retroductive, middle-range theories are often derived from ethnographic or qualitative studies with an inductive approach. An example of a middle-range theory is Hutchinson's (1987) grounded-theory study of chemical dependency among nurses.

Other examples of middle-range theories include Glaser and Strauss' classic studies *Awareness of Dying* (1965) and *Time for Dying* (1968), Wilson's study on *Deinstitutionalized Residential Care of the Mentally Disordered: The Soteria House Approach* (1982), and Hutchinson's study entitled *Survival Practices of Rescue Workers: Hidden Dimensions of Watchful Readiness* (1983). Middle-range theories, more so than grand theories, fit the empirical world from which they are derived and, as such, permit suggestions for nursing practice.

Middle-range theories are often developed by inductive methods (see Chapter 13) such as grounded-theory or ethnographic methods and require that the researcher be theoretically sensitive to the data. The researcher conceptualizes empirical data. Honigman (1976) makes it clear that data are

> . . . not reflections of facts or relationships, existing independently of the observer. In the process of knowing, external facts are sensorily perceived and immediately transferred into conceptualized experience, the observer being an active factor in the creation of knowledge, not a passive recipient or register [p. 245].

In Search of Paradigms

Using Kuhn's (1970) broad definition of paradigm, we can view nursing as having multiple paradigms that guide knowledge building. The notion of acquiring a dominant paradigm for a discipline, as Kuhn suggests, was at one time thought desirable, because the prevailing paradigm would provide a research tradition for the community of nurse scientists and accelerate scientific progress. However, as many scholars have since speculated, a dominant paradigm for nursing may be not only impossible but also undesirable for a practice discipline that focuses its research on human responses of enormously variable scope and complexity.

Feyerabend, a historian philosopher of science, warns of overcommitment to a paradigm: "Epistemologic prescriptions are not guarantees of the best way to discover a few isolated facts or secrets of nature and further, rigid scientific education cannot be reconciled with a humanitarian attitude—it maims by compression like a Chinese lady's foot" (1975 p. 20). Thus, although paradigms provide a rich foundation for generating research questions and are of value in advancing theory, an *unquestioning adherence* to a research tradition or a particular world view may blind us to new discoveries and delay scientific progress.

We need to develop and foster our ability to challenge conventional wisdoms and pose new approaches to the study of intractable problems: promotion of multiple paradigms for a discipline helps us develop creative approaches to old problems and puzzles. Pluralism in research will assist in the development and testing of middle-range practice theories. It will also help us contribute our fair share to the fundamental pool of science or produce knowledge for knowledge's sake.

Paradigm-transcending research, which Kuhn proposes as the basis for scientific revolutions, has the goal of discovering new theories and methods. And these new theories, or paradigms, will subsequently guide further inquiry. Meleis, Wilson, and Chater (1980) suggest the discovery of the oxygen theory of combustion as an example of paradigm-transcending research. This discovery significantly altered the paradigm of pneumatic chemistry. Examples of paradigm-transcending research in nursing include studies by Hutchinson (1983), Stern (1982), and Wilson (1982). Nursing needs more paradigm-transcending studies to develop theories that explain and predict empirical phenomena relevant to the discipline. The counterpart to the development of theories is the testing of existing theories (remember the double helix). Nursing is progressing in the testing of hypotheses derived from existing nursing theories that will expand the scope of nursing knowledge.

Whither Nursing Theories?

Let's now examine some issues surrounding the development of nursing theories. We have established that the discipline of nursing needs theories, but of what type, and for what purpose? Questions raised in the recent literature include:

1. Is nursing research basic or applied (Crawford, Dufault, and Rudy 1979; Donaldson and Crowley 1978)?

2. Is nursing theory borrowed or unique (Donaldson and Crowley 1978)?

3. Should we have grand theories of nursing or practice theories (Beckstrand 1978, 1980; Collins and Fielder 1981; Crawford, Dufault, and Rudy 1979; Wald and Leonard 1964)?

4. What paths to knowledge and development exist (Crawford, Dufault, and Rudy 1979)?

These issues were the dominant focus of past nursing theory conferences. Nurse theorists presented papers that examined the questions in detail. Although many diverse opinions and beliefs were evident, there appeared to be consensus on several points.

Basic or Applied Research?

Debating whether nursing knowledge is "basic" or "applied" raises the question of whether nursing research should aim to discover new knowledge (thus expanding the knowledge base for the sake of acquiring more knowledge) or to develop knowledge that can be used expressly to guide nursing practice. An example of research in nursing that contributes to our knowledge may be a physiological study about how respiratory exchange works with cardiopulmonary disease patients. Early on, this research may not have a clear application for practice, but ultimately its utility would be recognized once scientists understood the process. Such understanding surely would suggest appropriate nursing intervention measures.

This example illustrates a point that many nurse scientists make: It is foolish and wasteful to spend time discussing whether nursing research is basic or applied. Rather, nursing needs all kinds of research, basic and applied, and inevitably most basic research in nursing results in practical suggestions that affect patient care (see Chapter 2).

Borrowed or Unique Theory?

A second question is whether nursing theory is borrowed or unique. There is agreement among nurse scientists that *nursing theory is both borrowed and unique*. That is, nurses use knowledge from many disciplines (psychology, sociology, physics, physiology, education); however, this knowledge becomes integrated into nursing theory only if nurses adapt it and alter it to fit the unique needs and perspectives of nursing. Nursing theories are those that are systematically derived from studies of nursing practice and that reveal a unique nursing perspective.

Grand Theories or Practice Theories?

The nursing literature is replete with articles addressing the third question of whether we should seek one or several grand theories *of* nursing, or theories *for* practice. Grand theories of nursing concern the profession in general—what it is, what the responsibilities are, and how work is viewed. A **grand theory** is "a generalized theory capable of supporting an overall concept of a process of nursing . . ." (Putnam 1965 p. 430.) In contrast, practice, or prescriptive, theories offer nurses *direct guides for action*. Theories *for* rather than *of* nursing aim to improve practice so as to "help individuals cope with health problems when their own strength, will or knowledge is insufficient" (Ellis 1968 p. 218).

Efforts to develop grand theories for nursing are not as necessary as working toward middle-range, empirically based theories that can guide practice. Grand theories are less useful, because their large scale inevitably makes them vague and diffuse and, consequently, difficult to test. Beckstrand (1980) argues forcefully against a focus on grand theories of nursing: "Identifying the concepts relevant to nursing as an activity will not help nursing develop comprehensive scientific knowledge of its clients' problems and how to deal with them" (p. 76). Ultimately, perhaps, a grand theory could be developed if numerous practice theories could be synthesized and conceptualized clearly enough to suggest some overriding or transcending concepts and constructs that are unique to nursing.

Emphasis should be placed on generating multiple practice theories appropriate to specific problems and areas in nursing—for example, theories of pain alleviation or care of the dying (Jacox 1974). If some unity could ever be derived from a conglomeration of practice theories, then perhaps a general practice theory could be synthesized. At this time, the likelihood of achieving such a goal is remote. Furthermore, some nurse scientists question the worth of such a huge undertaking.

Beckstrand (1978, 1980), a solo voice, argues in a series of articles against practice theories at all. Instead, she believes that knowledge of science, ethics, metatheory, and philosophy is sufficient for nursing.

What Paths to Knowledge?

The fourth question concerns the appropriate paths for knowledge development for nursing science. Again, pluralism in methodology is recognized. Nurses need to generate theory inductively, test theory deductively, and also embrace the use of philosophical, phenomenological, and historical methods of research. The method chosen should not become an end in itself, but rather must be appropriate for answering the question. (See the discussion of study designs in Chapter 5.) Platt (1964) cautions us:

> Beware of the man who is method-oriented rather than problem-oriented. The method-oriented man is shackled; the problem-oriented man is at least reaching freely toward what is most important [p. 353].

A major goal for nursing is to decide what questions are relevant to and significant for nursing. Donaldson and Crowley (1978) warn us that we can no longer assume that we all have a tacit understanding of "the nursing perspective" and "the essence of nursing." Rather, we must be able to articulate our unique perspective so that our knowledge and our philosophy are made clear. We are aiming for refinement of the metaparadigm, "the broadest consensus within a discipline . . . which provides the general parameters of the field and gives scientists a broad orientation from which to work" (Hardy 1978b p. 38).

Nursing Paradigms: Some Exemplars

This section of the chapter offers you a brief encounter with 12 nursing theorists. This overview acquaints you with the major perspective of each model and gives you a feeling for the historical development of nursing theory. Perhaps one or more models will catch your interest, and you can read in more depth by going directly to the writings of the particular theorist or an authoritative source on nursing theory.

Florence Nightingale

Nightingale can be considered the first nursing theorist if we accept evidence that she offered a theoretical orientation to nursing without calling it one. Her focus was on the physical environment (as opposed to the psychosocial environment), which was appropriate for the difficult conditions of the Crimean War. Her table of contents in *Notes on Nursing: What It Is and What It Is Not* (1945) clearly illustrates her environmental approach: Ventilation and Warming, Health of Houses, Petty Management, Noise, Variety, Taking Food, What Food? Bed and Bedding, Light, Cleanliness of Rooms and Walls, Personal Cleanliness, Chattering Hopes and Advices, and Observation of the Sick (p. 5). Nightingale believed that if nurses altered the environment in a positive fashion, the reparative process could begin.

Lydia Hall

Hall's theory presents the three "aspects of nursing": the person (or the core of nursing), the disease (or the cure of nursing), and the body (the care of nursing) (see Figure 9–7). Her philosophy developed from her work at the Loeb Center of Montefiore Hospital in the Bronx. Patients had recovered from their acute illnesses and were recuperating in this long-term, patient-centered treatment center. Depending on the patient's problems, each of the three aspects of nursing might be emphasized or deemphasized, demonstrating the changing nature of their relationships.

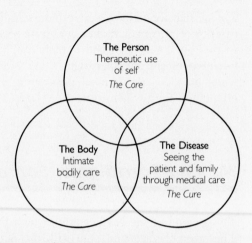

Figure 9–7   Hall's three aspects of nursing   Source: Nursing Theories Conference Group. *Nursing Theories: The Base for Professional Nursing Practice*, 1980, p. 44. Reprinted by permission of Prentice-Hall, Inc., Englewood Cliffs, N.J.

Virginia Henderson

Henderson wrote her famous definition of nursing in 1955:

> Nursing is primarily assisting the individual (sick or well) in the performance of those activities contributing to health or its recovery (or a peaceful death) that he would perform unaided if he had the necessary strength, will, or knowledge. It is likewise the unique contribution of nursing to help the individual to be independent of such assistance as soon as possible [1966 p. 4].

Following up her philosophical definition with concrete examples, Henderson listed 14 components of basic nursing care (see Box 9–1). These components focus on "helping the patient with the [listed] activities or providing conditions under which he can perform them unaided" (1966 pp. 16–17). You can see by her list that Henderson recognized physiological, psychological, and spiritual needs.

Hildegard Peplau

Peplau, a psychiatric nurse, presented her theoretical model in *Interpersonal Relations in Nursing* (1952). According to Peplau, nursing is a "significant therapeutic interpersonal process. . . . Nursing is an educative instrument, a maturing force, that aims to promote forward movement of personality in the direction of creative, constructive, productive, personal, and community living" (1952 p. 16) (see Figure 9–8).

Box 9–1   Henderson's Components of Basic Nursing Care

1. Breathe normally.

2. Eat and drink adequately.

3. Eliminate body wastes.

4. Move, and maintain desirable postures.

5. Sleep and rest.

6. Select suitable clothing—dress and undress.

7. Maintain body temperature within normal range by adjusting clothing and modifying the environment.

8. Keep the body clean and well groomed, and protect the integument.

9. Avoid dangers in the environment, and avoid injuring others.

10. Communicate with others in expressing emotions, needs, fears, or opinions.

11. Worship according to one's faith.

12. Work in such a way that there is a sense of accomplishment.

13. Play or participate in various forms of recreation.

14. Learn, discover, or satisfy the curiosity that leads to normal development and health and use of the available health facilities.

Source: V. Henderson, *The Nature of Nursing*, New York: Macmillan, 1966, pp. 16–17. Reprinted with permission of Macmillan Publishing Company. Copyright © 1966 by Virginia Henderson.

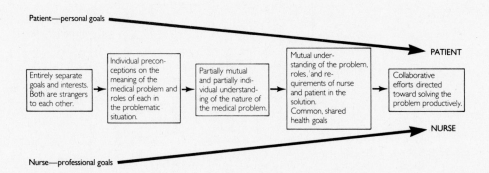

Patient—personal goals

| Entirely separate goals and interests. Both are strangers to each other. | Individual preconceptions on the meaning of the medical problem and roles of each in the problematic situation. | Partially mutual and partially individual understanding of the nature of the medical problem. | Mutual understanding of the problem, roles, and requirements of nurse and patient in the solution. Common, shared health goals | Collaborative efforts directed toward solving the problem productively. |

PATIENT

NURSE

Nurse—professional goals

Figure 9–8   A continuum of the changing nurse-patient relationship   Source: H. Peplau, *Interpersonal Relations in Nursing*, New York: Putnam's, 1952, p. 10. Reprinted with permission.

Peplau's theory focused on the four phases of the nurse-patient relationship (see Figure 9–9).

1. Orientation—the nurse and patient meet in response to the patient's "felt need" (p. 18).

2. Identification—the patient responds to the nurse if he or she offers needed help (p. 30).

3. Exploitation—the patient uses the nurse as a resource person (p. 37).

4. Resolution—when the patient's needs are met, he or she relinquishes ties to the nurse (p. 40).

Wilson and Kneisl (1988) say that Peplau's phases of the relationship represent precursors to the phases of the nursing process (assessment, planning, intervention, evaluation).

Fay Abdellah

Abdellah classifies nursing problems into 21 categories (see Box 9–2). She views the nurse as a problem solver whose goal is to identify and then remedy these

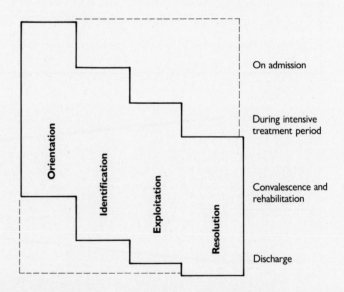

Figure 9–9 Overlapping phases in nurse-patient relationships   Source: H. Peplau, *Interpersonal Relations in Nursing*, New York: Putnam's, 1952, p. 21. Reprinted with permission.

Box 9–2   Abdellah's List of Nursing Problems

1. to maintain good hygiene and physical comfort

2. to promote optimal activity: exercise, rest, and sleep

3. to promote safety through the prevention of accidents, injury, or other trauma and through the prevention of the spread of infection

4. to maintain good body mechanics and prevent and correct deformities

5. to facilitate the maintenance of a supply of oxygen to all body cells

6. to facilitate the maintenance of nutrition of all body cells

7. to facilitate the maintenance of elimination

8. to facilitate the maintenance of fluid and electrolyte balance.

9. to recognize the physiological responses of the body to disease conditions—pathological, physiological, and compensatory

10. to facilitate the maintenance of regulatory mechanisms and functions

11. to facilitate the maintenance of sensory function

12. to identify and accept positive and negative expressions, feelings, and reactions

13. to identify and accept the interrelatedness of emotions and organic illness

14. to facilitate the maintenance of effective verbal and nonverbal communication

15. to promote the development of productive interpersonal relationships

16. to facilitate progress toward achievement of personal spiritual goals

17. to create and/or maintain a therapeutic environment

18. to facilitate awareness of self as an individual with varying physical, emotional, and developmental needs

19. to accept the optimum possible goals in the light of limitations, physical and emotional

20. to use community resources as an aid in resolving problems arising from illness

21. to understand the role of social problems as influencing factors in the cause of illness

Source: F. Abdellah et al., *Patient Centered Approaches to Nursing*, New York: Macmillan, 1960, p. 16. Reprinted with permission of Macmillan Publishing Company. Copyright © 1960 by Macmillan Publishing Company.

biopsychosocial problems. Abdellah's list is comparable both to Henderson's 14 nursing care components and Maslow's hierarchy of needs (Falco 1980).

Dorothea Orem

Orem's theory of self-care appeared in the nursing literature in 1959. Her theory centers on the individual and self-care. "Self-care, the practice of activities that individuals personally initiate and perform on their own behalf to maintain life, health, and well-being is the person's ongoing contribution to his own health and well-being" (1985). Orem proposes three categories of universal self-care requisites (see Box 9–3). If an individual cannot meet self-care needs because of illness, injury, or disease, the nurse enters and offers "health deviation self-care." The nurse assesses the patient's level of functioning and ability to care for himself or herself and then gives "wholly compensatory," "partially compensatory," or "supportive-educative" care. Orem calls these three types of assistance "nursing systems," and each one describes the patient's and nurse's role. Orem's theory is of great interest in contemporary nursing with its renewed focus on self-care.

Martha Rogers

Rogers published her book *An Introduction to the Theoretical Basis of Nursing* in 1970 (see Rogers 1983), drawing on knowledge from anthropology, sociology, religion, philosophy, mythology, and general systems theory. Her theory has changed somewhat and become clarified over the years. *At the present time, she views the "unitary" person as the basis of nursing's uniqueness.* The science of nursing is "the study of the nature and direction of unitary human development and the derivation of descriptive, explanatory, and predictive principles that are basic to nursing practice." The practice of nursing is "the use of the body of knowledge in service to people." The purpose of nursing is "to help individuals and groups achieve maximum well-being within the potential of each" (Rogers 1987).

Rogers views science as humanistic, not mechanistic. People and the environment are two energy fields that are always open, have pattern and organization, and change continuously and creatively (Rogers 1984). Rogers identifies three principles of homeodynamics that postulate the nature and direction of change. (See Box 9–4).

Myra Levine

Levine proposes four conservation principles that aim to alter a patient's adaptation processes in positive ways. Levine writes: "Conservation means 'keeping together' (L. *conservatio*), but it should not imply minimal activity. In nursing, to keep together means to maintain a proper balance between active nursing intervention

---

Box 9–3   Orem's Universal Self-Care Requisites

1. air, water, food, and other supportive life materials

2. conditions that promote developmental processes

3. prevention and control of genetic and constitutional defects

Source: From D. E. Orem, *Nursing: Concepts of Practice*, 2nd ed., New York: McGraw-Hill, 1985.

---

coupled with patient participation on the one hand, and the safe limits of the patients' ability on the other" (1967 p. 46). The nurse first identifies the patient's specific pattern of adaptation and then uses the following principles to plan nursing intervention:

1. the principle of the conservation of patient energy. Nursing intervention is based on conserving the individual patient's physiological and psychological resources.

2. the principle of the conservation of structural integrity. Nursing intervention is based on conserving the individual patient's body form and function.

3. the principle of conservation of personal integrity. Nursing intervention is based on conserving the individual patient's self-identity and self-respect.

Box 9–4   Rogers' Principles of Homeodynamics

1. Principle of resonancy	the continuous change from lower to higher frequency wave patterns in human and environmental fields
2. Principle of helicy	the continuous innovative, probabalistic increasing diversity of human and environmental field patterns characterized by nonrepeating rhythmicities
3. Principle of integrality[a]	the continuous mutual human field and environmental field process

[a]Formerly called the principle of complementarity. From the Second National Post-Master's Conference, April 5–6, 1984.

Source: M. Rogers, Department of Nursing, New York University, Handout, 1984.

4. the principle of conservation of social integrity. Nursing intervention is based on conserving the individual patient's ethnic, religious, and subcultural affiliations (1967 pp. 46–59).

Levine views her principles as offering new directions for holistic approaches to patient care.

Sister Callista Roy

Roy's adaptation theory views us as biopsychosocial beings who have to continually adapt to a variety of stimuli, which she labels as focal, contextual, and residual (1984 p. 43). The focal stimulus has to do with a degree of change (e.g., a temperature variation); contextual stimuli include other stimuli present (e.g., humidity); and residual stimuli involve beliefs and attitudes that affect a given situation. Roy identifies four adaptive modes that help people cope with the changing environment—basic physiological needs, self-concept, role function, and interdependence. These four adaptive modes are essentially methods of coping that appear between a need and a behavior. For example, if the environmental temperature changes, a person may be hot or cold, and these feelings elicit an adaptive mode. The person feels the need and acts to address the need. Roy views basic needs as underlying the adaptive modes. The nursing process is used to promote the patients' adaptation in each mode. In her book, Roy (1984) gives examples of nursing interventions for specific adaptation problems.

Imogene King

King proposed a general systems theory in 1978 about the human level of functioning. *People*, *environment*, *nursing*, and *health* are her four basic concepts. She postulates three dynamic interacting systems (see Figure 9–10). Each individual is a *personal system*. These individuals interact among one another to form *interpersonal systems*, such as dyads, triads, and groups. The interpersonal systems then form *social systems*, which are comprehensive levels of functions of human beings (1981 p. 11). A person's "personal system" is dependent largely on one's perception of self. These perceptions directly influence behavior. The nurse-patient nursing process is implemented in the interpersonal system. The social systems—family, religious, educational, and health care systems (King 1981)—provide a context in which nurses work. To help patients achieve goals, nurses must interact effectively with social systems. King views her theory as "organizing complexity and variety in nursing . . . [and] in looking for relationships within this complexity and variety" (p. 15).

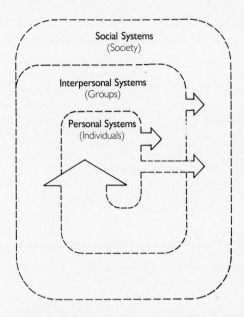

Figure 9–10   Conceptual framework for nursing   Source: I. King, *Toward a Theory for Nursing*, New York: John Wiley, 1981. Reprinted with permission.

Betty Neuman

Neuman (1982) proposes a health-care systems model, which views the person as a complete system with parts and subparts that interrelate. Neuman sees human beings as subject to stressors, which she identifies as intrapersonal, interpersonal, and extrapersonal, and as having flexible lines of resistance that help defend against these stressors (see Figure 9–11). Nursing assessment focuses on gaining information about the relationship among physiologic, psychologic, sociocultural, and developmental variables; nursing intervention can be primary, secondary, or tertiary. The nursing process, including nursing diagnosis, nursing goals, and nursing outcomes, is expected to facilitate the use of the model (1982 p. 119).

Rosemarie Rizzo Parse

Parse (1981, 1987) has developed a unique paradigm for nursing by synthesizing Martha Rogers's principles and concepts of the science of unitary human beings and the major tenets and concepts of existential-phenomenological thought. Parse drew primarily from Jean-Paul Sarte, Maurice Merleau-Ponty, and Martin Heidegger. The *Man-Living-Health* (Parse 1981) paradigm provides an explicit framework allowing nurses to uncover the meaning of phenomena experienced by human beings. In Parse's model, nursing science is a process whose significance lies in

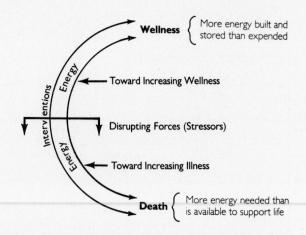

Figure 9–11 Neuman's wellness-illness continuum based on a systems model
Source: B. Neuman, *The Neuman Systems Model*, Norwalk, Conn.: Appleton-Lange, 1982, p. 11. Reprinted with permission.

dealings with the experiences of people: "Nursing, rooted in the human sciences, focuses on Man as a living unity and Man's qualitative participation with health experiences" (1981 p. 4). Parse's model is holistic in that it is a system of inter-related concepts describing "unitary man's" interrelating with the environment while cocreating health (1981 p. 13). Parse explicates Rogers's principles of hom-eodynamics, helicy, resonancy, integrality, and four-dimensionality. Other existen-tial-phenomenological tenets of the model are intentionality and human subjectivity and the concepts of coconstitution, coexistence, and situated freedom. Parse used the deductive method to derive nine explicit assumptions from the major concepts of the Rogers' model (see Box 9–5).

1. Man is coexisting while coconstituting rhythmical patterns with the environ-ment (concepts: coconstitution, coexistence, and pattern and organization)

2. Man is an open being, freely choosing meaning in situations and bearing re-sponsibility for decision (concepts: energy field, coconstitution, pattern and organization).

3. Man is a living unity continuously coconstituting patterns of relating (concepts: energy field, coconstitution, pattern and organization).

4. Man is transcending multidimensionally with the possibles (concepts: four-dimensionality, situated freedom, and openness).

5. Health is an open process of becoming, experienced by people (concepts: openness, coconstitution, and situated freedom).

6. Health is a rhythmically coconstituting process of the man-environment interrelationship (concepts: coconstitution, pattern and organization, and four-dimensionality)

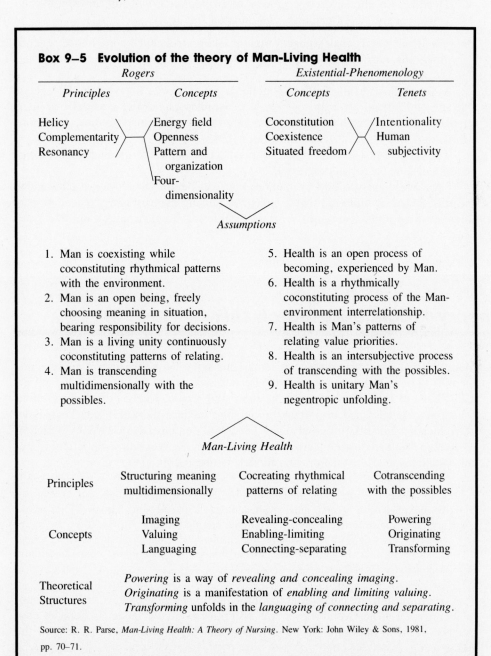

Box 9–5 Evolution of the theory of Man-Living Health

Rogers		Existential-Phenomenology	
Principles	*Concepts*	*Concepts*	*Tenets*
Helicy	Energy field	Coconstitution	Intentionality
Complementarity	Openness	Coexistence	Human
Resonancy	Pattern and organization	Situated freedom	subjectivity
	Four-dimensionality		

Assumptions

1. Man is coexisting while coconstituting rhythmical patterns with the environment.
2. Man is an open being, freely choosing meaning in situation, bearing responsibility for decisions.
3. Man is a living unity continuously coconstituting patterns of relating.
4. Man is transcending multidimensionally with the possibles.

5. Health is an open process of becoming, experienced by Man.
6. Health is a rhythmically coconstituting process of the Man-environment interrelationship.
7. Health is Man's patterns of relating value priorities.
8. Health is an intersubjective process of transcending with the possibles.
9. Health is unitary Man's negentropic unfolding.

Man-Living Health

Principles	Structuring meaning multidimensionally	Cocreating rhythmical patterns of relating	Cotranscending with the possibles
Concepts	Imaging Valuing Languaging	Revealing-concealing Enabling-limiting Connecting-separating	Powering Originating Transforming

Theoretical Structures

Powering is a way of *revealing and concealing imaging.*
Originating is a manifestation of *enabling and limiting valuing.*
Transforming unfolds in the *languaging of connecting and separating.*

Source: R. R. Parse, *Man-Living Health: A Theory of Nursing.* New York: John Wiley & Sons, 1981, pp. 70–71.

7. Health is man's patterns of relating value priorities (concepts: patterns and organization, openness, and situated freedom).

8. Health is an intersubjective process of transcending with the possibles (concepts: coexistence, openness, and situated freedom).

9. Health is unitary man's negentropic unfolding (concepts: coexistence, energy field, and four dimensionality).

A full understanding of Parse's model requires a prior knowledge of Rogers's (1983) model of unitary man and existential philosophy. Parse's model has been reported in the research literature in a number of qualitative studies. For more information, see Parse, Coyne, and Smith (1985).

The models just discussed offer a perspective on where nursing science originated and how far it has progressed.

Upon close analysis and evaluation, you will be able to recognize similarities and differences in philosophy and focus. As nursing evolves as a science, its paradigms will be refined to better serve as a guide for research, education, and practice.

The Theory-Practice-Research Link

Models guide us in our nursing practice and serve as a springboard for practice theories. Through research we can devise methods to test practice theories empirically and add to nursing's knowledge base. Wilson and Kneisl (1988) discuss four conceptual models used in psychiatric nursing: medical-biological, psychoanalytic, behavioristic, and social-interpersonal. Table 9–2 demonstrates clearly how each of these models affects patient care. Plans for nursing intervention with patients' specific problems are derived from the model. Gudmundsen (1982) says:

> One models nursing as one models all else: by proposing symbolic systems that can be identified with specific nursing phenomena in specific situations by means of observation and experimentation. . . . The criteria for judging all models are the same, however, deriving from their general role in the developing of nursing science: scope, adequacy to their chosen data base, extendability, predictive power, communicability, simplicity [p. 265].

When we link the conceptual model with the research process, it is important to identify the major world views and assumptions of the model to achieve congruence between philosophical beliefs about nursing practice and the aims of the study.

TABLE 9–2   *A Comparative Analysis of Major Features of Four Conceptual Models*

Conceptual Model	Assessment Base	Problem Statement	Goal	Dominant Intervention
Medical-biological	Individual client symptoms	Disease	Symptom control Cure	Somatotherapies
Psychoanalytic	Intrapsychic Unconscious	Conflict	Insight	Psychoanalysis
Behavioristic	Behavior	Learning deficit	Behavior change	Behavior modification or conditioning
Social-interpersonal	Interactions of individual and social context	Dysfunction	Enhanced awareness and quality of interactions	Group and milieu therapies

Source: H. Wilson and C. Kneisl, *Psychiatric Nursing*, 3rd ed. Menlo Park, Calif.: Addison-Wesley, 1988.

Nursing Paradigms in Research

During the late 1970s, nurse scholars were calling for researchers to provide a theoretical or conceptual model for research studies, and nurse-theorists were summoning practitioners and researchers to explore ways of testing nursing models through research and clinical applications. The prevailing belief was that the majority of nursing models had been developed through armchair theorizing, which is not to say that the models are not valuable. But the need was recognized to devise empirical means of testing the models or the hypotheses that could be generated from the models. The emphasis on the use of nursing models as paradigms for research was proposed to provide the researcher with the unique perspective of nursing in exploring the problem or research question.

After a cursory review of the nursing research journals of the last decade, you might be struck by several events related to knowledge building in nursing:

1. the notable increase in the use of the terms *theoretical framework/model* or *conceptual framework/model* in the published research articles

2. the fact that many of the studies do not actually test nursing theory or any theory but include the terms *theoretical model* or *conceptual framework* because most reviewers do not recommend publication unless this issue is addressed

3. the increasing use of nursing conceptual models over the last decade (Moody and Wilson 1987)

In 1986, Silva conducted an analysis of nursing research studies to determine the degree to which investigators have tested nursing theory through empirical research. Silva selected what she considered the five most commonly used nursing models (Johnson, Roy, Orem, Rogers, and Newman) and analyzed 62 studies that had in some way attempted to link the research to one of the five nursing models. Silva (1986 p. 4) classified the use of the models from the 62 studies according to three categories:

1. *minimal use of models for theory testing* (24 studies)

2. *insufficient use of models for theory testing* (29 studies)

3. *adequate use of models for theory testing* (9 studies)

Silva's analysis shows that nurse researchers have conducted few studies that have explicitly tested nursing theory but rather have used nursing models primarily as frameworks for research. Silva concludes that progress in the testing of nursing theory has been impeded by several factors: lack of investigator commitment; intolerance of methodological imperfections; and unsystematic retrieval strategies (1986 p. 10).

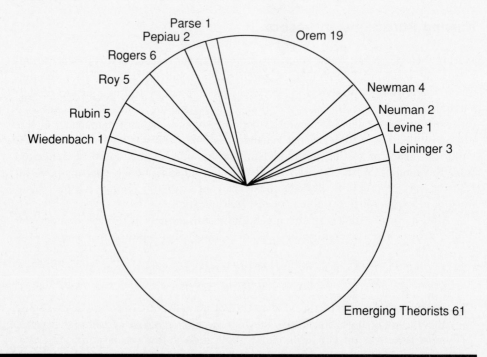

Figure 9–12 Nurse theorists cited in nursing practice research: 1977–1986 Source: As published in six major journals: *HAL, IJNS, JAN, NR, RINH, and WJNR*

Theory in Nursing Practice Research

How has nursing progressed over the last decade toward the use of theory-driven research or research that is based on a sound theoretical framework? In an effort to address that question, Moody and Wilson (1987) analyzed 720 research articles published in six of the major nursing research journals, focusing exclusively on "nursing practice research" in the period 1977–1986. The journals included: *Nursing Research*, *Western Journal of Nursing*, *Research in Nursing and Health*, *International Journal of Nursing Studies*, and *Journal of Advanced Nursing*. Moody and Wilson's findings were similar to those of Silva (1986). There was a link between the research design and the theory in 55% of the studies; of those, half were at the descriptive level of theory. The most commonly used conceptual models in nursing practice research during 1977–1986 are shown in Figure 9–12 (Moody and Wilson 1987).

The most frequently used nursing model was Orem's, followed by Rogers's Newman's and Roy's. Of the 720 studies, only 10% reported some level of usage of a nursing theory in the research. Less than 3% designed the research to test concepts or hypotheses of a theoretical nursing model. The proportion of research studies using nursing models increased significantly during the second half of the decade, by 5%. As we progress in our theory development, more and more research will derive from conceptual models.

Other Paradigms in Nursing Research

As with nursing practice, the conceptual model structures the entire research process. Nursing models or models from other disciplines can be used. Dickoff and his colleagues (1968b) make the following point about "borrowing" models from other disciplines: "Practically speaking, what is needed is for a nurse researcher to develop both her self-surveillance and her self-esteem so as to be able to take advantage of the help and securities of established disciplines without thereby sacrificing her nursing impetus or nursing identity" (p. 553).

As early as 1968, Myrtle Irene Brown wrote on the use of the concept of socialization (from sociology) in geriatric nursing research. She calls her early classifications "primitive" yet emphasizes that her work aimed "to describe the socializing behavior of nurses with the aged and to identify related variables" (p. 216). This is an appropriate first step in research and theory development, at least according to Dickoff and his associates' idea of levels.

Other nurse scientists have made efforts to adapt existing theories to nursing. For example, Ann Whall (1980) examines existing theories of family functioning and shows their relationship to nursing theories. She discusses the similarities between Peplau's (1952) approach and the psychoanalytic approach in family functioning, between King's (1978) theory and the communicationist approach, and between Rogers's (1983) theory and the family systems approach. Whall's work demonstrates her assertion that existing theory must "be examined and, if relevant,

be formulated or adapted in terms of nursing theory" (p. 67). After such refor-
mulations, propositions can yield hypotheses that can be tested, thus forming the
basis for nursing research.

In a similar quest for useful models for nursing research, Cronenwett and Brickman (1983) discuss four models of helping and coping in childbirth. After describing
each model and its assumptions and the pros and cons, they conclude the article
by raising some relevant questions for nursing research (pp. 87–88). Some or all of
these questions could be adapted and asked about many other models for nursing:

1. Are some helping models generally better than others?

2. Are different models best for different clients?

3. Are client-provider teams using the same (congruent) models most effectively?

4. Is it better to apply one method to a client consistently or to change as the
   client's needs, situations, and skills change?

5. Are some models better for providers?

6. Do organizational structures determine the choice of helping model?

7. Does professional role socialization determine the choice of helping model?

8. Has there been a historic evolution of the dominant helping models applied
   to childbearing families? (pp. 87–88)

The search for theories and models for helping and coping in many areas of nursing
is a most useful endeavor. Nursing research needs to use nursing conceptual models
as theoretical frameworks, but we must continue to discuss and evaluate all theories
to ensure that they are being interpreted correctly and offer a useful framework for
nursing research.

Moody and Wilson (1987) also identified the use of theory from other disciplines in nursing practice research, for the same journals and time period as for the
nursing models. Results are shown in Figure 9–13. Use of theories from other
disciplines remained fairly stable over the decade. In 1977, 52% of the studies used
a theory or framework from another discipline, compared to 49% in 1986. Theories
from psychology, physiology, and sociology were cited most frequently. The three
most frequently used theories from the social sciences were Lazarus's theory of
coping (27 studies), the health belief models of Becker or Rosenstock (25 studies),
and locus of control from social learning theory (12 studies). Physiologic theories
were represented fairly evenly across all biosystems. From education, various theories of learning were used, mostly adult learning theory.

Dickoff and James (1986) and others have been proponents of theoretical pluralism in nursing, meaning more than theoretical detente or a tolerance of other
ideas but a willingness to accept the notion that multiple paradigms are essential
in addressing the multiple realities of the complex nature of phenomena that need
to be studied in nursing.

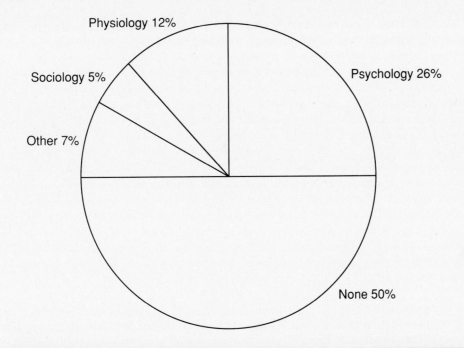

Figure 9–13   Use of nonnursing theories in research   Source: $N = 720$ as published in six major journals: *HAL, IJNS, JAN, NR, RINAH,* and *WJNR*

When nursing leaders were concerned about the autonomy of the discipline and called for a single nursing theory hoping to provide unity and direction for the discipline, it was believed that theoretical knowledge must evolve from nursing and nursing alone, and the idea of using theories from other disciplines was rejected.

The idea of developing "unique nursing theory" is now viewed as a necessary part of the evolutionary growth of nursing (Suppe and Jacox 1985). Over the last few decades, many nurse scholars have argued effectively that the goal of a single nursing theory was naive but proposed with good intentions. Leaders were saying, in effect, that theory in nursing or for nursing needed to focus more narrowly on improving nursing practice. When Ellis wrote her now classic article "Characteristics of Significant Theories" in 1968, she explained that it was in response to those in nursing who borrowed theories from other disciplines in an uncritical way, without making a linkage to improvement in nursing practice, and to the ambiguity surrounding many of the theory-related terms. Ellis explains further:

> The phrase *for nursing* implies that . . . only those theories that are relevant to that function which has to do with helping individuals to cope with health problems when their own strength, will or knowledge is insufficient. Improvement in the practice that achieves this function is the appropriate goal of theory development for nursing. . . . It determines what theories, or theories of what, are significant [1968 p. 217].

Therefore, it is more appropriate or correct to speak of theories for nursing, meaning that the theory is concerned with nursing practice, specifically the four metaparadigm concepts: nursing, person, environment, and health. Although Fawcett (1984) maintains that the more sophisticated theories for nursing would address all metaparadigm concepts, a theory that does not address the concept nursing could still be classified as a nursing theory. This view supports the notion that a theory that does not address the nursing concept might be useful to another discipline and therefore could not be classified as a nursing theory. If, however, "knowledge has no surname," it is part of nursing's obligation to society and the scientific community to contribute to the fundamental pool of knowledge. For example, if Freud's psychoanalytic theory is applicable to a nursing practice situation, should we conclude that his theory is not a psychoanalytic one? Of course not, and, as Fawcett (1984) argues, the utility of a nursing theory to another discipline is irrelevant in determining its status as a nursing theory. Internal criticism of nurse scholars has focused on the need for nursing to develop its own theory from an empirical base rather than relying on other disciplines. Stevens reminds us that most disciplines have ambiguous and overlapping knowledge boundaries:

> . . . borrowed theories remain borrowed as long as they are not adapted to the nursing milieu and the nursing image of man. Once such theories have been adapted to the nursing milieu, it is logical to refer to these boundary overlaps as shared knowledge rather than as borrowed theories [1984 p. 95].

Many theories used in nursing practice, education, and research are borrowed from other disciplines or shared with other fields. Yet, the point must be made that nursing has also developed theories that are applied uniquely to phenomena of concern in practice or research. Ellis expands this point, noting that the scope of nursing practice should provide the parameters appropriate to the development of nursing theory. In determining what is significant theory for nursing, we consider this: "Theory, whether begged, borrowed, derived, or originated by nurses, is significant for nursing if it can enlighten nursing practice" [or research] [1968 p. 222].

The hallmarks of the scientific growth of a discipline, according to Toulmin (1977) and Laudan (1977), are competition of multiple theories, creativity of thought, and innovation of ideas. In fact, the growth of knowledge in nursing cannot easily be classified as cumulative or revolutionary, but perhaps a combination of both. The exploration and encouragement of diverse theories and research traditions are highly desirable and conducive to knowledge production. The discipline of nursing, although young, has a notable, rich history and many nursing models to serve as heuristic devices for research and practice.

Theory Evaluation

Evaluation of theory can be classified as **metatheory**, a type of philosophy of science that studies the logical and methodological foundations of a discipline (Carnap

1966). A systematic approach to evaluation is needed in selecting a theory or theoretical framework to guide research and advance theory. Evaluation approaches or models for theory analysis, first introduced into the nursing literature in 1968, have become increasingly sophisticated. As a researcher, you need to know about theory evaluation models and understand how to select the evaluation model most appropriate to the stage of development of the theory. Although several evaluation approaches (from descriptive criteria to complex symbolic interactive models) exist, this discussion is limited to one of the most commonly used models for theory evaluation. The importance of finding the "best fit" between theory and research is discussed. Before we present the theory evaluation model, we review the process of theory description, analysis, and critique as well as some key terms.

Steps in Theory Evaluation

Stevens (1984), Meleis (1985), and Fawcett (1984) emphasize the need for a systematic method to describe, analyze, and critique the theory under consideration, thus narrowing the chance of biasing the evaluation process. Reducing bias in the evaluation enhances your appreciation for the process of theory development and augments the potential for further theory refinement. Although we can delineate certain objective criteria (e.g., *accuracy, consistency, broad scope, simplicity, and fruitfulness in research*) for evaluating competing theories, we must remember in the evaluation process to acknowledge our predilection for certain theories because of their novelty, their cognitive appeal, their congruence with our world views, or our disposition toward the theorist (positive or negative).

Theory Description   The first and crucial step in the evaluation process is an immersion in the works of the theorist and related works by others in the field to gain a full understanding of the structural and functional components of the theory. The *structural components* include assumptions, concepts, and propositions. The *functional components* consist of the domain concepts of the theory and the manner in which they are to be used (e.g., to describe, explain, predict, or control). Depending on the level of development of the theory and the degree of conceptual clarity of the concepts and propositions, the effort required in this phase will vary.

Theory Analysis   Theory analysis is a systematic process of examining the content and structure of a theory and suspending judgment regarding its value until the last phase, evaluation. Theory analysis is conducted if the theory or framework holds potential for being useful in practice or research. The purpose of theory analysis is to identify the theory's usefulness as a heuristic device to guide practice (clinical, evaluation, and administration). For research, the focus is on a theory's potential to guide the development of testable hypotheses or researchable questions. The key terms for theory analysis are *content* and *structure* examination.

The mode of analysis is usually holistic and particularistic. *Holism*, as an analytic approach, means that the theory is examined as a whole; the focus is on the generic property. A *particularistic* or reductionistic analysis disaggregates the theory for aspects that are of specific interest for description and analysis. Both approaches facilitate evaluation of the theory and foster an understanding of its focus and internal structure (Kim 1983 p. 15).

One of the major goals of theories is prediction and understanding of the phenomena under study. Understanding implies knowledge of the interaction of units in a system (Dubin 1978 p. 19). When the goal of the theory is prediction, the analytic focus of attention is directed toward research outcomes. A theorist-researcher perceives a portion of the world and attempts to understand and predict or possibly change beliefs within the theory or current world view. Thus, when a researcher considers a theory's utility for research, the analysis includes the focus of the theory, the world view of the theorist, and research outcomes. A systematic approach to development of analytic criteria establishes the foundation for the next phase, evaluation or critique.

Theory Critique or Evaluation Theory evaluation or critique is the next step after theory analysis. The purpose of the evaluation phase is to assess the potential contribution of the theory to scientific knowledge. Evaluation involves judgments of the worth of the theory. Strengths and weaknesses of a theory are assessed by examining the outcomes of theory testing in reality and by comparing the theory with other criteria (Walker and Avant 1983 p. 10).

When we conduct a systematic evaluation, regardless of how objective we strive to be in our assessment, we must make subjective judgments about the value and structure of a model. Yet this process helps us draw conclusions about the model's validity and usability and about future steps in developing or refining the theory.

Meleis (1985) and Laudan (1977) see the critique as the final component of the three-step process: description, analysis, and critique. Critique is a critical examination of the nature and limitations of the theory according to preestablished standards or criteria.

Throughout this chapter, the term *theory evaluation model* is used to mean a "blueprint" for evaluating theory and includes the three-step process: description, analysis, and critique. We include Stevens's (1984) model for theory evaluation because it is easy to apply and can be used for all levels of theory.

Criteria for Judging a Theory

Stevens* presents one set of standards for theory evaluation. She advocates internal and external criticism. "Internal criticism deals with how theory components fit with each other. Internal criticism asks (given the premise that a theory assumes), does the theory logically follow? Do its pieces relate in a logical pattern" (p. 50)? The following four criteria are used to judge internal construction:

1. *Clarity* means that a theory is presented in such a way that the definitions of concepts and propositions and their relationships are easily understood. Glaser

---

*From B. Stevens, *Nursing Theory: Analysis, Application, Evaluation.* Boston: Little, Brown, 1984.

and Strauss (1967) emphasize the crucial nature of this criterion and call it a theory's "grab" for the practitioner or actor in the social world under investigation.

2. *Consistency* requires that the theory be consistent in the meaning of terms, interpretations, principles, and methods of reasoning (Stevens 1984). A term used in one part of the theory must mean the same thing when used later on in the theory; and if a phenomenon is interpreted one way, it should be interpreted with the same meaning throughout the theory.

3. *Logical development* demands that the reasoning process be logical and lead logically to conclusions. The premises for the argument must be true and logically yield the conclusions. For example, "All patients are sick," "All mentally ill people are sick," and therefore "All patients are mentally ill" is an *illogical* sequence. Here, the premise may be wrong (patients may not be sick, depending on the definition), and the conclusions are surely wrong, based on illogical thinking.

4. The *level of theory development* must be assessed to understand the theory in a context of knowledge. You will assess whether it is a conceptual analysis, or a descriptive theory, or a situation-relating or more advanced situation-producing theory.

The next six criteria refer to *external criticism*; that is, how does a particular theory relate to the world of people, health, environment, and nursing (the four key variables in most nursing theories)?

1. *Adequacy* refers to the ability of the theory to deal satisfactorily with the nurse scientist's perspective of nursing. There must be adequacy of principles, interpretations, and methods. Do you accept the basic principles that are the foundation of the theory? Does the theorist's perception or interpretation of nursing make sense and accurately mirror the real world? Does the method of the theory permit research, and if so what types of research are appropriate (deductive, philosophical)?

2. *Utility* requires that a theory be useful in education, research, or practice. Glaser and Strauss (1967) talk of "fit," which means essentially the same thing as utility. The concepts and propositions must "fit" the work world of the nurse and must be operationalized so that they can be applied and tested.

3. *Significance* refers to the requirement that a theory address issues basic and relevant to nursing and aim toward increasing nursing knowledge. The theory's significance should be obvious and should lead to further discovery of knowledge through research.

4. *Discrimination* requires that the theory clearly define its boundaries so that its relatedness to nursing is obvious. The theory must discriminate between what nursing is and what it isn't.

5. *Scope* is an indication of whether the theory has a narrow or broad focus. Earlier in this chapter you read about different levels of theory (from "abstracted empiricism" to "grand" and from "factor-isolating" to "situation-producing"), and you are aware that there is some disagreement over how broad the scope of a theory should be. However, most nurse scientists recognize the current need for theories of limited scope to guide practice decisions.

6. *Complexity* and *parsimony* are two sides of a coin. **Parsimony** is a property of a theory, meaning that it explains as much as possible with the fewest possible variables. This is sometimes called the *power* of a theory. A powerful theory is one that makes few assumptions and that clearly separates the critical variables from the diffuse background. Some scientists believe that in aiming for parsimony, one may miss the essence. Rather, one should strive for complexity because it examines the relationships among many variables. In fact, the nature of the subject matter should dictate to what degree a theory is complex or parsimonious (Stevens 1984).

Theoretical models can be classified as developmental, interaction, or systems. Thibodeau elaborates, saying "developmental models use life-span physiological, cognitive, and psychosocial theories to define the four assertive components (people, environment, health, nursing) of the nursing paradigm. Systems models use general systems theory as the basis for defining the four components. Interaction models have symbolic interaction and role theories as their base" (1983 p. 43). An eclectic model combines several types, offering a diversified perspective. As you read theories, evaluate and analyze the theoretical perspective and determine if they are consistent throughout.

Other nurse scientists (Duffey and Muhlenkamp 1974, Ellis 1968, Hardy 1978a, Johnson 1974) have proposed some similar and different criteria for theory evaluation. Any or all of these criteria offer a useful structure for you to evaluate any theoretical model for nursing. Two final points are important regarding the evaluation of theoretical models:

1. Recognize that both internal and external criticism are necessary for a thorough understanding of a nursing model.

2. Criticize a model only after you fully understand it, because *unbiased* criticism is the only fair and helpful criticism. To criticize a model because you intuitively don't like it or because your values are different from those inherent in it is not appropriate. Rather, view it for what it is, and use theoretical rather than emotional criteria for your evaluation. Chapter 6 offers some useful points about the art of criticism of a research study; these are equally applicable to nursing theory evaluation.

Developing a Theoretical Framework

We have discussed the major issues in theory building, presented several paradigms and theories from nursing and other disciplines, and outlined a process for theory evaluation. An important next step for you, as researcher, is making the link between the research and the theoretical perspective explicit in the study. This is the topic of this last section.

Regardless of how descriptive or exploratory the research approach might be, our very ability to formulate problems and ask questions stems from our ability to conceptualize. Our conceptualizations are made possible by the fact that we hold a particular world view or theoretical perspective. From that we derive the language to observe, describe, and explain phenomena. We first discuss key questions you need to answer before you can develop the theoretical perspective for the study.

Where To Start?

The approach you take in developing a theoretical framework or model for the research depends on a number of factors. How much research has been conducted in the area under study is one important factor, if we are to build scientific theories based on cumulative knowledge in a discipline. For example, much research has been conducted about this persistent problem: prevention of decubitus ulcers. The researcher who wishes to build on past research in decubitus ulcer care needs to conduct an extensive review of the literature from various fields to search for the best theory or model to guide the research.

You may wonder how a researcher who is planning to do a qualitative study in an area where little research has been conducted proceeds to place the study in theoretical perspective. This process of linking the theory and research is often difficult even for the experienced researcher. Regardless of approach, the goal is really trifold: to develop a linkage between the *problem conceptualization*, *measurement operations*, and *data interpretation*. As a researcher, these questions will guide you in formally explaining the relationship between the theory and research.

1. What is the nature and scope of the research aims: exploratory, descriptive, explanatory (correlational), or predictive (hypotheses)?

2. Did an existing theory or model serve as a heuristic device for generating the idea for the research (deductive approach)?

3. Is the aim of the research to test *existing concepts* or *relational statements* from a theory, model, or paradigm (deductive approach)?

4. Were study *concepts or relational statements derived* from an existing theory, model, or paradigm (deductive approach)?

5. Is the purpose of the research to describe phenomena and from those phenomena to develop a descriptive or explanatory theory (an inductive or grounded-theory approach)?

6. What is the world view of the researcher?

Finding the Best Approach

After answering the preceding questions, you should have knowledge about the approach to be used (inductive or deductive), the level of the research question, the amount of past research on the problem posed for study, and the world view of the researcher. Now that you have a perspective on how to proceed, you should, if you have conducted an extensive review of the literature and talked with researchers in the area, have a fairly good idea of whether you will use a theory, a framework, a conceptual map or a paradigm from nursing or another field. In most cases, if the research design is descriptive, then the level of theory is factor-isolating (descriptive or exploratory). For correlational or experimental studies, a review of past research in the area usually helps you locate a prescriptive-level theory or theoretical model of "best fit" to guide conceptualization, measurement, and interpretation of findings.

Theory Testing

If the purpose of the research is to test concepts, constructs, or propositions from a theory, theoretical model, or paradigm, then the task of developing a theoretical framework is fairly straightforward: The theoretical and operational definitions of concepts must be linked to valid and reliable measurement operations and empirical referents. Regardless of the source of the theory, the goal is the same. In theory testing, the researcher deduces axioms and develops propositions that can be empirically tested. The theory or model is never tested directly, but the propositions or hypotheses derived from it are. Through this process the theoretical propositions are continually subjected to testing until some piece of evidence cannot be explained by the theory but can be explained by a new theory that also accounts for previous findings. The tentative nature of theories is recognized, and new theories are proposed in response to the empirical evidence.

For a theory to be considered testable, it must have the following components:

1. concepts that describe the empirical world

2. definitions of concepts (constitutive and operational)

3. constructs or propositions

4. links among the concepts and constructs that explain and predict phenomena

An example of theory testing is presented in Box 9–6. Weaver (1987) used factor analysis to test the construct "self-care agency" from Orem's (1985) self-care deficit theory in nursing.

Fawcett and Downs (1986) explain the deductive process of developing axioms, theorems, and hypotheses. Propositions that represent the starting points for deduction are called axioms, premises, or postulates; they are accepted as a given in a theory and do not have to be proved or tested. A proposition that is deduced from two or more axioms is called a theorem or conclusion. A theorem is a supposition whose logical and empirical adequacy must be determined. The transitive rule of relationships is used to deduce a theorem from axioms (p. 35).

Box 9–6   Perceived Self-Care Agency: A LISREL Factor Analysis of Bickel and Hanson's Questionnaire

Author: Michael T. Weaver (1987)

Source: *Nursing Research*, vol. 36, pp. 381–387

Abstract: The psychometric properties of Bickel and Hanson's Perceived Self-Care Agency Questionnaire (PSCAQ) were examined using a LISREL confirmatory factor analysis approach in a sample of 462 noninstitutionalized adults. Findings indicated that the factor structure of the PSCAQ is significantly different from that described by Bickel (1982) and does not appear to conform to the expected self-care power component structure. These findings call into question the construct validity of the PSCAQ as a measure of self-care agency in noninstitutionalized adults. It should be used only with extreme caution, if at all, for testing the self-care deficit theory.

Theoretical Framework: A central construct of the self-care deficit theory of nursing is self-care agency (SCA). Defined as a person's ability to engage in self-care, that is, perform actions to meet individual health care needs, SCA provides both rationale for and guidance of nursing interventions.

Discussion: As with any psychometric evaluation, observed measurement discrepancies may result from problems inherent in the measure itself, the theoretical basis from which the measure is derived, or a combination of the two. From the results of this study, one cannot assign culpability. From a theoretical standpoint, mixing concepts within a construct makes it difficult, if not impossible, to produce a clean measure and evaluate the constructual underpinnings. Alternatives to the PSCAQ (e.g., professional judgment, measures of SCA outcome, actual self-care practices observed) may be more appropriate for testing and refining self-care deficit theory concepts than the PSCAQ.

The format used to express sets of deductive propositions is shown here:

Axiom₁ If x is related to y, and
Axiom₂ if y is related to z,
Theorem then x is related to z.

Using this form of deduction, the researcher can develop hypotheses in this manner:

Axiom₁ If x is related to y, and
Axiom₂ if x is defined by x', and
Axiom₃ if y is defined by y'
Hypothesis then x' is related to y'.

The example below demonstrates the use of the deductive method to derive theorems and hypotheses:

Axiom₁ If self-actualization is inversely related to anxiety, and
Axiom₂ if there is a relationship between anxiety and depression,
Theorem then, there is an inverse relationship between self actualization and both anxiety and depression.

Axioms₃₋₅ and the following hypothesis identify the empirical indicators for the concepts that will be studied in the research:

Axiom₃ If self-actualization is measured by the Personal Orientation Inventory, and
Axiom₄ if anxiety is measured by the State-Trait Inventory, and
Axiom₅ if depression is measured by the Beck Depression Scale,
Hypothesis then, the higher the scores on the Personal Orientation Inventory, the lower the scores on the State-Trait Inventory and the Beck Depression Scale; and, the converse will hold.

This process, along with careful analysis of past research, aids the researcher in arriving at logically deduced hypotheses that can be submitted to testing. Fawcett and Downs point out that "it is unlikely that any one test of a hypothesis or theory will provide the definitive evidence needed to establish empirical adequacy" (1986 p. 65). Therefore, empirical evidence from all studies should be considered; the greater the number of tests that yield supporting evidence, the more credible the theory.

Theory Construction (Generation) or Grounded Theory

The method of induction is used in this approach to theory construction. The researcher moves by logical thought from fact to theory by means of a proposition stated as an empirical generalization. The process may be diagramed in this way:

RESEARCH

    FACT

        ↓ Empirically verifiable observations; the mind
           organizes the facts into concepts.

    PROPOSITION

        ↓ Statement of the interrelationships observed
           among the concepts (empirical generalization).

    EMPIRICAL GENERALIZATION

        ↓ Statement of the observed relationships between
           concepts.

    THEORY

        General statement that explains the
        interrelationships among propositions.

The method of grounded theory is explained more fully in Chapter 13. We include it here to show the process of linking the theory with the research. Numerous examples of the inductive approach to theory construction can be found in the literature. A few of these examples are illustrated in this chapter. See Box 9–7 for Hutchinson's (1987) grounded-theory study of chemical dependency in nurses. See Box 9–8 for Mishel and Murdaugh's (1987) grounded theory of family adjustment to heart transplantation. For a study of the bereaved elderly by Rigdon et al (1987) using the dialectic approach of hermeneutics, see Box 9–9.

Theory Derivation

Another approach to development of middle-range practice theories is that of theory derivation. The process of theory derivation uses analogy to obtain explanations or predictions about a phenomenon in one field from the explanations or predictions in another field (Walker and Avant 1983). There are five steps in the process of theory derivation:

1. immersion in the literature concerning the phenomenon/problems of interest in the primary field (field 2, nursing) and evaluating the suitability of current theories for explaining the phenomenon

2. analyzing the literature from other disciplines (field 1) to identify possible analogies

3. choosing a parent theory from field 1 to transpose and reformulate to explain the phenomenon of interest in field 2

4. identifying the content or structure from the parent theory that will be used in field 2

Box 9–7   Toward Self-Integration: The Recovery Process of Chemically Dependent Nurses

Author: Sally A. Hutchinson (1987)

Source: *Nursing Research*, vol. 36, pp. 339–343

Abstract: This qualitative field research explored and described the process of recovery for chemically dependent nurses. Data collection methods included participant observation in a chemically dependent nurses' self-help group for one year and in-depth interviews with 20 chemically dependent nurses who were in the process of recovery. Data analysis was done according to the grounded-theory method. In accordance with this method, a substantive theory was proposed that viewed the recovery process as a move from self-annihilation to self-integration. Stages and phases of self-integration are presented.

Grounded Theory:

Figure 1. The Substantive Theory: Major Theoretical Constructs

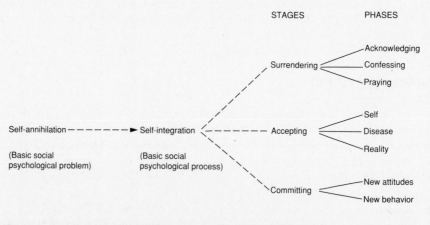

5. modifying the concepts or structure from the parent theory and restating the concepts in the form of relational statements or propositions to derive a theory for the primary field, nursing.

Box 9–8   Family Adjustment to Heart Transplantation: Redesigning the Dream

Authors: Merle H. Mishel and Carolyn L. Murdaugh (1987)

Source: *Nursing Research*, vol. 36, pp. 332–338

Abstract: The processes family members of heart transplant recipient use to manage the unpredictability evoked by the need for and receipt of heart transplantation were explored. Twenty family members were theoretically sampled using the grounded-theory approach. Three separate family support groups, each of 12 weeks duration, provided data for constant comparative analysis. Redesigning the dream was identified as the integrative theme in the substantive theory that described how family members gradually modify their beliefs about organ transplantation and develop attitudes and beliefs to meet the challenge of living with continual unpredictability. The theory consists of three concepts—immersion, passage, and negotiation—which parallel the stages of waiting for a donor, hospitalization, and recovery.

Grounded Theory:

Figure 1. Substantive Theory—Redesigning the Dream

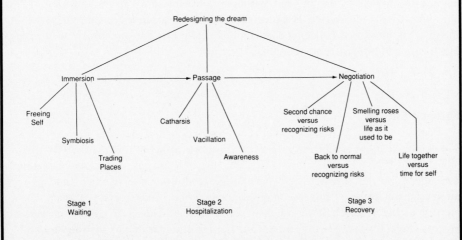

Box 9–9   Toward a Theory of Helpfulness for the Elderly Bereaved: An Invitation to a New Life

Authors: Imogene S. Rigdon, Bonnie C. Clayton, and Margaret Diamond (1987)

Source: *Advances in Nursing Science*, vol. 9, pp. 32–43

Abstract: The purpose of this study was to generate a theory of helpfulness for the elderly bereaved. The theory is grounded in data from responses of 30 participants concerning what advice they would give others who have lost a spouse and how others were helpful to them. Participants responded during six interviews following death of their spouses. A content analysis of responses was the basis of a dialectical theory of helpfulness: *An Invitation to a New Life.*

Dialectic Approach to Theory Development: The authors maintained that the issue of personal meaning cannot be ignored; the interpretive mode, of which hermeneutics is central, was used since nursing was viewed as a human science and bereavement is a subjective experience. Therefore, the bereavement study followed the canons of hermeneutic interpretation.

Wewers and Lenz (1987) demonstrate the use of theory derivation in their study of relapse among ex-smokers (Box 9–10), using an analogy from Cronkite and Moos's theory of recovery after alcohol abuse.

How does theory derivation differ from borrowed theory? Derivation is different in that it involves an alteration of the content or structure of an existing theory, whereas borrowed theory is used without modification. Wewers and Lenz (1987) note that theory derivation is especially useful when data are limited or when a theorist has identified concepts that may be related to the phenomenon of interest but has not identified their relational structure.

Theory Fitting

The process of theory fitting is somewhat more difficult to describe. In this approach, the researcher first formulates the research purpose or research questions. The ideas for the research may have originated from the practice field or from interactions with practitioners or colleagues. Then, the researcher becomes immersed in the research literature and searches for a theory to guide the research process. Selecting the theory, model, or framework that makes for the "best fit" is difficult in that it requires an extensive search of the literature and some understanding of theoretical progress in nursing and other fields. It also requires that you identify your own world view and belief system.

Box 9–10   Relapse among Ex-Smokers: An Example of Theory Derivation

Authors: Mary E. Wewers and Elizabeth R. Lenz (1987)

Source: *Advances in Nursing Science*, vol. 9, pp. 44–53

Abstract: Theory derivation, the use of analogous concepts from other disciplines to derive theory about a particular phenomenon, has been described as an effective strategy for building nursing theory, especially where existing theory bases are limited. This article provides a detailed, step-by-step description of how the theory derivation process was used to develop a theory of smoking relapse from an analogous theory of recovery after alcohol abuse. Empirical testing revealed partial support for the derived theory.

Derived Theory: The Cronkite and Moos theory of recovery after alcohol abuse was selected as the most appropriate parent theory since it had been tested, and each of the six factors had been studied separately in smoking research and put forth as a possible determinant of relapse. Finally, the model incorporated a multivariate structure deemed desirable for a theory of smoking relapse.

Next, scrutinize the research purpose and the research aims or questions. From those, explicate the major concepts of study. What is the level—descriptive, exploratory, explanatory, or predictive—of the research questions posed? Begin to identify the particular language used: What major concepts comprise the research questions, and how do they fit nursing's metaparadigm? Based on that, begin to determine what existing models or theories come to mind. Do the major research concepts fit an existing nursing paradigm, such as that of Orem or Rogers? Ask if perhaps an earlier exposure to a paradigm or theory served as a stimulus for the research or guided the development of the research questions. What propositional statements or hypotheses can be derived at this point?

At this juncture, you may be able to place the research questions within an appropriate paradigm or theoretical framework. Recall that, depending on the degree of past research in the area, you may have to construct your own theoretical framework or conceptual map to guide the research. There is a common misconception that only nursing models can be used to guide the research. Because of this misconception, many researchers fall into the trap of trying to force research questions into an existing framework or model, resulting in two undesirable outcomes: (1) the research questions are revised and retrofitted to the theory, causing the researcher to deviate from the original purpose or (2) research aims are not logically consistent with the theory or model, and thus the theory or framework cannot serve to guide data collection and interpretation of results. Box 9–11 depicts the process of identifying the concepts, operational definitions, and empirical referents of a research study. This process will help you build a conceptual map to guide your research. For more on this process, see Fawcett and Downs (1986) or Moody (in press).

Atheoretical Research?

Abstracted empiricism (Mills 1959) implies that the empirical phenomena or facts are in isolation from any theory. For example, some nurses go about their practice

---

Box 9–11   Preexisting Correlates of Hospital Stress

Author: B. Volicer (1977)

Source: *Nursing Research*, vol. 26, pp. 408–415.

Abstract: The purpose of this study was to "identify" (test) the relationship between hospital stress and life stress, seriousness of illness, prior hospitalizations, and demographics in a sample of 468 medical/surgical patients. Other study variables were age, education level, marital status, and gender.

The linkage of concepts to operational definitions and empirical indicators is shown below:

Concepts (refer to the properties of a phenomenon)	Hospital stress	Life stress		Seriousness of illness	
Operational Definitions (state how concepts are measured)	Hospital Stress Rating Scale (HSRS)	Social Readjustment Rating Scale (SRRS)		Serious Illness Rating Scale	Patient's perception of pain
Empirical Indicators (actual instrument or methods for measurement)	Patient's *mean* rank score for all events patient reported since hospitalization	*Sum* of stress value rating of life stress events for 1 year prior to hospitalization.	Sum of stress value rating of life stress events for 2 years prior to hospitalization	*Rating* of diagnosis on rank scale from least serious (dandruff) to most serious (leukemia)	Patient's *rating* of pain or discomfort on scale of 1–100, where 0 is no pain
				# of previous hospitalizations	
				# Years since last hospitalization	

without theory to guide them, functioning instead on the basis of facts or beliefs. In some hospitals, nurses use ice before giving heparin injections because they believe ice should decrease bruising since it causes vasoconstriction. In other hospitals, nurses don't use ice, either because they have never thought to use it or perhaps because they believe that vasoconstriction prevents the absorption of heparin, thereby encouraging bruising. These nurses are basing their care on authority or tradition rather than on theoretical protocols, derived from research. Jacox (1974) points out that the underlying assumption of the abstracted empiricist approach to theory development is that the accumulation of many pieces of data will ultimately and clearly suggest relationships among the data. She writes: "This is analogous to a collection of bricklayers, each making a brick in isolation from other bricklayers, and with no blueprint to follow. They throw these bricks together into a large pile, confident that, somehow, a house will emerge" (p. 11).

To prevent isolated fact collecting, research should be directly linked to either nursing theory or theory from other disciplines. If the state of knowledge or a particular study question makes this impossible, then it behooves a researcher (student, faculty member, or practicing nurse) to do level 1 studies (see Chapter 8) that aim at descriptions of subjects relevant to nursing. Only in this way can nurses formulate the theoretical base necessary to direct practice decisions. Other nurse scientists advocate the idea of groups of nurses working on research problems from different perspectives, and with different methods, so as to expand the knowledge base; or a nursing career can be built around a narrow focus, which over time yields depth. Anderson's work from 1975 to 1983 with sucking and newborns is an example of this in-depth approach. Speciality groups (cardiac care nurses, psychiatric nurses) in some areas can collaborate and specify specialty-linked research priorities that, when linked with theory, provide a scientific base for practice.

Summary

This chapter has emphasized the interdependence of nursing theory, research, and practice. Dickoff and his associates (1968a, b) offer a meaningful model and summary statement: "Theory is born in practice, is refined in research, and must and can return to practice if research is to be other than a draining-off of energy from the main business of nursing and theory more than idle speculation" (p. 415).

Practice ———————— Research

Practice ———————— Theorizing

Research ———————— Theorizing

Developing a body of knowledge about nursing and for nursing practice is critical if we are to move from a discipline based on tradition and conventional wisdoms to a discipline based on science. Placing nursing studies within the context of our evolving theoretical base is essential to that goal.

Guidelines for Critique

- Is the theoretical perspective of the research made explicit in the review of literature? If the research is atheoretical, was it appropriate?

- According to Silva's (1986) criteria, what was the purpose of the theory in relation to the research? Based on your assessment, was the theoretical perspective appropriate and relevant to the research, or was a theory or model "thrown in for good measure" and not linked to the research aims?

- Is the research designed to test a theory? If so, what type theory (model, paradigm, grand, middle-range, descriptive, explanatory, predictive, and so on)? Is the theory from nursing or another discipline? How much empirical evidence or empirical adequacy exists for the theory?

- Was the theory designed to derive a theory? If so, what parent theory was used, and was it used appropriately?

- Does the research report successsfully link the theory and the research?

- Does the research suggest additional areas for theory building or theory testing? If so, were the suggestions appropriate? If not, what recommendations would you make?

SUMMARY OF KEY IDEAS AND TERMS

✓ A *theory* is a set of interrelated constructs (concepts), definitions, or propositions that provide a view of reality for the purpose of describing, explaining, predicting or controlling the phenomena of interest.

✓ *Concepts* are the building blocks of theories, and may be concrete or abstract.

✓ A *conceptual framework* or model includes concepts or propositions that essentially structure or guide the conduct of the research.

✓ A *construct* is a group of concepts that are derived from a combination of academic and clinical knowledge and contribute meaning and scope to a theory.

✓ *Propositions* describe the relationship of two or more concepts.

✓ The empirical-theoretical continuum demonstrates the relationship between what is observed empirically and what is described theoretically.

✓ A *model* is a structural, pictorial, diagrammatic or mathematical depiction of structural or functional relationships.

✓ *Conceptual mapping* provides a theoretical orientation for understanding the relationship among variables in a study.

✓ Types of theories include grand, middle range, and abstracted empiricism. *Grand theories* are global and vague and attempt to explain almost everything about a subject. *Middle-range theories* focus on an empirical area, have clear propositions from which hypotheses can be derived, and have implications for practice. *Abstracted empiricism* focuses only on empirical phenomena, i.e., facts in isolation from theory.

✓ Looking at levels of theory is another way to categorize theories. *Factor-isolating theories* (factor-naming theories) involve the identification and classification of concepts or variables. *Factor-relating theories* (situation-depicting theories) relate factors to each other. *Situation-relating theories* (predictive and promoting or inhibiting theories) allow predictions that if *A* happens, *B* happens, and can suggest what factors influence the causal relationship and in what way. *Situation-producing* theory is prescriptive theory.

✓ According to Ellis, theories serve four purposes: (1) theory allows us to distinguish fact from pseudofact; (2) they help synthesize facts from many fields; (3) theoretical knowledge gives direction to practice; (4) theory acts as a framework for storing knowledge available in the literature.

✓ Prior to the 1980s, most nursing research was conducted without a theoretical structure. Rather, theories from other disciplines were used, or the researcher used no theoretical framework but rather chose specific research instruments to collect data on some variable.

✓ *Paradigms* specify the type of research questions to be asked and the appropriate methods for answering them. A *metaparadigm* is the most global world view held by a discipline.

✓ Nursing has multiple paradigms to guide practice and research. Nurse scientists continue to develop useful paradigms to guide nursing practice and research.

✓ *Paradigm-transcending research* has the goal of developing new theories and methods. Nursing needs more of these studies that explain and predict empirical phenomena relevant to our discipline.

✓ Nursing theory is both borrowed from many disciplines and unique in that some theories are derived systematically and directly from nursing practice.

✓ Nurses need to encourage pluralism in research methods and in theory testing and theory generation.

✓ A theory may be evaluated on four criteria that refer to the internal construction of a theory: (1) clarity; (2) consistency; (3) logical development; and (4) level of theory development.

✓ A theory may be evaluated on six criteria that refer to the external criticism of a theory: (1) adequacy; (2) validity; (3) significance; (4) discrimination; (5) scope; and (6) complexity/parsimony.

✓ Theoretical models can be classified as developmental, systems, or interaction. Developmental models use life span theories to define the four components of the nursing paradigm—people, environment, health, and nursing. Systems models use general systems theory, and interaction models are based in symbolic interaction and role theories.

✓ Conceptual models from nursing and from other disciplines can be used to guide nursing practice and nursing research.

✓ Nursing theory is dependent on nursing practice, practice is dependent on theory, and research is dependent on practice.

References

Abdellah F et al: *Patient Centered Approaches to Nursing.* New York: Macmillan, 1960.

Anderson G: Infant colic: A possible solution. *Am J Maternal Child Nurs* 1983; 8:185.

Anderson G: A preliminary report: Severe respiratory distress in two newborn lambs with recovery following nonnutritive sucking, *J Nurse Midwifery* 1975; 20:20–28.

Artinian B: Conceptual mapping: Development of the strategy. *West J Nurs Res* 1982; 4:379–393.

Beckstrand J: The notion of a practice theory and the relationship of scientific and ethical knowledge to practice. *Res Nurs Health* 1978; 1:131–136.

Beckstrand J: A critique of several conceptions of practice theory in nursing. *Res Nurs Health*, 1980; 3:69–79.

Brown M: Social theory in geriatric nursing research. *Nurs Res* 1968; 17:213–217.

Bush H: Models for nursing. *Advances Nurs Sci* 1979; 1: 13–21.

Carnap R: *Philosophical Foundations of Physics.* Gardner M (editor). New York: Basic Books, 1966.

Chinn P, Jacobs M: Theory development in nursing. Tape series. Denton: Nursing Sciences Tape Library, Texas Woman's University, 1987.

Clark P, Clark M: Therapeutic touch: Is there a scientific basis for the practice? *Nurs Res* 1984; 33:37–41.

Collins R, Fielder J: Beckstrand's concept of practice and theory: A critique. *Res Nurs Health* 1981; 4:317–321.

Cox CL, Roghmann KJ: Empirical test of the interaction model of client health behavior. *Res Nurs Health* 1984; 7:275–278.

Crawford G et al: Evolving issues in theory development. *Nurs Outlook* May 1979; 27:346–351.

Cronenwett L, Brickman P: Models of helping and coping in childbirth. *Nurs Res* 1983; 32:84–88.

Dickoff J, James P: A theory of theories: A position paper. *Nurs Res* May/June 1968; 17:197–203.

Dickoff J et al: Theory in a practice discipline: Part I Practice oriented theory. *Nurs Res* 1968a; 17:415–435.

Dickoff J et al: Theory in a practice discipline: Part II Practice oriented research. *Nurs Res* 1968b; 17:545–554.

Dickoff J, James P: *Outline: Theoretical pluralism as a direction for a practice discipline* (Unpublished handout). Presented at the 1986 Nursing Theory Congress, Toronto, Ryerson School of Nursing, 1986.

Diers D: *Research in Nursing Practice.* Philadelphia: Lippincott, 1979.

Donaldson S, Crowley D: The discipline of nursing. *Nurs Outlook* February 1978; 26:118–120.

Dubin R: *Theory Building*, rev ed. New York: Free Press, 1978.

Duffey M, Muhlenkamp A: A framework for theory analysis. *Nurs Outlook* 1974; 22:571.

Ellis R: Characteristics of significant theories. *Nurs Res* May/June 1968; 17:217–222.

Erikson E: *Childhood and Society.* New York: Norton, 1963.

Estes WK: Growth and function of mathematical models for learning. In: Marx M (editor), *Theoris in Contemporary Psychology.* New York: Macmillan, 1963.

Falco S: Faye Abdellah. In *Nursing Theories.* Nursing Theories Conference Group (editor). Englewood Cliffs, N.J.: Prentice-Hall, 1980.

Fawcett J: The relationship between theory and research: A double helix. *Advances Nurs Sci* 1978; 1:49–62.

Fawcett J: The "What" of theory development. Pages 17–33 in: *Theory Developments: What? Why? How?* New York: National League for Nursing, 1978b.

Fawcett J: *Analysis and Evaluation of Conceptual Models of Nursing.* Philadelphia: F. A. Davis, 1984.

Fawcett J, Downs F: *The Relationship of Theory and Research*. Norwalk, Conn.: Appleton-Century-Crofts, 1986.

Feyerabend P: *Against Method*. London: Verso Press, 1975.

Fitzpatrick et al: *Nursing Models and Their Psychiatric Mental Health Applications*. Bowie, Md.: Robert J Brady, 1982.

Flaskerud J, Holleran E: Areas of agreement in nursing theory development. *Adv Nurs Sci* 1980; 3:1–7.

Floyd J: Rhythm theory: Relationship to nursing conceptual models. In Fitzpatrick J et al: *Nursing Models and Their Psychiatric Mental Health Applications*. Bowie, Md.: Robert J Brady, 1982.

Forsyth G: Analysis of the concept of empathy: Illustrations of one approach. *Adv Nurs Sci* 1980; 2:33–42.

Glaser B, Strauss A: *Awareness of Dying*. Chicago: Aldine, 1965.

Glaser B, Strauss A: *Discovery of Grounded Theory*. Chicago: Aldine, 1967.

Glaser B, Strauss A: *Time for dying*. Chicago: Aldine, 1968.

Gudmundsen AM: Conceptualization of the Neuman model for nursing practice by nursing students. Pages 265–266 in Neuman B: *The Neuman Systems Model*. Norwalk, Conn.: Appleton-Century-Crofts, 1982.

Hardy M: Evaluating nursing theory. In: *Theory Development: What? Why? How?* New York: National League for Nursing, 1978a.

Hardy M: Perspectives in nursing theory. *Adv Nurs Sci* 1978b; 1:37–48.

Henderson V: *The Nature of Nursing*. New York: Macmillan, 1966.

Henkel R: *Tests of Significance*. Beverly Hills: Sage, 1976.

Honigman J: The personal approach in cultural anthropological research. *Curr Anthro* 1976; 17:243–261.

Hutchinson S: Humor: A link to life. In: *Current Issues and Trends in Psychiatric Nursing*. Kneisl C, Wilson H (editors). St. Louis: CV Mosby, 1976.

Hutchinson S: *Survival Practices of Rescue Workers: Hidden Dimensions of Watchful Readiness*. Lanham, Md.: University Press of America, 1983.

Hutchinson S: Creating meaning out of horror. *Nurs Outlook* 1984; 32:86–90.

Hutchinson S: The hospital of broken dreams: A systematic investigation of a moribund psychiatric hospital. *Issues Mental Health Nurs* November 1984b.

Hutchinson S: Toward self-integration: The recovery process of chemically dependent nurses. *Nurs Res* 1987; 36, 339–343.

Jacox A: Theory construction in nursing: An overview. *Nurs Res* 1974; 23:4–13.

Johnson D: Development of theory: A requisite for nursing as a primary health profession. *Nurs Res* September/October 1974; 23:372–377.

Kaplan A: *The Conduct of Inquiry*. San Francisco: Chandler, 1964.

Kerlinger N: *Foundations of Behavioral Research*. New York: Holt, Rinehart & Winston, 1973.

Kim HS: *The Nature of Theoretical Thinking in Nursing*. Norwalk, Conn.: Appleton-Century-Crofts, 1983.

King I: The "why" of theory development. *Theory Development: What? Why? How?* New York: National League for Nursing, 1978.

King I: *Toward a Theory for Nursing*. New York: John Wiley, 1981.

Kuhn TS: *The Structure of Scientific Revolutions*. Chicago: University of Chicago Press, 1970.

Laudan L: *Progress and its Problems: Toward a Theory of Scientific Growth*. Berkeley: University of California Press, 1977.

Levine M: The four conservation principles of nursing. *Nurs Forum* 1967; 6:45–59.

Levine M: Holistic nursing. *Nurs Clin North Am* 1971; 6:253–264.

Meleis A et al: Toward scholarliness in doctoral dissertations: An analytical model. *Res Nurs Health* 1980; 3:115–124.

Meleis A: *Theoretical Nursing: Development and Progress*. Philadelphia: Lippincott, 1985.

Mercer R: The process of maternal role attainment over the first year. *Nurs Res* 1985; 34, 198–203.

Merton R: *Social Theory and Social Structure*. New York: Free Press, 1968.

Mills CW: *The Social Imagination*. New York: Oxford University Press, 1959

Mishel M, Murdaugh M: Family adjustment to heart transplantation: Redesigning the dream. *Nurs Res* 1987; 36, 332–338.

Moody LE: *Advancing Nursing Theory Through Research*. In press.

Moody LE: Wilson M: *Analysis of a Decade of Nursing Practice Research*. Gainesville, Fla.: Summary grant report to the University of Florida, Division of Sponsored Research, 1987.

Neuman B: *The Neuman Systems Model*. Norwalk, Conn.: Appleton-Lange, 1982.

Nightingale F: *Notes on Nursing: What It Is and What It Is Not*. Philadelphia: Lippincott, 1946.

Norris C: Restlessness: A nursing phenomenon in search of meaning. *Nurs Outlook* February 1975; 23:103–107.

Orem D: *Nursing: Concepts of Practice*, 2nd ed. New York: McGraw-Hill, 1985.

Orlando IJ: *The Dynamic Nurse-Patient Relationship*. New York: Putnam, 1961.

Parse RR: *Man-Living-Health: A Theory of Nursing*. New York: John Wiley & Sons, 1981.

Parse RR: *Nursing Science Major Paradigms, Theories and Critiques*. Philadelphia: W. B. Saunders, 1987.

Parse RR, Coyne AB, Smith MJ: *Nursing Research: Qualitative Methods*. Bowie, Md.: Brady Communications, 1985.

Peplau H: *Interpersonal Relations in Nursing*. New York: Putnam, 1952.

Piaget J: *The Growth of Logical Thinking from Childhood to Adolescence*. New York: Basic Books, 1958.

Platt JR: Strong inference. *Science* 1964; 146:347–353.

Putnam P: Conceptual approach to nursing theory. *Nurs Sci* December 1965; 430–442.

Rawnsley M: The concept of privacy. *Adv Nurs Sci* 1980; 2:25–31.

Reilly D: Why a conceptual framework? *Nurs Outlook* September 1975; 23:556–567.

Rigdon IS, Clayton BC, Diamond M: Toward a theory of helpfulness for the elderly bereaved: an invitation to a new life. *Adv Nurs Sci.* 1987; 9, 32–43.

Rogers M: *An Introduction to the Theoretical Basis of Nursing*. Philadelphia: FA Davis, 1983.

Rogers M: *The Second Post-Masters' Nursing Conference*. Savannah, Ga., April 1984.

Rogers M: Roger's science of unitary human beings. In: RR Parse, *Nursing Science: Major Paradigms, Theories, and Critiques*. Philadelphia: WB Saunders, 1987.

Roy Sister C: *Introduction to Nusing: An Adaptation Model*, 2nd ed. Englewood Cliffs, N.J.: Prentice-Hall, 1984.

Silva M: Research testing nursing theory: State of the art. *Adv Nurs Sci* 1986; 96: 1–11.

Stern P: Affiliating in stepfather families: Teachable strategies leading to stepfather-child friendship. *West J Nurs Res* 1982; 4:74–83.

Stevens B: *Nursing Theory: Analysis, Application, Evaluation*. Boston: Little, Brown, 1984.

Suppe F, Jacox A: Philosophy of science and the development of nursing theory. In: Werley H, Fitzpatrick J (editors), *Annual Review of Nursing Research*. Boston: Springer, 1985.

The Nursing Theories Conference Group: *Nursing Theories: The Base for Professional Nursing Practice*. Englewood Cliffs, N.J.: Prentice-Hall, 1980.

Thibodeau J: *Nursing: Analysis and Evaluation*. Monterey, Calif.: Wadsworth Health Sciences Division, 1983.

Torgerson S: *Theory and Methods of Scaling*. New York: Wiley, 1958.

Toulmin S: *Human Understanding: The Collective Use and Evolution of Concepts*. Princeton, N.J.: Princeton Univ Press, 1977.

Volicer B: Preexisting correlates of hospital stress. *Nurs Res* 1977; 26, 408–415.

Wald F, Leonard R: Towards development of nursing practice theory. *Nurs Res* Fall 1964; 13:309–313.

Walker LO, Avant KC: *Strategies for Theory Construction in Nursing*. Norwalk, Conn.: Appleton-Century-Crofts, 1983.

Weaver M: Perceived self-care agency: A LISREL factor analysis of Bickel and Hanson's questionnaire. *Nurs Res* 1987; 36:381–387.

Wewers ME, Lenz ER: Relapse among ex-smokers: An example of theory derivation. *Adv Nus Sci* 1987; 9, 44–53.

Whall A: Congruence between existing theories of family functioning and nursing theories. *Adv Nurs Sci* 1980; 3:59–67.

Wilson H: *Deinstitutionalized Residential Care of the Mentally Disordered: The Soteria House Approach*. New York: Grune and Stratton, 1982.

Wilson H, Kneisl C: *Psychiatric Nursing*, 3rd ed. Menlo Park, Calif.: Addison-Wesley, 1988.

Yura H, Torres G: *Today's Conceptual Frameworks Within Baccalaureate Nursing Programs*. NLN publication #15-1558. New York: National League for Nursing, 1975, pp. 17–25.

C H A P T E R

10

The Selection and Development of Psychosocial Instruments

DIANE R. LAROCHELLE

Chapter Objectives

After reading this chapter the student should be able to:

- Identify sources where existing psychosocial instruments can be located

- Discuss the criteria for the selection of psychosocial instruments

- Discuss the use of psychosocial instruments in relation to the nursing process

- Decide when the development of a new psychosocial instrument is necessary

- Describe the instrument development process

- Explain the concepts of reliability and validity as they relate to instrument development

- Discuss the reasons for field-testing an instrument

- Describe the elements to look for in a good test item

- Discuss the advantages and disadvantages of each of the following rating scales: graphic, Likert, and semantic differential

- Explain the relationship of data coding and data cleaning to the format of the instrument.

There is no doubt about it: measurement works when the instruments work, and when you have a fairly clear idea of what is being measured, and when you know what to do with the numbers when they tumble out. (Lewis Thomas 1983)

In This Chapter . . .

Measurement in nursing, as in the other health and social sciences, provides the means for quantifying human behavior. Nurses have always recognized the value of identifying psychosocial variables and relating them to the patient's medical condition to obtain a complete assessment of the individual and his or her relationship to the environment and to others. What is new and different is that nurses are now systematically investigating the impact of psychosocial factors on health and illness through formal research. These investigations use either existing or newly designed psychosocial measures (instruments) that provide quantitative data on phenomena of concern to nurses.

Measurement of psychosocial variables is an extremely difficult process (Cunningham 1986, Kerlinger 1979). Psychological characteristics and the social behavior of human beings are so complex that numerical indexes fail to describe them adequately, and results may even be misleading. Yet, without measurement, there would be no universal language for describing phenomena, objects, and events. There would also be no reliable means of comparing individuals or groups on variables of interest. The assignment of numbers to variables (phenomena, objects, and events) according to predetermined rules makes it possible to quantify them in a uniform way. It also then becomes possible to determine the relationships that exist between variables as well as the magnitude of those relationships. Statistical tests can be applied to determine if significant differences exist between individuals and groups on the variables measured.

A major priority for nurse researchers is the identification and development of appropriate psychosocial instruments (tests and self-report measures) needed for research on nurse, client, and health system behavior (Ventura, Hinshaw, and Atwood 1981) and for clinical and administrative decision making. Use of instruments for the collection of relevant data, as opposed to other types of data-collection methods (e.g., direct observation), is advantageous because they permit the systematic collection of data in a controlled way. Also, instruments can be administered efficiently to large numbers of subjects and are objective, to the degree that they do not admit individual interpretation. Finally, psychosocial instruments provide empirical data that can be subjected to statistical analyses prior to decision making, thus enhancing one's ability to draw valid conclusions based on the significance of the data.

Instrument development is becoming a frequent practice among nurse researchers. Yet few of the psychosocial instruments developed by nurses meet the strict criteria for reliability and validity established by experts in the field of measurement. Thus, we must rely on established instruments from other disciplines for some studies. This reliance is quite appropriate and necessary if the instrument precisely measures the phenomenon of interest to nurses. However, it is inappropriate to use an instrument just because it is readily available. It is true that the development of quality instruments is a lengthy process that requires expertise in measurement theory (Allen and Yen 1979, Nunnally 1978), research design, and statistics. However, even novice researchers can develop a valid and reliable tool if they follow the major steps in the process systematically and meticulously.

One of the major decisions in every research project is which instruments to use. The goal is to obtain the most precise measurements of the identified variables with either existing or newly developed tools. The purpose of this chapter, therefore, is twofold: first, to present guidelines for selecting appropriate existing psychosocial instruments from nursing and other fields and, second, to describe the essential steps in developing psychosocial instruments. Since the concepts presented in each of these sections overlap, those researchers choosing an existing instrument will find the material on instrument development helpful in obtaining a better understanding of the properties of instruments (e.g., predictive validity). Researchers about to develop an instrument will also be interested in the first section on criteria for evaluation, because these are the identical criteria by which their instruments will be judged.

Psychosocial Testing: A Chronology

Psychosocial testing is essentially a twentieth-century phenomenon. Its development has its roots in the development of psychology as a science during an era when objectivity and precision of measurement differentiated science from non-science (Cunningham 1986). To gain recognition from established disciplines such as chemistry and physics, psychologists developed tests to assess behavior and measure human abilities. The first psychological tests were designed to test intelligence. The early work in this area by pioneers such as Alfred Binet (1905) laid the groundwork for the methods used in psychosocial testing today.

Prior to the development of quantitative tests "behavior was explained by means of descriptions in the form of a narrative, utilizing the techniques of a novelist or journalist" (Cunningham 1986 p. 2). This method of gathering data was not totally acceptable because the scientists of the day believed that quantification provided the only real proof that a phenomenon existed. In an attempt to meet this standard, psychologists began to quantify human behavior so that their work would also be accepted by the scientific community. This earlier focus on measurement continues to permeate not only psychological research but also research in the health and social sciences. It is important to note that the recognition of nursing as a science, like that of psychology, paralleled its empirical development. In nursing, however, knowledge development through theory building, the testing and validation of models of care delivery, and the validation of nursing interventions did not become a major thrust until the last decade.

Nursing is a human science and therefore draws heavily on the measurements developed in other fields, particularly psychology and sociology. Since nursing is essentially a newcomer to the scientific community, nurse researchers are only at the beginning stages of quantification. Phenomena of particular relevance to nursing practice are still being identified and operationalized for testing.

The development of psychosocial instruments is not a new activity for nurse researchers. After analyzing three decades of nursing research, Brown, Tanner, and Padrick (1984) documented some trends in the use of instruments by nurses. They noted that in 1952–1953, nurse researchers were likely to develop their own instruments, whereas in the 1970s they were more likely to borrow tests and measurements from other disciplines, particularly psychology. During the present decade nurse researchers are continuing to borrow instruments but also to design their own. What is different about the process of both selecting and developing instruments in today's research environment is an overriding concern with the psychometric properties of the instruments. This is a much-needed focus in nursing research. Knowledge of the psychometric properties of an existing instrument helps the researcher decide whether to use it or to design a new one. When a psychometrically sound and proven instrument from another field is available, it is inappropriate to waste precious resources in developing another tool that measures the same thing. However, if an appropriate instrument is not available, or if its conceptual meaning is not congruent with the conceptual meaning ascribed to the variable of interest by nurses, then it is more appropriate to develop a new instrument.

Data Collection with Psychosocial Instruments

In a study that relies on psychosocial measurements, the quality of the data-collection instrument is a major determinant of the overall quality of the study. For the data obtained on human attributes and behaviors to be reliable and useful, the measurements that represent those attributes and behaviors must be sound. Thus, it is useful to know and understand the criteria for the development and selection of psychosocial instruments that will provide the most valid and reliable data for your study.

The choice of a data-collection method is one of the most important steps in the research process. Gay (1981) points out that there are three major ways to collect research data: observation, the administration of a standardized or researcher-developed instrument, and the recording of naturally available data (e.g., a retrospective audit of patients' medical records). The very first step in the selection of a data-collection method is to review the various approaches that could be used. Next, through a systematic analysis, consider the strengths and weaknesses of each of the methods in relation to the research question, target population, and setting for the study. Now you are ready to select your method, or a combination of data-collection methods.

Most nurse researchers use questionnaires as the primary data-collection tool (Brown, Tanner, and Padrick 1984; Jacobsen and Meininger 1985). Questionnaires are very effective for obtaining measurements of people's attitudes, perceptions, and opinions. Self-report forms are most useful for measuring personal and social attributes and behaviors. Other data collection methods include:

. . . anecdotal notes; content analyses; critical incident technique; decision making exercises; Delphi technique; interviews, both structured and unstructured; tests of knowledge; audits; observation; paper and pencil approaches such as questionnaires, checklists, rating scales and semantic differentials; Q-sort; analysis of existing records such as nursing care plans, incident reports and nurses' notes; process recording; multimedia techniques; and recording of physiologic data (Ward 1986 p. 42–43).

Sources of Psychosocial Instruments

There are thousands of psychosocial instruments (Miller 1983) available for use by nurse researchers. Yet, there is no centralized source that can be used to locate instruments and obtain complete information on their properties. A considerable

TABLE 10–1   *Sources of Psychosocial Instruments*

Nursing	Other Fields
Compendia	Compendia
Instruments for Measuring Nursing Practice and Other Health Care Variables (vols. 1 and 2) (Ward and Lindeman 1979).	*Mental Measurement Yearbooks* (Buros 1944–1979)
Instruments for Use in Nursing Education Research (Ward and Fetler).	*Tests in Print* (Buros 1974)
Instruments for Nursing Research (Frank-Stromborg 1988).	Scales for the Measurement of Attitudes (Shaw and Wright 1967)
Major Research Journals	Handbook of Scales and Indices of Health Behavior (Reeder et al 1976)
Nursing Research	Handbook of Research Design and Social Measurement (Miller 1983)
Western Journal of Nursing Research	Measures for Psychological Assessment (Chun, Cobb, and French 1975)
Research in Nursing and Health	Major Research Journals
International Journal of Nursing Studies	Those selected depend on the field of interest (e.g., in sociology, *American Sociological Review*)
Advances in Nursing Science	
Computerized Data Bases	Computerized Data Bases
MEDLARS (Medical Literature Analysis and Retrieval System). Includes several on-line data bases including MEDLINE and BIOETHICSLINE. See Sparks (1984) for descriptions of these and others included in this system.	ERIC (Education Indexes and Abstracts. Includes published and unpublished research)
National Health Planning Information Center (NHPIC)	Other Sources
Other Sources	Psychological Abstracts
Dissertation Abstracts	Sociological Abstracts

amount of time and effort will be needed to find the best instrument for your particular study. The best way to start is to conduct a systematic review of published compilations of instruments with the assistance of a reference librarian. Some of these compilations in nursing and other fields are listed in Table 10–1. However, your search should not be limited to just these sources. There are many other compendia available, some of which are specific to an area of practice such as mental health (Comrey, Backer, and Glaser 1973) or child development (Johnson 1976). In addition there are other ways to locate instruments, such as by content area, in the indexes of research and specialty journals. Making personal contacts at professional meetings and writing to publishing houses for their test catalogs are additional ways of obtaining information about research instruments. It is often possible to discover just the right instrument through a computerized search. You can also contact the National Health Planning Information Center (NHPIC) in Hyattsville, Maryland, for a computerized search related to the variables identified for your study. These and other major sources of psychosocial instruments are listed in Table 10–1, which should provide a good start for your search.

Criteria for Instrument Selection

Instrument selection should be a three-step procedure: (1) Identify the type of instrument you need in relation to the purpose of your study and target population, (2) systematically search for and obtain all relevant and appropriate instruments, and (3) using predetermined selection criteria, conduct a comparative analysis of the instruments that appear to be appropriate, and then identify the best instrument for your study (Gay 1981).

It will be a great temptation to stop searching for additional instruments as soon as you find one that appears adequate. That would be a big mistake, since the overall quality of your research depends on the quality of the measurements obtained. Important criteria used to evaluate psychosocial instruments are presented in Table 10–2. For additional information, see Gay (1981) and Waltz et al (1984).

It is useful to keep several other points in mind during instrument selection. First, some instruments are copyrighted, and you must obtain the permission of the author before using them. This can be a long process if you have difficulty locating an author. Also, when new instruments are developed, they are typically reported in research journals with a few sample questions. If you decide that the instrument might be useful for your study, you need to write to the researcher directly for a copy of the entire instrument. Most researchers are willing to share their instruments, as well as additional information on the psychometric qualities of the instrument and reports of ongoing studies, with other researchers. However, it is not uncommon for a researcher to give permission to use an instrument, with the provision that you share the raw data from your study. This is a reasonable request, and one of the methods by which researchers accumulate data to contribute to the ongoing development of the psychometric properties of their instruments.

Some instruments can be purchased only from publishing houses and cannot be reproduced for personal research. If the instrument is particularly expensive,

TABLE 10–2 *Criteria for Instrument Selection*

1. The purpose of the instrument is stated, and the basis for the selection of items is described.
2. Individuals for whom the instrument is appropriate are specified.
3. Directions for administration and scoring are clear and complete.
4. Guidelines for interpreting individuals' scores are included.
5. The underlying theoretical-conceptual basis for the development of the instrument is described.
6. The development of psychometric properties is described, and both the testing procedures and the psychometrics obtained (validity and reliability data) are acceptable in terms of the purpose and population for which the instrument was designed.
7. The level of specificity (whether the instrument measures a single dimension or several aspects of the construct) is delineated and acceptable.
8. Items are well developed (clear and brief) and relevant to the construct they purport to measure.
9. Items are not obsolete with regard to the prevailing culture, technology, or environment.
10. Items are easy to interpret and are minimally intrusive.
11. Length, level of difficulty, and average amount of time needed to complete the instrument are acceptable for the intended subjects.
12. The cost of the instrument and of resources (personnel) needed to administer it is acceptable.

and some are, the study may have to be delayed until funding can be obtained. Finally, some instruments can be purchased only by qualified professionals, therefore students may need to send a letter explaining the nature of the research to the publisher, with the signature of a qualified researcher who will be supervising the study.

Even when high-quality instruments are available, questions invariably arise as to what the test scores really mean and how the data should be used. The answers to these questions are very complex and relate to the theoretical rationale for the design of the instrument, as well as its psychometric properties (reliability and validity), the conditions under which the instrument is administered, and the various errors in measurement. These concerns are addressed in the section on instrument development, later in this chapter.

Designing Psychosocial Instruments

We have already established the need for high-quality psychosocial instruments in nursing. Areas of special need include: (1) the development of measures for variables related to nursing interventions where no measures currently exist, (2) the adaptation of instruments developed by other scientists for health care settings, and (3) the design of multiple measures for the same construct (Ventura, Hinshaw, and Atwood 1981).

Psychosocial Instruments and the Nursing Process

Psychosocial testing is a major component of nursing research because most phenomena associated with nursing care involve a human dimension that is critical to understanding them. For example, the patient's pain experience can't be completely understood without assessing its subjective component (perceived duration and intensity), as well as its cultural component (usual response patterns and coping mechanisms) and biophysical and environmental components. Thus, to understand concepts like pain fully, we need to obtain measurements on each of these dimensions.

An individual's cognitive, affective, and behavioral characteristics covary with medical status (physiological factors) and environment in ways that affect health care outcomes. Thus, the measurement of each of these variables and their interconnections must be a clinical nursing priority. Green (1985) says:

> Current behaviors and attitudes should be interpreted in conjunction with the physical aspects of the presenting problem. The premorbid background of the patient must be delineated in an effort to clarify the historical context or pattern of the syndrome. Moreover, personality and environmental circumstances must be appraised to optimize therapeutic recommendations [p 202].

Few psychosocial instruments have been specifically developed to assess an individual's personal attributes and behaviors in relation to health and illness. One reason is that instruments developed for clinical assessments must be grounded in theory and meet the highest standards of reliability and validity to provide legitimate measures for clinical decision making. We also need instruments designed to measure individual and group reactions in the patient's immediate social environment, as well as instruments designed to provide specific data on environmental factors related to health. Many variables play a mediating role in how patients define health, interpret symptoms, and respond to medical procedures and conditions (Turk and Kerns 1985 p. 337). We are just beginning to appreciate the extent to which factors other than the patient's medical condition (e.g., social support) determine health care outcomes.

Psychosocial data are typically obtained from patients through self-report inventories and questionnaires (Strickland and Waltz 1986), and the data obtained are predominantly used to test hypotheses in formal research studies. There is little evidence that nurses use psychosocial data for clinical decision making. However, this situation is likely to change as a result of the recent focus on clinical nursing studies, and the corresponding efforts of nurse researchers to develop instruments tailored to help nurses implement and validate the nursing process.

Table 10–3 presents some nursing instruments that, with additional testing, could prove useful in the assessment, planning, intervention, and evaluation phases of the nursing process. The few instruments selected are not the only ones available, however. They were chosen to point out some of the different types of instruments that could be used for clinical decision making in the context of the nursing process.

This discussion of psychosocial testing would not be complete without a warning about some of its hazards. First, testing procedures, especially structured questionnaires, do not provide direct measurements of human characteristics, traits, or behaviors. At best, they provide an accurate description of subjects, to the extent that the instrument itself is sound, and to the extent that subjects are willing and able to reveal themselves (Cunningham 1986). Second, interpretation of psychosocial instruments tends to be difficult and should not extend beyond the purpose for which the instrument was designed. The one most common error in the interpretation of psychosocial data is to measure attitudes and then report the results as though they were representative of the subjects' actual behavior. Attitude surveys only measure a subject's preferences for certain behaviors, or intentions to act in a specific way. Third, psychosocial instruments can be inadvertently misused. For example, some instruments expressly developed to obtain measurements on groups have been used to assess individuals. Another misuse of psychosocial instruments is to predict behavior from them when this property of the instrument has not been established through appropriate psychometric testing.

Deciding When To Develop a Psychosocial Instrument

When a particular measurement is needed and an appropriate psychosocial instrument cannot be found, it can be developed. For example, Fenton (1987) believed

---

TABLE 10–3   *Psychosocial Instruments and the Nursing Process*

Assessment
  "Value Orientations as an Assessment Tool in Cultural Diversity" (Brink 1984). Used the Kluckhohn and Strodtbeck instrument, which consists of 22 situations, and three solutions for each.
Planning
  (None Found for Use in Clinical Decision Making)
Implementation
  "Comparison of Two Group Interventions for the Bereaved" (Constantino 1988). Used the Beck Depression Inventory and the Depression Adjective Checklist Form E.
Evaluation
  "Psychiatric Inpatients' Perceptions of the Seclusion-Room Experience" (Richardson 1987). Used an 88-item semistructured interview schedule derived from Gutheil's theory of seclusion.

that if humanistic care contributed positively to patients' health care outcomes, then it should be measured. Since an instrument had not yet been developed to measure this component of nursing care, Fenton (1987) developed the Scale of Humanistic Nursing Behaviors to be used in hospital settings.

It is important for nurses who develop instruments to be aware that the current standard is to design and test instruments in accordance with psychometric theory (Cattell and Johnson 1986). Fenton's (1987) work is an excellent example of the use of psychometric theory to guide instrument development. Other models developed in accordance with psychometric theory include the Time Experience Scales (TES), which resulted in the identification of six modes in which individuals experience an awareness of time (Sanders 1986) and the Nurse Practitioner Rating Form (NPRF), Part I (Prescott, Jacox, Collar, and Goodwin 1981) and Part II (Goodwin, Prescott, Jacox, and Collar 1981). The NPRF measures both the medical and nursing components of the nurse practitioner role.

Instrument development is both a time-consuming and complex process. It should be undertaken only by those who already possess the requisite knowledge and resources or are willing to learn. Thus, whenever feasible, existing instruments should be used for psychosocial measurements. As evidenced by comprehensive reviews of the research literature, most of us are likely to use instruments that have already been developed. Since these tend to be from other disciplines (psychology, sociology), it is critical to determine whether they will, in fact, provide acceptable measures for the constructs that we need to measure (e.g., quality of life) with patients. In addition, you need to show that the instruments you borrow are reliable and valid for the target population in your study. A common misconception about reliability and validity is that once these properties are developed for an instrument, those properties will hold for all further testing. This, of course, is an erroneous assumption. Each time an instrument is used with a different target population, or for purposes other than originally designed, the psychometric properties must be reestablished.

A final caveat pertains to psychosocial instruments that have been widely used yet do not meet the current standards for quality because they have not been designed according to psychometric theory. Use of these instruments in research is extremely difficult to justify, although there may be an occasional exception.

With regard to the psychometric properties of an instrument, the following problems have been identified from an analysis of published studies: inconsistencies between the conceptual framework for the instrument and the conceptual framework of the study; the use of only one instrument to measure a complex construct, when multiple indicators were called for; and citing inappropriate evidence for validity and reliability (Strickland and Waltz 1986).

An Overview of the Research Development Process

The development of a psychosocial instrument is integrally tied to the research design. Each affects the other in both subtle and obvious ways. The research or clinical question that needs to be answered determines the kind of data that are needed. The researcher must then determine the type of instrument that is best suited to obtain the data needed. For example, if the researcher is interested in measuring patients' perceptions of their postoperative pain, he or she could administer a self-report measure that utilizes a visual analog scale (the patient responds by relating the degree of pain felt to a numerical scale). An alternative instrument for obtaining measurements is a questionnaire with selected questions about the pain. The patient responds on a Likert scale, which consists of gradations of agreement from "strongly disagree" to "strongly agree." If the clinical question has to do with the relationship of pain intensity to other physiological measures (e.g., pulse rate), the visual analog scale will probably be the instrument of choice. It is a more direct and more precise method of assessment than a questionnaire.

When designing the instrument, the researcher takes into consideration the characteristics of the respondents. Age, type and severity of illness, and educational level, as well as the intended setting in which the instrument will be administered, are some important characteristics to consider. The item, structure format, and complexity of the instrument must all be designed with the target population in mind.

In the next stage of the process, the researcher seeks clarification about the construct to be measured from the literature, colleagues, and sometimes others (e.g., individuals from the population of interest). The researcher must carefully select variables that represent the construct of interest, because constructs cannot be directly measured. A concept is a term that "expresses an abstraction formed by generalization from particulars" (e.g., pain) (Kerlinger 1973 p. 28). A construct is a concept that is "deliberately and consciously invented or adopted for a special scientific purpose" (e.g., administrative support) (Kerlinger 1973 p. 29). The researcher's primary task is to find or develop an instrument(s) to measure the construct/variable of interest. A second concern is to identify and measure other variables (antecedents, mediators, and outcomes) related to the major construct (see Figure 10–1).

The final stage of instrument development includes the formulation of items that represent the construct/variable of interest, the development of directions for administration and scoring, and the testing, refinement and development of the instrument's psychometric properties. After the entire process is completed, the instrument is ready to be evaluated and field-tested for use in research and/or clinical decision making. This process is summarized in Table 10–4.

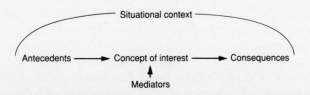

Figure 10–1   Situational context

TABLE 10–4 *Overview of Instrument Development*

---

1. Delineate the content area.
2. Identify the various dimensions of the content area that need to be measured.
3. Search the literature and draw upon the professional expertise of colleagues/others to generate item stems.
4. Determine the types of questions to be asked (e.g., multiple choice).
5. Develop each item (question/statement) to convey one idea, and aim for brevity and clarity.
6. Decide on the response format best suited to obtain the type of data needed.
7. Select a panel of experts to critique the instrument.
8. Refine the instrument and begin testing for reliability and validity.
9. Refine the instrument again if necessary and repeat tests for reliability and validity. This process continues until the instrument meets established criteria.

Steps in Instrument Development

This section describes how to develop a psychosocial instrument, starting with the identification of the construct/variable of interest. Also included are sections on item construction, scale construction, and the administration and scoring of instruments.

Content Area Identification   The first step in instrument development is to identify the content area that needs to be measured. It is very important to delineate the exact nature of the construct and its boundaries (content area) clearly. Once this is accomplished, items that will adequately represent the content area can be developed. In some instances, a construct has several dimensions (domains). It then becomes essential to identify every dimension that the instrument will measure. For example, there are several different mental status questionnaires, and each taps a somewhat different dimension of this construct (Foreman 1987). The various components of mental status include state of consciousness; orientation; attention; memory; calculation; abstraction; judgment; insight; thought form, content, and processes; use of language; constructional ability; personal appearance; and general knowledge (Foreman 1987). In a validity and reliability check of three mental status questionnaires (the Short Portable Mental Status Questionnaire, Mini-Mental State Examination, and Cognitive Screening Examination), Foreman (1987) found that each did, in fact, differ in psychometric properties, but the instrument of choice depended on the characteristics of the target population and setting.

Unless the researcher constructs items that relate specifically to one or more of the various dimensions of a construct and communicates this information to potential users, there will always be some uncertainty about what the instrument is actually measuring. Such uncertainty also makes it difficult to interpret the measurements and to compare the results obtained with those of other studies. If, however, items are developed to represent fully each of the construct dimensions that the instrument is supposed to measure, then the instrument will have good content validity. Content validity reflects an adequate sampling of the content area (specified dimensions) of the construct of interest.

Number of Items. The number of items in an instrument varies with the complexity of the construct being measured. It generally takes five to ten items to sample each dimension of a construct adequately. These separate dimensions, once tested and validated, often become the subscales of the instrument. For example, Hemphill's Index of Group Dimensions (Miller 1983) is built upon 13 independent group dimensions that became the subscales of this instrument. The dimensions are: autonomy, control, flexibility, hedonic tone, homogeneity, intimacy, participation, permeability, polarization, potency, stability, stratification, and viscidity.

It is not necessary to create subscales for the measurement of every complex construct. Even though the researcher systematically taps several dimensions of a construct/variable of interest during item generation, the development of subscales might not be relevant to the overall purpose of the instrument. If so, only one score is calculated for the instrument. For example, the Miller Hope Scale (Miller and Powers 1988), was developed after a comprehensive review of the literature and an exploratory study of hope in individuals who survived a critical illness. Only one score is calculated for each individual. However, this total score is interpreted in light of the three factors that emerged during factor analysis (satisfaction with self, others, and life; avoidance of hope threats; and anticipation of a future).

Table of Specifications. To be absolutely sure that the content of the instrument reflects its purpose, some researchers find it helpful to develop a table of specifications prior to item generation. Such a table is merely a breakdown of the construct/ variable of interest into domains (content areas). Item stems appropriate to each domain are then inserted into the table (see Table 10–5). Gay (1985) recommends using a table of specifications for item generation. He claims that it becomes the blueprint for the instrument, specifying its content and ensuring that all intended factors (characteristics and behaviors) are included.

TABLE 10–5 *Table of Specifications for Item Generation*

Construct	Dimensions	Representative Item Stems
Organizational commitment	Innovative behaviors	1. Recommends changes to improve patient care 2. Volunteers for new projects

Test specification tables can be very simple, as in Table 10–5, or can be embellished. For example, an additional column for comments could be added. Some researchers might also like to add a column reflecting the source from which the item stems were drawn. A carefully developed table of specifications, although yet another step in a very complex and lengthy process, will prove its worth in contributing to the validity of the instrument. This step should definitely not be skipped if the instrument is to be used for clinical decision making. In clinical situations, we depend on instruments to discriminate among subjects who possess various amounts of the characteristic/behavior being measured, such as level of coping. It is important to have assurances, therefore, that instruments designed for clinical use adequately measure the construct of interest.

Item Construction   The way a particular test item is constructed depends on the nature of the test and the intended audience. Thus, a test developed for patients is usually quite different from one developed for health care practitioners, even though they are essentially measuring the same thing. However, in the construction of individual test items, the following goals should be achieved regardless of the intended audience:

- The item should clearly communicate one, and only one, idea from the content area/domain of interest.

- The item should be understood in the same way by all members of the target population.

- The item should be worded in a way that does not bias the response (lead the subject to respond in a certain way).

- Avoid sensitive and negative items that discourage subjects from responding.

- Include enough items to tap all relevant dimensions in the construct/variable of interest.

- Limit the items to one or two types (e.g., multiple choice and rank order).

- Group the same types of items together to facilitate subjects' responses.

- Different individuals should be able to score the items objectively without disagreement over the correctness of the response.

One question frequently asked about instrument development is whether to include items containing universals such as never and always. There is no straightforward answer to this question. However, experienced instrument developers prefer not to use items containing universals and do not recommend their use. Such items are often misunderstood by subjects. It is also difficult to figure out the intent of a negative question. For example, the statement "Pregnant women should never take excessive vitamin supplements" is not meant to refer to those women whose physicians have prescribed higher than average doses of certain vitamins, but this is not evident from the statement.

Another question pertains to items' reverse scoring. **Reverse-scored items** are those in which the direction of the response is the opposite of most other items. They should discourage individuals from responding to all questions either positively or negatively. An example of such an item is "Team members perceive their roles as competitive." On a five point Likert scale from strongly disagree to strongly agree, the desired response to this question would be strongly disagree (and five points as opposed to only one would be given for this response). The idea is for team members to view their roles as cooperative. An individual who responds positively to reverse-scored items has probably developed a "response set" (a tendency to respond is one way, in this case positively to all items on the questionnaire). When a "response set" is identified, the entire questionnaire is usually considered unusable for data analysis.

The last comment relates to the use of screen questions. A screen question does just what it implies: It screens subjects to determine which questions are appropriate for them to answer. An example of a screen question is "Have you ever had eye surgery?" If the response is yes, the subject is then instructed to answer a set of questions that pertain to the eye surgery. If the response is no, the subject is instructed to skip the next five questions (e.g., 3 through 7) and move to another item (e.g., number 8). Screen questions are a useful mechanism to use when it is necessary to prevent subjects from responding to questions that they do not have the knowledge, experience, or information to answer. When used appropriately, screen questions help to increase the internal validity of the instrument.

To summarize, sensitive, complex, and confusing items contribute to dishonest responses, nonresponses, and response errors due to incorrect interpretation of the item. Therefore, every effort should be made to perfect the wording and design of questionnaire items. A complete cycle of item review, revision, and refinement should take place prior to the field-testing of an instrument to minimize the inclusion of poor items. Also any word or phrase that is open to different interpretations or is used in a specific way should be defined for the respondent. Finally, the use of negative items is not recommended. Reverse-scored items and screen items should be used when needed to enhance the collection of valid and reliable data.

Scale Construction   The selection of an appropriate scale for a psychosocial instrument depends on three things, the construct/variable being measured, the level of measurement (nominal, ordinal, or interval), and the capacity of the target population to respond as desired. Two types of questions are used in psychosocial testing, open-ended (unstructured) and structured (also called closed-ended or fixed alternative). An example of an open-ended question is "Would you please tell us what the pain you're feeling is like?" An example of a fixed alternative question is "Would you be willing to work the night shift if the pay differential is increased substantially?" ("yes" or "no") The problems inherent in open-ended questions are immediately evident. First, such a question will be interpreted differently by different patients, and second, there are so many possible responses that analyzing them will be difficult.

Structured questions provide respondents with a fixed number of options from which to choose, thus overcoming the problems posed by open-ended questions.

TABLE 10–6 *Major Types of Scales*

Categorical Response Scale

Yes	No	Don't Know	Not Applicable

Summative Scale (Likert)

Definitely true	Mostly true	Don't know	Mostly false	Definitely false
_____	_____	_____	_____	_____

Graphic Rating Scale

Unfair_____Very fair
         1   2   3   4   5   6   7

Semantic Differential

Good _____:_____:_____:_____:_____:_____:_____:Bad

Several different types of fixed alternative scales are available for this purpose (see Table 10–6). None of these is difficult to create. Each consists of only three parts: (1) an item stem that states the main idea or behavior and serves as the stimulus for the subject's response, (2) a series of scale steps, and (3) labels or anchors that give meaning to the scale steps (Waltz, Strickland, and Lenz 1984). The goal is to determine gradations of responses that are sensitive enough to discriminate among respondents who possess the characteristic/behavior and those who do not. One way of ensuring the discriminatory power of the instrument is to eliminate items most individuals would respond to in a similar way, for example, "Every American has a right to health care." Other major considerations in scale construction include ease of response and the inclusion of enough alternatives to incorporate a full range of options for subjects to respond to.

A major disadvantage of measurement scales is that individuals who do not find an option that truly reflects their opinion may be discouraged from answering the question at all. Some may even refuse to complete the remaining questions as well. Also, some researchers consider fixed response scales too superficial in their ability to shed light on the true meaning of complex psychosocial variables. One way to overcome this is to add depth to the instrument through the inclusion of screening questions, followed by a series of very specific items.

Scale Data.   Most researchers consider scale data to be at the interval level of measurement. Those who disagree view scale data as ordinal. In this chapter, we consider scale data as interval. Interval scales (e.g., Likert scales, which provide gradations of responses) provide more precise measurements than ordinal scales (e.g., check-lists that indicate the presence or absence of characteristics/behaviors). More pow-erful statistical analyses are possible with interval data (Cunningham 1986).

Four different types of fixed alternative scales are shown in Table 10–6. The first is a categorical response scale providing ordinal data for analysis. Each of the remaining scales provides interval data for analysis. Subjects' responses vary in in-tensity according to a numerical value assigned by the researcher. The **Likert scale**, a summated rating scale, is the most widely used scale (Cattell and Johnson 1986). The sum of all responses are calculated to arrive at a total score. The magnitude of the score (high or low) is usually indicative of the degree to which an individual possesses the attribute measured (e.g., autonomy).

Likert scales range from 3 to 7 points, and there is disagreement as to whether a middle or neutral ground should be provided. Scales both with and without the neutral ground have proved effective in research. However, use of the Likert scale may pose problems with certain groups. Flaskerud (1988) recently pointed out the potential for cultual bias in the scale's format. She noted that in one study with Central American refugee clients, one third of the subjects were unable to make a choice on a four-point scale. They provided "yes" or "no" responses instead. This was also true in a study with Vietnamese refugees. Fifty percent of the subjects coud not grasp the format of the Likert scale despite the fact that semantic integrity had been established. These individuals were unable to respond to gradations in feeling, and therefore substituted a "yes" or "no," instead of selecting a position from the scale on the questionnaire.

The third scale in Table 10–6 is a graphic scale consisting of a series of num-bered scale steps. Subjects tend to like graphic scales because of the flexibility of the response format. In general, the more steps graphic scales have, the greater their reliability (Cunningham 1986). After 7 steps, the increase in reliability is neg-ligible, and it declines after 20 steps (Cunningham 1986). Graphic scales are es-pecially useful in studies that assess biopsychosocial variables (e.g., pain). In nurs-ing administration studies, graphic scales can be quite valuable in measuring organizational variables (e.g., organizational climate) and human interactions (e.g., collaboration).

The last scale is the **semantic differential** scale, designed to quantify concepts in terms of their word meanings (semantic properties). Cunningham (1986) reports that the scale was developed by C. E. Osgood in 1962. In using this scale, the researcher first chooses a concept, then selects a set (several pairs) of bipolar ad-jectives (e.g., good/bad, sharp/dull) to elicit a range of responses. Subjects respond by marking one of a number of undefined positions on a fixed scale anchored by one pair of the bipolar adjectives. Subjects respond to several pairs of bipolar ad-jectives for each construct/variable of interest. See Cunningham (1986) for more detailed information about this scale. Major advantages of semantic scales are that they are easy to construct, are simple to administer, and provide large amounts of data. In addition, they do not need to be field-tested (Cunningham 1986). The major disadvantages are that data analysis is complex and that interpretation of results requires skill.

The Sociodemographic Questionnaire. The sociodemographic questionnaire is a specialized instrument designed to obtain personal, social, and environmental data about subjects. When developed properly, sociodemographic questionnaires provide data that are useful in hypothesis testing and in determining the effect of mediating factors, such as amount of work experience or educational level, on a construct/variable of interest, such as job satisfaction.

A variety of scales are often seen on sociodemographic questionnaires. These include: checklists, fill-in-the-blanks scales, rank-order scales, and rating scales. As a general rule, interval level sociodemographic data are more useful in analyses than ordinal level data. Therefore, ask for the subjects' actual birth dates as opposed to having them merely check a category (e.g., under 40, or 41 and older). Remember, it is always possible to collapse data into meaningful categories if this becomes necessary later.

The literature provides increasing evidence that researchers are carefully selecting and measuring those social and demographic variables that could have an effect on the observed variance in the dependent measures. For example, Northouse (1988) incorporated a wide array of social and demographic variables in her analysis of the relationship between social support and the adjustment of mastectomy patients and their husbands immediately after surgery and one month later. Some of these variables were age, length of marriage, marital history, and employment status. In nursing administration research, it is important to include organizational and environmental as well as sociodemographic data in analyses. For example, in their study on the consequences of turnover among newly hired nurses, Lowery and Jacobsen (1984) included the following job factors in their analysis: overall performance, job knowledge, quality of work, quantity of work, planning and organization, leadership skills, human relations skills, adaptability and dependability, interest and motivation, communication skills, and equipment and supplies used. This study made an important contribution to nursing in beginning to explain the consequences of turnover by using a variety of job-relevant variables.

Cognitive Instruments. Cognitive instruments are typically designed to obtain information about an individual's knowledge of a particular subject. The most frequently used scales to measure knowledge are multiple choice and fill in the blanks, although other methods such as checklists and rating scales are also appropriate. With the current emphasis on health teaching, one possible application of the cognitive scale is to test patients' level of knowledge and understanding before and after instruction to determine if learning has occurred. One researcher used two different scales on the same instrument to obtain data on older adults' knowledge and attitudes about sexuality and aging (Steinke 1988). The research instrument (Sexual Behavior Questionnaire and the Aging Sexual Knowledge and Attitudes Scale) contained 35 true, false, and don't know questions to assess subjects' knowledge about sex and aging. A Likert scale was incorporated into this same instrument to measure attitudes.

Affective Instruments. Affective instruments are often developed to measure attitudes, values, and perceptions. These tests are the ones most commonly administered by nurses. The most frequently used scale for affective measurements is the Likert scale because of its gradations of response options. Other useful scales to measure variables in the affective domain include the semantic differential and graphic scales. For example, Strumpf and Evans (1988) conducted a study to determine the impact of physical restraints on elderly patients and the perceptions of both patients and nurses about the use of restraints. These researchers used several instruments to obtain their data and a semistructured interview guide (Subjective Experience of Being Restrained) to elicit patients' perceptions. They also administered the Perceptions of Restraint Use Questionnnaire (PRUQ) to the patient's primary nurse and interviewed the same nurse using a semistructured guide. The PRUQ is a three-point Likert scale, with measurements ranging from least important (1) to most important (3). Data on several predetermined variables (e.g., restraint documentation, assessed mental status, and medications) were also obtained from the patient's chart as a validity check on both patients' and nurses' subjective responses. These authors are to be commended for their use of multiple data sources.

Behavioral Instruments.   Behavioral measurements are the most difficult to obtain because it is rarely possible to observe subjects on a continuous basis or to be available at specific time intervals to sample behavior adequately. It is usually necessary to rely on subjects' self-reports of their behavior as obtained through self-report inventories, checklists, and diaries. It is also possible, but not easy, to use a Likert scale to construct an instrument to measure health behaviors. These instruments have the disadvantage of asking subjects to recall behavior, instead of recording actual behavior about the time it occurs. In a comprehensive study, Heitkemper, Shaver, and Mitchell (1988) used several instruments to obtain women's retrospective assessments of their gastrointestinal symptoms and bowel patterns across the menstrual cycle (after they were screened for inclusion through a telephone interview). Subjects maintained a GI Health Diary that contained a checklist of six symptoms (stomach pain, nausea, diarrhea, constipation, increased food intake, and decreased food intake) and used a four-point rating scale to assess each symptom (not present to extreme). The diary was also used to record daily self-reports of GI function. The subjects used the MDQ, a six-point Likert scale containing 47 symptoms grouped into eight factors (including one that contained control symptoms to reveal general tendency to complain about a variety of symptoms) to assess their premenstrual symptoms retrospectively. From this brief description, it is evident that the reliability of the data for this study weighs heavily on the ability of the subject not only to remember events but also to provide accurate accounts of them.

Formatting the Instrument   Subjects should perceive the instrument as having a professional appearance. The initial impression could make a difference in how effectively subjects respond to the instrument or whether they respond at all. It is worth the time and effort to create a final product of professional quality. It is relatively inexpensive to develop an instrument on a microcomputer and use a laser printer to obtain a professional master copy, which can then be taken to a copy center for reproduction.

What are some of the formatting features that not only affect the appearance of an instrument but can also damage its validity? First is the number and spacing of items. An instrument with items crowded together is both unappealing and confusing. A wide space should be left between items and between directions and items. Second, like items (those from the same domain) should be grouped together to avoid the frustration and fatigue that results when subjects must constantly shift their "train of thought" to respond. This grouping also facilitates subjects' responses when each new group of questions is introduced, for example, with the phrase "The next set of questions relates to your experiences while you were hospitalized." Write your questions on 3-by-5 cards, one to a card, so that it will be easy to sort and rearrange them until you are satisfied with the logic of the arrangement. Third, number items consecutively. If you include screen items, provide extra directions to ensure that all subjects will respond accurately and completely. The likelihood of obtaining incomplete data with screen questions is fairly high, especially if answering yes to a screen question entails completing an extra five or six questions and answering no entails skipping to a new section of the test. Some subjects will respond negatively just to finish quickly. This will bias the results. Fourth, the portion of the instrument reserved for recording responses should be spaced so that item scales are not squeezed together. Item responses that run together and cannot be easily deciphered bias the results. Fifth, ask several different individuals to proofread the test for clarity, flow, grammatical errors, and colloquialisms. As previously mentioned, such errors should be corrected prior to field-testing.

Instrument Length It is better to create a lengthy instrument that adequately measures the construct of interest than to sacrifice quality for brevity. The final length of an instrument is the result of many independent judgments during the process of development. For example, should one repeat a question using slightly different terminology as an internal check on the honesty of responses? The ability, interest, and motivation of the target population should be assessed to answer this question. It is possible to obtain accurate and complete data, even on a particularly long instrument, if it is of some special benefit to the respondents. As a general rule, an instrument can be shortened by eliminating redundant and unnecessary questions. It is also possible to develop short forms of a long test, but this requires additional knowledge of test development and statistics (Gay 1986). To be useful, a shortened version of the test must meet the same rigorous criteria for development and testing as the long form of the same test. It is unwise to use a short form of a test unless it can be shown to have adequate psychometric properties.

Instrument Directions Information about the nature of the instrument and complete directions for responding to the questions should be provided. Even if this information can be inferred from the title of the instrument, information should be provided on the construct being measured and the type of response expected (e.g.,

---

TABLE 10–7   *Sample Instrument Directions*

Primary Nursing Questionnaire

In order to obtain the data we need to evaluate the effect of Primary Nursing at University Medical Center, we would appreciate your cooperation in completing the following questionnaire.

Please respond to each item with a check ($\sqrt{}$) in the column that best represents your opinion. You may take as much time as you need.

1. Planning a unit schedule should be the responsibility of unit staff nurses.

Never	Seldom	Sometimes	Usually	Always
_____	_____	_____	_____	_____

"Circle the response that best represents your opinion"). Any special instructions (e.g., "There are no right or wrong answers") and the time allowed to complete the instrument (e.g., "You may take as much time as you need to complete this questionnaire") should be explicitly stated. Clear and complete directions provide each respondent with a common frame of reference from which to respond. See Table 10–7 for an example of instrument directions.

Instrument Administration   The researcher will choose the method of administration (e.g., mailed instrument for self-administration versus distribution to a group for simultaneous administration) based on the characteristics of the target population and the amount of control needed to obtain the desired data. If questionnaires are mailed, subjects do not have the opportunity to request clarification. Group administration of an instrument allows for interaction with the researcher, but is somewhat restrictive in terms of the timing and limits on privacy and anonymity. The researcher's goal should be to choose the method that is most likely to be accepted by subjects, achieve a high rate of participation in the study, and provide quality data (complete, accurate, and usable).

Scoring and Coding Instruments   Instruments should be coded and scored in ways that facilitate computer analysis of the data. There are several options from which the researcher can choose. Each, of course, has its advantages and disadvantages. The instrument can be constructed with information needed for coding (e.g., column numbers) so that data can be entered directly into the computer from the original instrument. This is a convenient method when all data must be handled by the researcher. Second, pressure-sensitive response sheets that are sent out for machine scoring can be used. This method is usually expensive. However, for instruments that require complex scoring procedures (e.g., instruments with weighted items and reverse-scored items), it is money well spent. Third, the instrument can be scored, the data transferred to code sheets, and the data then entered into the computer.

Whenever instruments are being hand scored and coded, it is advisable to have a second rater check a predetermined percentage of the instruments for accuracy. Sometimes the rater must make decisions pertaining to the scoring or coding of data that are not covered in the general directions provided by the instrument developer. These should be written in a special log for later reference. For example, in one instrument, an error in the numbering sequence (one number was inadvertently skipped) was found. Had this problem not been written in the researcher's data log and accounted for in the coding of data, the computer-generated listing of item scores would not have corresponded with the items on the questionnaire.

A different example is a decision that has to do with the scoring of a subject's response. Although the subject was instructed to check only one response for each item, two were checked for several statements. There are several ways to handle this problem. One option is to throw the question out. Usually this isn't necessary, however, because the scoring procedures that accompany the instrument usually include a system for handling missing values. If not, a mean of the subject's responses to all of the other questions on the instrument could be computed. That value could then be inserted where data were missing. When a subject fails to respond to a large number of items on an instrument, the entire instrument should be considered unusable. Before data collection, the researcher should determine and annotate in the data log the point at which missing data make an instrument unusable. It is important to record beforehand this and any other decision made about anticipated problems. Also, when an unanticipated problem is encountered, the researcher should record the nature of the problem and how it was handled in the data log.

Unless such decisions are recorded, it is possible for the researcher to make a different decision when the problem recurs later in the data-handling process. Also, different individuals scoring and coding the same set of data need written guidelines to make consistent decisions. This is the method of choice to maintain the integrity of the data set and the reliability of the data.

Data Cleaning Data cleaning refers to the verification and correction of errors in your data prior to analysis. Some of the problems to look for are missing data, improperly coded data, and errors in data entry (which will most likely occur during the creation of a data file on a microcomputer).

Suter (1987) points out that several sources of error (e.g., improper coding) can be managed if the data-collection tool is developed to facilitate data cleaning. Suter recommends the technique of "chunking data" (grouping four or five items together followed by a blank field) on questionnaires to identify missing data quickly and easily. Additionally, this technique makes it very easy to transfer subjects' responses directly from the instrument to the computer in "chunks." This speeds the process of data entry and cuts down on entry errors. When a Likert format is used in questionnaires, Suter recommends that subjects circle responses on a numbered scale. This again facilitates data entry directly from the questionnaire. It also eliminates the counting that must occur when subjects check an undefined position in a scale, e.g.:

Disagree |—|—|—|—| Agree

Barhyte and Bacon (1985) discuss several approaches to cleaning data sets in detail. The goal in data cleaning is simply to make your data set as error free as you can. The first method is visual inspection of the data. To accomplish this, run a printout of your entire data set and visually inspect it to verify that the values for each participant begin and end in the same columns (assuming a fixed variable format). Next, check each of the cells for missing data and go back to the original questionnaires to determine if there was a recording error or if subjects failed to respond.

Other methods of data cleaning involve the generation of frequency distributions for each variable to determine if the values for each fall within the expected range. Use cross-tabulations to determine if the specified combinations of values for pairs of variables are illegitimate. Another method involves verification of subjects' responses using the original questionnaire. To accomplish this, another person should be recruited to read all of the responses of a specified sample of subjects while the researcher verifies the data on the computer printout. Barhyte and Bacon (1985) recommend that the researcher decide in advance how many records with errors need to be found before the entire sample of records would need to be verified.

Development of Psychometric Properties

Instruments are typically tested, revised, and retested several times to develop their psychometric properties sufficiently. When a researcher or clinician has confidence in an instrument, he or she is satisfied with the psychometric properties (validity and reliability) and the methods by which they were obtained. **Validity** means that the instrument actually measures what it purports to measure (e.g., stress). **Reliability** means that the instrument measures the same thing consistently (e.g., across all subjects in the target population).

Several types of reliability and validity can be developed for psychosocial tests. The most common forms of validity are content, construct, and criterion related. The most common forms of reliability are test-retest, internal consistency and split-half. The combination of validity and reliability testing actually chosen for a particular instrument depends on the purpose for which the instrument was developed. As a general rule, instruments that provide individual assessments to be used in clinical decision making are held to a more rigorous standard than those used for general research and administrative decision making. Minimal psychometric standards for published instruments have been suggested by Norbeck (1985 p. 380), including:

- one type of content validity
- test-retest reliability
- internal consistency reliability
- at least one type of criterion-related or construct validity

It is useful to consult a biostatistician or psychometrician prior to testing an instrument to obtain advice on the specific testing procedures that should be used (e.g., criterion-related validity), sampling techniques, and statistics. Since the validity and reliability data that need to be generated depend on the nature and purpose of the instrument, there is no specific set of rules to aid in decision making. However, reference to one of the established texts in this area should prove helpful (Allen and Yen 1979, Gay 1985, Nunnally 1978, Waltz et al 1984).

Existing instruments, even if they have been widely used, need to be evaluated for their validity and reliability in your particular study. Additionally, if subjects will be selected from a different target population, the instrument should also be field-tested prior to use (Fox and Ventura 1983). At minimum, internal consistency reliability and content validity should be obtained on an existing instrument. If these estimates prove inadequate for the purpose of your study, the instrument should be revised and reevaluated until acceptable psychometric properties are obtained. Remember, instruments are not valid for all situations; they are valid for certain groups under certain conditions.

Validity

An instrument which has validity is able to achieve its purpose. Thus, researchers must provide evidence that the instruments they use meet the standards established by psychometricians for validity. The validity of most instruments is established by providing evidence of content validity, construct validity, and/or criterion-related validity.

Content Validity   To establish the content validity of a new or existing instrument, the researcher must show that the items selected adequately represent the entire content area/domains that the instrument claims to measure. Lynn (1986) emphasizes that content validity is not face validity. She points out that **face validity** is an assumption, "a non-statistical assessment of the logical tie between the elements or items of an instrument and its purpose" (p. 382), whereas **content validity** is a rigorous assessment based on quantitative evidence. See Lynn (1986) for a complete description of a two-stage process (developmental stage and judgment quantification stage) for establishing the content validity of instruments. In the developmental stage, each content area/domain is carefully defined, and representative behaviors are identified. In the next stage (judgment quantification) a structured procedure is used with five to ten expert judges to quantitatively verify (through the use of rating scales) that all items as well as the entire instrument adequately represent the content area/domains specified.

Construct Validity   **Construct validity** is more difficult to establish than content validity. The goal is to demonstrate the extent to which the instrument will discriminate between those who possess and those who do not possess the characteristic/attribute of interest (e.g., hope). Construct validation of an instrument is an ongoing process that utilizes several different procedures. In their review of 17 articles reporting on instrument development or modification, Rew, Stuppy, and Becker (1988) identified 14 methods used to demonstrate construct validity, including:

> . . . factor analysis, expert review, principal-component factor analysis with varimax rotation, correlation with scores from another tool, known groups or multitrait-multi-method analysis, Tucker's Coefficient of Congruence, readability, and correlation with literature review [pp. 13–14].

Referring to statements issued by the American Psychological Association, Rew et al (1988) point out that ideal validation includes several types of evidence from each of the traditional categories (content, criterion, and construct). Because of this, they recommend that all researchers reporting on instrument development interpret the meaning of their studies for other researchers and recommend additional steps for validation. Also, limitations in the methods used during the validation process should be made explicit.

Criterion-Related Validity   There are two types of **criterion-related validity**: predictive validity and concurrent validity. With each, an individual's performance on one measure is used to infer his or her probable standing on another measure (a criterion) (American Psychological Association 1974). With *predictive validity*, a current measure is used to predict future performance (e.g., a high score on a leadership test is used to predict successful leadership on the job). The American Psychological Association's (1974) standards for psychological tests clearly state that instruments intended for prediction must have established criterion-related validity (based on at least one but preferably on multiple studies) and that there is no substitute for criterion-related validity.

Concurrent validity indicates an individual's present standing on a criterion. For example, individuals who respond to an instrument on leadership style might also be asked to complete a measure on the management of people, to determine if high scores on one are indicative of high scores on the other, more established instrument. From this example, it is evident that criterion validity is dependent on the quality of the criterion measure selected by the researcher. Thus, the instrument used to obtain measures on the criterion variable must also have sound psychometric properties.

Reliability

Instruments that are reliable measure the construct/variable of interest in a consistent manner. Therefore, an instrument is reliable to the extent that it provides consistent measurements across subjects and is stable over time. Reliability is expressed as a coefficient. An instrument with perfect reliability has a coefficient of 1.00. If an instrument is composed of several subscales, the reliability of each must be assessed (Gay 1985). Gay provides guidelines for the interpretation of the coefficients of **correlation**. Gay notes that a coefficient of over .90 is acceptable for any instrument. A coefficient of at least .90 is recommended for achievement and aptitude tests, whereas a coefficient of .80–.89 is acceptable for personality measures. Gay points out that researchers using attitude scales usually report correlation coefficients in the range .60–.80.

The major types of reliability tests used by researchers include test-retest reliability, internal consistency reliability, and split-half reliability. It is recommended that researchers obtain at least two reliability measures for each instrument because each method involves different sources of error (American Psychological Association 1974). **Test-retest reliability** is a measure of the stability of an instrument over time, thus a high coefficient is desirable. This measurement is very easy to obtain. You simply administer the instrument to a representative sample of your target population; administer the instrument again after about a two-week lapse in time; and correlate the two sets of scores. There is no set standard for the interval of time between testings, but it should be long enough so that subjects are not able to recall their responses from the first administration. The **internal consistency reliability** is a measure of how well all of the items in the instrument relate to each other and to the total instrument. To obtain this coefficient, you need to administer the instrument only once to a representative sample of subjects and then apply a statistical test. Alpha is the most widely used measure of internal consistency; it provides an indicator of how a subject's performance on one item on the instrument relates to all other items. Waltz et al (1984) claim that the alpha coefficient is the preferred measure of internal consistency because it provides one value for an entire set of data, and "is equal in value to the distribution of all possible split-half coefficients associated with a particular set of test data" (p. 136). **Split-half reliability** is also an indicator of the internal consistency of an instrument, based on administration of the instrument to a representative sample of subjects from the target population. A split-half reliability coefficient is computed by dividing the instrument in half (into even numbers and odd numbers); computing a score for each half (for every subject); and correlating the two sets of scores.

Field-testing Instruments

Field-testing (pretesting) an instrument usually consists of a trial run with 10–20 subjects unless the instrument is complex (Fox and Ventura 1983). The purpose of field-testing is to reveal problems related to the administration and scoring of the instrument, which if corrected, will increase the validity and reliability of the measure. For example, you may find out that a particular item is constantly being skipped, or that subjects are writing N/A (not applicable) on key items. It is also possible that some subjects will not have the information to answer a particular question (e.g., staff nurses might not know if the hospital administrator involves the vice-president for nursing in strategic planning meetings).

Fox and Ventura (1983) provide a useful list of suggestions for field-testing instruments. Those with particular relevance for this discussion include trying several methods of data collection, if necessary, before making a final decision about the instrument and conducting a second or third trial run if major changes in procedures are made after each field test.

At this stage of instrument development it is also worthwhile to analyze the responses from a small number of completed instruments in relation to the research questions (if a study), or total patient profile (for clinical decision making), to determine the adequacy and usefulness of the data obtained. As a result of this analysis you may find it necessary to alter some of the questions, add new questions, or perhaps alter the time of testing.

Conclusion

Three common errors in instrument selection can affect the quality of nursing studies: use of instruments without established psychometric properties, use of established instruments without retesting for validity and reliability, use of instruments that do not truly measure the variable(s) of interest. The first two errors are likely to occur when the researcher is in a rush to develop an instrument and skips some of the basic and necessary steps to ensure the instrument's validity and reliability. The third error, not obtaining a true measurement on the variable of interest, occurs when an instrument is selected in haste. A systematic search is always needed to find an instrument that measures the construct of interest with precision. It would be interesting to know the degree to which these errors alone contribute to the number of studies that produce nonsignificant results.

The goal of every researcher should be to select the best instrument available, as opposed to one that is merely adequate (Gay 1981). As a general rule, it is best to use an existing instrument with appropriate psychometric properties, which also meets all of the criteria for your study, thus enabling you to compare your results with the results of other studies. It will also facilitate the replication of studies. To test the generalizability of findings over time and with a variety of subjects, replication studies that use the same instrumentation are needed. In their survey of published research, Jacobsen and Meininger (1985) reported that less than 10% of the 434 studies they reviewed were replications, yet these are a nursing priority. Finally, the use of existing instruments will expand our understanding of particular constructs and provide data for the ongoing evaluation of the psychometric properties of the instruments themselves.

Experienced researchers concur that it is never worth the time or effort to conduct a study with instruments known to be poorly constructed or inadequately tested. It is especially unfair to employ volunteers, especially if they are patients, in studies that will never produce valid data because of poor instrumentation. Also, findings of published studies in which poor measurement instruments were used can be very misleading. The average nurse is not an expert in instrumentation and therefore must depend on the researcher to be objective and honest in choosing instruments with psychometric properties that are appropriate for the study. The researcher should report the psychometric properties of the instrument obtained during its initial development and testing. If it is an existing instrument, the psychometric properties established for the current study should be reported. An extensive review of published nursing studies (Brown, Tanner, and Padrick 1984) revealed that most nurses (more than 50%) fail to report on the reliability and validity of their instruments.

To avoid these errors, researchers need to use a systematic process for instrument selection. Once a potential instrument is found, a set of selection criteria, such as that presented in Table 10–2, should be applied. If an appropriate instrument cannot be located, none of the four options left is ideal:

1. Modify the operational definition to conform to the instrument and establish its reliability and validity for your study.

2. Modify and test an existing instrument to make it acceptable.

3. Change the research question and/or the variable to be measured, and begin the search for an appropriate instrument.

4. Develop and test a new instrument to fit the purpose and target population of your study.

The first option, modification of your operational definition to conform to the instrument you would like to use, is the most efficient of the four available. If the nature and purpose of the research permit such a change, then you need only establish the validity and reliability of the instrument selected for your study. If option two is your choice, take into consideration the extent of the modifications needed. For example, it is relatively simple to change the wording in the item stems to make them more relevant to the target population (e.g., by substituting the word *medical center* for *institution*). However, if you want to modify an instrument designed for one target population (e.g., lung cancer patients) for patients in a different target population (e.g., women with breast cancer), you could be taking on a major project. You need to follow all of the principles of instrument development to have confidence in the final product, which could turn out to be a new instrument.

If, in the researcher's total assessment of the situation, the best thing to do is change the nature of the variable to be studied (option 3) and start again, then, as tough as it may seem at the time, this is the appropriate action to take. The fourth option involves a substantial commitment of time and resources, and requires advanced knowledge of measurement principles and statistics. However, if the researcher decides that the development of a new instrument is the best option, then he or she should proceed in this direction. The key to success is to follow the procedures described in this chapter rigorously and systematically.

Guidelines for Critique

- What psychosocial variables were measured in the study?

- What were the levels of measurement for the variables?

- What types of instruments were developed or used to measure the psychosocial variables?

- Was the instrument appropriate for the study purpose and target population?

- What types of measurement scales were used?

- If sample items were provided, what types of items were used, and do they meet the goals for item construction?

- Were the reliability and validity tests appropriate for the instruments described?

SUMMARY OF KEY IDEAS AND TERMS

✓   Construct validity is an estimate of how well an instrument measures a theoretical construct, as determined by hypothesis testing. For example, an instrument designed to measure creativity should differentiate creative and noncreative individuals.

✓   Content area refers to the circumscribed area of content that an instrument measures.

✔ Content validity is a systematic assessment (qualitative and quantitative) used to establish that an instrument adequately represents the entire content area/domains specified.

✔ Criterion-related validity can be either concurrent or predictive, where predictive validity is a current score on an instrument used to predict future performance. Concurrent validity indicates an individual's current standing on a criterion measure related to the construct of interest.

✔ Face validity is an individual's personal opinion that an instrument adequately represents a specified content area.

✔ Internal consistency reliability is the statistical determination of how well each item on an instrument relates to all other items. It provides an indication of how consistently individuals respond to all items on an instrument.

✔ Measurement scale is the options on a psychosocial instrument to which subjects respond (e.g., strongly agree to strongly disagree). These options are usually assigned a numerical value for analysis.

✔ Psychometric properties refer to the validity and reliability of the instrument.

✔ Reliability is the property/characteristic of an instrument that means the instrument measures the same theory consistently (e.g., across all subjects in the target population).

✔ Semantic differential scale is a psychosocial scale designed to quantify concepts in terms of their word meanings (semantic properties).

✔ Split-half reliability is an indicator of the internal consistency of an instrument. It is determined by dividing an instrument in half, computing a score for each half and correlating the two sets of scores.

✔ Sociodemographic questionnaire is a specialized instrument designed to obtain personal, social and environmental data about subjects.

✔ Test-retest reliability is the administration of an instrument to the same individuals at two different times to determine if scores are consistent over time.

✔ Validity is the property/characteristic of a psychosocial instrument that means the instrument measures what it purports to measure (e.g., stress).

References

Allen MJ, Yen W: *Introduction to Measurement Theory*. Monterey, Calif.: Brooks/Cole, 1979.

American Psychological Association: *Standards for Educational and Psychological Tests*. Washington, D.C.: American Psychological Association, 1974.

Barhyte DY, Bacon LD: Approaches to cleaning data sets: A technical comment. *Nurs Res* 1985; 34, 62–64.

Brink P: Value orientations as an assessment tool in cultural diversity. *Nurs Res* 1984; 33, 198–203.

Brown JS, Tanner CA, Padrick KP: Nursing's search for scientific knowledge. *Nurs Res* 1984; 33, 26–32.

Buros OK: *The Eighth Mental Measurement Yearbook*. Highland Park, N.J.: Gryphon, 1979 (the latest publication in a series that began in 1944).

Buros OK: *Tests in Print*. Highland Park, N.J.: Gryphon, 1974 (a supplementary volume to the yearbook).

Chun K, Cobb S, French J: *Measures for Psychological Assessment: A Guide to 3,000 Original Sources and Their Applications*. Ann Arbor: University of Michigan Institute for Social Research, 1975.

Comrey A, Backer T, Glaser E: *A Sourcebook of Mental Health Measures*. Los Angeles: Human Interaction Research Institute, 1973.

Constantino RE: Comparison of two group interventions for the bereaved. *Image* 1988; 20, 83–87.

Cunningham GK: *Educational and Psychological Measurement*. New York: Macmillan, 1986.

Fenton MV: Development of the scale of humanistic nursing behaviors. *Nurs Res* 1987; 36, 82–87.

Flaskerud JH: Is the Likert Scale format culturally biased? *Nurs Res* 1988; 37, 185–186.

Foreman MD: Reliability and validity of mental statistics questionnaires in elderly hospitalized patients. *Nurs Res* 1987; 36, 216–220.

Fox RN, Ventura MR: Small-scale administration of instruments and procedures. *Nurs Res* 1983; 32, 122–125.

Frank-Stromborg: *Instruments for Nursing Research*. Norwalk, Conn.: Appleton-Lange, 1988.

Gay LR: *Educational Research: Competencies for Analysis and Application*, 2nd ed. Columbus, Ohio: Charles E. Merrill, 1981.

Gay LR: *Educational Evaluation and Measurement*, 2nd ed. Columbus, Ohio: Charles E. Merrill, 1985.

Goodwin L et al: Nurse practitioner rating form part II: Methodological development. *Nurs Res* 1981; 30: 270–276.

Green CJ: The use of psychodiagnostic questionnaires in predicting risk factors and health outcomes. Pages 301–333 in Karoly P (editor), *Management Strategies in Health Psychology*. New York: Wiley, 1985.

Jacobsen BS, Meininger JC: The designs of published nursing research: 1956–1983. *Nurs Res* 1985; 34, 306–312.

Johnson O: *Tests and Measurements in Child Development: Handbooks I & II*. San Francisco: Jossey-Bass, 1976.

Karoly P (editor): *Measurement Strategies in Health Psychology*. New York: Wiley, 1985.

Kerlinger FN: *Foundations of Behavioral Research*. New York: Holt, Rinehart and Winston, 1973.

Kerlinger FN: *Behavioral Research, A Conceptual Approach*. New York: Holt, Rinehart and Winston, 1979.

Lowery BJ, Jacobsen BS: On the consequences of overturning turnover: A study of performance and turnover. *Nurs Res* 1984; 33, 363–367.

Lynn MR: Determination and quantification of content validity *Nurs Res* 1986; 35, 382–385.

Miller DC: *Handbook of Research Design and Social Measurement*, 4th ed. New York: Longman, 1983.

Miller J, Powers M: Development of an instrument to measure hope. *Nurs Res* 1988; 37, 6–10.

Norbeck JS: What constitutes a publishable report of instrument development? *Nurs Res* 1985; 34:380–382.

Northouse L: Social support in patients' and husbands' adjustment to breast cancer. *Nurs Res* 1988; 37, 91–95.

Nunnally JC: *Psychometric Theory*. New York: McGraw-Hill, 1978.

Prescott PA et al: The nurse practitioner rating form, part I: Conceptual development and potential uses. *Nurs Res* 1981; 34:223–228.

Reeder L, Ramacher L, Gorelnik S: *Handbook of Scales and Indices of Health Behavior*. Pacific Palisades, Calif.: Goodyear Publishing, 1976.

Rew L, Stuppy D, Becker H: Construct validity in instrument development: A vital link between nursing practice, research and theory. *Adv Nurs Sci* 1988; 10, 10–22.

Richardson BK: Psychiatric inpatients' perceptions of the seclusion-room experience. *Nurs Res* 1987; 36, 234–238.

Shaw ME, Wright JM: *Scales for the Measurement of Attitudes*. New York: McGraw Hill, 1967.

Sparks S: The National Library of Medicine's bibliographic databases: Tools for nursing research. *Image* 1984; 16, 24–27.

Steinke E: Elder adults' knowledge and attitudes about sexuality and aging. *Image* 1988; 20, 93–95.

Stinson SM, Ken JC (editors): *International Issues in Nursing Research* Philadelphia: Charles Press Publishers, 1986.

Strickland OL, Waltz C: Measurement of research variables in nursing. Pages 70–90 in Chinn PL (editor), *Nursing Research Methodology, Issues and Implementation*. Rockville, Md.: Aspen, 1986.

Strumpf NE, Evans LK: Physical restraint of the hospitalized elderly: Perceptions of patients and nurses. *Nurs Res* 1988; 37, 132–137.

Suter WN: Approaches to avoiding errors in data sets: A technical note. *Nurs Res* 1987; 36, 262–263.

Turk DC, Kerns RD: Assessment in health psychology: A cognitive behavioral perspective. Chapter 9 in: *Measurement Strategies in Health Psychology*. Karvly, P (editor). New York: John Wiley & Sons, 1985.

Ventura MR, Henshaw AS, Atwood JR: Instrumentation: The next step. *Nurs Res* 1981; 30, 257.

Waltz CF, Strickland OL, Lenz E: *Measurement in Nursing Research*. Philadelphia: F. A. Davis, 1984.

Ward MJ, Fetler M: *Instruments for Use in Nursing Education Research*. WICHE, 1979.

Ward MJ, Lindeman C: *Instruments for Measuring Nursing Practice and other Health Care Variables*. Superintendent of Documents, Washington, D.C., Vols 1 and 2, 1979.

Ward MJ: Nursing research instruments: Some considerations and recommendations. Pages 41–60 in Stinson SM, Ken JC (editors), *International Issues in Nursing Research*. Philadelphia: Charles Press Publishers, 1986.

11

Collecting Data on Biophysiological Variables

ADA M. LINDSEY ▪ NANCY A. STOTTS

Chapter Objectives

After reading this chapter, the student should be able to:

- Propose a plan to identify the biophysiological variables that have been studied and the measurement techniques used

- List available resources for gaining information about biophysiological instruments that can be used for measurement of variables

- Discuss analytically the guidelines for selecting an instrument to manipulate or measure a biophysiological variable

- Compare and contrast at least one direct and one indirect measurement for a selected biophysiological variable

- Compare and contrast the criteria for selection of a paper-and-pencil versus other measures of biophysiological variables

- Give at least two examples of biophysiological variables for which measurement will yield interval-level data

- Give two examples of equipment/instruments used in measuring a biophysiological variable of interest

(Continued)

- Explain how reliability of equipment may be tested

- When given a research study that includes biophysiological variables, evaluate the instrumentation used for the independent and the dependent variables

- Critique the methods section of research reports relative to inclusion of information about instrumentation used for measuring biophysiological variables

In This Chapter . . .

Is it common practice to withhold iced beverages from patients with a myocardial infarct? Do you know what effects the drinking of ice water or some other iced, noncaffeinated beverage will have on the myocardium of patients with a myocardial infarction? Do the degree of coldness, the volume consumed, the time over which it is consumed, and the position assumed for drinking the fluid make a difference in the effects? How would you determine or measure these effects?

Do you know what effects the provision of sucking opportunities for premature infants during tube feedings will have on their weight or the length of time until they can be bottle fed? Will the sucking opportunities adversely affect these infants? How much energy is required for sucking? How would you determine or measure these variables?

Do you know what effects therapeutic touch or conversation about the patient's condition will have on the intracranial pressure of unconscious head-injured patients? How can you define therapeutic touch? When should you measure intracranial pressure? How many data points are needed? Is a mean pressure over some specified period of time sufficient to capture the nature of change in the dependent variable, intracranial pressure?

These are only a few of the examples and questions that can be addressed in collecting data on biophysiological variables. This is an exciting and challenging area for nurse researchers, and the findings may have a significant impact on patient outcomes.

Because nurses are concerned with human responses, nurse researchers frequently combine biophysiological, psychological, and sociological variables in a study. Many psychosocial variables, e.g., depression and anxiety, can be measured indirectly by biophysiological measures. Nursing research often includes variables that must be measured by means of physiological instrumentation. (**Instrumentation** is the process of using a device or combination of equipment for measurement.) For example, if you want to determine the effects of some specific nursing activity, such as turning, on the intracranial pressure of head-injured patients, instrumentation is necessary to quantify changes in the dependent variable (intracranial pressure) as influenced by the independent variable (turning). If you want to examine the effect of use of the bedside commode on oxygen consumption and heart rate in myocardial infarct patients, you also need instrumentation to quantify those dependent variables.

In this chapter, we address the measurement of biophysiological variables from the perspective of the research process. Conceptualization of these variables is acknowledged as being critical to the selection of instruments for measurement. Prior research frequently provides the foundation for further study. Thus, we emphasize the areas of evaluation of the conceptualization, operationalization of the variables, instruments used for measurement, and analysis of the findings, specifically in relation to measurement. We propose a method of summarizing prior research to help you identify existing knowledge in the field and conceptualize the area of your research interest. The wide array of instruments available as well as the strengths and limitations of some of the instruments are explored. We address practical issues, such as whether the "ideal" instrument is available, whether a noninvasive measure can be used instead of an invasive one, and how issues of cost affect various measurement techniques. Threats to validity and reliability of instruments are repeatedly emphasized. These themes are illustrated with examples of nursing research.

Specifically, we use five major content areas of concern to nursing as the scheme for organizing the review of research examples. These five areas are feeding alterations, activity and position, patient education, healing and infection, and environmental stimuli. These problem areas were selected because they are research areas of particular interest to nursing, as evidenced by several studies reported recently in the nursing literature. The process of measuring biophysiological variables, from conceptualization to interpretation of findings, is presented and illustrated with examples from these five conceptual areas.

Preparing for Your Study

Background literature and research reports relevant to the problem area help you conceptualize the specific research questions you want to study and determine which variables are of greatest importance to your problem area. Once you identify the variables of interest, from the theoretical, empirical, and clinical perspective of the research problem, you need to develop an operational definition for each of them (see Chapters 4 and 8). These operational definitions provide specific information about how the variables will be measured.

Read Broadly

Knowing how other investigators have defined and measured the same or similar variables helps you select measurement instruments. Initially, as you begin to address your problem area, it is useful to read broadly. Determine what questions others have addressed, identify problems in the design or measures used previously, and think about what remains unknown.

Use Summary Charts

In our experience with reviewing previous work, it has been particularly helpful to develop summary charts (Lindsey et al 1981; Lindsey 1982, 1983). Table 11–1 is an example of such a chart. A summary of studies in which the effects of activity on intracranial pressure were examined is another example of this kind of review (Mitchell 1980). On the summary chart, always identify the following information:

- Authors
- Source of their report
- Purpose(s) of the study
- Research questions or hypotheses
- Independent and dependent variables
- Measures and equipment used to quantify the variables
- Study sample
- Specific procedures described for the data collection
- Major findings and conclusions

Preparing the information from each related study in this manner makes it easier for you to evaluate studies, to analyze designs and data-collection techniques, and, if possible, to compare findings across studies. It is absolutely essential to do this review of prior work in your problem area and to integrate and synthesize the ideas about what is known and what remains unknown.

Make Decisions Based on Information from Prior Studies

From this review, you should be able to determine the focus for subsequent research in your problem area. The review also helps you make decisions about the measurement of the variables you have selected for your study.

Discuss Your Study with Others

Once you have formulated your study, talk to other clinicians and researchers about it. Specifically, discuss the questions you will be attempting to examine and the measurement aspects of your research problem. Others may help you refine your

TABLE 11–1   *Chart for Summarizing Studies in a Problem Area*

Authors Source of report Purpose of study	Research questions or hypotheses	Variables: independent and dependent	Instruments or equipment	Sample and procedure	Major findings and conclusions
1.					
2.					
3.					

work and identify potential problems. It is much better to troubleshoot all possible contingencies *before* you begin your data collection. Think, talk, read, rethink, continue to talk, and reread. These activities are most frequently associated with better research outcomes.

Biophysiological Instruments

An enormous array of biophysiological phenomena and variables are of interest to nurse researchers. A considerable range of equipment has been used, and it varies widely in sophistication. In some situations, the equipment is used to create the independent variable, such as equipment for oxygen administration, for suctioning, or for administering tube feedings. In other cases, the equipment and instruments are used to measure the dependent variables of interest, such as a thermometer, a scale, a sound-level meter, or an **electroencephalograph** (EEG) or **electrocardi-**

```
┌─────────────────────────────────────────────────────────────────┐
│                                                                   │
│   Box 11–1   Four Biophysiological Instruments and What They Measure │
│                                                                   │
│   Cardiac monitor:        Sphygmomanometer:       Flow meter:     │
│     Rate                    Systolic blood pressure   Blood pressure │
│     Rhythm                  Diastolic blood           Volume       │
│     Conduction pattern        pressure                Rate         │
│                             Mean blood pressure                    │
│   Infusion pump:            Pulse pressure                         │
│     Volume                                                         │
│     Pressure                                                       │
│     Rate                                                           │
│                                                                   │
└─────────────────────────────────────────────────────────────────┘
```

ograph (ECG). Whether equipment is used for the independent or the dependent variable depends entirely on the research design and the research questions or hypotheses to be examined.

Examples of equipment used include the cardiac monitor, sphygmomanometer, stopwatch, protractor, treadmill, strain gauge, infusion pump, femoral arteriovenous shunt flow meter, thermometer, gastric motility recording device, scale, tape measure, motorized rocking hammock, rocking bed, audio tape player, wrist accelerometer, electric surface stimulator, hand positioning device, transcutaneous oxygen monitor, Holter monitor, Douglas bag, and biofeedback equipment. And the list goes on. A few biophysiological instruments and the parameters they measure are given in Box 11–1.

Information about biophysiological instruments and their characteristics, such as usability, validity, and reliability, has not been organized into a single source like those available for psychosocial instruments. Available resources that describe biophysiological instruments are not as comprehensive as those in other fields, but the following may be of help to you:

- instrument compilation texts

- review articles

- published research reports

- equipment catalogs from manufacturers

- exhibits at major meetings

The second volume of *Instruments for Measuring Nursing Practice and Other Health Care Variables* (Ward and Lindeman 1978) includes a few descriptions of instruments used for measuring biophysiological variables. Very few of the nursing research texts address measurements of biophysiological variables in any detail. Content about such instruments is usually so well integrated that it is not readily accessible. Lindsey (1982, 1983, 1984) identifies biophysiological phenomena and variables studied by nurse investigators from 1970 to 1980. Reviews are an important source of information; in addition, you should read the original articles. Reviews provide a compilation of research, allowing you to compare specific instruments. Most investigators are willing to share information about the equipment they used. Another source for information about instruments is catalogs from manufacturers of equipment; these may be obtained directly from the company or from sales representatives. Information about equipment can also be obtained by visiting the exhibits at major nursing meetings. Using a combination of these resources will supplement your review of studies and will help you select the most appropriate instrument.

Guidelines for Selecting Biophysiological Measures

In making decisions about measuring variables, you must consider several factors. Consideration of these areas facilitates your selection of the optimal instrument(s).

Availability

Availability is a major factor. From your clinical experience you will have some idea of the equipment used in the patient population from which you will select your sample. If the desired equipment is not used routinely in the settings where you plan to collect data, it may be possible to obtain it from other sources. You may be able to borrow it from another setting or obtain it on loan from the company that manufactures it. Perhaps it will be necessary to purchase it.

Direct or Indirect Measure

Another factor to consider is whether or not it is possible to obtain a direct measure of the variables. Whenever a direct measure is available, it is ideal to use it. For example, if you are interested in the effect of body position on blood pressure, an arterial line (not a cuff sphygmomanometer) is the most direct measure of blood pressure.

In some cases you may have to use an indirect measure of the variable. If you are interested in comparing the energy expended in two types of bathing—for example, a bed bath versus a standing shower—you must select an indirect measure of energy expenditure, such as oxygen consumption. If you are interested in determining the stress response to some stressor, such as observing resuscitation of other patients in the coronary care unit, you must select several indirect measures to quantify the response. Examples include heart rate, blood pressure, plasma cortisol levels, and urinary excretion of catecholamines.

Single versus Multiple Measures

This last example illustrates another important notion. For some variables, you may need to use multiple measures to assess the effect of the independent variable on changes in the outcome variable(s) of interest. One measure may not be adequate to demonstrate change; it may not be sufficiently sensitive to show the effects of the independent variable. With a single measure, the changes observed also could be due to other events; multiple measures help control for this possible problem. The uncontrolled existence of these other factors poses competing hypotheses and reduces the strength of the study findings. For example, caffeine consumption and body position, as well as the introduction of some independent variable stressor such as a treadmill, influence heart rate and blood pressure. Your findings are less credible unless all the other major factors that influence the dependent variables (e.g., heart rate and blood pressure) are held constant or accounted for. When you make the final decision about the operational definitions, you should have taken the potential threats into account. The definitions that emerge direct the instrumentation. For this reason, creating the operational definitions for the variables is a critical step in the research process. If measurement of the variables is not sufficient to capture the phenomena, it is impossible for others to believe or to use the findings.

Sensitivity, Validity, and Reliability

The instruments selected to measure the study variables should be the most appropriate ones available. They should be sufficiently sensitive to show changes in the parameter being measured, and they should be valid and reliable. Issues related to the use of the transcutaneous oxygen monitor illustrate this point. The more traditional and accurate approach for measuring change in the blood gases has been via collection of arterial blood samples. Obtaining arterial blood for gas analysis is considered an invasive procedure, and multiple samplings may adversely influence an already compromised patient. Transcutaneous oxygen and carbon dioxide monitors have been developed to alleviate this problem; a heated electrode is used as a noninvasive sensing device. These monitoring devices are used frequently for the short-term gestation infant because the blood gas values obtained from the monitors and from the actual blood samples are more nearly identical (except at hypoxic levels) than those values obtained when the monitors are used for adults.

Invasive versus Noninvasive Measures

This example also illustrates several other issues involved in selecting instruments to quantify changes in biophysiological variables. One issue is that of selecting **invasive** versus **noninvasive** techniques. The only true or credible measure for a variable may require an invasive procedure. In some patient populations the clinical state of the desired study population may preclude the use of such techniques. However, these subjects may already have undergone the necessary invasive procedure. For example, if you want to determine the effects of the patient's position on central venous pressures, it is possible to do this study in subjects who already have a central venous line connected to a monitor with either a polygraph tracing or a digital readout.

Level of Data Obtained

Another consideration in instrument selection is the type of data that can be obtained. Measurement of many biophysiological variables yields interval-level data, because values for the variables usually lie along some continuum (see Chapter 14). For example, heart rate, respiratory rate, temperature, oxygen consumption, body weight, serum albumin, urinary output, and age yield data points distributed at equal intervals. Such continuous data points allow the use of more powerful statistical analyses. (See Chapter 14 for the benefits of collecting interval-level or ratio-level data.) With some paper-and-pencil measures you are unable to get interval-level data, but in some circumstances these measures must be used nonetheless, because they best capture the variable of interest.

Cost

The last issue influencing equipment selection is cost. Of course, it is essential to select an instrument that is both affordable and appropriate. You may need to find a source of funds—for example, working with another researcher who has grant or institutional support, submitting an application to a funding source to obtain your own support, or obtaining assistance from the manufacturer whose equipment you will be using in your study. It is also possible to conduct studies without incurring additional costs for instrumentation. See later sections of this chapter.

You should also give serious consideration to the cost of the research to the subjects—that is, cost of equipment, cost ot time, cost of privacy, and attendant risks—and the potential benefits to be gained. When you make these costs and the benefits explicit, most subjects willingly consent to participate in research that they perceive to have merit.

Summary of Guidelines

All these issues must be examined in determining the measurements to be made for all the study variables. Major questions to ask yourself when selecting an instrument are summarized below:

■   What instruments are routinely used in your setting to measure the variable of interest?

- Are the instruments you want to use readily available?

- Which is more meaningful and practical—direct or indirect measurement?

- Will the instrument be sensitive enough to detect changes in the variable?

- Are multiple measures needed to capture the breadth of the variable(s) of interest?

- Do the measures yield interval-level data?

- Are the instruments considered valid and reliable?

- If invasive measures are needed, are they a routine part of the care for the patient population of interest?

- What is the cost of the instruments you are planning to use?

The selected instruments must be (1) able to measure the variables(s), (2) sensitive to changes in the variable(s), (3) valid and reliable, and (4) affordable.

Paper-and-Pencil Instruments to Measure Biophysiological Variables

Some biophysiological phenomena are more subjective than objective; pain, fatigue, and nausea are three examples. To quantify these phenomena, the investigator must rely on the subject's perception and evaluation of the magnitude or changes in the sensation experienced. In these instances, paper-and-pencil instruments are used frequently to measure the sensation. The McGill-Melzack Pain Questionnaire (Melzack 1975), the Fatigue Symptom Checklist (Yoshitake 1971), and the Symptom Distress Scale (McCorkle and Young 1978) are examples of paper-and-pencil instruments that have achieved some measure of validity and reliability. In addition, visual analog scales have been devised for subjects to rate the magnitude of the perceived sensation. These have a straight line with anchoring words placed at either end of the line. At one end the phrase might be "the worst I have ever had"; at the opposite end, "the least I have ever had." The subjects are told to place a mark along the line to convey what they feel with respect to the dimension being assessed, for example, pain or nausea. An example is shown in Figure 11–1.

Some biophysiological phenomena are assessed according to written criteria developed to quantify the status (or change in status) of individuals. The criteria were determined with respect to the accepted range of normal values. An example is the Glascow Coma Scale; it is used to evaluate an individual's responsiveness to specific graded stimuli (Teasdale and Jennett 1974). After the subject's responses to the listed items are evaluated, a composite score is determined by summing the

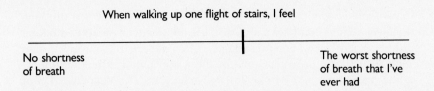

When walking up one flight of stairs, I feel

| No shortness of breath | | The worst shortness of breath that I've ever had |

Figure 11–1 Visual analog scale for measuring one dimension of the biophysiological variable breathlessness. The distance from the left end of the scale to the vertical cross line, as measured with a ruler, is the measurement.

ratings. Three areas in which the responses are rated are eye opening, best verbal response, and best motor response. The scale is short, and the responses are rated according to well-defined criteria, such as eyes open spontaneously = 4; eyes open to speech = 3; eyes open to pain = 2; and eyes don't open = 1. This scale is used clinically as well as for research to assess level of consciousness. Another example is the Short Portable Mental Status Questionnaire; it is frequently used to assess the mental status of elderly subjects (Pfeiffer 1975). Ten questions are asked. If fewer than six correct answers are given, the elderly subject is considered to be unreliable in providing accurate information. In essence, this instrument is a measure of cognitive function.

The foremost determinant of instrument selection, in all cases, must be the conceptualization of the phenomena to be studied. There is no inherent value in using a sophisticated invasive measure, such as serum level of lactic acid, if it does not capture the real effect of the variables being studied. Do not dismiss paper-and-pencil instruments to measure phenomena just because the variable is physiological. Remember the guideline of appropriateness; the instrument must measure the phenomena of concern sensitively, reliably, and validly.

Instrumentation: Independent and Dependent Variables

Some equipment is used to create and specify the independent variable. An example is the **treadmill**, a platform covered with a moving surface on which the subject walks. The speed of the moving surface and the angle of the platform can be altered to produce a known physiological demand. The treadmill is used frequently in research. It is set at certain speeds and at certain gradients to establish variable levels of activity as the independent variable; thus, the effects of various levels of activity can be studied.

Other equipment is used to quantify changes in the dependent variables. For example, the cardiac monitor (ECG tracing) is used to determine changes in cardiac rhythm, rate, and conduction patterns in response to varying activity levels. These same dependent-variable parameters could be used to assess the effects of drinking ice water on the myocardium in infarct patients. The independent variable, drinking ice water, could be varied by temperature (degree of coldness), amount given, and position assumed for ingestion of the water. In these two rather different studies, the same outcome measures could be used to show changes. The determination of what parameters to quantify is based on the operational definitions of the study variables.

The considerations for selecting instruments to manipulate the independent variable are really the same as those for choosing instruments to measure the dependent variable. Thus, of concern is the ability of that equipment to manipulate or affect, under the specified experimental conditions, the phenomena of concern. For example, if you want to assess the effects of the temperature of dressings (independent variable) on wound healing (dependent variable), you need to be sure that your equipment provides the specific temperature required for the dressing. Material to provide insulation for the dressing would also be necessary to prevent an influence of environmental temperature on the temperature of the dressing. These conditions have the potential of influencing the dependent variable, wound healing. Conceptual considerations and the operational definitions for the independent variable also provide direction for selection and use of the instruments.

Biophysiological Phenomena: Measurement of Variables

There are diverse types of measures to quantify biophysiological variables. The researcher's conceptualization of the variable provides the referent frame for determining the measurement strategy and for selecting the measurement instrument(s). Some variables, such as body temperature, are physical, whereas others, such as serum albumin, are biochemical. It is possible to use a number of diverse measures as a composite to quantify changes in some variable(s). For example, if the outcome variable of interest is nutritional status, a composite of anatomical, physical, and biochemical measures may be used; these include temperature, weight, caloric intake, activity, nitrogen balance, and serum albumin. Although it is possible to categorize the measures as physical, anatomical, or biochemical, it is more useful from a research perspective to select the appropriate measures on the basis of how variables are conceptualized and defined operationally for the specific study.

Instrument selection is based on conceptualization of the research questions. Biophysiological phenomena studied previously by nurse investigators have been reviewed by Lindsey (1982, 1983, 1984), Kinney (1984), and Foster, Kloner, and Stengrevics (1984). The number of these phenomena examined in nursing studies is large and quite varied. Within the limits of this chapter, it is possible to address only five of these research areas. For each problem area included, one or more studies will be used to show how nurse researchers have measured some of the variables and to address some salient points about the selection and use of instruments to quantify the study variables. The five phenomena to be included are *feeding alterations, activity and position, patient education, healing and infection, and environmental stimuli.*

Feeding Alterations: Instrumentation and Measurement Issues

The majority of the reported research on feeding alterations has addressed two problem areas: the effects of tube feedings, and nausea and vomiting associated with anticancer therapy. Several studies representative of these problem areas are used to illustrate the measurement techniques selected to quantify the variables of interest.

Tube Feeding

Tube feeding can be an uncomfortable experience for many patients. By altering the variables of tube feeding (such as temperature, rate, and volume) and studying the effects, researchers may be able to determine the optimal conditions that will cause the least discomfort.

Using six paid volunteers, Kagawa-Busby and colleagues (1980) conducted a study to "evaluate the effects of nasogastric tube feedings (NGTF) administered at three different temperatures on gastric motility, total gastrointestinal transit time, diarrhea and adverse subjective symptoms" (p. 277). The independent variable was the temperature of the tube feeding, and the dependent variables quantified were the gastric pressure (used as an indirect measure of gastric motility), stool transit time, intragastric temperature, and subjective symptoms reported by the subjects. The materials and equipment required to conduct this study included nasogastric tubes, liquid diet, an infusion pump, a nonabsorbable stool marker, a thermistor, gastric strain gauge and pressure-recording device, and a system for the subjects to indicate their subjective sensations during the tube feedings.

Two similar studies had been reported previously; one using five adult volunteers (Hanson 1973) and one using two rhesus monkeys (Williams and Walike 1975). In each of these reports, the instruments used and the procedures are well described.

Heitkemper and colleagues (1977) conducted a study to determine the effects of rate and volume of tube feeding on tolerance of subjects to the feedings. Rate, as one independent variable, was set at 30, 60, and 85 ml/min, and volume, as the second independent variable, was given as 200, 350, and 500 ml. Tolerance was operationalized to include frequency of subjects' subjective responses, frequency and severity of observed adverse effects, and gastrointestinal disturbances (indirectly assessed by measuring pressure changes within the gastrointestinal tract). This study also used six paid volunteers, and materials and equipment similar to those described above were used for data collection. The instruments and procedure are described in the report.

In these studies, the number of subjects included was inadequate, but the studies represent preliminary work. They provide examples of questions about biophysiological phenomena of interest to nurses.

Nonnutritive Sucking

Feeding alterations of another kind occur in premature infants. The sucking reflex of a premature infant is poorly coordinated, and the general weakness of these vulnerable infants may preclude them from obtaining sufficient formula via sucking. Usually these infants (gestation 34 weeks or less) are given tube feedings, and few to no opportunities for sucking are provided during this period.

Nurse researchers designed a study to test the effects of nonnutritive sucking (using a pacifier nipple) on the clinical course of premature infants (Measel and Anderson 1979). Opportunities for nonnutritive sucking were provided during and for 5 minutes after every tube feeding. Operational definition of the dependent variable, clinical course, included morbidity, time of initiation of bottle feeding, weight, and time of discharge. Fifty-nine premature infants were alternately assigned to the experimental or to the control group. Exclusion criteria and description of the sample are described in the research report.

The equipment needed to create the independent variable, sucking, was made by the investigators. The equipment is not expensive and is readily available. The report includes a description of the construction of the pacifiers as well as the manipulation. Although not used in this study, an electronic suckometer has been developed and can be attached to a research nipple so that sucking can be quantified.

These investigators also developed a feeding evaluation scale that was used at the time of the first bottle feeding. The remainder of the data were collected from the chart or from observation. Unfortunately, from the perspective of the research design, infants in both groups were allowed to have pacifiers at any time, and the frequency and duration of these extra sucking opportunities were not reported.

Another limitation to credibility of the findings acknowledged by the investigators is that complications between the two groups were different. It is difficult to control confounding variables in clinical research; however, attempts to control or account for these variables should be made. The researchers did report that the infants in the experimental group gained more weight (2.6 g/day), that bottle feeding was initiated earlier (3.4 days), and that they were discharged earlier (4 days).

Nausea and Vomiting

Studies in which nausea and vomiting are examined primarily have been conducted with cancer patients. Several different examples illustrating different measurement issues are given.

Zook and Yasko (1983) investigated the relationship between anxiety, hopelessness, pain, specific demographic characteristics, and the degree of nausea and vomiting experienced by 26 cancer patients receiving chemotherapy for the first time. The subjects were receiving a variety of cytotoxic agents and a variety of antiemetics; the study could have been strengthened if both of these confounding variables had been controlled by sample selection criteria. (This is important, because different chemotherapy agents have a different potential for causing nausea and vomiting.) Standardized instruments were used to measure some of the specified variables—for example, the Spielberger State-Trait Inventory, the Beck Hopelessness Scale, and the McGill-Melzack Pain Questionnaire. A nausea and vomiting scale was developed specifically for this study.

When investigators develop instruments for a study, validity and reliability data are usually not established (see Chapters 4, 6, and 10). Lack of these data always creates a question about the findings, because one cannot assume that the scale is, in fact, measuring accurately and reliably what it is purported to measure. This study, however, is a good example of the use of paper-and-pencil instruments to quantify the subject's perception of biophysiologically related sensations.

Cotanch (1983) tested the use of progressive muscle relaxation (PMR) in reducing nausea and vomiting and psychological averseness associated with cancer chemotherapy. The nine subjects were all experiencing refractory drug-induced nausea and vomiting. They were being treated aggressively with a variety of experimental cytotoxic agents, and all were receiving antiemetic agents. Again, control of these confounding variables could have strengthened the study. Progressive muscle relaxation was the independent variable. The investigator provided the PMR training individually to each subject, and they were given audiotapes to take home to practice PMR twice a day and while receiving chemotherapy. One question that remains unanswered is the extent to which each subject achieved PMR. This is an important question, because PMR (the independent variable) was being tested for its influence on the outcome variables (nausea and vomiting) of interest. Baseline values were obtained, and then data were collected at subsequent cycles of chemotherapy administration. However, the study was not initiated at the first cycle of therapy. Data for several variables were collected. They include physiological arousal (operationally defined as blood pressure, pulse, and respiration), state-trait anxiety (Spielberger's inventory), food and fluid intake for two days after therapy, change in weight, and degree and frequency of nausea and vomiting. The use of antiemetics for 48 hours was recorded.

This is an example of a quasi-experimental study (no randomization and no control group, see Chapter 5) in which the intervention had a biophysiological component, and the effects of the PMR were assessed by measuring nausea and vomiting as the dependent variables.

Because anxiety as a state or trait and food and fluid intake may also influence the nausea and vomiting experienced, measurement of these moderating, or intervening, variables was included in the study design. Accounting for or measuring the extent or existence of other variables that may have some potential contribution in influencing the magnitude of the outcome variables is of critical importance in research. If it is known or suspected that food and fluid intake would contribute to nausea and vomiting, the dependent variables of interest, then control of or measurement of food and fluid intake becomes important in explaining the findings obtained. Think about all the major possible explanations that could account for the findings other than the independent variable being tested (such as PMR), and attempt to control for or to measure those other variables. This will increase the credibility of the results obtained (see Chapter 5).

Nutritional Status

Nurses have become more interested in determining the nutritional status of various populations. From clinical observations, it is apparent that the patient's nutritional status may influence the health outcome. Those with less than an adequate nutritional status are at risk for a variety of effects, such as prolonged hospitalization, increased incidence of infection or other complication, and decreased tolerance of therapy. Assessment of nutritional status is particularly important for elderly or obese patients and patients with cancer or anorexia nervosa. Nutritional status is one of those biophysiological variables, like the stress response, that requires measurement of multiple parameters. Because there is no one best measure, researchers must use several.

Layton and colleagues (1981) evaluated, over a three-month period, the nutritional status of eight allogeneic bone marrow recipients who were given total parenteral nutrition. The laboratory tests and the other parameters monitored are well described in this research report.

This is an example of a study in which measurement of the biophysiological parameters requires obtaining blood and urine samples and sending them to a laboratory for analysis.

Each laboratory establishes the normal values for each parameter based on the specific analytical procedures used in making the determination. These normal values may vary from laboratory to laboratory. Usually, the investigator reports the normal range of values as established by the laboratory that performed the analyses. You need to consider this fact when reading and comparing findings from several research reports and in designing and conducting your own study. In the study by Layton et al, the parameters for which laboratory analysis was used included serum albumin and 24-hour urinary creatinine and nitrogen.

In addition to using lab values, Layton et al used other measures, including body weight, triceps skinfold thickness, and arm muscle circumference, to determine the subject's nutritional status. Using established formulas, they calculated nitrogen balance from intake and output measures of nitrogen, and the creatinine height index from the 24-hour urinary creatinine excretion. Several pieces of equipment were used: a scale, a plastic tape measure, and calipers designed to measure skinfold thickness.

Because this study was longitudinal and thus data were collected at several points in time, it was important to determine the reliability of the equipment in collecting these values over time. For example, the same scale should be used for all weight determinations, or prior to weighing the subject, an object of a known weight should be weighed and the scale adjusted accordingly. This is one way to achieve reliability of measurement over time. This same attention to reliability is necessary for the skinfold measurement. Although one manufacturer of calipers reports an accuracy of measurement within a 1-mm error range, a small metal block with specified varying thicknesses can be used to calibrate the calipers to ensure reliability. This is important when measuring parameters at several different times, particularly if you are interested in determining changes over time.

As you are aware, determining the reliability of an instrument is different from determining **interrater reliability** (see Chapter 10). Establishing interrater reliability is essential if more than one individual will collect data. For instance, if your study requires data on skinfold thickness as measured by calipers, all those measuring skinfold thickness should practice repeatedly on several different individuals and record their measurements. Comparison of the values obtained will provide evidence of the similarity or dissimilarity in the measurements made by the raters.

TABLE 11–2 *Feeding Alterations: Four Examples with Variables and Instrumentation*

Variables		Instrumentation	
Independent	**Dependent**	**Independent**	**Dependent**
1. Temperature, volume, and rate of liquid diet (tube feeding)	Subjective sensations Stool transit time Gastric motility Intraluminal temperature	Method of maintaining temperature and flow rate of tube feeding	Assessment tool for sensations Nonabsorbable stool marker Strain gauge Thermistor
2. Sucking Opportunities	Weight change Time to first bottle feeding Success with first bottle Time to discharge	Nipples Electronic suckometer	Scale Medical record Evaluation instrument for bottle feeding
3.	Nausea Vomiting		Instruments to quantify incidence, frequency, duration, and amount
4.	Nutritional status		Scale Tape measure Skinfold thickness calipers Laboratory analysis of selected serum and urine components Diet intake records

If different raters report different measurement for the same individual (that is, if the difference is statistically significant), there is obviously a problem in interrater reliability. The point is that both reliability of the instrument in measuring the parameter as well as reliability across raters in obtaining the measurements must be established. Both of these reliability issues influence data collection. This information should be included in research reports and clearly must be part of the research plan.

Nurse researchers have conducted a number of other studies to examine various aspects of feeding alterations. Some of the variables and instruments used are listed in Table 11–2. The studies just cited where selected to illustrate a variety of considerations that are important to the conduct of research in which biophysiological variables are measured.

Activity and Position: Instrumentation and Measurement Issues

Studies in the area of activity and position have focused on the effects of increases or decreases in activity and the effects of various positions or of changing position. Examples are the effects of ankle flexion against a footboard, an activity regimen in a stroke rehabilitation program, or the mobilization of a patient after surgery. Dependent variables in this type of study have included electrocardiographic responses, various vascular pressures, energy expenditure, fatigue, and intracranial pressure. Understanding the approaches used to measure the effects of activity and position help you formulate your own research or appreciate studies that have been conducted to determine the effects of daily patient activities and the measurements used to quantify the magnitude of the effects. Examples of the variables studied and instruments used are given in Table 11–3.

Energy Expenditure

Oxygen consumption is one of the variables frequently used to measure the effects of activity. It is often used to measure energy expenditure.

Johnston, Watt, and Fletcher (1981) used oxygen consumption to examine the effect of standard in-hospital bathing practices on patients who had recently had a myocardial infarction. Twelve patients with documented transmural infarctions were the convenience sample for the study. The independent variable, standard bathing techniques, included three levels of bathing activity—standing shower, bed bath, and tub shower. The dependent variables were oxygen consumption as well as other responses determined by hemodynamic and electro-cardiographic changes observed in response to the bathing treatment. The variable oxygen consumption was operationalized as the volume of oxygen consumed per kilogram of weight per minute (V_{02}), the total ventilation of expired air at ambient temperature pressure saturated (VE_{atps}), metabolic equivalent units (METS), and respiratory quotient (RQ). Oxygen consumption was measured using the Max Planck respirometer technique. The method of calibration of the gas meter was described, and a known reference gas was used.

The validity of the technique was established by comparing the **Douglas bag technique** with the **Max Planck respirometer technique**. Equations were not ex-

TABLE 11–3 *Activity and Position: Four Examples with Variables and Instrumentation*

Variables		Instrumentation	
Independent	**Dependent**	**Independent**	**Dependent**

1. In-hospital bathing	Oxygen consumption
	Hemodynamic
	    responses
	EKG responses
		Thermometer	Portable EKG
			    recorder
			Cuff
			    sphygmomanometer
			Stethoscope
			Stopwatch
			Max Planck
			    respirometer
			Beckmann automatic
			    gas analyzer

2. Arm extension
Hip flexion
Turning supine to
    right
Turing right to
    supine
Turning supine to
    left
Turning left to
    supine
Head rotated right
Head rotated left
	Intracranial pressure		Ventriculostomy
			    drainage with #8
			    French tube
			Open bore
			    manometer
			Ruler

3. Backrest position:
    Flat and 20°
	Cardiac output	Carbon dioxide
		    injector
		Protractor
			Thermodilution
			    catheter
			Cardiac output
			    computer

4. Backrest position:
    0°, 20°, 30°, 45°
	Pulmonary artery
	    pressure (systolic,
	    diastolic, mean)
	Pulmonary capillary
	    wedge pressure
		Ruler	Strain guage
			Thermodilution
			    catheter
			Gould brush recorder

plicitly stated for the oxygen calculations, but a reference giving those calculations was cited. The reported detail of the methodology permits replication of the study. Oxygen consumption is a complex and expensive measure to obtain but an accurate way to quantify an important variable.

In a study of the effects of various lifting techniques on the energy expenditure of subjects being lifted, (Geden 1982) investigated the mechanical lift, rocking axillary, self-lift, shoulder assist, and straight pull.

Geden was interested in determining the effects on normal subjects lifted by nurses using each of these techniques. The dependent variables were energy expenditure, heart rate, respiratory rate, and blood pressure. Energy expenditure was operationally defined as oxygen consumption; the Waters MRM-I Oxygen Consumption Computer was used to measure it in this study. The authors noted that this instrument is comparable to Douglas bag gas sampling.

It is important to recognize that there are many instruments available to measure oxygen consumption. The Douglas bag technique is considered the "gold standard"—that is, the ideal against which all other measures are evaluated. When you are reading or planning a study and the techniques noted by others for measuring a physiologic variable are not familiar to you, you need to consult a reputable source to increase your understanding of the technique. Normally, authors cite references they have used for instrumentation, and this is a good place to begin your search for further information. In addition, the validity of that instrument—that is, how accurately it measures the variable under consideration—is a critical consideration. The reliability of the instrument also is important, because it tells you how reproducible the findings are. Information about both of these aspects of an instrument should be noted in a study report or found in the references cited in the article.

Hathaway and Geden (1983) built on this work when they studied the effect of various types of leg exercises on energy expenditure. They used a convenience sample (see Chapter 8) of 36 healthy adults, 18 men and 18 women. The independent variable of various types of leg exercise was divided into three levels—passive range-of-motion exercises, active range-of-motion exercises, and isometric exercises. Hathaway and Geden measured energy expenditure by oxygen consumption, respiratory rate, heart rate, and blood pressure. The type of instrument used to collect each variable is described. The model number is given; this detail about instrumentation adds credibility to the findings.

Position The effects of position and activity on other aspects of biophysical functions also have been reported. Intracranial pressure is one of those areas.

Mitchell, Ozuna, and Lipe (1981) examined what effects turning patients in bed to four positions had on intracranial pressure. The independent variables were two activities—arm extension, hip flexion—

and the four positions—supine to right, right to supine, supine to left, left to supine. Also, the effects of head rotation left and head rotation right were evaluated. The dependent variable of intracranial pressure was operationalized as ventricular fluid pressure (VFP). The authors describe its normal variations and the effects that various maneuvers have on VFP. Lengthy descriptions are provided of the VFP system used, its insertion, associated equipment, and the technique for measuring intracranial pressure. The authors discuss the assets and limitations of this system in producing valid and reliable data. They include a discussion of why these data could be used to accomplish the purpose of the study.

This study is an excellent model for the new researcher to follow in describing his or her instruments and for the critical consumer of research findings to use in evaluating studies.

Backrest position has been studied to determine its effect on parameters obtained from a pulmonary artery catheter. For the critical care nurse, such studies add to the scientific basis of nursing practice.

Grose, Woods, and Laurent (1981) reported one of the first studies in which the effect of backrest position on cardiac output measured by the thermodilution technique was examined. The two positions evaluated were flat and 20-degree backrest elevation. Instrumentation for both the independent variable and the dependent variable is important in this study. A protractor was used to determine the angle of the backrest accurately and consistently.

Although studies in which physiological variables are measured are sometimes quite technologically complex, the operationalization of this independent variable illustrates that the instrumentation selected must be appropriate to the purpose of the study and need not always be expensive or complex.

The **thermodilution technique** for determination of cardiac output is well described. Measurement of cardiac output with a pulmonary artery catheter requires the injection of a solution and the distal measurement of its temperature to calculate the flow through the heart, that is, the cardiac output. The authors controlled extraneous contamination from other variables when they standardized the pressure, timing, and volume of injectant. They achieved this control by the use of a carbon dioxide injector, which provided a uniform rate and volume of injectant. In addition, cardiac output was measured two times, and the average of these two samples was used for the study (see Chapter 5). Also, when the cardiac output was read from the digital readout, it was checked by two investigators. The authors planned these various details of the design to increase internal validity of the measures and reported them so that readers could know what precautions had been taken. The detailed descriptions that Grose, Woods, and Laurent provided allow others to build on their work.

Backrest elevation was also addressed by Chulay and Miller (1984). They investigated its effect on pulmonary artery and pulmonary capillary wedge pressure measurements in cardiac surgery patients. They had an interesting way to operationalize the four angles of backrest—0, 20, 30, and 45 degrees. They used basic geometry and defined the distance of elevation of the backrest by the sine of the angle (for example, sine 20 degrees = 11/32). In other words, they elevated the head of the bed 11 inches vertically if they wanted the sloping portion of the bed to be 32 inches long (see Figure 11–2).

Again, the authors provide detailed information about all of the instrumentation. It includes use of the phlebostatic axis, placement of the transducer, and the types, models, and brands of the various pieces of equipment used. A brush recorder was used to record the **waveform** from which the dependent variables of pulmonary artery pressure and pulmonary capillary wedge pressure were derived. Although the authors indicate that data were read at end-expiration and that data were rounded off to the nearest torr (millimeter of mercury), they could have further strengthened the instrumentation (internal validity) if they had indicated who had interpreted the waveforms and who had validated the readings that the first person obtained.

The effects of a lateral position compared with a supine position on pulmonary artery pressures also have been explored (Kennedy, Bryant, and Crawford 1984). The dependent variable of pulmonary artery pressure was measured using instruments comparable to those in the Chulay and Miller study. These authors, however, had to solve the problem of how to keep the transducer at the level of the left atrium when patients were in the lateral position.

From the consumer's perspective, this study shows that although instruments such as the pulmonary artery catheter have a high degree of validity and reliability,

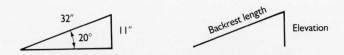

Figure 11–2   Example of use of geometry to determine angle of elevation for backrest.

consideration must be given to appropriate use so that the data generated are meaningful. You, therefore, must understand the underlying physiological conditions/principles when using instruments to measure biophysiological variables if you want to make the best use of the quantitative data they are capable of producing.

Activity and position have been examined in a variety of other studies, and data on the physiological effects of activity and position are being accumulated. Sufficient replication of these studies will help provide a scientific base for nursing care related to activity and position in various patient populations.

Patient Education Outcomes: Instrumentation and Measurement Issues

The value of patient education is frequently measured by multiple dependent variables. These variables often include measures of knowledge gained, psychological adjustment, and physiological function. The focus of this section is the biological measures used to examine some outcomes of patient education.

The content of a teaching program dictates the measures that can logically be used to measure the effectiveness of education provided. To some extent, the nature of the content also determines the manner in which, as well as the instruments by which, the independent variable is delivered.

For example, when King and Tarsitano (1982) compared the effects of structured and unstructured preoperative education, part of the content of the structured program focused on coughing and deep breathing. Thus, the authors selected pulmonary function measures to evaluate the effectiveness of the program. The selection of pulmonary function tests in this case was decided, in part, by the fact that this study was a replication of a study by Lindeman and Van Aernam (1971). Measures of the dependent variable of pulmonary function included vital capacity, maximum midexpiratory flow rate, and forced expiratory volume. King and Tarsitano added another pulmonary function test, expiratory reserve volume, because of a recommendation arising from the original study. Length of hospital stay was the second dependent variable.

Duration of hospital stay is frequently used as a general category to evaluate the complete status of biological variables. It is a gross measure of sickness and is often used because data to calculate the length of hospitalization are easy to collect, inexpensive to obtain, and positively correlated with the cost of hospitalization.

The conceptual framework of the study usually indicates the theoretical considerations dictate the nature of the instruments to be used. This is an important point for consumers of research, because it means that part of your decision to use data from a study will be based on whether there is logical consistency between the conceptual framework and the instruments selected to measure the selected variables. If the instrument measures the variable under consideration, either directly or indirectly, you have some assurance that the correct instrument was selected. When the conceptual framework and the operationalization of the variables, and thus the instruments, are not congruent, or the measurement is a remote approximation of the variable under consideration, then there is a possibility that the instrument cannot measure what the researcher intended it to measure. King and Tarsitano's study (1982) is an example of a good fit between the conceptual framework and the instrumentation.

In Hill's study (1982) of the effect of providing various methods of preoperative information on the recovery of older people undergoing cataract surgery, the independent variable was type of information. The four types were behavioral information, sensory information, both behavioral and sensory information, and general information. The dependent variables were postoperative orientation, mood states, and performance. Performance was operationalized with physiological measures, such as ambulation, length of postoperative hospitalization, and time of first venture from home after discharge.

It is somewhat difficult to standardize the instrumentation for the independent variable in educational studies where people deliver the content. However, reliability among nurses can be established and needs to be addressed to minimize the confounding variables. Hill (1982) could have strengthened this study by addressing the interrater reliability of the nurses in applying the independent variable (type of information). A strength of this study, however, is the cluster of physiological and psychological measures used to capture the essence of recovery.

The effectiveness of the educational component of a rehabilitation program was examined in Perry's study (1981). Perry operationally defined effectiveness as subjective evaluation by the patient that the day was "good"; the reported number of symptoms experienced; the symptoms treated by the patient; the appropriateness of the treatment for the symptom; and a change in the number of and types of treatment used by patients. Thus, in this study, self-report is used to determine the effectiveness of education on physiological functioning.

Because of its subjectivity, self-report is fraught with the potential for threats to validity. It is possible that the use of more objective measures for some of the physiological data would have strengthened the measurement portion of the study—for example, the addition of measures of changes in pulmonary function values or changes in blood levels of drugs used.

Janson-Bjerklie and Clarke (1982) used another set of pulmonary parameters to determine whether asthmatics could learn to control bronchial diameter by the use of biofeedback. Whole body **plethysmography** was used to obtain measures of thoracic gas volume, total respiratory resistance, and change in airway resistance. This involved putting the patient in a box that looked like a telephone booth, in which respiratory gas volume and composition were controlled. Dependent variable values were obtained by measuring the pressure and flow of the gases.

This measurement provides information about bronchial diameter. As bronchial diameter increases, airway resistance decreases; thus, airway resistance is a direct measure of airway diameter and, as a part of airway diameter, bronchial diameter. Although the research topic seems simple, the instrumentation needed to answer the question is complex and expensive. The researchers selected an appropriate instrument to measure the dependent variable to assess the effectiveness of use of biofeedback to control bronchial diameter.

The effects of teaching various types of relaxation to patients have also been explored. A wide range of biophysical responses has been used as the dependent variable.

Wells (1982) examined the effects of a relaxation technique on postoperative muscle tension and pain. Using a two-group, pretest-posttest design (see Chapter 5), the author compared relaxation with routine preoperative instructions. She used a surface **electromyograph** (EMG) and a visual analog scale to measure pain intensity and distress. There was a separate scale for pain intensity and distress. (See Figure 11–1 for an example of a visual analog scale.) Both of these instruments are described.

For the EMG, the accuracy of the measurement is said to have been 1%. This small percentage of error makes the data generated more credible. But it would be helpful to know how the validity of the EMG was tested. In addition, the validity of the analog scale is said to have been investigated in the author's laboratory, but how the author concluded that it would distinguish the two components of the pain experience is not stated. As a consumer of research, you must look for the validity and reliability of the tools used for measurement and for specific descriptions of how those conclusions were reached (see Chapter 6.)

The effects of relaxation therapy also were addressed by Nath and Rinehart (1979). They investigated the effect of teaching relaxation individually and in groups on the blood pressure of subjects with essential hypertension. Blood pressure was measured with an aneroid sphygmomanometer, with the cuff placed 2.5 cm above the antecubital space; the bag was deflated at 2–3 mmHg per second.

The blood pressure cuff is commonly used in the clinical area and is considered an accurate instrument. It does need to be calibrated periodically, and the authors make no mention of whether calibration was done, whether the same sphygmomanometer was used for all subjects, or whether blood pressure was consistently measured by a single individual on all of the subjects. Statements about these aspects of instrumentation would have strengthened the measurement portion of the study. Knowing what the researcher did to ensure the validity of the instruments adds credibility to the findings obtained.

Measurement of the physiological effects of patient education may be of interest in a study you are reading or designing. Examples of measures that investigators have used to examine the specific effects of patient education are found in Table 11–4. Serious attention must continue to be focused on identifying and using measures that are sensitive to physiological effects produced by patient education and on clustering those measures to capture the full impact that such education may have.

Infection and Wound Healing: Instrumentation and Measurement Issues

Studies by nurse researchers in the area of healing and infection have focused largely on care of invasive lines or local wounds. The independent variable(s) of concern have included various skin preparation techniques and products, various dressings, and administration of drug therapy. The dependent variables in these studies have focused on infection rate, phlebitis, and healing. Instrumentation is a challenge when these areas are studied, and appreciation of the equipment needed to ma-

TABLE 11–4   *Patient Education: Four Examples of Variables and Instrumentation*

Variables		Instrumentation	
Independent	**Dependent**	**Independent**	**Dependent**
1. Level of structure of the teaching program	Pulmonary function (vital capacity, maximum midexpiratory flow rate, forced expiratory volume, expiratory reserve volume)		Spirometer
	Length of hospital stay		
2. Types of information: Sensory Behavioral Sensory and behavioral General	Ambulation Length of postoperative hospitalization First venture from home after discharge		Chart Self-report
3. Bronchial diameter	Total respiratory resistance Functional residual capacity Airway resistance	Computer with analog to digital converter Oscilloscope	Respiratory resistance unit Whole-body plethysmography
4. Educational component of a rehabilitation program	Number of "good" days Changes in number of symptoms Whether symptoms were treated by the patient		Self-report

nipulate the independent variable(s) and assess the dependent variable will allow you to plan your study design and critique related studies. Examples of variables and instruments used in the area of healing and infection are given in Table 11–5.

Infection

Antibiotics are frequently prescribed prophylactically and as therapeutic treatment for infection. The nursing responsibility inherent in this medically prescribed regimen lies in the manner in which the antibiotic is administered.

TABLE 11–5   *Wound Healing and Infection: Four Examples with Variables and Instrumentation*

Variables		Instrumentation	
Independent	**Dependent**	**Independent**	**Dependent**
1. Methods of administration of antibiotic	Quantity of antibiotic administered	IV sets with and without volume control chamber	Spectrophotometer
2. Frequency of changing intravenous tubing and percutaneous site	Incidence of phlebitis		Subjective evaluation of pain, erythema, elevated temperature
3. Site and type of thermometer	Temperature reading		Electronic and mercury thermometers Calibration plug for electronic thermometer Water bath NBS certified thermometer
4. Epidermal growth factor	Migration of keratinocytes Rate of differentiation of keratinocytes Rate of healing	Dermatome Grading of ulcers	Biopsy equipment Histologic slides Kundin wound tool

Kerr and her colleagues (1979) examined two commonly used methods of administering antibiotics to see if there was a difference in the quantity of the antibiotic remaining in the tubing between the primary bottle and the volume control chamber when the tubing was clamped and when it was unclamped. The quantity of antibiotic was simulated with the dye methylene blue, which has the same pH as ampicillin and was provided in concentrations approximating those used for ampicillin administration. The color comparisons between the various concentrations of the dye administered by the two different methods was evaluated using a **spectrophotometer**, an instrument that measures the relative intensities of light in different parts of a spectrum. The more concentrated the solution, the greater the intensity of the blue light. The dilutions and the readings from the spectrophotometer were checked by two investigators. A visual evaluation was also completed.

This rather elaborate laboratory study is a fine example of testing a clinical problem in the laboratory. In this case, there is direct applicability of the findings to the clinical area. The instrument used to quantify the dependent variable is a well-accepted measure of color intensity, but the question of the relative adherence of antibiotics and methylene blue to the inside of the IV equipment raises another problem. That is, solutions of varying molecular weight and composition have different affinities to adhere to surfaces, and these differences between the two solutions were not addressed. Nevertheless, the researchers demonstrated ingenuity in approaching a clinical problem using the more controlled laboratory environment with its sophisticated instruments.

Some problems, however, are examined in the clinical setting. When the study design is well controlled, findings can be generalized to the population in question.

In one such study, Nichols, Barstow, and Cooper (1983) sought to determine the relationship between the incidence of phlebitis and the frequency of changing the intravenous tubing and the percutaneous site. The dependent variable in this study was the incidence of phlebitis, with the operational definition for phlebitis being the presence of two of the three classic signs of inflammation: pain, erythema, and elevated temperature.

It is not clear from the narrative in the study whether the elevated temperature was a local or systemic phenomenon. Such details in operational definitions have implications for both the validity and reliability of the measures selected and used. These authors have provided a model for the clustering of symptoms to measure a dependent variable. The strength of their definition of phlebitis lies in its conceptual basis, which is made explicit in the conceptual framework of the study (see Chapter 9). Here is another example in which the test of internal consistency shows a logical link between the theoretical underpinnings of the study and the measurement technique.

An interesting series of studies has been conducted on the validity and reliability of thermometers as a measure of temperature. These studies are included here because one cardinal sign of infection is elevated temperature. These studies as a whole are presented because they illustrate the variability of a single instrument when used under different environmental conditions and when applied using different techniques. The research consumer must be constantly alert to what precautions the investigator has taken to minimize these threats to instrument validity and reliability (see Chapter 5).

Erickson (1980) examined the effect of sublingual site and type of thermometer on oral temperature. The three sublingual sites were the right and left sublingual pockets and the front sublingual area. The two types of thermometers were electronic and mercury in glass. A second purpose of the study was to examine the effect of insertion technique on temperature readings and thermometer response time. This researcher compared the thermometers to be used in the study against a bath of a known temperature to establish their validity. The electronic thermometers were then calibrated, and the amount of error of the mercury-in-glass thermometers was noted.

This researcher used acceptable methods to ensure the validity of her measuring tool. Without this information, the data would not be meaningful. The rigor in this approach is important.

Schiffman (1982), who examined the difference between axillary and rectal temperatures in neonates, used the same method to establish the validity of measurement by the thermometers. The researcher and three additional data collectors took the temperatures of the neonates, and the researcher noted that interrater reliability in reading the thermometers was established when the validity of the thermometers was evaluated.

Description of the validity and reliability of instruments was critical to this study. The procedures used to establish validity and reliability make the data believable.

Hasler and Cohen (1982) examined the effects of various means of oxygen administration on oral temperature readings in healthy subjects. They compared subjects' temperatures before oxygen administration with those during oxygen administration. They built on the work of Erickson (1980) in selecting their thermometer placement. No check was made on the validity of measurement by the thermometer, although the investigators did standardize the thermometer used. Because of the failure to check the accuracy of the thermometer, the findings must be questioned.

When you evaluate a study, you must consider what role establishing the validity of measures of physiological variables plays in drawing implications for practice application (see Chapter 2). Appreciating the need to establish the validity of such a simple measure as taking a temperature suggests that validity procedures must also be undertaken for more sophisticated instruments.

Wound Healing

Several studies of wound healing are of interest from an instrumentation perspective. Instruments used to manipulate the independent variable(s) as well as to measure the dependent variable(s) must be considered.

Gill and Atwood (1981) reported a study that sought to establish a dose-response curve for epidermal growth factor and wound healing in the pig model. Specifically, they were intested in the effect of epidermal growth factor on migration of keratinocytes over the wound, the mitotic index, and rate of differentiation of keratinocytes. The independent variable was the epidermal growth factor, and the dependent variable was histologic evaluation of keratinocytes.

This study is an example of a nursing research study that combines a basic science framework with a nursing science framework (see Chapters 1 and 9). Gill and Atwood manipulated a factor that influences cell growth—that is, epidermal growth factor—and described this manipulation from the nursing science framework of Rogers, specifically in terms of the principles of reciprocy and helicy. The interpretation of this model has been criticized (Kim 1983), and the authors have replied to this criticism (Atwood and Gill-Rogers 1984). This debate increases our understanding of their perspective of the conceptual framework for the study. The use of a combination of frameworks is an important model for nursing to acknowledge and use. The framework for a study need not arise from one discipline. It must, however, be logical and internally consistent. Again, it is important that the conceptual perspective drive the choice of the independent variable and the instruments used to measure it.

Instruments are an important part of manipulating the independent variable as well as measuring the dependent variable in this study. The choice of instrument used to make wounds on the pig's back was critical. The wounds had to be of uniform depth (not all of the layers of the skin were removed) so that the effects of the various concentrations of growth factor could be examined. A standard approach to creating such wounds is to use a **dermatome**, an instrument for cutting thin slices of skin, but in this case the instrument employed is not described. The authors performed tissue biopsies to measure the dependent variable, yet they describe neither the specific technique and instrument they used nor the manner in which the cells were prepared for histologic examination. Interpretation of the microscopic evaluation of the cells is also critical to the credibility of the findings of the study, yet the authors do not mention who did the evaluation or whether it was confirmed by an independent rater. The authors did take steps to control for bias in that they randomly selected the wounds to be biopsied. Another strength is the authors' acknowledgment that it was a pilot study.

Two treatments for decubitus ulcers were evaluated in a consortium study directed by Roesler (1983). The independent variable in this study was type of treatment for decubitus ulcers. The specific dressings evaluated were Op-Site, which was used on all stages of decubitus ulcers, and Vigilon Primary Wound Dressing, which was used on stage III and IV ulcers. Subjects with a stage I–IV ulcer were included in the study. The stages of ulcers were defined, and these categories were mutually exclusive. Training of nurses in use of the wound care products is described.

How or whether reliability was established among the nurses in staging the ulcer or applying the treatments is not stated. Incorrect staging would cast serious doubt on the findings, as would inconsistent application of the wound care agents. Description of the steps used to control for this variation would have strengthened the study. When multiple care givers are involved and multiple research sites are used, consideration must be given to the reliability of the instruments and to the people who use them.

The dependent variables for this study were the rate of healing, nursing time required to perform the treatments, and cost effectiveness. Rate of healing was measured with the **Kundin wound tool**, which assesses volume of missing tissue by measuring the depth and circumference of the wound. Stage I ulcers were defined as reddened skin that is intact, and Stage II ulcers as reddened and broken skin that may be excoriated or vesiculated. The nurses were taught to use the tool, but how reliability between raters was evaluated is not described.

It is difficult to measure healing in the clinical area because the available tools are indirect, disrupt healing, or are not sensitive to subtle daily changes in healing. Some currently used measures of wound healing have the potential of disrupting the healing process, for example, tissue biopsy by punch or scraping. This is a threat to subsequent measures in terms of validity and reliability in assessing healing of those disrupted wounds. Repeated sampling may delay healing. Stotts and Cooper (1984) report a Wound Assessment Instrument to assess healing that allows evaluation of the physical attributes of the wound, such as color of tissue and adherence of exudate. Once reliability of this instrument has been established in a patient population, it may be used in studies to improve measurement of healing without disrupting the healing process.

Nursing time in the Roesler study (1983) was operationally defined as the amount of time recorded by nurses to complete the treatment. The author notes that nursing time did not include the time it took to turn and position the patient. The nurses kept a flowsheet for this purpose. Six hospital sites and clients of one visiting nurses association were used for this study, and a self-report method was a practical approach to determining the time it took for the daily care. Cost effectiveness was quantified as the cost of the products for the three treatments and additional supplies needed for that treatment. All the variables are operationally defined, which makes replication of the study possible.

The areas of healing and infection are often under the control of the nurse. Appreciation of the instrumentation needed to manipulate variables and assess their effects will facilitate mounting of studies in this area and improve the interpretation of findings.

Environmental Stimuli: Instrumentation Measurement Issues

Nurse investigators have been interested in the effects of different environmental stimuli on a variety of dependent biophysiological variables. In some cases, the effects of naturally occurring environmental stimuli have been examined. In other studies, the investigators have created diverse environmental stimuli as the independent variables (see Table 11–6 for examples).

Sound

A study of naturally occurring stimuli was reported by Helton and colleagues (1980). They examined the mental effects of sleep deprivation on 62 critically ill subjects. In another study, Woods and Falk (1974) used a sound meter to measure naturally occurring sounds in two different hospital units.

In another descriptive study, the relationship between selected sounds in a coronary care unit (CCU) and the heart rate responses of subjects in the CCU was determined (Marshall 1972). An audiotape recorder was used, and the ECG recordings of the subjects yielded the heart rate.

The major problem with the instrumentation in the Marshall study was that the tape recorder and ECG system were not synchronized for the simultaneous recording of unit sounds and ECG tracings. This coordination of timing of the data collection is necessary for moment-to-moment analysis in determining the effects of specific environmental sounds on heart rate responses.

Therapeutic Application of Stimuli

Nurse investigators have also manipulated environmental stimuli. Short-gestation infants are used as the subjects in a number of such studies. Examples of the stimuli used include cycling-motion exercise of upper and lower limbs (Porter 1972), auditory stimulation (playing the recording of a heartbeat), and kinesthetic stimulation (using a motorized hammock or a rocking water bed) (Barnard 1973, Neal 1977). The outcome measures included growth and development and neurological func-

TABLE 11–6 *Environmental Stimuli: Four Examples with Variables and Instrumentation*

Variables		Instrumentation	
Independent	**Dependent**	**Independent**	**Dependent**
1. Kinesthetic stimulation	Growth Development Neurological function	Motorized hammock Rocking bed Movement of limbs	
2. Suctioning	Oxygen tension	Suctioning equipment	Transcutaneous oxygen monitor Blood gas analyzer
3.	Sleep		Observation records Videotape recording EEG, EMG tracings
4. Touch Therapeutic or physical		Person trained in techniques of touch	Cardiac monitor Intracranial pressure monitor Thermistor Thermograph Dermograph Electrodes

tion. Several nurse investigators, using **animal models** (studies conducted on animals), studied the effects of thermal applications to the abdomen on local and systemic tissue temperatures (Dyer and Bagnell 1970, Martinson and Anderson 1978). The question these studies raise is the extent to which animal findings can be applicable to humans. Beyond access to animals and training in the techniques of handling, the equipment needed for these two studies was rather simple. It included equipment for quantifying and maintaining the temperature specified for the thermal application. The outcome, or dependent, variable was local and systemic tissue temperature change. The major piece of equipment needed was a sensitive and reliable thermometer. In another study, the association between insertion of a rectal thermometer and changes in heart rate and rhythm was examined in 19 acute myocardial infarct patients (Gruber 1974). Again, the equipment needed to conduct this study was readily available.

As shown in these studies, measurement of some biophysiological variables is not complicated. The important considerations are whether the instruments selected do, in fact, measure the variables under study directly or indirectly, whether they are sensitive to the changes expected, and whether they are reliable. If measurement must be indirect, an additional consideration is consensus on whether the instruments provide the best indirect measure of the variables.

Coronary Precautions

Many commonly accepted nursing practices are not based on empirical data. Specific procedures described in older editions of nursing fundamentals texts and some that have been passed along by tradition need to be subjected to empirical testing (see Chapters 1 and 2). A number of nursing practices, referred to as coronary precautions, are believed to control environmental stimuli that might adversely affect the individual with a myocardial infarct—for example, prohibiting the drinking of ice water (Kirchhoff 1981). The effects of some of these environmental stimuli are being examined by nurse investigators. These studies need to be replicated to determine if the findings are consistent. If the reported findings are confirmed, they will form the basis for change in nursing practice, and some of these coronary precautions will be retired as myths.

The effects of commonly used clinical nursing therapies need to be studied, and more than one study is needed to justify changes in practice. Similar studies—using similar patient populations, addressing similar questions, and using similar instrumentation—need to be conducted to confirm or refute findings across studies. Findings from only one study, regardless of the quality of the study, are insufficient as a basis for change in practice.

Kirchhoff (1982) conducted a national survey using 240 hospitals with critical care units to determine the restrictions imposed on myocardial infarct patients. She reported that "despite findings that cast doubt on the practices of restricting ice water and rectal temperature measurement, coronary precautions are commonly practiced" (p. 196). Two recent research reports illustrate the study of one of the coronary precautions, oral temperature.

To determine the effect of oxygen inhalation by a nasal cannula on oral temperatures, 100 healthy adults were randomly assigned to four groups—a control group and three groups to which oxygen was administered for 30 minutes at 2, 4, or 6 liters per minute (Lim-Levy 1982). The oral temperature of each subject was measured before oxygen was administered and after 30 minutes of exposure while oxygen was still being given. No significant effects of oxygen administration on oral temperature were found.

Because of these findings, the investigator suggests that there is a need to review the practice of using less acceptable sites (axillary or rectal) for obtaining the temperature of patients receiving oxygen. However, several critical questions must be addressed before these findings can be used to change practice. One question is whether findings in a healthy adult population are similar to those in a clinically ill population. Another question is whether changes would be found if the subjects received oxygen over a period of time greater than 30 minutes, which is the case in a clinical population.

An adequate description of the instruments used is included in the research report. A single electronic solid-state thermometer capable of registering 94 to 108°F $\pm$ .2° was used for measuring the dependent variable, the oral temperature of each subject. When the subject's maximum temperature was reached, a red light and an audible tone signaled the investigator. The investigator describes the placement of the probe well. To eliminate possible differences in temperature due to placement of the probe in different sublingual areas, the investigators placed it in the same area in each subject. Attention to the placement and use of the same probe for each subject is an important aspect of controlling factors that could affect the findings. There was no report, however, that the thermometer readings obtained with the single probe were compared with readings from another thermometer. This simple check of reliability of instruments used to measure biophysiological variables would strengthen the credibility of the findings. The other equipment used to manipulate the independent variable, oxygen administration, included compressed oxygen tanks, a flow meter to establish the desired liter flow per minute, a humidifier, and a nasal cannula for each subject.

The investigator also addressed control of several factors that are known to influence one's temperature; these include gum chewing, ingesting food or fluid, and smoking. Identification and control of other factors that may influence either the independent or the outcome variables are especially critical steps in designing and conducting studies in which biophysiological variables are measured. How the researcher accounts for these confounding variables must be specified in the research plan and included in the report of the findings. For example, if the investigator does not report that the subjects refrained from eating, drinking, and smoking before and during the experimental procedure, you would have to question the findings, because these factors influence the dependent variable (oral temperature). Having or acquiring knowledge about the topic area of the research problem and reading numerous studies relevant to the area is of tremendous value in helping you to become aware of the potential influencing factors, special characteristics of the equipment used, and the important measurement issues that need to be addressed to ensure credibility of the findings.

In another study, Hasler and Cohen (1982) examined the effect on oral temperature of 15-minute periods of oxygen administration by aerosol, venti-mask, or nasal prongs in 40 healthy adult volunteers. This is an example of a counterbalanced design; the effects of each method of oxygen administration were tested on each subject. Equipment similar to that described in the last example was required to conduct this study. These investigators conducted a reliability check of the electronic thermometer and found a variability range of 0.4°F. Consequently, they decided that, to be clinically significant, the observed change in temperature after an experimental treatment would have to be greater than 0.5°F. This caution illustrates yet another important point in studying biophysiological variables. Although it may be possible to show statistically significant differences, these differences may not be clinically significant. Unless the equipment is tested for reliability and the variation taken into account (as it was in this study), the observed changes could be due to variation in measurement by the instruments used.

Suctioning

Suctioning and heel stick (to obtain a blood sample) are environmental stimuli that are part of the routine care of premature infants. Measurement issues are presented for several of these studies.

Norris and colleagues (1982) examined the effects of these procedures on blood oxygen levels in 25 premature infants with respiratory distress syndrome. No additional equipment or instruments were re-quired; the subjects were hospitalized, and everything needed to collect the desired data was already available and being used in the routine care of the infants.

This may be the case for a number of studies in which biophysiological variables are measured. To measure the dependent variable of blood oxygen level, a transcutaneous oxygen monitor was used. Baseline measures were obatined before the experimental treatments were begun, and rest periods were provided between the treatments. In studies where some experimental treatment is used as the independent variable (in this case, suctioning), a commonly used research design includes obtaining baseline values for the dependent variable (blood oxygen level) before subjects are given the experimental treatment. Without this baseline measure, it is difficult or impossible to demonstrate the effects of the treatment, that is, to show change in the outcome variable as a result of the experimental treatment.

It is also critical for the experimental treatment to be carried out in some well-defined standard way for each subject. The following are examples of procedural issues that need to be specified:

1. Will different nurses be carrying out the suctioning?

2. Will continuous suctioning or will intermittent suctioning be used?

3. What amount of normal saline (if any) will be instilled before suctioning?

4. For what period of time will suction be applied?

5. Will nurses turn the infant's head in each direction for a different pass of the suction catheter?

6. Will the endotracheal tubes have a side port through which oxygen administration will be continued throughout the suctioning procedure?

All of these possible variations in the independent variable might influence the dependent variable (blood oxygen levels). Another influencing factor is whether hyperoxygenation or hyperinflation is to be part of the procedure, and if so, how similarities in delivery will be determined. To avoid this kind of problem, reseachers must make decisions about the conditions for the experimental treatment and specify precisely how it will be administered to all subjects. Again, this care and precision in the research process make the findings more credible and allow others to replicate or to extend the work.

Several studies have been conducted to determine the effects of suctioning. Most of them have been conducted to determine techniques to decrease tracheobronchial trauma or to prevent a fall in the arterial oxygen tension as a consequence of suctioning. Studies have been conducted on animals as well as on humans of varying ages. When these studies are conducted in adults, if the dependent variable of interest is the arterial oxygen tension, it is necessary to obtain blood samples for blood gas analysis. Although the suction equipment is available and being used clinically, for purposes of research, the type to be used and the precise technique for suctioning need to be specified. Examples of this kind of information are found in the reports of the suctioning studies (Adlkofer and Powaser 1978; Belling, Kelley, and Simon 1978; Skelley, Deeren, and Powaser 1980).

Measurement of **transcutaneous oxygen tension** has also been used to determine the effects of nonnutritive sucking in premature infants (Burroughs et al 1978). This monitor is used clinically, and in the premature infant it has been shown to be reasonably reliable as an indirect measure of blood oxygen levels. Thus, it is possible to design studies to determine the effects of a variety of environmental stimuli or clinical interventions, using this piece of equipment to measure a clinically important parameter, oxygen levels. Clinical availability of equipment and the clinical importance of the dependent variable are major considerations in designing a study in which changes in biophysiological variables are to be quantified.

Sleep

A variety of approaches can be used to measure sleep; they range from indirect, subjective measures to direct, objective measures. Examples are:

- Self-report (from interview or questionnaire)
- Participant-observer technique
- Activity rating scale

- Television recordings

- EEG tracings

Sleep has been examined by nurse investigators primarily as a dependent variable.

You need to consider the approach to measurement as you read the research reports. One approach has been to ask the subjects their perception of their sleep; descriptors such as quality and duration, frequency and duration of periods of wakefulness, and identification of factors that promote or impede sleep have been included. In such an approach, the data collection instrument (whether interview or paper-and-pencil, self-administered technique) is not standardized; that is, no validity or reliability data are accumulated. There are also acknowledged problems with self-reported data. The credibility of findings is a function of the veracity and accuracy of the subjects' reports.

Another approach to collecting data on sleep is the participant-observer technique. Someone observes the subjects over specified periods of time, or a television camera and recorder are used. The videotape recording can then be viewed by a panel of expert observers, and the periods of sleep rated. These are still indirect and imprecise measures of sleep, but they are more objective than self-reports. However, you may be more interested in obtaining the subjects' perceptions about the quality of their sleep than in actually documenting the precise minutes and hours of sleep or wakefulness.

EEG and EMG recordings are a more direct measure of sleep. Certain EEG and EMG patterns characterize the various stages of sleep. From these tracings it is possible not only to distinguish periods of sleep from periods of wakefulness but also to determine the stage of sleep and the time spent in each stage. The equipment required to obtain this more precise objective measurement of sleep, although rather commonly used for diagnostic purposes, may not be readily available for research purposes. In addition, training and skill in interpreting the tracings are requisite.

Perceived changes in the sleep-awake patterns three months after cerebral concussion were studied using self-report data from an adapted version of an investigator-developed questionnaire (Parsons and Ver Beek 1982). Effects of noise in intensive care units and number of interruptions to sleep have been studied using the participant-observer technique (Walker 1972). An activity scale for recording sleep observations was developed and used to determine the effects of auditory (recording of a heartbeat) and kinesthetic (rocker bed) stimulation on general maturation, weight gain, and sleep-awake behavior in premature infants (Barnard 1973). Television recordings were used to assess time of sleep onset (and incidence of regurgitation) in relation to specified feeding practices in newborn infants (unpublished thesis). The relationship between breathing patterns and stability of sleep was determined in six chronic obstructive pulmonary disease patients; the investigator had access to a well-equipped laboratory (Smyth 1980).

The purpose of the study, the research questions, and the state of the art of the measurement techniques should be the primary criteria used in determining the measurement strategies. Practicality, availability, and cost to the investigator and to the subjects also need to be considered in making the selection.

Surgery

Hypothermia has been observed to occur in the immediate postoperative period. In this instance, surgery and its attendant procedures are the environmental stimuli. However, other factors may influence the frequency, magnitude, and duration of postoperative hypothermia.

For example, the relationship of age, anesthesia, and shivering to rewarming was examined in 198 adult postsurgical patients (Vaughan, Vaughan, and Cork 1981). These are all biophysiological variables. In this study, the outcome variable, body core temperature, was measured with a disposable tympanic membrane sensor that had a battery-operated monitoring unit. The measurement and calibration procedures used are described in the research report. Observations were used to determine the presence or absence of shivering; thus, the shivering data were dichotomous (present or absent). There was considerable variety in the surgical procedures, in the range of duration of anesthesia, and in the characteristics of the study sample.

This, too, represents a study in which the equipment needed to assess the biophysiological variables was not elaborate. Data were collected by instrumentation (temperature), from the medical record (age, surgical procedure, anesthesia), and from observation (shivering). Data for a variety of variables can be obtained from the medical record and from observation. Collecting data for biophysiological variables does not have to involve complex equipment or great cost.

Touch

The effects of touch have been studied by nurse researchers. Touch, as an environmental stimulus, or as a therapeutic intervention, is not yet well defined operationally.

The effect of pulse palpation (touch) on cardiac arrhythmia in 62 patients hospitalized in a coronary care unit was examined (Mills et al 1976). The investigators concluded that autonomic responses to human contact (pulse palpation) can affect the rate of ectopic impulse generation. In 31 of their subjects who exhibited cardiac arrhythmia, ectopic beat frequency changed when the pulse was palpated.

This study required no equipment not already used for routine care; the subjects were connected to electrocardiographic monitoring equipment, tracings were available, and pulse palpation was done routinely at least every four hours. To evaluate the findings of this study, you need to raise questions about sample selection, exclusion and inclusion criteria, sample characteristics (such as medication regimen), and other circumstances occurring in the environment simultaneously during the periods of data collection. Acquiring extensive knowledge about the topic area will help you to critique the studies.

Touch, in the form of a stroking motion to the side of the face and to the back of the hand, was used as an independent variable in a study of 30 patients who were connected to an intracranial pressure monitoring device (Wallech 1983). A counterbalanced design was used; the subjects were assigned randomly to have either the side of the face or the back of the hand stroked first, followed by a four-minute period of rest and then stroking (two minutes) the other site (hand or face). This information is given in an abstract, and no information is given about the subjects, such as type of condition (head injury versus some other state) or state of consciousness. No data are reported, but the investigator concluded that stroking did lower the intracranial pressure.

Without baseline values of the intracranial pressure and the values obtained during and after the stroking, the magnitude and duration of the decrease in intracranial pressure remain unknown to the reader. More information is needed to evaluate this study. The study does represent an experimental approach to quantifying the effect of touch (stroking) on intracranial pressure. Again, most of the equipment needed was already in use; extra equipment needed to conduct this study is a stopwatch or clock to time the periods of touch and rest accurately. Data for the dependent variable, intracranial pressure, were obtained from the monitors already being used to evaluate the patients' clinical progress.

In a more recent study, an attempt was made to differentiate between therapeutic touch and physical touch (Randolph 1984). The effect of these two types of touch on physiological response to stressful stimuli was evaluated in 60 female college students. The stressful stimulus was viewing a 13-minute silent film depicting a ceremony of an Australian Aboriginal tribe. "A sequence of operations performed with a sharp stone on the genitals of adolescent boys" was shown (p. 34). Therapeutic touch was given to the experimental group of subjects by eight nurses who had completed a course on therapeutic touch and who had at least a year of experience using the technique. Application of this kind of touch is described in the report. Directing energy and attention to the subjects, the nurses touched the subjects' abdomens and backs. For the control group, eight other nurses applied physical touch; this involved light placement of hands on the subject's abdomen and lower back. Physiological response was operationalized to encompass several measures, including skin conductance, muscle tension, and peripheral skin temperature. These measures of physiological response were selected as being reflective of central, autonomic, and peripheral nervous system function.

This study required a variety of equipment, which is detailed in the research report. A 16-mm film projector to deliver the stressful stimulus, an Autogenic 2000 Feedback Thermograph and a **thermistor** to measure peripheral skin temperature, and an Autogenic 3400 Feedback Dermograph and silver/silver chloride electrodes to measure skin conductance are examples. Specific information about equipment is useful to those who want to compare findings across studies, offer possible explanations for any differences or similarities found, or design and conduct a study. Although not of great interest to all readers, this kind of information should be included in sufficient detail in research reports, because it is important to those who are intensely interested in the topic area. Reporting of this information makes possible the replication of the study or identification of problems in the instrumentation.

The differences in the physiological responses of the two groups in this study were not statistically significant. The experimental group (therapeutic touch) did not remain more relaxed than the control group (physical touch). One interesting possibility that might account for the findings is that touch alone could evoke a physiological response. To account for this possibility, a third group of subjects could have been subjected only to therapeutic touch (not the film) for 13 minutes. When designing a study, it is important to think about what alternative explanations could also influence the findings and to design the study so that the major factors are controlled or studied.

Slow-stroke back massage has been used in combination with guided imagery as a therapeutic intervention for chemotherapy-induced nausea and vomiting in cancer patients. Touch, although variously defined, is an environmental stimulus that has been studied in different populations. In addition to the examples just cited, the effects of touch have been explored using very different biophysiological measures as the dependent or outcome variables. We can include only a few representative studies in this chapter.

Pain

External or internal environmental conditions may result in pain. Although the sensation of pain is a subjective phenomenon, nurses are concerned with the relief of pain and the promotion of comfort. Because pain is subjective, it is difficult to quantify precisely. Pain, in the human model, has been measured primarily as the dependent variable. A variety of clinical therapies have been tested as the independent variable, with their effects on pain reduction assessed.

For example, Bafford (1975) used progressive relaxation as an intervention to control pain in open-heart surgery patients. Thirty subjects were assigned to three groups. The dependent variables were the direct pain response, related patient behavior, and mental status disturbance. Direct pain response was operationalized by the count of medications (as recorded on patient charts) that each subject received for pain, sleep, or tension and by self-reports from each subject estimating the amount of pain experienced. A visual analog scale was used for this self-report. The subjects drew a horizontal line across a 10-inch vertical line to indicate the total amount of pain they had experienced since surgery. The bottom of the vertical line represented no pain and the top of the line represented the most pain possible. The distance from the bottom of the line to the location of the horizontal line drawn by the subjects was measured; this length was used as the subject's score of total pain experienced since surgery.

Descriptions of the other dependent variables are provided in the report; although they are of interest, they are not included here because they are not specifically related to the measurement of pain. Little difference was found between the three experimental groups on the dependent variables. Several questions could be raised. The extent to which the one experimental group practiced and achieved relaxation is unknown. The extent to which the subjects were able to assess the "total amount" of pain experienced over a 9-day period remains elusive. The extent to which "count" of medications received for sleep and tension (in addition to pain medications) reflects pain is open to debate. These are all examples of issues that readers of research as well as researchers need to address because these factors may influence the findings obtained.

Another study was conducted to determine the effectiveness of a relaxation technique in increasing the comfort level of postoperative patients in their first attempt to get out of bed (Flaherty and Fitzpatrick 1977). Forty-two subjects were assigned to the experimental group (relaxation technique) or to the control group. After their first attempt to get out of bed, self-report pain and distress scales were used to assess the subjects' incisional pain and body distress. The pain and distress scales used had been developed and tested previously by Johnson (1972, 1973). The investigators determined the amount of analgesics used and compared values obtained for blood pressure, pulse, and respiratory rates before surgery and after the first attempt to get out of bed. From the findings obtained, these investigators concluded that use of the relaxation technique to reduce muscular tension did increase the subjects' comfort levels.

Operational definitions for each of the variables, including the relaxation technique, are well defined in the research report. For example, comfort level was assessed from the responses on the pain and distress scales, the total amount of analgesics used in the first 24 hours after surgery, and changes in the vital signs; thus, a composite of measures was used in quantifying the dependent variable, comfort level.

Electrical surface stimulation (ESS) has been used as a therapeutic intervention for the control of pain. It involves low-level controlled electricity being administered through the skin.

In one study the efficacy of ESS in controlling acute postoperative pain and preventing ileus and atelectasis was determined in a group of subjects having abdominal surgery (Menzel and Martinson 1975). From their study of 27 subjects, the investigators concluded that ESS was not effective in reducing postoperative pain nor in preventing the two complications. The group was assigned randomly to the experimental or control group. One transcutaneous electric surface device was designed to operate without giving stimulation; this was used for those assigned to the control group. A double-blind design was used, so neither the subject nor the nurse using the device knew who was receiving the experimental treatment.

In this example the manufacturer of the instrument cooperated with the nurse researchers in providing the device to be used for the control group. A description of how the electric surface stimulator was applied is provided in the report. Measurement of pain was achieved by interviewing the subjects 24 hours after the surgery. Their subjective reports were rated on an ordinal scale (see Chapter 14). The range of possible responses was *none, a little, some, quite a bit*, or *a lot*. The investigators acknowledged the lack of validity and reliability for this instrument.

These studies did not require any elaborate equipment; they did require careful definition of the variables. Most of the data were collected from the chart or from the subjects. In each of these studies, the subjects were asked to rate their perception of their pain, and the amount of analgesic used was accounted for. In each example, different scales were used for assessing the pain experience. Because pain is a subjective variable, precise quantification in the human model remains problematic. However, pain is a biophysiological variable of considerable interest to both clinicians and researchers.

Nursing Research and Measurement of Biophysiological Variables

The studies included in this chapter were selected to illustrate a range of important issues to be considered in reading research reports and in designing and conducting studies that measure biophysiological variables. To achieve a sense of order in the diverse body of content of these studies, we categorized and presented them within five broad biophysiological phenomena—feeding alterations, activity and position, patient education outcomes, healing and infection, and environmental stimuli. Comments pertinent to specific problem areas were included to illustrate important factors that need to be considered to strengthen the studies and thus enhance the credibility of the findings.

Many additional examples could have been included; they are so numerous that it is not possible to provide a definitive list. Some have been used as the independent variable, whereas others have been studied as the dependent, or outcome, variables. How these variables are measured is diverse because there are many instruments and equipment available for measurement. Some of the instruments provide indirect measures of the variable; others provide a direct, precise measurement. Determining measurement reliability of the instruments is essential. The biophysiological phenomena, variables, and instruments included in this chapter were selected because they represent the possible range and reflect the current state of the art of this type of nursing research.

Some biophysiological variables require subjective assessment, but most can be quantified by some objective measure. For some variables, a battery of several measures is necessary, because there is no single best measure. Quantification of many biophysiological variables yields interval-level data, and ratio-level data can be obtained frequently. Biophysiological variables can be influenced by factors other than experimental treatment, and these other factors need to be identified and accounted for in the research design.

There are many clinical situations in which the instruments or equipment needed for research are already available and being used for monitoring purposes. Extensive knowledge of the problem area and familiarity with the clinical management of the population of interest are invaluable assets for the researcher. It is from this perspective that the most credible research evolves.

Guidelines for Critique

- What type of biophysiological variables were examined in the study?
- What type of instruments were selected to measure the biophysiological variables?
- Were the instruments selected congruent with the conceptualization of the study problem?
- Are the instruments direct or indirect measures of the variables?
- Were single or multiple measures used to quantify the variable(s)?
- Were the sensitivity, validity, and reliability of the instruments described?

- Were the instruments selected invasive or noninvasive?
- What level of data do the biophysiological instruments generate?

SUMMARY OF KEY IDEAS AND TERMS

✓   There are diverse types of measures to quantify physiological variables.

✓   Information about instrumentation must be provided in detail by the researcher.

✓   Findings from only one study are insufficient to use as a basis for change in practice.

✓   A combination of resources helps you to select the most appropriate instrument for your research.

✓   Availability, direct or indirect measures, single or multiple measures, sensitivity, validity, reliability, invasive versus noninvasive measures, and levels of data and cost are all considerations in selecting a biphysiological instrument.

✓   For some biological variables a battery of measures must be used.

✓   The guiding force for instrument selection must be the conceptualization of the phenomenon being studied.

✓   Which instrumentation one uses and how one uses it depend on the research question and research design.

References

Adlkofer R, Powaser M: The effect of endotracheal suctioning on arterial blood gases in patients after cardiac surgery. *Heat Lung* 1978; 7:1011–1014.

(Continued)

Atwood JR, Gill-Rogers BP: Metatheory, methodology, and practicality: Issues in research uses of Roger's science of unitary man. *Nur Res* 1984; 33:88–91.

Bafford DC: Progressive relaxation as a nursing intervention: A method of controlling pain for open-heart surgery patients. *Commun Nurs Res* 1975; 8:284–290.

Barnard K: The effect of stimulation on the sleep behavior of the premature infant. *Commun Nurs Res* 1973; 6:12–33.

Belling D et al: Use of the swivel adaptor aperture during suctioning to prevent hypoxemia in the mechanically ventilated patient. *Heart Lung* 1978; 7:320–322.

Burroughs A et al: The effect of nonnutritive sucking on transcutaneous oxygen tension in noncrying preterm neonates. *Res Nurs Health* 1978; 1:69–75.

Chulay M, Miller T: The effect of backrest elevation on pulmonary artery and pulmonary capillary wedge pressures in patients after cardiac surgery. *Heart Lung* 1984; 13:138–140.

Cotanch PH: Relaxation training for control of nausea and vomiting in patients receiving chemotherapy. *Cancer Nurs* 1983; 6:277–283.

Dyer ED, Bagnell HK: Local tissue and general temperature changes in dogs produced by temperature applications. *Nurs Res* 1970; 19:37–41.

Erickson R: Oral temperature differences in relation to thermometer technique. *Nurs Res* 1980; 29:157–164.

Flaherty GG, Fitzpatrick JJ: Relaxation technique to increase comfort level of postoperative patients: A preliminary study. *Nurs Res* 1977; 27:352–355.

Foster SB et al: Cardiovascular nursing research: Past, present and future. *Heart Lung* 1984; 13:111–116.

Geden EA: Effects of lifting techniques on energy expenditure: A preliminary investigation. *Nurs Res* 1982; 31:214–218.

Gill BP, Atwood JR: Reciprocity and helicy used to relate mEGF and wound healing. *Nurs Res* 1981; 30:68–72.

Grose BL et al: Effect of backrest position on cardiac output measured by the thermodilution method in acutely ill patients. *Heart Lung* 1981; 10:661–665.

Gruber PA: Changes in cardiac rate associated with the use of the rectal thermometer in the patient with acute myocardial infarction. *Heart Lung* 1974; 3:288–292.

Hanson RL: Effects of administering cold and warmed tube feedings. *Commun Nurs Res* 1973; 6:136–140.

Hasler ME, Cohen JA: The effect of oxygen administration on oral temperature assessment. *Nurs Res* 1982; 31:265–268.

Hathaway D, Geden EA: Energy expenditure during leg exercise programs. *Nurs Res* 1983; 32:147–150.

Heitkemper M et al: Effects of rate and volume of tube feeding in normal human subjects. *Commun Nurs Res* 1977; 10:71–95.

Helton MC et al: The correlation between sleep deprivation and the intensive care unit syndrome. *Heart Lung* 1980; 9:464–468.

Hill BJ: Sensory information, behavioral instructions and coping with sensory alteration surgery. *Nurs Res* 1982; 31:17–21.

Janson-Bjerklie S, Clarke E: The effects of biofeedback training on bronchial diameter in asthma. *Heart Lung* 1982; 11:200–207.

Johnson JE: Effects of structuring patients' expectations on their reactions to threatening events. *Nurs Res* 1972; 21:499–504.

Johnson JE: Effects of accurate expectations about sensations on the sensory and distress components of pain. *J Pers Soc Psychol* 1973; 27:261–275.

Johnston BL et al: Oxygen consumption and hemodynamic and electrocardiographic responses to bathing in recent post-myocardial infarction patients. *Heart Lung* 1981; 10:666–671.

Kagawa-Busby KS et al: Effects of diet temperature on tolerance of enteral feedings. *Nurs Res* 1980; 29:276–280.

Kennedy GT et al: The effects of lateral body positioning on measurements of pulmonary artery and pulmonary artery wedge pressures. *Heart Lung* 1984; 13:155–158.

Kerr JC et al: A comparison of the effectiveness of two methods of intravenous antibiotic administration. *West J Nurs Res* 1979; 1:101–110.

Kim HS: Use of Rogers' conceptual system research: Comments. *Nurs Res* 1983; 32:89–91.

King I, Tarsitano B: The effect of structured and unstructured pre-operative teaching: A replication. *Nurs Res* 1982; 31:324–329.

Kinney M: The scientific basis for critical care nursing practice: 1972 to 1982. *Heart Lung* 1984; 13:116–123.

Kirchoff KT: An examination of physiologic basis for "coronary precautions." *Heart Lung* 1981; 10:874–879.

Kirchoff KT: A diffusion survey of coronary precautions. *Nurs Res* 1982; 31:196–201.

Layton P et al: Nutritional assessment of allogeneic bone marrow recipients. *Cancer Nurs* 1981; 4:127–135.

Lim-Levy F: The effect of oxygen inhalation on oral temperature. *Nurs Res* 1982; 31:150–152.

Lindeman CA, Van Aernam BV: Nursing intervention with the presurgical patient—The effects of structured and unstructured pre-operative teaching. *Nurs Res* 1971; 20:319–332.

Lindsey AM: Phenomena and physiological variables of relevance to nursing, review of a decade of work: Part I. *West J Nurs Res* 1982; 4:343–364.

Lindsey AM: Phenomena and physiological variables of relevance to nursing, review of a decade of work: Part 2. *West J Nurs Res* 1983; 5:41–63.

Lindsey AM: Research for clinical practice: Physiological phenomena. *Heart Lung* 1984; 13:496–507.

Lindsey AM, et al: Social support as a moderator of health outcomes in post-mastectomy women: A review. *Cancer Nurs* 1981; 4:377–384.

Marshall LA: Patient reaction to sound in an intensive care unit. *Commun Nurs Res* 1972; 5:81–92.

Martinson IM, Anderson SE: Effects of thermal applications on the abdominal temperature of rats. *Res Nurs Health* 1978; 1:123–130.

McCorkle R, Young K: Development of a symptom distress scale. *Cancer Nurs* 1978; 1:373–378.

Measel CP, Anderson GC: Nonnutritive sucking during tube feedings: Effect on clinical course in premature infants. *J Obstet Gyn Neonatal Nurs* 1979; 8:265–272.

Melzack R: The McGill Pain Questionnaire: Major properties and scoring methods. *Pain* 1975; 1:277–299.

Menzel NJ, Martinson IM: Effects of electrical surface stimulation on control of acute postoperative pain and prevention of atelectasis and ileus in patients having abdominal surgery. *Commun Nurs Res* 1975; 8:273–283.

Mills M et al: Effect of pulse palpation on cardiac arrhythmia in coronary care patients. *Nurs Res* 1976; 25:378–382.

Mitchell P: Intracranial hypertension: Implications of research for nursing care. *J Neurosurg Nurs* 1980; 12:145–154.

Mitchell PH et al: Moving the patient in bed: Effects on intracranial pressure. *Nurs Res* 1981; 30:212–218.

Nath C, Rinehart J: Effects of individual and group relaxation therapy on blood pressure in essential hypertensives. *Res Nurs Health* 1979; 2:119–126.

Neal MV: Vestibular stimulation and development of the small premature infant. *Commun Nurs Res* 1977; 8:291–302.

Nichols EG et al: Relationship between incidence of phlebitis and frequency of changing IV tubing and percutaneous site. *Nurs Res* 1983; 32:247–252.

Norris S et al: Nursing procedures and alterations in transcutaneous oxygen tension in premature infants. *Nurs Res* 1982; 31:330–336.

Parsons L, Ver Beek D: Sleep-awake patterns following cerebral concussion. *Nurs Res* 1982; 31:260–264.

Perry JA: Effectiveness of teaching in the rehabilitation of patients with chronic bronchitis and emphysema. *Nurs Res* 1981; 30:219–222.

Pfeiffer E: A short portable mental status questionnaire for the assessment of organic brain deficit in elderly patients. *J Am Geriatr Soc* 1975; 23:433–441.

Porter LS: The impact of physical-physiological activity on infants' growth and development. *Nurs Res* 1972; 21:210–219.

Randolph G: Therapeutic and physical touch: Physiological response to stressful stimuli. *Nurs Res* 1984; 33:33–36.

Roesler LD: A comparison of two treatments of decubitus ulcers: Op-Site and Bard products. *Final Report, Department of Nursing Research, Stanford University Hospital* September 28, 1983.

Schiffman RF: Temperature monitoring in the neonate: A comparison of axillary and rectal temperatures. *Nurs Res* 1982; 31:274–277.

Skelley B et al: The effectiveness of two preoxygenation methods to prevent endotracheal suction-induced hypoxemia. *Heart Lung* 1980; 9:316–323.

Smyth ML: Alterations in respiratory patterns in sleeping subjects with chronic obstructive pulmonary disease. *Commun Nurs Res* 1980; 13:25.

Stotts NA, Cooper DM: *Development of an Instrument to Measure Wound Healing.* 12th Annual Nursing Research Conference, University of Arizona, Tucson, Arizona, 1984.

Teasdale G, Jennett B: Assessment of coma and impaired consciousness: A practical scale. *Lancet* 1974; 2:81–83.

Vaughan MS et al: Postoperative hypothermia in adults: Relationship of age, anesthesia and shivering to rewarming. *Anesth Analg* 1981; 60:746–751.

Walker BB: The postsurgery heart patient: Amount of uninterrupted time for sleep and rest during the first, second and third postoperative days in a teaching hospital. *Nurs Res* 1972; 21:164–169.

Wallech C: The effect of purposeful touch on intracranial pressure. Abstract. *Proceedings of the American Association of Critical-Care Nurses National Teaching Institute.* Newport Beach, Calif.: American Association of Critical-Care Nurses, 1983, p. 335.

Ward MJ, Lindeman C (editors): *Instruments for Measuring Nursing Practice and Other Health Care Variables.* Vols 1 and 2. Washington, D.C.: U.S. Department of Health, Education, and Welfare, 1978.

Wells N: The effect of relaxation on postoperative muscle tension and pain. *Nurs Res* 1982; 31:236–238.

Williams KR, Walike BC: Effect of the temperature of tube feeding on gastric motility in monkeys. *Nurs Res* 1975; 24:4–9.

Woods NF, Falk SA: Noise stimuli in the acute care area. *Nurs Res* 1974; 23:144–149.

Yoshitake H: Relations between the symptoms and the feelings of fatigue. *Ergonomics* 1971; 14:175–196.

Zook DJ, Yasko JM: Psychologic factors: Their effect on nausea and vomiting experienced by clients receiving chemotherapy. *Oncol Nurs Forum* 1983; 10:76–81.

12

Strategies of Field Research

HOLLY SKODOL WILSON

Chapter Objectives

After reading this chapter, the student should be able to:

- Discuss the intellectual roots of field methods

- Explain why nursing science can profit from carefully documented field studies

- Enumerate three characteristics of field research

- Compare and contrast the logic of inquiry in field research with traditional, deductive research

- Describe strategies useful in the five major stages of fieldwork: (1) locating the field, (2) gaining entrée and access, (3) bargaining for a role, (4) collecting and recording data, and (5) leaving the field

- Recognize the advantages and disadvantages of the roles of complete participant, participant as observer, observer as participant, and complete observer

- Demonstrate the ability to solve practical and ethical issues related to each fieldwork stage

(Continued)

- Evaluate the balance in types of data according to the criteria of information adequacy and efficiency

- Formulate a plan for observing based on four guidelines

- Organize observations into the recording system of observational notes (ONs), theoretical notes (TNs), methodological notes (MNs), and personal notes (PNs)

- Comprehend the characteristics of partially structured and unstructured interviews

- List the advantages and disadvantages of interviews vis-à-vis questionnaires

- Pose clarifying questions that reflect active listening

- Distinguish between case histories and case studies as sources of data

- Distinguish between scientific and artistic modes of analyzing qualitative data

In This Chapter...

Fieldwork is data-collection strategies, including observation, interviewing, case studies, case histories, and document review, that rely on "firsthand knowing" under natural conditions. Field research grew out of a combination of traditions in cultural anthropology and the social philosophy of symbolic interactions (see Chapter 1). These traditions have taught us that experience is defined differently in different places. The field-worker's philosophy of science is based on the belief that people have not only different customs, language conventions, kinship patterns, religious practices, and expectations of their lives but also different worlds with different realities. *Ethnography* requires the special skill of entering such an alien world and discovering its own logic. The very best field-workers do this kind of science with their hearts as well as their intellects. *The Teachings of Don Juan* is a story by the anthropologist Carlos Castaneda of a Yaqui Indian from Sonora, Mexico—a *brujo* (medicine man). It describes the five years that these two men spent together, in which Don Juan taught Castaneda the uses of peyote, jimson weed, and other plants in achieving mastery over a nonordinary reality (Castaneda 1968). Although some would reasonably argue that this study and subsequent successful trade books based on it were merely products of the 1960s, timely in topic and style, others believe that it is among the best portrayals of human reality divested of intellectual detachment, eroding jargon, and officiousness. How to use field research methods and how to decide whether such a rendering is *true* by scientific as well as pragmatic criteria are the subjects of this chapter. Our emphasis here is on doing fieldwork. Analyzing the data collected is covered in detail in Chapter 13.

Intellectual Roots of Field Research

The Growth of Anthropology

Anthropology, one of the youngest disciplines in the social sciences, comes from the Greek words *anthropos*, meaning "man," and *logos*, meaning "study." It can be divided into three branches.

In the late nineteenth century, anthropologists concerned themselves with what is now called *physical anthropology*—the study of human anatomy, physiology, and the biological bases of behavior. A. C. Haddon organized and led the Torres Straits expedition from Britain in 1889 to "find out possible physiological or racial bases for cultural differences in primitive cultures on islands near Australia and New Guinea." This first "field study" was considered the original purely anthropological expedition. Haddon and his associates concluded, by the way, that "islanders hardly differed from Europeans in their perceptions, and that the differences that were found were personal rather than racial" (Penniman 1965 p. 99).

The second major type of anthropological problem is the study of ancient objects and the remains of former civilizations. The emphasis here is on discovering major lines of development and paths of influence on contemporary society. This branch of anthropology is called *archaeology*.

Ethnology, the third division of anthropology, is concerned with individual human beings as social or cultural actors, thinkers, and communicators rather than exclusively as physical organisms. It focuses on cultures and societies as systems of rules, rights, roles, language customs, and established relationships rather than as physical remains of ancient environments.

Early ethnologists were strongly influenced by a tradition in Europe in the nineteenth century called sociology, particularly the works of Herbert Spencer, Auguste Comte, Max Weber, George Simmel, and Emile Durkheim. These thinkers considered culture or society a unit of study in and of itself that was not reducible to its parts or members. Spencer called this concept *civilization*, and Comte called it *social principle*. The word for the idea became *culture* in Germany and the United States, and scholars in England and France called it *society*. From these early thinkers came a philosophic attitude about studying people summarized by Leaf:

> It is the idea that the actions of an individual are relative to his cultural surroundings . . . and have to be evaluated in terms of the moral principles and beliefs of his society or culture. . . . One cannot arrive at a proper evaluation of the actions of persons in another culture by imposing the values or beliefs or meanings of one's own culture upon them [1974 p. 28].

Ethnography

Social scientists of the 1940s and 1950s sought a fair-minded, universal research method that would avoid imposing their own values and ideas upon the cultures they studied yet would result in a balanced, comparative analysis. *Ethnology* was dubbed the "whole science of man." Its focus was observable individuals and their setting or environment. **Ethnography** is a systematic methodology for studying cultures, subcultures, and life-styles. According to Leininger (1985 pp. 35–36), a nurse anthropologist who used ethnography in studying the phenomenon of "caring" and in transcultural research, ethnography is the "process of observing, detailing, describing, documenting and analyzing the . . . particular patterns of a culture." Important early scientific works included Clyde Kluckhohn's *Navaho Witchcraft*, Ruth Benedict's *The Chrysanthemum and the Sword*, Max Weber's *The Protestant Ethic and the Spirit of Capitalism*, Claude Lévi-Strauss's *Elementary Structures of Kinship*, and Edmund Leach's *Political Systems of Highland Burma*. In 1943 William Foote Whyte published a study of an Italian slum society in North Boston that has become a fieldwork classic. In a section he entitled "Reflections on Field Research," Whyte made the following observations about the method he used to produce this important and influential work:

> As I carried through the Cornerville study, I was also learning how to do field research. . . . I learned to understand a group by observing how it changed through time. This familiarity gave rise to the ideas in this book. I did not develop these ideas by any strictly logical process. They dawned on me out of what I was seeing, hearing, doing—and feeling. They grew out of an effort to organize a confusing welter of experience. . . . I had to try to get outside of my participating self and struggle again to explain the things that seemed obvious. . . . I was seeking to build a study based upon observed interpersonal events. That to me is the chief methodological and theoretical meaning of *Street Corner Society* [1955 pp. 357–358].

The burgeoning scientific tradition called field research expanded to guide the work of scientists in related disciplines. In the 1960s the psychologist Kenneth Keniston published two brilliant studies of alienated youth and the New Left in American society, *The Uncommitted* and *Young Radicals*. The psychiatrist Robert Coles reported on nonviolent youth in the South in his paper "Serpents and Doves." Howard Becker explained the process of becoming a marijuana user in a monograph called *Outsiders*. In an effort to make the management of dying more rational and compassionate, the medical sociologists Barney Glaser and Anselm Strauss, in collaboration with a team of nurse researchers at the University of California, San Francisco, published their works *Awareness of Dying* (1965) and *Time for Dying* (1968). In the world of physical science, the geneticist James D. Watson (1968) revealed the human side of his discovery of the structure of DNA when he expressed a view in *The Double Helix* that science proceeds in a far less logical manner than is imagined by nonscientists. Personalities and human events play major parts in scientific discovery. Nurse scientists, usually trained in anthropology, have made important contributions to knowledge using the process of ethnography. Here are a few examples: Aamodt (1986) studied a child's view of alopecia. Field (1983) studied public health nurses' perspectives. Kus (1985) studied phases of coming out. Parse and colleagues (1985) studied the experience of aging. Stern (1981) studied the Filipino childbearing family, and Tripp-Reimer (1983) studied faith-healing practice among Greek immigrants. In studies that emphasize theory testing, issues of measurement, sample size, validity and reliability of instruments, and appropriateness of statistical analysis are the important ones. But as a nurse scientist studying the subculture of a neonatal intensive care unit, these issues are not the useful guidelines. Instead, you need to design a study that allows you to learn about a world you don't understand by encountering it firsthand and making sense out of it. In Agar's (1987) words, "Ethnographers set out to show how social action in one world makes sense from the point of view of another. Such work requires an intensive personal involvement, an abandonment of traditional scientific control, an improvisational style . . . and an ability to learn from a long series of mistakes." Ethnography is at its core a process of mediating frames or meaning. It offers a way of seeing different worlds. It requires an interpretive approach to data analysis (see Chapter 13) and uses strategies of field research for data collection. The nurse researcher becomes the data collection "instrument" in order to discover what is presented to us rather than what is created through scientific controls. In such studies, methods of theory-testing and verifying are not appropriate.

Field Research and Nursing Science

In 1970 the National Commission for the Study of Nursing and Nursing Education put forward as its first recommended priority the study of problems in nursing practice. Scholars and scientists at Yale University defined *nursing practice research* as problems in patient care where either direct or indirect nursing care is given to people and their significant others. They advocated the position that the essence of research is in everyday nursing practice and that the business of nursing research is to examine, describe, define, explain, and predict that practice. Diers summarized the ideas of scholars and scientists: "The closer the relationship between nursing practice and nursing research, the better the research and the better the practice" (1979 p. 5). Research questions about everyday nursing practice are waiting around every corner and down every corridor: "What keeps staff nurses going when they confront the stresses of working in a neonatal intensive care unit?" "How do elderly indigent patients with emphysema get around?" "How do patients manage to live with incurable pain?" "What is the influence of 'high tech' equipment on compassionate nursing care?" "How do nurses provide culturally sensitive postpartum care to Mexican-American mothers?" "How do Arab immigrants define their health care needs?" "What is the nature of usual inpatient treatment in a community mental health center's locked unit?" "How do the chronically ill view their world?" "How can a diabetic diet be best taught to an adolescent patient?" "What can a nurse do to ease the trauma of pain during 'tubbing' of burned children?" "Why do intensive care unit patients feel exhausted?" "How do relaxation techniques assist in the management of hypertension?" "What efforts will positioning a patient have on his or her intracranial pressure?" "What's the proper length for insertion of a nasogastric tube for feeding?"

Finding answers to such questions is the goal of clinical nursing research. The answers can improve patient care. Clinical research generates the knowledge necessary to guide patient-care practices based on science, not trial and error or tradition. It considers the whole patient in relationship to his or her environment. The knowledge gained is valued for the use it may have in the real world of decisions, judgments, and human encounters. Given all of this, we are not surprised to learn that research strategies originated by sociologists and anthropologists in their field studies hold considerable interest for nurse researchers.

Characteristics of Field Research

Fieldwork as a mode of scientific inquiry immerses the researcher in processes of day-to-day life that may be as novel as living with an isolated Eskimo band or as tense as spending many months incarcerated with inmates on death row in a maximum security prison. Wherever it may be, the **field** is the social-psychological area where the investigator gathers data to find answers in the central area of inquiry. In a pain study, the field might be hospital wards; in a study of face-to-face interaction with disfigured or handicapped persons, it might be bureaus or agencies. Field studies have been conducted by nurses in prenatal classes, labor rooms, nursing homes, self-help-group meetings, herbal pharmacies, pot parties, and rock concerts. The features that characterize such studies, whatever their location, are these:

1. The researcher, through face-to-face interviewing or participant observation, is the primary "instrument" for data collection.

2. Data collection and analysis go on in the natural setting. The investigator tries to learn about how variables vary under usual and unusual conditions rather than trying to control all variables except for the few under scrutiny.

3. The logical progression of field research contrasts with more traditional research in the ways summarized in Table 12–1.

4. Field researchers must make particular accommodations to the ethical principles discussed in Chapter 3. They usually conduct their work in close association with the people and situations they study. The potential for conflicts of interest, deception, exploitation, invasion of privacy, inconvenience to the subjects, and loss of confidentiality are all particularly intense. If you learn in a study of prior child abusers and their children that a new incident has occurred, should you report it? Should you make your field notes accessible to the police? What should you tell subjects about such matters from the start? No matter how unobtrusive, field research always pries into the lives of informants, usually with little personal gain to them. It can be used, however,

TABLE 12–1 *Comparison of Traditional Research with Field Research*

Traditional Deductive Research	Field Research
Start with hypotheses derived from reading existing literature—for example, independent variable yields dependent variable ($x \rightarrow y$)	Look at the data first. Then come up with your own multiple tentative hypotheses
Study a few propositions	Study many propositions
Proceed through a linear process	Proceed through a multidimensional process resembling a Rubic's cube or a spiral
Comply with precise steps for correct data collection and analysis	Gather data and analyze it simultaneously based on a general principle of being pragmatic and evolving the analytic scheme
Test, confirm, or refute hypotheses	Develop concepts, propositions, and middle-range theories

Source: S. Fagerhaugh, Presentation at Qualitative Research Conference, San Francisco, California, 1983.

to affirm their rights, interests, and sensitivities, and all informants have the right to know the researcher's aims, to remain anonymous, to refuse to participate, and to withdraw at any time without penalty.

The heart of the fieldwork enterprise, according to the sociologist Herbert Blumer, is "getting close to the people involved in it, seeing it in a variety of situations they meet, noting their problems and observing how they handle them, being party to their conversations and watching their way of life as it flows along" (1969 p. 37). As you can surmise, fieldwork commits the researcher to learning to define the world from the perspective of those being studied and requires that he or she gain as intimate an understanding as possible about their way of life. Methodological techniques in field research include observation, informal interviews, life histories, document analysis, and other nonintrusive, nonstructured methods. The following section clarifies the procedures and general rules that are available for locating the field, learning how to enter it, maintaining working relationships with subjects, collecting and recording data, and making a smooth exit. Most field researchers would admit, however, that the canons of fieldwork must frequently be bent and twisted to accommodate the particular demands and requirements of the study situation and the personal characteristics of the field-worker. The exact recipe for doing field research, as Shaffir, Stebbins, and Turowetz (1980) conclude, can at best only be suggested.

Stages of Fieldwork

Stage 1: Locating the Field

Any place or area of activity can become the field for research on a study question. A bus station where strangers wait aimlessly in one another's presence, a gay bar, the waiting room of an intensive care unit, a city hospital's emergency room, a running track, an Alcoholics Anonymous meeting. You can select a single social situation and expand it to many to acquire contrasts and variations. When Glaser and Strauss studied dying patients, they made observations in emergency rooms, hospice care units, neonatal intensive care units, operating rooms, nursing homes, and elsewhere, to grasp the full range of variation relevant to their emerging concepts *awareness contexts* and *the dying trajectory* (1965, 1968, 1970).

Appraising the suitability of the setting or field is a first stage in doing fieldwork. Researchers examine the setting to determine if it will yield data bearing on the purpose or research question that focuses their study. The success of a field study often depends on the attention paid to this preresearch phase. Familiarity with the routines, realities, and structure of the proposed setting facilitate not only the negotiations that follow but also the qualitative data that you can collect.

One nursing doctoral dissertation focused on psychiatric nurses' styles of communicating with psychiatric patients. The investigator was forced to abandon her original hospital unit in favor of another one because the patient population rarely if ever presented the psychotic language patterns that she wished to investigate. This discovery consumed many weeks of negotiation and observation and served as an early source of frustration for her in an already difficult and challenging scientific undertaking.

When planning a field study, never underestimate the importance of background interviewing and document research before you adopt a setting.

Stage 2: Gaining Entrée and Access

You proceed in field research by clearing the initial hurdle of getting into the selected setting or situation so that you can observe and talk to people about your research question. Then you must build rapport and trust so that subjects will willingly serve as informants and respondents. Barriers to getting in abound, and success depends on your ability to determine the wisest approach to the situation and cultivate the various "gatekeepers."

EXAMPLE: Covert Research in "Tearooms"

Humphreys's (1975) research investigated impersonal homosexual encounters in public restrooms (called "tearooms") in St. Louis from 1965 to 1968. The study required Humphreys to assume a phony role as "lookout" in these public facilities. Thus, he began with disguised observation in that he did not make his identity as a social researcher known to the participants. His sampling techniques furthermore involved tracing automobile license numbers in order to track down the names and addresses of the men who engaged in these encounters. When interviewing the respondents at their homes, he explained only that they had been chosen as part of a sample of men for a "social health survey" of the community. Respondents were not told the true purpose of the study, and the reseacher disguised his appearance so as to avoid recognition. The ethics of such subterfuge have been both criticized and defended in a long list of subsequent publications.

Study subjects did not give informed consent

An example of deception

The ethics of field research are an important consideration

Covert and Overt Research Problems of and strategies for "getting in" are influenced in part by the decision of whether to engage in covert or overt field research. The covert approach obviously eliminates the need to explain and justify the research or your presence. Here the investigator poses as an authentic participant in the setting—a diabetic, a hospital worker, a single parent, a drug abuser—to look at the social life of the subjects without any influence on them from knowing that they are under study. Such undercover research, although done in the past, is being subjected to serious ethical criticisms.

Degree of Accessibility Obviously, social situations or settings offer varying degrees of accessibility. On the one hand, you can enter a hospital lobby and observe easily. Observing transactions at the admissions desk, on the other hand, would probably require the permission of the hospital's administration. The operating room could in some cases prove to be completely inaccessible. Hospital board meetings are less accessible for a nurse researcher than unit change-of-shift reports. Intensive care units (ICUs) are less accessible than well-child clinics. Delivery rooms are less accessible than prenatal classes. All these settings offer opportunities for conducting field research, but the greater the accessibility and the freer the entry to the social situation, the less complicated and time-consuming is this stage of the research.

Strategies to Use With "Gatekeepers" When you elect to conduct overt research in a limited or restricted situation, you must convince those in charge as well as the subjects to cooperate with you. Strategies that have worked for other field researchers include the following:

First, attempt to serve the interests of the research setting in some way through your research. In Hutchinson's study of neonatal intensive care units (NICUs), one director of nurses urged her to study this unit because:

> She had never seen so much anger in her life! Nurses were quitting left and right and everyone said they were under a lot of stress. Doctors were blaming the nurses for infants' deaths. People had various explanations; the physical space was small, it was very crowded, there were no windows; the nurses were all suffering from depression and burnout [1983 field notes].

Hutchinson's field study was designed to examine and dissect the facts in this nursing care situation so as to discover the unarticulated problems and formulate solutions to them. Thus, the value of her research project influenced her initial acceptance in a positive way.

A second entry strategy is to "cultivate" the good will of the subjects by "contouring" one's own behavior to fit in with them. Here, the researcher attempts to present a personal style that enlists the help and support of others. In my own Soteria study (Wilson 1982), the suspicious, slightly antiestablishment, nonprofessional staff caring for psychotics in an antipsychiatric community found field methods to be more congruent with their own humanistic ideology than questionnaires or psychometric tests. They believed that the latter reduced their reality to a numerical score. How others define the field-worker's research and role influences the trust and confidence a field researcher needs to obtain data. And even experienced researchers attest to experiencing feelings of uncertainty and self-doubt when entering the field. As acceptance increases and anxiety decreases, the quality of the work invariably improves.

The two preceding suggestions notwithstanding, nothing seems as important in gaining entrée as a genuine appreciative interest in the subjects. Even the most impressive credentials will open only certain doors (and may even close others). Genuine rapport, in contrast, is established when the subjects accept the investigator for personal qualities rather than formal status, suggesting that research imitates life. A few principles to keep in mind when you try to achieve rapport include:

1. Reducing social distance and other interpersonal barriers increases trust in the researcher.

2. What you reveal about yourself becomes a factor in establishing the kinds of interaction you establish.

3. You always take a certain risk when presenting your research and yourself to potential informants.

4. Putting yourself in the other person's shoes improves cooperation and the quality of data.

All these principles are illustrated in the field note excerpt below:

R. asks who is going to see my stuff and whether I'm working for the project director, being paid, etc. She expresses concern about everything becoming public knowledge. I explain that I'm writing a dissertation but that I hope the findings will be helpful to Soteria people in explaining and understanding what is going on. I assure her that my findings will be abstract enough to protect specific identities. I feel challenged and uncertain about how to portray my work because I don't know how R. and the rest of the staff feel about the project directors. I tell W. that I won't write things that they ask me not to (i.e., various forms of "making out" like picking up receipts in supermarket for reimbursement). I mention that the management of work through humor interests me. They nod acceptingly at this kind of focus.

Most field-workers agree with Schatzman and Strauss when they point out that "entrée is a continuous process of establishing and developing relationships not only with a chief host but with a variety of on-site persons. . . . Successful negotiation through the front door is not always sufficient to open other doors" (1982 p. 22).

Issues that ought to be considered during entry negotiations include:

1. the researcher's right to publish material in his or her own scholarly community, given protection of the subjects' confidentiality

2. the extent of the researcher's freedom of access to documents, people, and situations

3. the expectations the hosts may have of the researcher for performance of work of some kind, copies, or final study reports, formal presentations of findings, and so forth.

Stage 3: Bargaining for a Role

Gold (1958) proposes that a field researcher can opt for any one of four roles, ranging on a continuum from complete participant to complete observer (see Figure 12–1). Between these two extremes are the participant-as-observer and observer-as-participant roles. Schatzman and Strauss (1982) refine these four into six types. The researcher's decision on the nature of his or her role influences how entrée and access are obtained and what kind of data are collected.

The Complete Participant   In the role of complete participant, the field researcher joins an organization or takes a job to learn about the inner workings of a

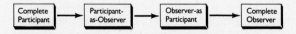

Figure 12–1   Fieldwork role continuum.

situation. In many such studies, the true identity and purpose of the field researcher are not known to those being observed, and "role pretense" is a basic although ethically questionable theme (see Chapter 3). Goffman's classic sociological study on life in a mental hospital, *Asylums* (1961), was based on data he collected while working as an attendant. All complete-participant roles have three potential problems:

1. The investigator may become so self-conscious about revealing his or her true identity that both the participant and observer role performances are hampered.

2. The researcher may "go native" and lose the intellectual distance required to analyze the how and why of study data and instead begin thinking in terms of should or shouldn't, right or wrong.

3. The demands of participation on the investigator for performing work may use time, energy, and flexibility needed for data collection.

Many experts now agree that the combination of these problems along with ethical questions about the propriety of doing "undercover" research outweigh the potential benefit of learning about aspects of behavior that otherwise might not be accessible to the field-worker. The exception, of course, might be in the case of research conducted in a free-access setting, such as a subway station or supermarket.

The Participant as Observer   Although basically similar to the complete-participant role, the participant-as-observer role differs in that both the field-worker and the informants are aware of the research process. The advantage of this role is that the researcher not only watches what others do but also learns from doing it. The major problem of this role is that participants may come to expect the field-worker to become more of a colleague and participant than he or she is capable of being without jeopardizing the research. Nurses are particularly vulnerable to these conflicting demands when conducting research in a health care setting where they possess the skills to intervene in situations and, in fact, are accustomed to doing so. If a patient asks for a glass of water or help to the bathroom, do you ask her to wait while you call a nurse? Do you suggest she call the nurse herself? Or do you do it and lose data potential?

The Observer as Participant   The role of observer as participant calls for more formal observation and entails less risk of getting overly involved in the work of the setting. The researcher limits his or her interaction to seeking clarification of events going on. This approach diminishes intrusion, conveys interest, and gets at meaningful data. In some cases, however, brief relations with a greater variety of people over shorter periods of time lead to fundamental misperceptions and misunderstandings of the social worlds under investigation.

The Complete Observer   In the role of complete observer, the field researcher attempts to observe people in ways that make it unnecessary for them to take him or her into account. Examples include systematic eavesdropping, loitering, bystanding, and spectating in free-access public places. This role also can involve analysis of cultural artifacts and secondary sources, such as patients' charts, case histories, or diaries. Obviously, this approach decreases the chances of losing intellectual distance as well as the impact of the investigator's presence on natural conditions in the field. But its drawbacks include the inability of the researcher to collect focused data from informants by interacting with them and the risk of never getting to understand their point of view. Complete observers watching the world go by risk less and are probably less anxious about rejection from others. But they also often wish that they could interrupt and ask questions about the meaning of what is going on. Many studies that begin with a completely passive role—for example, observing from outside the window of a hospital nursery to see how nurses hold infants and how long they allow them to cry—move on to a more active form of involvement by the researcher.

Shaffir and colleagues (1980) summarize their ideas concerning the stage of bargaining for a role with a list of questions or issues that most field researchers must thoughtfully answer, whatever the role assumed, based on (1) a sense of pragmatism about what stance will best serve the interests of the research project and (2) ethical considerations.

Fundamental Questions in Bargaining for a Role

Q.   How do I identify myself to others in the research setting?

A.   Honesty is probably the best policy here. Simply state that you are a nurse doing a study of what it's like to be in this kind of setting or activity (self-help group, diabetic clinic, emergency room, prenatal class). This identification is usually legitimate enough to allow you to stay yet vague enough to keep your focus open and avoid making the subjects self-conscious about their behavior.

Q.   After becoming a "regular," how do I avoid being entirely assimilated?

A.   Be wise enough to take personal notes (PNs) and write memos on your own impressions, behavior, and feelings during the research process. Periodically withdraw from the field for theoretical reflection to move concrete descriptions to an abstract theoretical level. Be wary of abandoning the excitement of developing your *ideas* about the study setting or situation for the excitement of being *a part* of the setting per se, no matter how interesting it may become for you.

Q.   How actively involved can one get as a participant without jeopardizing either the research, the subjects, or one's personal and professional ethics?

A.   As you become secure about your acceptance in the study setting, feel free to continue to interpret your role. In a study of juvenile delinquents you may dress like them to keep from standing out, but you should also indicate your preference not to participate in crimes, buy "hot" merchandise, or "do drugs." Be as clear and consistent as possible about what you will and will not do, keeping in mind that some of these decisions will influence the kinds of data that you collect. If you are studying tolerance ranges, cutting points, and the like on the subject of how long nurses will let a patient go before administering a pain medication, giving it yourself will obviously prevent you from obtaining indicators on the research question. But as a nurse and humane individual, you may well be willing to make such a choice.*

Dealing with these questions satisfactorily and presenting oneself in field research typically make even seasoned field-workers feel edgy, uncomfortable, uncertain, and anxious. Sometimes we feel awkward about prying into other people's private lives. Fears of rejection from either the officials of an organization or the day-to-day participants remind us to go through channels, cultivate relationships, contour our appearance, withhold evaluative judgments, and be as unobtrusive and charming as possible.

Finally the absence of a questionnaire, psychometric test, blood-pressure cuff, or other "tool of the research trade" often makes the field researcher extremely self-conscious. Recalling his study of Boston's North End, Whyte relates an instance early in his research when he attempted to enter into the small talk of the corner bars by blurting out a string of obscenities and profanities. The gang members looked at him in surprise and said, "You're not supposed to talk like that. That doesn't sound like you" (Whyte 1955 p. 304). Learning the ropes often reveals that study participants realize that the investigator *is* different and that they don't expect the investigator to behave just as they do. Such a discovery can relieve, in part, the burden of feeling self-conscious. The researcher who shows a respect for those being studied and is willing to consider their points of view and rights to confidentiality and privacy has already got a solid basis for becoming attuned to the social world under investigation. Bargaining for a role and learning the ropes are continuous processes that must allow enough flexibility to modify your role and cope with unanticipated developments. Rosalie Wax (1971) suggests that any researcher who feels embarrassed or out of place in unfamiliar circumstances ought to think twice before trying to do participant observation.

Stage 4: Collecting and Recording Data

The objective of field research is to spend an intense period of time in an arena of social interaction and record the ongoing experiences of its participants. This requires that the field researcher gain an understanding about others' ways of perceiving life. Data collection is shaped by the emerging themes and hypotheses that

---

*Adapted from W. B. Shaffir, R. A. Stebbins, and A. Turowetz, *Fieldwork Experience: Qualitative Approaches to Social Research*, New York: St. Martin's Press, 1980.

> **Box 12–1   Qualitative Data Sources in a Study of American Widows**
>
> 1. a content analysis of two sets of letters (74) directed to the author in response to a television program and the announcement of her study in the newspaper
>
> 2. interviews of half an hour with ten of the letter authors
>
> 3. an examination of the literature on aging, grief, divorce, single status, ethnic family construction, and the like with an eye toward their effects on widowhood
>
> 4. reinterviews of 35 previously contacted widows, attempting to cover all combinations of living situations
>
> 5. interviews with various groups of women to learn about racial and economic factors
>
> 6. interviews with mothers and daughters or other kin members with respect to relationship strains
>
> 7. attendance at and field notes on meetings of organizations for widows or single women and an analysis of their publications
>
> 8. attendance at meetings of groups that by nature attracted widows though did not focus on helping them per se, like the YWCA and church groups
>
> 9. attendance at meetings and tours of facilities, interviews with people and reviews of the publications from Home-Delivered Meals, the Mayor's Commission on Senior Citizens, and the like to determine their perceptions of problems of widowhood
>
> 10. collections and analysis of diaries and histories of events
>
> 11. interviews with friends and relatives of widows focusing observations on the process by which someone is selected to assume responsibility for a widowed mother
>
> Source: H. Z. Lopata, *Women as Widows: Support Systems*. New York: Elsevier, 1979.

develop in the course of doing qualitative analyses (see Chapter 13). Thus, in most field studies, data collection and analysis go on simultaneously.

Data collection begins with the question "What shall I look at?" Douglas (1976 p. 195) suggests that we begin by "casting a wide net." This means talking to all kinds of people and investigating all kinds of settings associated with the phenomenon in question. Polsky says that the initial rule for field researchers is "keep your eyes and ears open but keep your mouth shut" (1969 p. 12). In short, submerge yourself in everyday social life. This initial approach ought not be continued for too long, however, because you run the risk of simply generating an unmanageable explosion of irrelevant data. In Box 12–1 Lopata (1979) gives us a sense of the breadth of data-collection strategies she used to develop her analyses of role modifications and support systems of American urban widows.

Clearly, the initial data-collection principle in a field study is to record everything that might be vaguely or remotely relevant to your unfolding analyses, because you don't know until your focus narrows what might be useful. This process is loosely called "hanging around" (but I discourage using the phrase itself to describe your methodology in a thesis or grant proposal). It seems that observation is particularly arbitrary at the beginning of a field study. As the study progresses, however, you begin to accumulate more detailed information. Hypotheses present themselves, and your analyses and observations become more purposeful and focused. Field researchers often search documents in the exploration phase and then use unstructured interviews to raise specific questions and to supplement data gathered initially from published and archival sources. The interviews allow you to test hypotheses, fill in blank spots, and seek interpretations and clarifications. In an unstructured interview, the interviewer:

1. stresses the interviewee's definition of the situation

2. encourages the interviewee to structure the account of the situation

3. lets the interviewee introduce the notions of what he or she considers relevant instead of relying on the investigator's notions of relevance

The major methods of collecting data in the field, including participant observation and interviewing, are examined in detail later in the chapter (also see Appendix C).

Stage 5: Leaving the Field

Although many view the fieldwork experience as more of a continuous process than a series of separate stages, all agree that a wise field researcher attends to closure and leaving the field at some point in the process. Ultimately, the investigator must gracefully withdraw from the study setting and from most, if not all, of the personal relationships that have for a time been relatively intense. Clearly, if one researcher is insensitive or is viewed unfavorably upon departure from the field, future investigators' efforts to gain entrée and access will be handicapped.

Problems that have developed may need to be addressed, entrée bargains reappraised, and personal relationships resolved. If a nurse has been a complete participant on a hospital unit, he or she may need to redefine this role once the study is completed. The following checklist offers some basic and general guides for leaving the field:

1. Be prepared for some respondents to feel abandoned, misrepresented, or even duped. The transition from personal involvement and intense concern for

those in the field to preoccupation with analyses and publication of findings may come as an abrupt shock to some who expected on some level that you would live out your involvement with the study setting. When study subjects become aware of your diminished interest in their lives and situation, some may come to feel cheated.

2. Because of the considerations just mentioned, withdraw gradually if at all possible, clearly defining your timetable of diminishing contacts. Junker (1960 p. 11) calls this strategy "easing out."

3. If norms for leaving the situation or setting exist, such as a farewell wine-and-cheese party or an exchange of gifts, allow these norms and customs to facilitate your withdrawal or role redefinition as well. Sometimes, however, there are no formal good-byes, just drifting off and returning intermittently to talk less and less frequently. This alternative, termed "suspended" rather than "terminated" research, leaves room to drift back and resume data collection at a later date.

4. Fulfill the commitments you made in order to gain access and entrée. If you promised a hospital staff a preliminary presentation of your findings once your analysis began to solidify, schedule a date and time to make that presentation as a closure ritual. If you promised to provide a copy of your final report to subjects in recognition of their contributions, do so. But be prepared for some to greet their anonymity with less than enthusiasm and others to feel that confidentiality was only thinly protected.

5. Be prepared to have become so involved and attached that you don't want to make your exit and find yourself thinking up excuses to extend your stay. It is usually advisable to make clear from the outset, to yourself and to others, how long you plan to remain in the field. Even then be prepared to experience some feelings of alienation, guilt, and melancholy when relationships are ended. This is particularly likely when the research project depended a lot on trust and friendship between investigator and respondents or informants.

6. Impersonal, structural factors sometimes offer a convenient (and honest) explanation for terminating a field study relationship. The expiration of a research grant, termination of a visa, completion of a degree, or a geographic move all help the process of easing out without offending setting participants.

Major Methods of Field Research

Fieldwork experts classify the methods for obtaining data in the field into either three or four types, depending upon the author's point of view. All agree that type 1 consists of participant observation, that type 2 is the interviewing of informants, and that type 3 involves accumulating countable data through surveys or psycho-metric tests. (This last type of data collection was the subject of Chapter 10.) Proponents for limiting the types to these three argue that the analysis of documents really represents results or combinations of the three primary types of data collection. For example, documents such as diaries and logs are basically an informant's *written* account of his or her experience and should be treated just like any other evidence of perspectives or occurrences. Other documents, such as hospital staffing patterns, the books of a nursing service department, or the membership rolls of a state nurses' association, are essentially enumerations.

Some authorities, however, choose to categorize as type 4 the analysis of documents, case studies, case histories, videotapes, and the like, grouping them under the term *unobtrusive*, or *nonreactive*, *methods*. An unobtrusive measure is any method of observation that directly removes the observer from the interactions or events being studied. Archival document analysis includes chart audits, observation of play therapy for disabled children from behind a one-way glass, viewing audiotapes of psychiatric intake interviews, and physical trace analysis that involves the study of signs people leave behind (personal objects the elderly take with them when they move into nursing homes, special toys 2-year-olds bring to the hospital, and the like). Such techniques allow researchers to make inferences about people while minimizing the influence that the investigator might have on behavior. For example, just knowing that a field-worker is studying nonprofessional behavior among professional staff can have a reactive influence on the people in the field and create doubt in the investigator about how typical the data collected really are.

Criteria for Balancing Types of Data

Answers to certain kinds of question are most efficiently and accurately obtained with one data-collection method. In making decisions about which strategies you should plan to use as a field-worker, use two important criteria to guide your choice:

1. *information adequacy*—that is, precision and completeness of the data

2. *efficiency*, meaning the cost of obtaining the information

Such criteria notwithstanding, most experienced field researchers also agree that a study's validity is enhanced when you *triangulate* your data-collection methods. **Triangulation** means using several different collection methods to obtain different "slices of data" on the same study question and then cross-checking accounts against one another for consistency and comparability. In short, triangulation requires that a researcher examine the study question from as many different perspectives as possible. The sociologist Norman Denzin (1970) also uses the term *triangulation* to refer to:

1. including a wide variety of data sources (individuals, families, groups)

2. involving a variety of investigators working individually and in teams

3. combining a range of theoretical orientations on the same situation—for example, approaching a study of hospice care for dying patients from psychological, biological, and sociocultural theory

Methodological triangulation is, however, the most conventional meaning for the term. In a discussion of nursing studies on the concept of stress, for example, Muhlenkamp (1978) writes that it was important to use a variety of stress indicators, particuarly ones that did not share the same bias and measurement error.

Each of the major types of data-collection strategy used in field research is discussed in the sections that follow, with the exception of type 3, to which Chapter 10 is devoted.

Observation

If you elect to emphasize participant observation in a specific study setting rather than interviews about a social experience, here are some guidelines to help you get started.

Guidelines for Observing

1. Begin by orienting yourself to what Schatzman and Strauss (1982) call "the various social, spatial and temporal maps of the setting." If you are studying an institution, you may obtain organizational charts, a schedule of meetings and routines, even a blueprint or floor plan. In a study of burn units, you might take notes on the physical layout, routines and emergencies, pacing of work, division of labor, status relationships, treatment ideologies, ideals and values, and problems and concerns.

2. Take a "tour of limited discovery"—a first extensive (not intensive) look at things, persons, and activities that constitute "the site" (Schatzman and Strauss 1982). Don't be concerned about missing things. Underlying patterns will occur over and over. Use this step to identify informants, meet and cultivate people, establish your legitimacy, and figure out what your next steps will be.

3. Selectively sample people, places, events, and any other categories that are suggested by the initial mapping and beginning analysis. Typically, if you are studying a hospital or police system that is on a 24-hour day, you will selectively sample all times of the day, all days of the week, activities such as routines and shifts, and special occasions and events.

4. Decide on locations from which to observe. Select these based on where events and information will come within your line of sight. Sometimes you may follow one person around; at other times you may sit in the corner of a nurses' station or clinic waiting room. Schatzman and Strauss suggest the use

of single, multiple, and mobile positioning. *Single positioning* is staying put for a period of time to gain a greater familiarity with one station. *Multiple positioning* means moving around the setting to observe in different locations. *Mobile positioning* is the term for actually following someone—a woman in labor, a nursing student, a chemotherapy patient—through the course of a day or an experience. You can maximize your variety of perspectives by seeking out people who you anticipate might have different points of view, such as oldtimers versus newcomers, patients versus staff, or advocates versus critics. Most field researchers learn that they can ultimately listen for what they didn't see. One's continuous presence and repeated visits over a relatively long period result in the regulars telling the researcher what was missed between visits.

> You should have been here on Saturday night. It was a really heavy time! We admitted this guy who tried to shoot the governor (from field notes).

Recording Field Notes A field researcher needs a system for remembering observations and, even more importantly, retrieving and analyzing them. If your identity and general purposes are known, you may take notes on a notepad or small clipboard in the presence of participants. Most of the time, field researchers jot a key word or phrase or cue down and then periodically leave the scene briefly to fill in full notes. Some field researchers dictate their observations into a tape recorder and later have a transcriber type them. The danger of the latter approach is that weeks and months of observing can yield a veritable ocean of disorganized data, and its continuous flow can be as overwhelming to a researcher as the original experience of entering the field.

Writing and then typing one's own field notes (or entering them using a computer program for qualitative data, such as Ethnograph) increase the likelihood that the notes will be legible years later and will include sufficient detail and context to serve as a fund for future analyses, yet not be so voluminous as to be unapproachable. Each researcher tends to develop an individual format and approach for recording field notes. Schatzman and Strauss (1982) offer the following model as a starting point.

Observational notes (ONs) are descriptions of events experienced through watching and listening. They contain the who, what, where, and how of a situation and contain as little interpretation as possible. An example of an ON from a field study of a burn unit follows:

ON: The burn unit is laid out with a central nursing station that faces three glassed-in wards. Male and female patients are in the same ward. The treatment room has a big tub shaped so that arms and legs can be spread out. The tub has a whirlpool mechanism. The ratio of staff to patients seems to be one staff member to three patients. Staff members seem to work in groups of two's and three's, and the atmosphere is one of tremendous hustle and bustle.

Theoretical notes (TNs) are purposeful attempts to derive meaning from the observational notes. Here you interpret, infer, conjecture, and hypothesize to build your analytic scheme. Here is a TN from Fagerhaugh and Strauss's (1977) burn study:*

TN: There is a cocoon-like effect on the unit. Patients spend weeks and months there. Visitors are limited to the family. There are no mirrors or windows. Four patients could tell me about the day they came into the hospital but *none* knew what day it was today. They state that the days all "run together," that thinking about how long they'd been in didn't matter. It was the excruciating treatment pain that consumed them. The pain is absolutely indescribable in its intensity. S said it reduces him to a blubbering baby, something that he never was.

Methodological notes (MNs) are instructions to oneself, critiques of one's tactics, and reminders about methodological approaches that might be fruitful.

MN: I decided to spend one day observing the varieties of painful treatments. There seem to be plenty of them! I decide to look for situations in which staff members actually talk about the god-awful pain these people are experiencing instead of the technical matters related to burn management.

Personal notes (PNs) (not a component of the original Schatzman and Strauss format) are notes about one's own reactions and reflections and experiences. Field-

---

*This and other quotations from S. Fagerhaugh and A. Strauss, *Politics of Pain Management*, Menlo Park, Calif.: Addison-Wesley, 1977.

work relies on the investigator's ability to "take the role of the other" and be introspective. A final illustration from the burn study presents a PN.

PN: I had a somewhat unnerving morning. There's so much pain and misery on the unit yet the light-heartedness of the staff and the lack of pain expression among the patients except during treatments creates in me a sense of horror and awe! My friends and husband don't want to hear about working with burn patients. It's too horrible! I feel isolated and wonder if other nurses avoid the nurses on the burn unit or keep shop talk to superficial social "chit-chat."

After ONs, TNs, MNs, and PNs are recorded, they are customarily typed, paginated, labeled and dated, duplicated, and filed and become the basis for analytic memos (see Chapter 13). If you are not using a computer, remember to use headings and subheadings for ease of data retrieval and to leave wide margins around the edges for penciled codes.

A good set of field notes not only relieves the investigator of some of the burdens of remembering events but also constitutes a written record of the development of observations and ideas to be used in future publications of the research findings and method.

Interviewing

Interviews depend on the respondents' verbal report about experiences, perceptions, preferences, problems, feelings, attitudes, or whatever other phenomena may be relevant to the study question. Some interviews may be highly structured, in the sense that the wording of each question, the sequence in which they are asked, and the possible responses are planned by developing an interview schedule (a lot like a script). Interviewers are trained to use it. Structured interviews are akin to questionnaires, with the exception that the interviewer and the respondent are in each other's presence when the interview is used.

The next sections of this chapter address the use of partially structured and unstructured interviews, because these two types are generally preferred by nurses doing field research.

Focused or Partially Structured Interviews   A *partially structured interview*, or **focused interview**, begins with at least an outline of topics the investigator intends to cover with each subject; but both the interviewer and the subject are free to deviate from the prepared agenda and introduce thoughts or observations that are particularly relevant to their personal perspective as the conversation unfolds. (See

---

Box 12–2   Guidelines for Assessing the Sexual Needs of the Aged

1. When you were growing up, did people you knew discuss sex and romance?

2. How do you feel about discussing it now?

3. What do you think about romance at this stage in your life?

4. What were you told about sex when you were a child?

5. Do you think it is a very important part of life satisfaction for people of all ages?

6. How important has sexual activity been in your life?

7. What were you told about masturbation?

8. What does sexuality mean to you?

9. Does your present living situation give you opportunities to express your sexuality?

10. What values and morals influence your feelings about sex now?

11. How are your needs of intimacy being met now?

Source: H. Wilson and C. Kneisl, *Psychiatric Nursing*, 2nd ed., Menlo Park, Calif.: Addison-Wesley, 1983.

Box 12–2 for a progression of questions for assessing the sexual needs of the aged.) Partially structured interviews offer the interviewer latitude to move from content area to content area, to follow up on cues suggested by the respondent, and to spend various amounts of time interviewing one subject or another. Such interviews, however, require that by the end of the interview *all of the predetermined topics or questions have indeed been covered in some sequence and in some form with each interviewee.*

Clinical interviews are basically a subtype of focused interview. They are used when the interviewer is a clinician, the respondent is a patient or client, the circumstances involve a health care problem, and the purpose of the interview is to collect data to formulate a nursing diagnosis or health care problem assessment. Nursing histories, psychiatric intake interviews, and verbal mental status examinations are all used by clinicians to identify problems, make nursing diagnoses, and plan nursing care. Box 12–3 presents an example of a psychosocial clinical interview guide (Wilson and Kneisl 1988). Clinical interviews can also provide data that are valuable to nurses conducting research. McCorkle (1977) used such interviews to study the impact of a diagnosis of inoperable lung cancer on a person's attachments and goals as the illness progressed. Data from clinical interviews helped reestablish the subjects' disease state and clarify their perception of their illness as well as to discover the differences and similarities in the quality of living for subjects with terminal cancer. Most researchers who use partially structured interviews believe

Box 12–3 Psychosocial Interview Guide

1. *Physical and Intellectual Factors*
   a. Presence of physical illness and/or disability
   b. Appearance and energy level
   c. Current and potential levels of intellectual functioning
   d. How client sees personal world, translates events around self; client's perceptual abilities
   e. Cause and effect reasoning, ability to focus

2. *Socioeconomic Factors*
   a. Economic factors—level of income, adequacy of subsistence; how this affects life-style, sense of adequacy, self-worth
   b. Employment and attitudes about it
   c. Racial, cultural, and ethnic identification; sense of identity and belonging
   d. Religious identification and link to significant value systems, norms, and practices

3. *Personal Values and Goals*
   a. Presence or absence of congruence between values and their expression in action; meaning of values to individual
   b. Congruence between individual's values and goals and the immediate systems with which client interacts
   c. Congruence between individual's values and assessor's values; meaning of this for intervention process

4. *Adaptive Functioning and Response to Present Involvement*
   a. Manner in which individual presents self to others—grooming, appearance, posture
   b. Emotional tone and change or constancy of levels
   c. Style of communication—verbal and nonverbal; ability to express appropriate emotion, follow train of thought; factors of dissonance, confusion, uncertainty
   d. Symptoms or symptomatic behavior
   e. Quality of relationship individual seeks to establish—direction, purposes, and uses of such relationships for individual
   f. Perception of self
   g. Social roles that are assumed or ascribed; compentence in fulfilling these roles
   h. Relational behavior
      • Capacity for intimacy

(Continued)

Box 12–3 Psychosocial Interview Guide (Continued)

- Dependence-independence balance
- Power and control conflicts
- Exploitiveness
- Openness

5. *Developmental Factors*
   a. Role performance equated with life stage
   b. How developmental experiences have been interpreted and used

   c. How individual has dealt with past conflicts, tasks, and problems
   d. Uniqueness of present problem in life experience

Source: H. Wilson and C. Kneisl, *Psychiatric Nursing*, 3rd ed., Menlo Park, Calif.: Addison-Wesley, 1988. Adapted from B. Compton and B. Galloway, *Social Work Processes*, 2nd ed. Homewood, Ill.: Dorsey Press, 1979, pp. 250–251.

---

that they are effective for exploration and hypotheses formulation but not appropriate or practical for hypothesis testing.

Unstructured Interviews The **unstructured interview** may be either spontaneous or scheduled, but its identifying characteristic is that respondents are encouraged to talk about whatever they wish that is relevant to the researcher's interest. Many such interviews begin with open-ended questions or statements, such as: "Tell me something about what it was like when you and your husband first learned that Stephen was retarded." or "What concerns you most when you think about managing your life, knowing what you do about your illness?" Some unstructured interviews begin by just inviting the interviewee to talk about whatever he or she wishes. The intent of the unstructured interview is to get to the subject's perception of the meanings in his or her world without introducing the investigator's conception of it. In fact, it is the method of choice among field researchers, and most researchers intentionally avoid structuring their interviews. Structure limits in advance what topics are important to ask about and often what the possible categories of response from interviewees might be. Unstructured interviews, in contrast, allow the interviewer a great deal of freedom in exploring whatever seems important to the respondent and promote what Brink and Wood (1988) call the likelihood that responses will be spontaneous, self-revealing, and personal.

Advantages of Interviewing Listening to people talk about their perceptions and experiences has a number of important advantages as a data-collection strategy:

1. Inviting subjects to tell their story face to face to an empathic person usually gets a better response rate than mailing them an impersonal questionnaire or structured data form.

2. Interviews allow you to collect data from people who either because of their literacy level or some other communication barrier such as paralysis following a stroke, bandages after burns, or immobilizing tubes or traction, simply can't write.

3. Interviews are usually more effective in getting at people's complex feelings or perceptions. In describing the burden of implementing the recommended regimen for their diabetic children, interviewed mothers in one nursing study spoke of a period of being overwhelmed as they tried to understand the "whats" and "whys" of food management for their children. One mother told the nurse researcher when describing the tensions of carrying this responsibility, "I felt like I was holding a stick of dynamite."

4. Interviews allow you to clarify responses that you don't understand fully, to probe certain responses in more depth, and to reword and rephrase questions so that the interviewee can understand them.

5. Unstructured interviews, particularly, allow you to discover the unexpected. In Lopata's (1979) study of American widows she commented:

My clumsiness with the tape recorder in the exploratory stages of my study proved to be a boon, preventing me from making some of the mistakes of new researchers not familiar with the world of their subjects. I knew what I wanted to ask these women.... My reading had filled me with questions and anticipated responses. The mechanical problems of using the recorder and the accompanying non-directed interaction finally forced me to listen to what the widows *wanted to talk about* before I had a chance to ask questions. Their monologues often focused on subjects very different from what I assumed would be important to them.... These interviews contributed to my increasing awareness that role modifications and support systems of widows contain a variety of realities which my lack of familiarity with their lives had not anticipated [p. 71].

Interviews used in field studies, although they may focus on pinpointing the development of one analytic idea or another, are essentially conversations in situ, which vary widely in style and type. The authors of a study of pain management, after two years of fieldwork in two clinics, twenty wards, and nine hospitals, had this to say:

We did no interviewing that involved asking identical questions of a pre-selected number of people, even when interviewing patients with similar disorders.... Even prearranged interviews followed no particular format, but the interviewer followed through on areas deemed relevant or on leads offered by the interviewee [Fagerhaugh and Strauss 1977 p. 306].

These kinds of interviews are most often done when checking hypotheses developed from extensive field notes or the analysis of case studies. For example, about an interview with one informant, the investigators wrote:

Mrs. Noble taught us, rather early in the study, to think about unfamiliar technology as a condition that might affect the patient's ability to get the staff to accept her pain as truly legitimate and thus influence the staff's handling of pain-relief tasks. The in-depth, free-response questioning usually used in fieldwork grows not only from the investigator's philosophy of science [see Chapter 1], but also from the fact that the research question at hand is one for which the investigators don't necessarily know the full range of possible responses [Fagerhaugh and Strauss 1977 p. 309].

Disadvantages of Interviewing As you might imagine, such free-response, unstructured interviews also have disadvantages, according to their critics:

1. In nursing studies, particularly, interviewees often expect some sort of direct help as a result of participating in the interview—a solution to their problems or even a complete change in their life. They may assume that the nurse interviewer can put them in touch with some special resources or benefits, unless he or she is careful in addressing with all candor the personal benefits section of the consent process (see Chapter 3).

2. It is time-consuming to collect data during open-ended, nonstructured, or semistructured interviews, and it is similarly time-consuming to analyze these data word by word, phrase by phrase (see Chapte 13).

3. It is difficult to make conventional quantitative comparisons across interviews in the absence of an interview schedule that ensures that all interviewees are asked the same set of questions in the same terminology.

4. If a substantial number of interviews are to be conducted, interviewers must be trained, particularly in using clear, nonleading language, expanding or clarifying a respondent's initial response, and developing listening skills.

5. Subjects may be self-conscious about being recorded on tape or about notes being taken about their replies. Thus, they may not give responses as freely as they would on an anonymous questionnaire.

Listening: An Essential Research Skill Listening is perhaps more crucial in unstructured interviews than questioning. Listening involves an active process of responding to words and body language. Parsons and Sanford (1979), two nurses writing about interpersonal interaction, encourage us to use Egan's (1970) definition: "Listening for our purposes means becoming aware of all the cues that the other emits and this implies an openness to the totality of the communication of the other" (Egan 1970 p. 248).

Effective listening requires the following steps:

1. coding what is said into something that makes sense for you, the interviewer

2. interpreting the meaning in the respondent's framework or perspective

3. responding by conveying to the interviewee that she or he is being heard and understood

Brammer (1973 pp. 81–87) developed some strategies for making listening more effective and applied them to the research interview. They include:

1. establishing eye contact with the interviewee (The difficulty of accomplishing this while writing notes is one of the reasons some field researchers prefer to tape record interviews.)

2. clarifying and checking perceptions by restating a summary of the basic message, asking for a repetition, but not interrupting

3. using clarifying questions that ask for elaboration, examples, and extensions of the original message

Most nurses are well acquainted with the principles of effective communication with patients. However, communicating with patients with the major objective of helping them directly is different from interviewing people to obtain data bearing on a research question and an analysis that may not offer them any direct benefit. For some nurse researchers, interviewing for research purposes rather than clinical ones presents something of a barrier. For others, it's an intellectual challenge.

Analysis of Documents, Case Studies, and Case Histories

Documents and Records Nursing research has tended to use document and record analysis more often than the other types of unobtrusive measure mentioned earlier in this chapter. An agency's perspective often emerges from analysis of statistics, reports of medication errors, nursing notes, policy statements, and procedure manuals. Field researchers realize that through such official documents they learn the agency's interpretation of what has gone or is going on and what is valued. Sudnow (1967), in studies of birth and death statistics, has commented on some of the ambiguities of relying exclusively on such official documents. His observations suggest that similar organizations processing the same sets of events may not generate comparable data on those events. Variations in delinquency rates, for example, may often really represent only differences in organizational bookkeeping. Because of this possibility, field researchers must always report document analysis as data obtained within a particular, situated context. In my qualitative field study of Soteria House, a nonconventional residential care setting for psychotic adults, documents revealed a pattern of limited and partial disclosures based on the audience for which a particular document was intended. The accompanying example memo summarizes my analysis.

Documents such as diaries, books, letters, newspapers, meeting minutes, legal documents, and reports as well as photographs, films, and drawings are also used as sources of data. Analysis procedures for documents and records used as data in field studies are described in Chapter 13).

EXAMPLE: Memo on Documents

Self-portrayals of Soteria share two general properties: ambiguity and a tendency toward chameleon-like protective coloration. Keeping Soteria ambiguous . . . limits a potential critic's ability to evaluate its success or failure. Self-portrayals in documents take on different characteristics depending on the audience. A manual called "The Care and Feeding of a Soteria" professes as its purpose: "to provide some examples of how various types of behavior gave rise to problems dealt with at Soteria." Its informal, atheoretical style is almost unrecognizable in a letter written to solicit financial support from federal funding agencies: "Soteria is a residential treatment program for first-episode schizophrenics utilizing a developmental crisis model. Six specifically trained nonprofessional staff work with the resident patients under the supervision of a psychiatrist and a social worker." Here the presentation attempted to link Soteria to the language of conventional, mainstream psychiatry. Professionals at Soteria recognize that to portray Soteria as a "good space" or "high energy" in the rhetoric and ideology of the staff is to risk being dismissed as naive or ostracized as outrageous. Thus to the professional community documents present it as an experimental research project in psychiatric residential care . . . which in my point of view, it is.

Analysis of properties

Limited, variable, and partial disclosures characterized self-portrayals in documents

Case Studies and Case Histories   The **case study** has a long and valued history in the sphere of clinical practice research. Here the clinician or researcher conducts an in-depth investigation of a patient, a community group or aggregate, or an institution, such as a hospital or clinic. Some clinicians have used literature, studying Tennessee Williams's *The Glass Menagerie* to learn more about a physical handicap or Eugene O'Neill's *Long Day's Journey Into Night* to learn about destructive family dynamics. Sylvia Plath's poignant *The Bell Jar* may be of greater value in learning to understand severe depression than more conventional quantified scientific modes.

Whether fictional or not, case studies offer information that is rich and sometimes difficult to come by. Obviously, Freud developed his psychoanalytic theory and methods primarily from careful case studies conducted in turn-of-the-century Vienna. Critics of sole reliance on case study data underscore their lack of generalizability. The methodology for compiling such data is not as rigorously prescribed as that for collecting survey or even participant observation field notes. Some say there is considerable freedom, if not outright ambiguity, in devising the data-collection strategies. The main principle is once again pragmatism in addressing the study question. And, of course, case study data must be analyzed and interpreted according to one of the qualitative analyses presented in Chapter 13.

Glaser and Strauss (1970) distinguish between a case history and a case study. They believe that the goal in a case history is to get the fullest possible story for its own sake. A *case study* focuses on description, verification, or developing of theory. A **case history**, on the one hand, provides highly readable imagery that can be explained and interpreted within theory. It is a way of demonstrating how theory can be used to understand human experience. A case study, on the other hand, generally exists for the purpose of comparative analysis and the generation of data and grounded theories. Even though Glaser and Strauss try to emphasize this distinction, they also recognize that for the most part the distinction is subtle and often blurred.

When trying to decide which is which, it is important to determine whether theory is being used to place the case within a more general context, as is done with a case history, or whether theory is actually being developed from the comparative analysis of multiple case studies. One of the most famous of case histories is the classic one by Thomas and Znaniecki (1918), which begins with a threefold typology of Polish emigrant men and then offers the personal history of one. Blau (1955) and Crozier (1964), in contrast, used case studies to correct and amplify Max Weber's theory of bureaucracy.

The potential of both case studies and case histories in nursing is wide open if we can overcome the accusation that such work fails to uphold the canons of science and is more properly categorized as journalism or art. Nurse authors have made substantial contributions to the professional literature, often in case histories.

In 1970 two medical sociologists in collaboration with a team of nurses involved in field research published a book entitled *Anguish: A Case History of a* *Dying Trajectory.* It was the story of a woman's protracted death in the hospital. According to its authors, the case demonstrated two major features; it was of long duration and it moved slowly but steadily downward. In presenting the case history of this lingering trajectory, Glaser and Strauss (1970) told the life story, or biography, of the patient; the story of how a hospital's staff related to her slow decline on their turf; the case history of the two nursing students who served as informants for the study; and, finally, the story of a final stage of a research project that had addressed the topic of dying and lasted over five years.

The interweaving of these four substories illustrates the rich detail and complex information that a case history can produce. Its authors remind us, however, that case history is not a novel or merely exciting informative description. It is deliberately intended to highlight and explicate theoretical explanations that can be more broadly generalizable.

Do Field Studies Yield Scientific Truth?

In a critique of Wolanin's (1977) study on confusion, Jackson began with the following comment: "Poor research is the art of drawing sufficient conclusions from insufficient data gathered by faulty methodology and inadequate instruments" (1977 p. 76). Field studies in general are open to criticism on these grounds. Overcoming the implicit and explicit criticisms of field research begins with avoiding a strict and narrow conception of what is science. It moves on to developing a research narrative that proves its credibility by explaining through a linear, logical process the problems, methods, and findings. Finally, it acknowledges the responsibility of the researcher to provide sufficient detail about the steps of the research process to enable a reader to evaluate the results. Table 12–2 summarizes Eisner's (1981) distinctions between studying something in a *scientific* mode and an *artistic* mode. On Eisner's grounds, most field research would be excluded as a valid scientific approach. But as for its ability to inform and enrich nursing practice, even he argues for seeking "a binocular approach" that includes both artistic and scientific approaches. "Looking through one eye never did provide much depth of field" (1981 p. 9).

Others acknowledge that field research is indeed a valid approach to the discovery of conceptual models. Some require that a particular analysis procedure be followed if a study is to be judged as credible (see Chapter 13), but all critics emphasize that the reader must be given sufficient data to judge whether a sample was homogeneous and to know the specifics of data collection and analysis. Brink (1975), criticizing Schuster's (1975) privacy study, writes: "I remain puzzled as to how inductive methodologists analyze their data. . . . I would be hard-pressed to duplicate what she did on the basis of the information presented" (p. 177).

TABLE 12–2 *Scientific and Artistic Ways of Knowing*

Criterion	Scientific Approach	Artistic Approach
Forms of representation employed	Formal, literal language	Idiosyncratic and figurative language
Criteria for appraisal	Whether conclusions are supported by the evidence and whether methods bias the conclusions (canons of sampling and test reliability)	How persuasive and informative the personal vision of the author is
Points of focus	Manifest behavior of the individual or group; experimental approach in search of law	The experience of individuals and the meaning their actions have for others; interpretive approach in search of meaning
Nature of generalization	Trends, central tendencies, and statistical differences	Belief that the general resides in the particular
Role of form	Standardization of style	Various styles
Degree of license allowed	Attempt to avoid bias, be objective, and present the facts	Avoidance of a facade of objectivity; selective use of informants; emphasis on what the author needs to say
Interest in prediction and control	Emphasis on prediction, explication, and control of future events	Emphasis on forms of understanding conveyed through the artistic image
Sources of data	Standardized tests and procedures	The investigator's experience of what he or she attends to
Basis for knowing	A positivistic view in which only formal propositions can provide knowledge	Central role of emotion ("To know a rose by its Latin name and yet to miss its fragrance is to miss much of the rose's meaning.")
Ultimate aims	Making true statements about the world—the laws of nature	Creation of images that people will find meaningful; implication that truth is relative, and diverse

Source: E. W. Eisner, "On the Differences Between Scientific and Artistic Approaches to Qualitative Research," *Educational Researcher*, April 1981, pp. 5–9.

We can conclude from Brink's critique, as well as those of many others, that field studies will receive a more favorable regard among nurse researchers when their results are presented with a clear, concise description of the process that led to the findings presented.

Guidelines for Critique

- Does the researcher fully describe the way in which field research was conducted?

- What data-collection strategies were used? Why were they chosen?

- If the data were collected by a participant observer, was the observer able to develop rapport with the subjects?

- Were interviews partially structured or unstructured? What procedures were used to record responses?

SUMMARY OF KEY IDEAS AND TERMS

✓ *Field research* is a mode of inquiry that grew out of anthropology and sociology. It relies on firsthand knowing under natural conditions and unstructured data-collection methods in which the investigator is the primary instrument or tool.

✓ *Ethnography* is the systematic study of cultures, subcultures, and life-styles.

✓ *Field studies* that examine, describe, define, and explain everyday nursing practice and have practical uses can make valuable contributions, particularly to factor-isolating and factor-relating types of clinical nursing research.

✓ The major characteristics of field studies are:

- *face-to-face interviewing or observation* by the investigator

- *data collection and analysis* of complex sets of variables that go on simultaneously and in the natural setting

✓ Field research emphasizes data-collection strategies that are designed to learn about the perspective, or world view, of those who are being studied. It includes participant and nonparticipant observation; unstructured interviewing; analysis of documents, case studies, and case histories; and other unobtrusive measures.

✓ Appraising the field is a strategy for locating a field that is suitable for conducting research on a study question. Any place or set of activities can be considered "the field" for a study.

✓ Serving the interests of the setting through your study, cultivating relationships, and contouring your presence to avoid being obviously intrusive are useful strategies in the second stage of field studies. Difficulties vary according to whether your research is overt or covert and to how accessible the study setting is.

✓ The role of observer can range along a continuum from complete participant to complete observer. Each role has advantages and disadvantages.

✓ Data collection in field research begins with casting a wide net and initial mapping of the setting to orient yourself to its various social, spatial, and temporal dimensions. Then it is guided by categories and ideas that are emerging in your analysis.

✓ Guidelines for gracefully leaving the field once your data collection is completed include:

- Be prepared for some subjects to feel abandoned or taken advantage of.

- Ease out gradually, based on a timetable of diminishing contacts.

- Take advantage of any typical exit rituals.

- Fulfill any commitments you have made.

✓ *Single, multiple,* and *mobile positioning* are all options for observing in a study setting.

✓ One model for recording field notes is to use a system that organizes them into *observational notes* (ONs), *theoretical notes* (TNs), *methodological notes* (MNs), and *personal notes* (PNs).

✓ Partially structured and unstructured interviews are preferred by field researchers, because the emphasis is on freedom in exploring whatever is important to the interviewee and stimulating responses that are spontaneous and revealing.

✓ The advantages of interviews over written questionnaires include:

- The response rate is usually better.

- They can be used with people who are unable to read and write.

- They allow for probing and clarification of complex ideas.

- They allow you to discover the unexpected.

✓ Disadvantages of interviews include:

- They do not directly benefit the respondent in most instances.

- They are time-consuming.

- It is hard to make quantitative comparisons of respondents.

- Interviewers must be trained.

- Subjects may be self-conscious and concerned about their loss of anonymity.

✓ Effective listening strategies in field research include:

- attending to the respondent by maintaining eye contact

- clarifying and perception checking by restating summaries of the basic message and asking for repetitions

- using clarifying questions that elicit examples and extensions of the original message

✓ Documents such as diaries, books, letters, meeting minutes, legal papers, reports, films, photographs, and nursing notes are all excellent sources of data in field studies.

✓ *Case studies* are used to develop and verify theory; *case histories* are ways of demonstrating how a theory can be used to understand human experiences.

✓ Some critics argue that field methods correspond more to the artistic rather than the scientific mode of inquiry. Others propose that as long as a field study conveys its logic, methods, and findings in sufficient detail, only a narrow conception of science would exclude it as a route to scientific truth.

References

Aamodt AM: Discovering the child's view of alopecia: Doing ethnography. In: Munhall PL, Oiler CJ (Editors), *Nursing Research: A Qualitative Perspective*. Norwalk, Conn.: Appleton-Century-Crofts, 1986.

Agan RD: Intuitive knowing as a dimension of nursing. *Adv Nurs Sci* 1987; 10, 63–70.

Agar MH: *Speaking of Ethnography*. Beverly Hills: Sage, 1986.

Blau P: *The Dynamics of Bureaucracy*. Chicago: The University of Chicago Press, 1955.

Blumer H: *Symbolic Interactionism*. Englewood Cliffs, N.J.: Prentice-Hall, 1969.

Brammer LM: *The Helping Relationship*. Englewood Cliffs, N.J.: Prentice-Hall, 1973.

Brink PJ: Critique of "Privacy and the hospitalization experience," pp. 172–80 in *Communicating Nursing Research*, Vol. 7. Boulder, Colo.: WICHE, 1975.

Brink P and Wood MJ: *Basic Steps in Planning Nursing Research*. Boston: Jones and Bartlett, 1980.

Castaneda C: *The Teachings of Don Juan: A Yaqui Way of Knowledge*. New York: Simon and Schuster, 1968.

Crozier M: *The Bureaucratic Phenomenon*. Chicago: The University of Chicago Press, 1964.

Denzin NK: *The Research Act*. Chicago: Aldine, 1970.

Diers D: *Research in Nursing Practice*. Philadelphia: Lippincott, 1979.

Douglas JD: *Investigative Social Research: Individual and Team Field Research*. Beverly HIlls, Calif.: Sage, 1976.

Egan G: *Encounter: Group Processes for Interpersonal Growth*. Monterey, Calif.: Brooks/Cole, 1970.

Eisner EW: On the differences between scientific and artistic approaches to qualitative research. *Educational Researcher* April 1981: 5–9.

Fagerhaugh S, Strauss A: *Politics of Pain Management*. Menlo Park, Calif.: Addison-Wesley, 1977.

Field P: An ethnography: Four public health nurses' perspectives of nursing. *J Adv Nurs* 1983; 8, 3–12.

Glaser BG, Strauss A: *Awareness of Dying*. Chicago, Aldine, 1965.

Glaser BG, Strauss A: *Time for Dying*. Chicago, Aldine, 1968.

Glaser BG, Strauss A: *Anguish: A Case History of a Dying Trajectory*. Mill Valley, Calif.: Sociology Press, 1970.

Goffman E: *Asylums*. Garden City, N.Y.: Doubleday, 1961.

Gold RL: Roles in sociological field observations. *Social Forces* March 1958; 36:217–223.

Humphreys L: *Tearoom Trade: Impersonal Sex in Public Places*. Chicago: Aldine, 1975.

Hutchinson SA: Creating meaning out of horror. *Nurs Outlook* 1984; 32, 86–90.

Jackson RK: Discussion: Alienation, confusion and disorientation and stress factors—Implications for health care delivery, pp. 76–81 in *Communicating Nursing Research*. Vol. 8. Boulder, Colo.: WICHE, 1977.

Junker BH: *Field Work: an Introduction to the Social Sciences*. Chicago: University of Chicago Press, 1960.

Kus R: Stages of coming out: An ethnographic approach. *West J Nurs* 1985; 7, 177–198.

Leaf MJ: *Frontiers of Anthropology*. New York: D. Van Nostrand, 1974.

Leininger MM: *Qualitative Research Methods in Nursing*. Orlando, Fla.: Grune and Stratton, 1985.

Lopata HZ: *Women as Widows: Support Systems*. New York: Elsevier, 1979.

McCorkle R: Terminal illness: Human attachments and intended goals, pp. 207–221 in *Communicating Nursing Research*, Vol. 9. Boulder, Colo.: WICHE, 1977.

Muhlenkamp AF: Stress: Conceptualization and measurement for nursing, pp. 74–76 in *Communicating Nursing Research*, Vol. 11. Boulder, Colo.: WICHE, 1978.

Parse RR et al: The experiences of aging: An ethnographic study, in Parse RR, Coyne AB, Smith MJ (editors), *Nursing Research: Qualitative Methods*, Bowie, Md.: Brady, 1985.

Parsons V, Sanford N: *Interpersonal Interaction in Nursing*. Menlo Park, Calif.: Addison-Wesley, 1979.

Penniman TK: *A Hundred Years of Anthropology*. London: Gerald Duckworth, 1965.

Polsky N: *Hustlers, Beats and Others*. Garden City, N.Y.: Doubleday, 1969.

Schatzman L, Strauss A: *Field Research: Strategies for a Natural Sociology*, 2nd ed. Englewood Cliffs, N.J.: Prentice-Hall, 1982.

Schuster EA: Privacy and the hospitalization experience, pp. 153–171 in *Communicating Nursing Research*, Vol. 7. Boulder, Colo.: WICHE, 1975.

Shaffir WB et al: *Fieldwork Experience: Qualitative*

Approaches to Social Research. New York: St. Martin's Press, 1980.

Spradley JP: *The Ethnographic Interview.* New York: Holt, Rinehart and Winston, 1979.

Stern RN: Solving problems of cross-cultural health teaching: The Filipino childbearing family. *Image* 1981; 13, 47–50.

Sudnow D: *Passing On: The Social Organization of Dying.* Englewood Cliffs, N.J.: Prentice-Hall, 1967.

Thomas WI, Znaniecki F: *The Polish Peasant in Poland and America.* New York: Knopf, 1918.

Tripp-Reimer T: Retention of a folk-healing practice (natiasma) among four generations of urban Greek immigrants. *Nurs Res* 1983; 32, 97–101.

Watson JD: *The Double Helix.* New York: New American Library, 1968.

Wax R: *Doing Field Work: Warnings and Advice.* Chicago: University of Chicago Press, 1971.

Whyte WF: *Street Corner Society.* Chicago: University of Chicago Press, 1955.

Wilson HS: *Deinstitutionalized Residential Care for the Mentally Ill: The Soteria House Approach.* New York: Grune & Stratton, 1982.

Wilson HS, Kneisl CR: *Psychiatric Nursing* 3rd ed. Menlo Park, Calif.: Addison-Wesley, 1988.

Wolanin MO: Confusion study: Use of grounded theory as methodology, pp. 68–75 in *Communicating Nursing Research.* Vol. 8. Boulder, Colo.: WICHE, 1977.

C H A P T E R

13

The Craft of Qualitative Analysis

HOLLY SKODOL WILSON

Chapter Objectives

After reading this chapter, the student should be able to:

- Define the term *qualitative analysis*

- Explain the qualitative analyst's philosophy of science

- Relate the major purposes of qualitative analysis

- Enumerate the steps involved in labeling, indexing, and filing data in preparation for analysis

- Differentiate among three kinds of data file

- Explain the procedures for types of qualitative analysis

- Apply these procedures to analyze qualitative data

- Identify criteria appropriate for evaluating the credibility of a grounded theory and a phenomenological interpretation

- Discuss the relevance of qualitative research to nursing practice and knowledge development in the discipline

(Continued)

- Comprehend the meaning of the terms *theoretical sampling, coding, saturation, basic social process, analytical induction, nominal scale, grounded theory, hermeneutics, paradigm case, exemplar,* and *phenomenology*

- Discuss the areas of controversy regarding qualitative versus quantitative approaches

In This Chapter...

Qualitative analysis is something that you probably do every day in your clinical practice. Each time that you collect patient information that is not numerical—not a blood pressure reading, a temperature reading, or a laboratory test value—you have to conceptualize, compare, combine, and categorize to arrive at a clinical interpretation. Whenever you use the nursing process to arrive at a nursing diagnosis, you have to make some meaning out of qualitative data. After all, a patient's acuity, adaptive functioning, self-care abilities, support systems, attitude toward health, and so on usually involve more than scores or measurements that can be plotted on a scale and subjected to statistical procedures. One expectant father whom you meet in the labor room is "involved," and a second is "detached." One recovery room patient is "stable," and another is "unstable." One family uses "open" communication, and another engages in "disturbed" communication patterns. Nurses are experts in grasping the significance of data acquired through observing and talking to patients about their subjective, real-world experiences. We may be inclined to call this skill sensitivity, insight, intuition, or perceptiveness, but in fact it involves a form of qualitative analysis.

Despite nurses' familiarity with these analytical operations in clinical practice, the term *qualitative analysis* in the research world evades conclusive definition. The lexicon of diverse terminology associated with qualitative analysis includes *content analysis, descriptive statistics, quasi-statistics, unstructured methods, induction, grounded theory, discovery method, themes, coding, categories, field methods, process analysis, hypothesis generating, case studies, ethnomethodology, intersubjectivity, phenomenology,* and *soft science*. Some authorities use the term *qualitative analysis* to denote the summarizing procedures performed on data that are gathered exclusively through unstructured methods, such as participant observation and interviewing. Others view it as an outright misnomer and even a myth, pointing out that statistical operations such as factor analysis (see Chapter 14) are frequently used to categorize nominal or qualitative data. Still others think of it as basically journalism or art, but definitely not science. The meaning of qualitative analysis is but one area around which controversy exists.

This chapter clarifies the varied definitions by giving both the consumer and the conductor of qualitative research a clear understanding of the full array of strategies that an investigator can use to move from observations to explanations and from practice to theory. Such an understanding can offer a basis for interpreting, evaluating, and using qualitative research findings in nursing practice and a technology for doing research that not too long ago relied on "immersing oneself in the data" and "having insight" as its major strategies. Topics considered include the qualitative researcher's philosophy of science, strategies for establishing files in preparation for analysis, and examples of major qualitative analysis procedures. Finally, pointers on evaluating the credibility of a study using qualitative analysis offer you a framework for critiquing and applying your own or someone else's research.

What Is Qualitative Analysis?

Analysis is the separation of data into parts for the purpose of answering a research question and communicating that answer to others. A research report that contained no analysis would be a chronological record of everything that happened during a specified time. Reading this report would be something like watching an Andy Warhol movie in which an actor did nothing but sleep for eight hours or reading a trunkful of computer printouts that showed the entire data set. By thinking analytically, researchers impose order on a large body of data to answer study questions and avoid overwhelming a research consumer with detail when reporting the findings.

Chapter 14 addresses descriptive and inferential statistical methods of analyzing data. Such analysis is often called quantitative because data must be collected in or converted to numbers before they can be analyzed. **Qualitative analysis** is the *non*numerical organization and interpretation of data in order to discover patterns, themes, forms, exemplars and qualities found in field notes, interview transcripts, open-ended questionnaires, journals, diaries, documents, case studies, and other texts.

Classic and Modern Examples

Classic and modern studies in the social sciences have served as prototypes for more contemporary nursing research employing qualitative analysis. These early studies include Anderson's *The Hobo*, Goffman's *Asylums*, Whyte's *Street Corner Society*, Roth's *Timetables*, Becker and colleagues' *Boys in White*, Cavan's *Liquor License*, Olesen and Whittaker's *The Silent Dialogue*, and Glaser and Strauss's *Time for Dying* and *Awareness of Dying*, to name but a few. Nurses working in this scientific tradition at a time when our profession was relatively new to the world of research and science had to resist pressures to equate respectable and legitimate science with quantification of data and statistical analysis methods. Yet recognizing, as Berkeley sociologist Herbert Blumer (1969) did, that "the study of human life calls for a wide range of variables" and that nursing research had to be a basis for improved practice in the real world, an increasing number of nurses have demonstrated the use of qualitative analysis methods in the research literature. Among their studies are Archibald's "Impact of Parent-Caring on Middle Aged Offspring," Bozett's "Gay Fathers: How They Disclose Homosexuality to Children," Chenitz's "Entry into a Nursing Home as Status Passage," Davis's *Living with Multiple Sclerosis*, Fagerhaugh and Strauss's *Politics of Pain Management*, May's "Three Phases in the Development of Father Involvement in Pregnancy," Quint's "Awareness of Death and the Nurse's Composure," Reif's "Ulcerative Colitis: Strategies for Managing Life," Stern's "Stepfather Families: Integration around Child Discipline," Hutchinson's *Survival Practices of Rescue Workers: Hidden Dimensions of Watchful Readiness* and "Chemically Dependent Nurses: The Trajectory toward Self-Annihilation," and Wilson's studies *The Soteria House Approach* and "The Process of Family Caregiving for a Demented Relative."

The Qualitative Analyst's Philosophy of Science

Qualitative analysis, like field research (see Chapter 12), is based on the belief that to know *about* people is not enough. Instead, face-to-face knowing is required for the fullest possible comprehension of another's world. The qualitative researcher aspires to capture what other people and their lives are about without preconceiving the categories into which information will fit. To understand others, the qualitative analyst and field researcher try to put themselves in others' shoes to discern how they think, feel, act, and behave. Anthropologists, such as Margaret Mead, have based their research on this notion for decades. In sociology, this belief is called "taking the role of the other." It was originally developed by George Herbert Mead and formally named by Herbert Blumer (1969). It is one of the central tenets of a social philosophy called symbolic interactionism. **Symbolic interactionism** is a perspective on society and people that emphasizes the need to conduct research in natural settings and to focus on the way people define their reality and construct their actions over time. Reality, or "the truth," is always viewed as emerging and relative rather than "all out there" waiting to be located and measured with a questionnaire or test. One patient swoons with fear in anticipation of the pain associated with a simple injection. Another dies of cancer never having asked for medication other than aspirin. One person perceives her miscarriage as but one in a long series of signs that she is inadequate. Another person sees her miscarriage as her liberation from an unwanted future.

The symbolic-interactionist philosophy underpinning most qualitative research is based on three simple premises:

1. Human beings act toward things on the basis of the meaning these things have for them.

2. The meaning of things in life is developed from the interactions a person has with others.

3. People handle and modify meaning through an interpretive process.

Qualitative research based on these premises has two main characteristics in common. It concerns itself with the natural, everyday, experienced world of human group life and thus uses methods of data collection and analysis designed to yield complex and diversified explanations. It also views the research process itself as a form of symbolic interaction, wherein the investigator is the "tool" or "technique" in both data collection and analysis. This notion follows a tradition developed by Alfred Schutz (1967), in which investigators acknowledge that they register not objective fact but rather "intersubjectivity," *verstehen*, or "subjective interpretation." Embracing these ideas, researchers carefully examine their own perspectives and interactions as both a source of data and as an analytic strategy. Validity, accordingly, comes from clarity about one's perspective and its influence on the study, not distance, objectivity, and control of variables. Corbin describes her awareness of how her nursing background began to influence her analysis of data in a study of high-risk pregnant mothers with serious illnesses:*

Initially I was convinced that the pregnant women's strategies for controlling the risk would intensify with the severity of risk. I expected the woman with lupus, for example, to use highly controlling strategies because her illness created a more severe risk than some of the others. I faced the fact that I had to reformulate this proposition when it didn't hold up in the data. The strategies didn't vary consistently with what I, a nurse clinician, assessed as "high risk." In-stead it had to do with the mother's own calculations or definitions of her risk severity based on cues of different types. My analysis began to fit the data when I went back into the field and began to sample for this. I ended up with an analytic scheme called *Protective Governing* that included all the ways these women control their illness and their treatment to try to govern the outcome of their pregnancy.

Such self-examination is critical to evaluating the rigor and credibility of interpretive qualitative research. Imposition of validity and reliability criteria from theory-testing research is, however, not appropriate.

Diagrammatically rendered, hypotheses in qualitative interpretive studies are molecular rather than linear, like the linear linking of a few variables. Swanson's (1980) study of men's perception of their role in family planning revealed that each

---

*From J. Corbin, "Coding Data," in *Qualitative Research in Nursing: From Practice to Grounded Theory*, W. C. Chenitz and J. Swanson (editors), Menlo Park, Calif.: Addison-Wesley, 1986.

respondent understood or perceived a contraceptive regimen differently, based on his own information and previous sexual practices. Qualitative methods allowed her to construct explanations that went far beyond the frequency and distribution of the simple variable *contraceptive use* found in most of the literature in her field. Haase (1987) used a systematic analytical process to generate themes and clusters of themes that allowed a phenomenological rendering of the components of courage in chronically ill adolescents.

Purposes of Qualitative Analysis

When a study involves open-ended, nonnumerical data collected through formal or informal interviewing, participant observation, documents, diaries, and case studies, the researcher is faced sooner or later with the challenge of making sense of this mass of heterogeneous data in relationship to the study's central questions. In Lofland's words, "The researcher of a qualitative-humanistic bent . . . seeks neither purely novelistic reportage nor purely abstract conceptualizing. . . . The aim is judiciously to combine them, providing the vividness of 'what it is like' and an appropriate degree of economy and clarity" (1971 p. 7). You as an intelligent reader of this kind of research must similarly be prepared to evaluate the credibility of a study's findings when they are based on qualitative data. If a study purports to test hypotheses, establish causal relations, summarize numerical patterns, or demonstrate statistical significance according to the laws of probability, the quantitative methods discussed in Chapters 14 and 15 should be used. If, however, a study has different purposes and raises different questions, particularly questions about people's experiences under natural conditions, qualitative methods will be used to analyze the data. The major purposes that can be served by using qualitative techniques are the following: exploration, description and interpretation of experienced processes in their personal and social contexts, accounting for and illustrating quantitative findings, discovery, explanation, and extension of theory.

Exploration and Description: Purpose 1   Sometimes a research study is designed to look for answers to questions in a field where a great deal of scientific work has already been done. A study about early childhood development and the differential responses to hospitalization based on a child's developmental level is one example. In this instance, the nurse investigator builds his or her study on prior work in the area, perhaps by measuring variables that others have reported as important or using instruments or findings developed by others. Bowers (1987) points out, however, that theory-generating interpretive methodologies can also be used to challenge inaccurate or inadequate knowledge in a well-studied area. Nonetheless, when a reseacher is tackling a study question about which very little is known, and the study is intended to gain insight about a particular group of patients or health conditions, a qualitative, interpretive approach is usually the design of choice. In this kind of research the investigator tries to collect and present rich and diverse accounts of findings so that any promising leads and ideas can be developed. Questions include "What is going on?" "How does something work?" "What is important here?" "What variations exist?"

An interesting area of debate in the nursing research literature surrounds the issue of whether the nature of the study question or the investigator's world view and philosophy of science determine method selection (DeGroot 1988). Yet another debate concerns whether nonexperimental (descriptive) designs are "compromise designs" or highly desirable in a human science. Nurses need to agree that the progress of good science depends on creative ideas and intellectual freedom. Allowing methodological conformity to become the unquestioned status quo "disables nursing's scientific progress" (DeGroot 1987 p. 15).

Throughout history important scientific advances have begun with *careful observation and description* of the nature of events as they occurred. Examples include Darwin's theory of evolution, Einstein's theory of relativity, Freud's psychoanalytic theory, and the discovery of penicillin, to name a few. Analyzing qualitative data for the purpose of description allows you to accurately and even insightfully characterize an event, a patient population, a process, or a setting. Dickoff and James (1968), scholars formerly at Yale University School of Nursing, call this factor-isolating research.

According to Schatzman and Strauss (1983), **description** can be done in one of two ways. First, the analyst may use categories or organizational schemes that already exist in the literature of a discipline and simply find classes or cases in the data that correspond to the classification scheme taken from the literature. This is called *straight description*. Describing a unit's patient population by diagnosis or social class is an example. In the second instance, the analyst attempts to think up novel classes or categories suggested by an active inspection of the data. This is called *analytic description*. May's (1986) typology of detachment and involvement styles of first-time fathers is an example of the originality that characterizes analytic description.

Accounting for and Illustrating Quantitative Findings: Purpose 2   Qualitative anecdotes are often used to answer "why" and "how" questions associated with quantitative study findings. For example, Mosher and Menn (1978) conducted a longitudinal comparative-outcome study of two modes of residential treatment for first-break schizophrenics. They relied on standardized scales like the Ward Atmosphere Scale and a global psychopathology rating before and after treatment to collect data about the settings and patients. Their two-year follow-up study findings supported the effectiveness of the experimental setting (Soteria House). They used my own qualitative field study (Wilson 1982) to explain how the Soteria approach worked. My theory of *infracontrolling* explained how social order was possible under the conditions of espoused freedom at Soteria House. My concepts of *presencing*, *fairing*, and *limiting intrusion* explained how patients, staff, and outsiders are managed.

Some nurse scientists argue that combining the qualitative and quantitative paradigms is essential to the development of nursing science (Bargagliotti and Trygstad 1987, Goodwin and Goodwin 1984). Jones (1987) notes that use of quantitative in *combination* with qualitative methodologies offers a form of *triangulation* (using more than one measure or method) that can only enhance the validity of a study's findings. Hinds and Young (1987) concur on the benefits of such "triangulation" in their work on the study of nurse-given wellness care.

On the other side of this philosophical and methodological issue are those who point out that qualitative and quantitative approaches are more than just different data collection and analysis techniques. They represent *fundamentally different philosophies of science and assumptions* (Powers 1987). "Quantitative data can be used descriptively or to project the extent to which the interpretation of phenomena might apply to a larger population. However, the idea that quantitative measures in qualitative research *strengthen* the interpretations is derived in an ideological imposition of one paradigm over another" (Powers 1987 p. 122). Resolving this issue for your own research requires awareness and thoughtful consideration of both points of view.

EXAMPLE: Norris's Study of Restlessness

Norris, in a clinical study entitled "Restlessness: A Nursing Phenomenon in Search of Meaning," traced the behavioral manifestations of restlessness and related her observations to a theory of rhythmicity. She began with questions like "Who is restless?" "When does it occur?" "How do people experience restlessness?" "How does it differ from rest?" She concluded her study with what she described as a sense of urgency "for all nurses who are at the bedside to observe and describe nursing events until nurses wherever and however they work have the data they need to recognize and assign meaning to the phenomena of nursing" [Norris 1975].

The research questions

The value of describing and explaining nursing phenomena

EXAMPLE: Swanson's Study of Men's Roles in Family Planning

Swanson's study of men's perceptions of their role in family planning represents an example of research done in an area that prior to her work was largely limited to counting men and their preferred method of birth control. Swanson used in-depth interviews and fieldwork to go beyond anecdotes and description toward theory development [Swanson 1980].

Interviews as a field method

Anecdotes as a basis for generating a theory grounded in data

EXAMPLE: Fagerhaugh's Study of Getting Around with Emphysema

Fagerhaugh's study of elderly indigents with advanced emphysema is one example of a grounded theory conducted by a nurse researcher. She explained how these patients juggled and balanced their time, energy, and money to achieve physical mobility and sociability. The outcome of her qualitative study was a diagram or model that linked the categories in relation to one another and explained how the patients in her study "got around with emphysema" (see Figure 13–1 later in this chapter). She described her model as analogous to a Rubik's cube that has to be written up linearly [Fagerhaugh 1973].

Key concepts in an explanatory scheme

Visual model of a grounded theory (sometimes called a conceptual map)

Discovery and Explanation: Purpose 3   Sometimes a reseacher wants to go beyond even abstract analytic description to discover in the data core patterns, variables, and categories that provide the basis for developing and then validating hypotheses about relationships. Once relationships are discovered, the analyst attempts to weave what Schatzman and Strauss (1983) call "these key linkages" into an explanatory scheme sometimes termed a paradigm, paradigm case, exemplar, conceptual map, model, or grounded substantive theory. Some of these study outcomes represent the discovery or generation of theory. Others are the "stories" that result from phenomenological interpretation.

The analyst attempting to develop a **grounded theory** uses a method of constant comparison and coding to develop a complex explanation of conditions, consequences, strategies, phases, stages, ranges, and other relationships among the classes of variable discovered in the data. The phenomenologist uses theme analysis, discovery of exemplars, and identification of paradigm cases to capture the practices and meanings of a lived experience through each description.

Extension of Theory: Purpose 4   Sometimes a reseacher has developed a theoretical explanation under one set of conditions and wants to extend it, refine it, or even move it from a middle range *substantive theory* that explains something under a specific set of conditions to a **grand**, or **formal**, **theory** that explains how something occurs under a great variety of conditions. In such a study, questions might include: "Is the original substantive theory correct?" "Does it fit other circumstances?" "Are there additional categories or relationships?" Glaser and Strauss's (1971) theory of *status passages* to explain transitions that dying patients experience has been extended to explain a wide variety of situations. Weivers and Lenz (1987) used theory from alcohol recovery to explain smoking relapse. Theory extending and theory derivation are, however, quite different processes with different assumptions and outcomes, the details of which exceed this chapter's scope.

Table 13–1 summarizes some distinctions associated with the four major purposes of qualitative analysis.

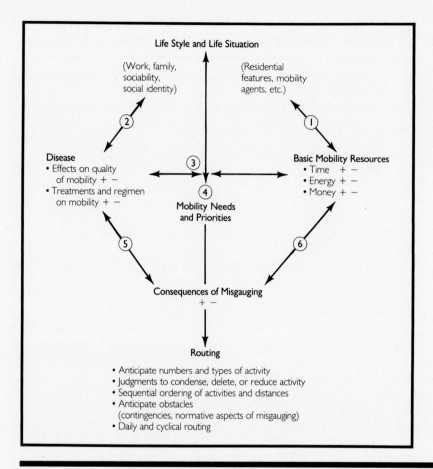

Figure 13–1 A model of how elderly indigents with emphysema get around. Source: Adapted from Fagerhaugh, S. "Getting Around with Emphysema," *American Journal of Nursing*, January 1973, 73:94–99. Copyright © 1973 American Journal of Nursing Company. Reprinted with permission.

Preparing Qualitative Data for Analysis

Just as the quantitative researcher must develop a code book and must enter data into a computer's memory and storage units, the qualitative analyst must develop a system for keeping track of data and retrieving them as needed. Hundreds of hours of field notes and typescripts of interviews can fill endless cardboard boxes and create a chaotic sea of paper.

Observational research produces an immense amount of detailed description. The records of field notes and interviews in a classic study of medical school education called *Boys in White* occupied 5000 single-spaced typed pages. The qualitative analyst faces the task of analyzing a diverse and seemingly unsystematic mass

TABLE 13–1 *Purposes of Qualitative Analysis*

Purpose	Research Questions	Methods	Outcomes
1. *Exploration and description*	1. What is going on? 2. How does it work? 3. What is important here? 4. What variations exist? 5. What meanings and practices occur in a lived experience?	1. Straight description using categories from existing literature 2. Analytical description generating novel categories from data 3. Content analysis 4. Quasi-statistics 5. Phenomenological interpretation	1. Case studies 2. Ethnographies 3. Frequency reports 4. Descriptive narrative 5. Typologies/themes 6. Cross-tabulations 7. Thick description 8. Paradigm cases
2. *Accounting for and illustrating quantitative findings*	1. How did something occur? 2. Why did something occur? 3. What are the characteristics, conditions, and consequences involved?	1. Analytic induction 2. Constant comparison	1. Anecdotes 2. Grounded substantive theory
3. *Discovery and Explanation*	1. What is the basic social psychological process here (BSP)? 2. What meanings and practices occur in a lived experience?	1. Constant comparison 2. Phenomenological interpretation	1. Grounded substantive theory 2. Paradigm cases 3. Conceptual maps 4. Thick descriptions
4. *Extension of theory*	1. Is the original substantive theory correct? 2. Does it fit other circumstances? 3. Are there additional categories or relationships?	1. Comparative analysis 2. Content analysis 3. Theory derivation	1. Formal theory 2. Adaptations of existing theory

of data usually collected over many months or even years of fieldwork. One technical problem is being sure that all 5000 pages of evidence are considered each time a related analytic idea or proposition is advanced. To avoid searching through all 5000 pages of notes over and over again, qualitative analysts develop a system for labeling, indexing, filing, sorting, and retrieving their field notes, documents, and interview transcripts.

Code numbers can be assigned to them that refer to the major topics under which a given episode or item might be considered. Entries can then be reassembled by code number so that all items might be considered and all observations on given topics can be located in one place. Each entry is put into as many conceptual categories as it might represent. Finally, the analyst establishes a set of differentiated files. The following steps offer guidelines for hand indexing and filing data in preparation for analysis. The major principles hold true when you use a computer program such as Ethnograph to analyze qualitative data.

Steps in Labeling, Indexing, and Filing Data

1. Transcribe all handwritten field notes, taped interviews, and documents onto 8½ × 11 typing paper, doubled spaced. Leave wide margins, especially on the right side of the paper, where you will later write codes.

2. Label each page with identifying information—for example: "Friday, May 13, 1989, Observation in City Hospital. Neonatal Intensive Care Unit, 7:00 A.M.– 3:00 P.M. First Day in the Field, p. 1." Be certain to use code names or numbers to protect the confidentiality of respondents and settings. A typical typed, labeled field note appears in Box 13–1.

3. Make at least three duplicate sets of your data. Keep one complete set locked up in a safe place apart from your original. Make the third set so that you can cut it up and file information if needed in separate files. (As Chapter 16 suggests, the manual system for sorting and retrieving files described here is being replaced by computers to accomplish the same goals. A printout of your data and backup diskettes should be kept in a safe place, because a power outage always poses the risk of your work being erased.) McCall and Simmons (1969) recommend typing field notes onto ditto spirit, mimeograph, or other inexpensive duplicating masters. Then you can make whatever number of copies you need to have maximum flexibility in manipulating the materials.

4. Establish files. The goal of a filing system is to get your data out of the chronological narrative of your field notes into a flexible storage, ordering, and retrieval format. Some qualitative analysts file their material in file folders and keep them in metal file cabinets, reserving different drawers for different types of file. Others use hanging files with metal "ears" that slide on rails in file drawers. Another possibility is to use boxes like the kind that hold 5000 sheets of ream-wrapped typing paper and can be purchased empty in bulk from

---

Box 13–1   Sample Field Note with Label*

H. Wilson   Friday 9:45 A.M.
Soteria Study   12:45 P.M.
Feb. 9, 1973   Visit #5

Situation: I arrive at House 15 min. before weekly meeting is to begin. *There's no sign of its beginning on time.* T. and C. are up but D. is asleep in livingroom, H. is in shower, T. and M. are out, and S. is using the phone re: his Real Estate Business stuff. A. hasn't yet arrived.

ON T., H., S., and I sit around kitchen table drinking coffee. T. talks constantly. Asks S. how Kingsley Hall got their money. H. answers with the joke that the residents "work really hard." *They are all in the basement turning out Kinsley Hall souvenirs.* S. says the residents pay and the staff volunteer.

ON A. arrives. I tell her things are going well . . . that I have some germs of ideas. I ask about papers written about S. She suggests that I come up to MRI to see all written documents from various periods in the past year. Ex. A newsletter type thing that was done in the beginning and staff's journals.

ON At 10:30 their meeting still hasn't started. M. and T. come back. They've been to Welfare and T. had a traumatic time because she had to fill out forms about her "disability." T. asks M. to take her out for breakfast and then to Jack LaLaine's gym. M. tells A. she'll do the former thing but doesn't think that latter will be very good for T. and *just doesn't want to be part of it.* A. says she thinks it might be fun but A. doesn't try to convince M. to change her mind. H. agrees to take T. after breakfast.

TN The staff seem permitted to make decisions about patients based on their own personal feelings. This is legitimate at Soteria and unusual in conventional psychiatric treatment.

ON A. begins the meeting without saying, "Well, let's get started, etc." She inquires if there have been any more problems with the police about drugs. Apparently the police had been snooping around the House. T. tells about being stopped by the police with B. and using the occasion to reassure the police that S. was clean. He mentions as an aside that the police asked him what he did (occupation) and he jokingly responded, *"I'm crazy."*

TN Despite the normalizing that goes on about mental illness in the house there are occasions when it is brought into awareness through contacts with the outside. T.'s experience is one example. While sitting at the table another occurred when C. asked what kind of place S. was called. "A home for the mentally disabled." S. *normalizes* by calling it "a board and care house." C. asked because she was filling out a form. (Welfare?)

*Words italicized here were underlined in my notes. H.W.

wholesale paper dealers. You can use a three-hole punch and keep your notes in three-ring binders. A computer's files serve the same purpose. Whatever physical setup you use, you need at least to establish three types of file and be prepared to disassemble copies of your notes for the purpose of cutting them up and refiling or block-moving them into various categories. If you are limited in the number of copies you can make, you can cross-reference to information in other files by entering a cross-reference page in a file. (See Chapter 16 for details on how to prepare data files for Ethnograph software.)

Types of File

Organizational Files   You must create one file to keep track of people, documents, places, organizations, phone numbers, and so on. In this file you put material under the most pragmatic category. For example, the transcript of an interview with a particular patient would be filed under his or her code number or code name. Field notes collected in different settings would be grouped together under the code name of the setting. The sociologist John Lofland (1971) calls these organizational files "mundane files," because they help you keep practical matters straight. They make it easier to locate something that happened months in the past, precluding a search through chronological notes or analytical files that might take hours. See Box 13–2 for a sample page from an organizational file.

Analytical Files   Files are crucial to the analytical process. The aim is to set up as many separate folders as you have codes or categories developing in your analysis. It doesn't matter if every category you use in the beginning becomes a part of your explanatory scheme in the long run. The important points are:

1. Continually think about your data in terms of the categories, concepts, or themes they may eventually serve as indicators or exemplars for.

2. Keep track of accumulating theoretical notes (TNs) (see Chapter 12) as they occur to you.

3. Summarize TNs and associated anecdotes or episodes in your data in a growing set of "analytical memos," (explained in detail later in this chapter).

In any case, analytical files are where you keep track of your emerging analytical scheme and the data related to it. Additional pieces of information can be added to each of your existing file folders, or new files can be started as your ideas for categories expand. Most importantly, remind yourself that your analytical files represent your emergent coding scheme, encouraging you to develop ideas about the clinical reality represented in your field work. They are flexible, collapsible, expandable, and stimulating and help you avoid getting too engrossed in the details of your data or becoming too closely involved with the setting for your study.

Box 13–2   Sample Page from an Organizational File (Wilson 1977)

List of Documents Used in Study Analysis

Community Alternatives for Treatment of Schizophrenia. Research proposal submitted to the U.S. Department of Health, Education, and Welfare, to expand Soteria House, May 1, 1973, to April 30, 1978.

*Community Alternatives for Treatment of Schizophrenia.*Research proposal submitted to the U.S. Department of Health, Education, and Welfare, to continue Soteria House from Nov. 1, 1974, to Nov. 1, 1979. (Submitted January 31, 1974)

Copes-Scale Profile for Soteria House Staff. Handout prepared by Soteria House professionals for National Institute of Mental Health site visit.

Essential Therapeutic Ingredients of Soteria. Outline prepared by research project staff for site visit, April 8, 1974.

IMPS Profile Sheet for Combined Rates Male and Female Acute Patients. Graph comparing Soteria House patients with control group.

Mosher, L. R. *New Treatment for Schizophrenia: Does it Work?* Paper presented at the meeting of the American Orthopsychiatric Association, held at San Francisco, May 1974.

_____, and Others, *Indigenous Nonprofessionals as Primary Therapists for Acute Schizophrenia.* Paper presented at the Eightieth Annual

Convention of the American Psychological Association, held at Honolulu, Hawaii, September 1972.

_____. *Schizophrenia and Crisis Theory.* Paper presented at the Annual Meeting of American Orthopsychiatric Association, Detroit, April 1972.

Research Design to Evaluate Psychosocial Treatments of Schizophrenia. Paper delivered at the Fourth International Symposium on the Psychotherapy of Schizophrenia. Turku, Finland, August 1971.

Soteria House. *The Care and Feeding of a Soteria: Our First Manual.* San Jose. The House. December 1972.

Methodological Files   Lofland (1971) calls methodological files his "fieldwork files," because in them you accumulate descriptions of *how* you conducted the research. These files allow you to bring together the methodological notes (MNs) and personal notes (PNs) (see Chapter 12) from your field notes and give you the basis for writing up your account of the methods used in your study. Reflections on methodological problems, such as gaining entry into a study setting or establishing rapport with an informant, can also become valuable articles in and of themselves once your research is complete. After completing my own qualitative study of Soteria House, I published an article in *Nursing Research* using part of my analysis to illustrate the method of discovering theory with the constant comparison method. On the problem of recording field notes openly, I wrote:

> My problems with recording were more interpersonal than technical. The decision to take notes in full view of the interactants was in part a consequence of the structure of the Soteria setting and in part a consequence of my attempt to avoid the social psychological risks of secretive behavior on my part. Unlike a hospital, a sixteen-room house full of people offered little opportunity for slipping off to a cafeteria or restroom to record from memory [Wilson 1982 p. 109].

The system for filing qualitative data just described is being transformed as more field researchers elect to substitute a small personal computer, diskette storage, and printer for the file folders and cardboard boxes cluttering their offices. The computer's capabilities to duplicate, to move whole sections of material around, to pull out all data related to specified codes, and to store volumes of information in a small toaster-sized space may well make the cut-and-paste, file-folder operation traditionally used by qualitative researchers obsolete (see Chapter 16).

How to Analyze Qualitative Data

Data gathered through fieldwork methods can occasionally be collected in a standardized form and transformed into statistical data. An observational checklist of a psychiatric unit's dominant philosophy might be an example. But usually the qualitative data we have been discussing are not collected in a form that conforms to the assumptions of statistical tests. Consequently, some critics question the scientific merit of conclusions drawn from qualitative data because they are often presented to readers with the comment, "We have gone over our data and find that they support this conclusion." Consumers may find it difficult to accept the findings without being told what exactly that "going over" consisted of. They feel uncomfortable having to accept research conclusions on faith.

This section considers five major procedures for systematically making sense out of transcriptions of open-ended interviews, field notes, documents, and other texts. These are (1) converting qualitative data to quantitative data, (2) doing a content analysis, (3) analytic induction, (4) discovering grounded theory, and (5) conducting a phenomenological interpretive analysis.

Converting Qualitative Data to Quantitative Data

In some studies, particularly those whose purpose is exclusively descriptive, an investigator elects to report the frequency and distribution of categories assigned to the data or to correlate their frequency or distribution with some other variables. In these cases, the study reports some numerical conclusions but not with the precision evident in most statistical studies. For this reason Becker (1958) calls such an attempt an application of **quasi-statistics**. The essential objective of quasi-statistics is to decide if the concepts or categories in your analysis represent typical and widespread patterns distributed in the data, thereby giving the analytical scheme more credibility. The analysts who combine quantitative methods with qualitative work usually engage in three processes to conclude that their final analysis is likely to be an accurate representation of the data or to depict the frequency and distribution of analytical categories. These processes are:

1. searching for *negative cases* to reformulate propositions that don't account for them (**Negative cases** are bits of data that run counter to your propositions.)

2. counting numbers of cases (not necessarily subjects) in each category and, when possible, running descriptive statistics that give you information about the frequency with which certain themes are supported in the data

3. constructing scales for nominal data

A scale for nominal data consists of a number of discrete, mutually exclusive categories of a variable. Data are then summarized in terms of the percentage of subjects in each of the categories. Sometimes numbers are assigned to represent different categories. The number *1* might represent married, *2* single, *3* divorced or separated, and *4* widowed for the variable *marital status*. The numbers are merely labels that serve as a shorthand method of reporting data. They, in and of themselves, have no other quantitative meaning. In some instances, investigators correlate nominal data by cross-tabulating them with other variables. (See Table 13–2).

The limitations of basing an analysis of qualitative data exclusively on converting the data to some quantified form are probably obvious to you.

- Although searching for negative cases might force revisions in your analysis, there are no hard-and-fast rules to guide you in answering questions such as "How long should I look?" "How many negative cases are too many?"

- The generation of analytical descriptions depends in part on the theoretical sensitivity of the analyst. Field research is designed to allow for the flexibility and creativity required to develop classes, categories, and propositions that are grounded in observational data. There is no guarantee that two analysts working independently with the same data will achieve the same results. Counting the number of incidents that appear in observational data collected using purposeful

TABLE 13–2   *Cross Tabulation of Marital Status and Number of Depressive Symptoms among a Nursing Home Population*

Marital Status	Percentage	Mean Number of Depressive Symptoms ($T = 20$)
Married	22%	5
Single	18%	12
Divorced or separated	30%	15
Widowed	30%	8
	100%	

rather than probability sampling methods seems like an exercise in "number mystification," particularly given the other characteristics of qualitative analysis.

- Scales for nominal data are sorting devices that might help an analyst group subjects into pigeonholes. But because there is no underlying continuum for the scale that links the categories together, they may hinder the rich portrayal of findings that a qualitative analyst seeks.

Doing a Content Analysis

One of the earliest specific procedures for analyzing unstructured qualitative data is called a **content analysis**. It is one way of categorizing verbal or behavioral data, and it shares with the other procedures in this section a requirement for analytical thinking and creativity in the researcher. The first studies that used the method of content analysis simply counted words or their synonyms when analyzing an interview or a document. If, for example, you were studying sexist stereotypes in journal recruitment advertisements for nursing positions, you might do the following:

1. Make a list of all the relevant terms that reflect sexist stereotypes.

2. Read a randomly selected sample of recruitment ads from journals.

3. Count the frequency with which each of the key indicators (terms) appeared in the data.

Later content analysis studies coded for latent feeling tone (akin to connotation) as well as the actual appearance of the terms themselves. Both of these types of content analysis were the prototypes for the two types used in contemporary nursing research: (1) *semantic content analysis* and (2) *feeling tone, or inferred, content analysis*. Some authorities differentiate these two types by making a distinction between content analysis done at the obvious, or manifest, level and content analysis at the implication, or latent, level. Semantic content analysis, simply coding and counting responses in a transcription, is an example of manifest content analysis. Feeling content analysis is an example of latent content analysis. Because in the latter the researcher goes beyond what was said directly to infer the meaning of something, research consumers usually require more evidence of a study's validity in this case. Some studies involve both manifest and latent analyses.

Steps Involved in a Content Analysis   The basic techniques for a content analysis are three: (1) deciding what the unit of analysis will be, (2) borrowing or developing the set of categories, and (3) developing the rationale and illustrations to guide the coding of data into categories.

1. *Deciding on the unit of analysis*. Deciding on the unit of analysis simply means deciding whether to use a whole response or to break down responses into separate words, phrases, or sentences.

2. *Borrowing or developing the set of categories*. If your study is concerned with concepts imported from an existing theory, you can set up your classifications in advance and then merely read through your data, code them into the existing categories, and ultimately report the frequency with which responses appeared in the various categories. For example, if you want to study a tentative classification system for psychosocial nursing diagnoses such as that published in the 1982 *Standards of Psychiatric Nursing Practice and Professional Performance*, you might read a large sample of nursing notes and code the nursing problem statement into one of the categories listed in Box 13–3. If, however, you discover in the course of your research that statements of nursing problems rather frequently fell outside of the preestablished categories, you would need to devise a set of categories based on themes appearing in the data. Ultimately, you would want to formulate a set of categories sufficiently detailed and mutually exclusive to allow you to code all of the notes in your sample. Researchers who use this method of analyzing qualitative data are quick to point out that it is complex, time-consuming, and sometimes quite difficult.

3. *Developing the rationale and illustrations to guide coding of data into categories*. The coding of data into categories requires that the analyst or coder make a judgment on the right category for every response or unit of analysis. It is important to define the categories as fully and clearly as you can. Typical examples from the data help to illustrate the properties a response should have if it is to be coded into a particular category. In my own master's thesis, focusing on the meaning of rock 'n' roll dancing to delinquent adolescents in an urban ghetto, I coded interview responses into one of the categories in Box 13–4 and then asked an independent judge to code the same data (Kelly 1968). Instructions for each were as precise as I could make them. For ex-

---

Box 13–3   Tentative Nursing Diagnoses

1. self-care limitations or impaired functioning whose general etiology is mental and emotional distress, deficits, in the ways significant systems are functioning, and internal psychic or developmental issues

2. emotional stress or crisis components of illness, pain, self-concept changes, and life-process changes

3. emotional problems related to daily experiences, such as anxiety, aggression, loss, loneliness, and grief

4. physical symptoms that occur simultaneously with altered psychic functioning, such as altered intestinal functioning and anorexia

5. alterations, in thinking, perceiving, symbolizing, communicating, and decision-making abilities

6. impaired abilities to relate to others

7. behaviors and mental states that indicate the client is a danger to self or others or is gravely disabled

---

ample, to code a response as an indicator of "creativity" it had to (1) reflect that the teenager thought kids had "made up" the current dances themselves, (2) report that the respondent had made up a dance once, and (3) include an illustrative example of an experience of creating a dance. If someone other

---

Box 13–4   Categories for Coding Responses on the Meaning of Current Dances

1. conformity to peer-group expectations

2. means of creative expression

3. indicator or adolescents' search for identity

4. route to success, status, and prestige

5. form of socialized sexual and aggressive impulses

6. outlet for rebellion against adult authority

Source: Kelly, H. S., "The Meaning of Current Dance Forms to Adolescent Girls: An Exploratory Study," *Nursing Research*, November/December 1968, vol. 17, pp. 513–519. Reprinted with permission. Copyright 1968 American Journal of Nursing Company.

than the primary investigator in a study is to code the data, coders must be well trained and have opportunities to practice coding data into categories with supervision or discussion among a team of researchers.

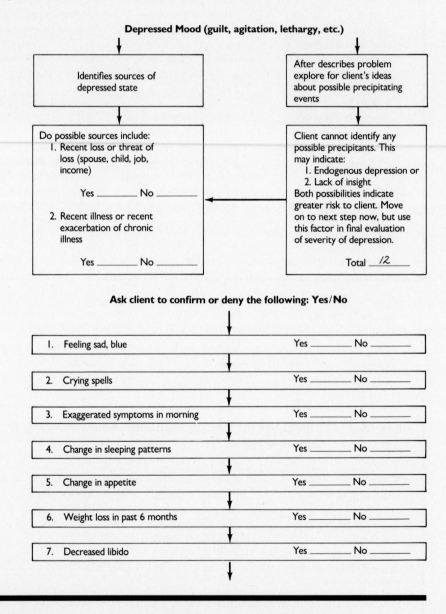

Figure 13–2 One page of a decision tree for depression. Source: Adapted from M. Orsolits and M. Morphy, "A Depression Algorithm for Psychiatric Emergencies," *J Psych Treat Eval* 1982; 4:37–145 (now defunct).

The "Unfolding Tributary" Method of Evolving Categories   Some content analysts apply what might be called the "unfolding tributary" method of extracting categories from the data rather than borrowing them from existing theory. This method proceeds systematically from two broad categories to more specific ones. If diagrammed, the process might look something like the decision trees nurses use in clinical practice (see Figure 13–2).

For example, if you decide to study hospitalized patients' awareness of and attitude toward the part that nursing services had played in their recovery from surgery, you might begin by coding your interview data in one of two major categories:

1. mentioned nursing services

2. did not mention nursing services

You would then reread the interview data and separate the data initially coded as belonging to the first category (having mentioned nursing services) into more precise feeling-tone codes (this second process is a semantic content analysis):

1. mentioned nursing services positively

2. mentioned nursing services negatively

3. mentioned nursing services neutrally

TABLE 13–3   *Cross Tabulation of Positive Awareness of Role of Nursing in Recovering, by Age*

Positive Awareness Frequency	Age of Patient
1%	1–6 years
3%	7–13 years
2%	14–20 years
10%	21–30 years
12%	31–50 years
34%	51–65 years
38%	66 years and older
$T = 100\%$	

This branching evolution can continue until the researcher has achieved a degree of precision that adequately summarizes the meaning discovered in the qualitative data in relation to the original study question. Cross-tabulations might then be run correlating the frequencies of responses in these nominal categories with other data of interest. For example, if an investigator suspected that the elderly patients were more likely to express positive awareness of the role nursing had played in their hospital experience, frequencies in this content analysis code could be cross-tabulated by age group (see Table 13–3).

A careful reading of the case illustration below gives you a sense of how qualitative data analyzed using a form of content analysis are presented in published research reports. It also allows you to tease out the indicators that were used to code a response into one of the four categories of orientation.

Example Evaluation of a Nursing Program: An Illustration of Content Analysis

In the late 1970s a team of educational and nursing researchers completed an evaluation study of the first bachelor of science program for RNs accredited by the National League for Nursing, at Sonoma State University in California. The task required that the team analyze qualitative responses to some open-ended questions collected during entry interviews with successive classes of students. In this case, data were coded into four categories that reflected the students' attitudes toward their intended role in the profession of nursing. The four concepts, or categories were (1) traditional, (2) academic, (3) leadership, and (4) frontiering. The findings were reported in the following way in the study's final report, giving you an idea of how the results of content analyses appear in a published document.

Frequency of cases

Over one third (35%) of the students were categorized as predominantly *traditional* in their outlook, seeking to maintain or to further their positions in nursing but without volunteering any particular dissatisfactions with the hospital as a practice setting. One responded, "My husband and I separated and I began to think of my profession as a lifetime career." Another said, "The handwriting is on the wall, if one wants to work in nursing, you need that degree!"

Traditional orientations was one category

Far fewer entering students indicated an *academic* orientation, but those who did (11%) were so categorized because they spoke of scholastic aspirations, usually including plans for graduate school and a career in teaching and/or research. For example: "At the age of 32 and with family responsibilities I couldn't pursue my interests. Now my children are no longer dependent on me, and I want variety, mobility, and intellectual stimulation. I'd like to prepare myself to teach and do research in nursing."

Academic orientation was one category

A somewhat larger group (24%) had a clear *leadership* orientation and came back to school seeking avenues to power and status. One respondent whose long-range objective was the presidency of the American Nurses' Association stated, "I'm convinced that change evolves from the top. To elicit change, you have to be involved at the top!"

Leadership orientation was one category

The most intriguing of the orientations is the one that earned the label *frontiering*. More than 4 out of every 16 entering students were so categorized. Their responses in the interviews reflected an interest in nontraditional positions and careers, a questioning of established health care delivery, and a willingness to pioneer or even create new and autonomous nursing roles. Many looked forward to functioning as independent practitioners, particularly in remote rural areas. Others hoped to "set up new programs, develop new ideas for health care in the community, participate in the management of an out-patient health service organization, set up programs for mental health and nutrition, to improve the current system, to be creative, innovative and constructive." One respondent characterized his intended role as "to joust with the system."

Frontiering orientation was one category

Indicators for coding data into the frontiering category

From M.W. Searight, et al., *Demonstration Study of a Second Step Nursing Program.* Rohnert Park, Calif.: Sonoma State College, unpublished Final Report, 1978.

Reliability and Validity of Content Analysis   Content analysis, although ostensibly rigorous in its procedure and certainly arduous in its conduct, is still accused by its critics of being prone to problems of validity and reliability. Some of the critical questions directed toward studies that use content analysis are the following:

1. How personal and idiosyncratic are the categories?

2. Would another researcher independently come up with the same ones?

3. How clear are the instructions for placing a response into a code?

4. How reliable is the coding?

5. What checks did the researcher include on the reliability and thoroughness of coding?

6. Do the categories have at least face validity?

7. What kind of evidence is presented to establish face validity?

8. Do the content analysis categories meet other necessary criteria such as homogeneity, inclusiveness, usefulness, mutual exclusiveness, and clarity and specificity?

    ■ *Homogeneity* means that all categories are variations of the same thing. Are all the categories on similar levels of abstraction?

    ■ *Inclusiveness* means that the categories include every possible aspect of the variable without reverting to a catchall category such as *mixed* or *miscellaneous*.

    ■ *Usefulness* means that each category serves a purpose and relates to an important question under study. Proliferating too many categories detracts from a category's usefulness.

- *Mutual exclusiveness* means that the categories are separate and independent. If responses can reasonably be coded into more than one place, the reliability of the coding is suspect.

- *Clarity* and *specificity* simply mean that the categories are stated in clear, direct terms that other people can understand.

Ultimate validity for your content analysis relies on:

- your ability to develop a rationale for your categories

- your ability to define the categories

- your ability to show how the categories are appropriate to your data

- your ability to illustrate the fit with which the data can be coded into the categories

- your ability to demonstrate relevance of the categories to the research question

Analytical Induction

Analytical induction and a cluster of approaches resembling it depart from the two methods discussed previously in this chapter in that reliance on frequency and on the hope of quantifying qualitative data, even using scales for nominal data, is no longer the key to discovering the truth. Instead, the analyst attempts to search for concepts and propositions in the data that apply to all cases of a question under analysis. This approach assumes the careful consideration of all analytical evidence, the intensive analysis of individual cases, and the comparison of cases to one another. According to Norman Denzin (1970), a sociologist whose name has become linked with this method in the social science literature, analytical induction involves the following steps:

1. Formulate a rough definition of the phenomenon to be explained. What is the study problem?

2. Based on files of qualitative data, formulate concepts and hypothetical explanations about what is going on (e.g., identify general categories).

3. Examine cases in the data to see if emerging propositions fit the facts.

4. Search for negative cases, and reformulate your hypotheses based on them.

5. Continue this process until a universal pattern of relationships or set of propositions is identified, explained, and supported with data.

6. Compare with other groups or conditions to develop an even more abstract and generalizable explanatory scheme.

Some Practical Questions

Q. How does an analyst using the induction method arrive at the classes, categories, or concepts?

A. If you don't use classes, concepts, or constructs from existing literature (for instance, assessing, planning, problem identification, goal setting, implementing, evaluation, or power structure, communication network or decision linkages), you must come up with original concepts by reading and thinking about the data. According to Schatzman and Strauss (1983), you have succeeded in devising a category when you can identify its properties or characteristics, know its boundaries, and can give it a name.

Lofland (1971) suggests "interrogating" your data according to three beginning research questions:

1. What are the characteristics of what is going on here? What forms does it assume? What variations can I find out about?

2. What are the conditions that preceded its occurrence, and what variations exist in them?

3. What are the consequences of a social phenomenon I can find here?

He believes that almost all qualitative analyses using a variation of analytical induction can be reduced to attempts to answer these three basic questions (Lofland 1971). He goes on to offer six *units of analysis*, ranging from microscopic to macroscopic, that can help you begin to classify your data:

1. acts—action in a situation that is temporary and brief

2. activities—action of major duration in a setting, consuming people's involvement as well as time

3. meanings—the verbal productions of participants that direct action

4. participation—people's involvement in or adaptation to the setting under study

5. relationships—interactions among different people

6. settings—the entire setting under analysis

Q. Once I can divide my data into Lofland's categories and maybe even find a novel name for what I observe in each category, then what?

A. Within each of Lofland's six units, a researcher can conduct either a static analysis or a phase (or sequence) analysis. This distinction is similar to that between a photograph of the phenomenon under study and a motion picture that captures processes evolving over time.

Typologies often result from *static analysis* of the six units of analysis. If, for example, we look at Alvin Gouldner's (1958) classic analysis of the different "types" employed in college teaching, we find that he identifies:

1. *cosmopolitans*—those low on loyalty to the employing organization but high on commitment to specialized skills and likely to use an outside reference group orientation. These are further divided into:

   - the outsiders
   - the empire builders

2. *locals*—those high on loyalty to the employing institution, low on commitment to specialized skills, and likely to use an interior reference group orientation. They were further subdivided into:

   - the dedicated
   - the true bureaucrat
   - the homeguard
   - the elders

An illustration of *phase analysis* can be found in Fred Davis's (1968) stages experienced by nursing students who are undergoing what he named *doctrinal conversion*—a social-psychological process whereby students come to exchange their own lay views and images of the nursing profession for those that the profession ascribes to itself. He identified this status passage as consisting of six stages:

1. initial innocence

2. labeled recognition of incongruity

3. psyching out

4. role simulation

5. provisional internalization

6. stable internalization

Q. Once you establish classes and relationships, how do you use the data?

A. Once classes, subclasses, and relationships are discovered, specific vignettes in the data are coded as indicators of them in order to further develop their properties and ultimately formulate an overall integrative scheme. Unfortunately, "hearing" meaning in the data is a major difficulty for many researchers who try to work with qualitative data. Data, as Schatzman and Strauss (1983) suggest, "do not leap off the page to speak for themselves" and fall into some insightful interpretive scheme. Every investigator must either eventually confront his or her own ability to make some sense out of notebooks full of field notes and hear their meaning in a complex explanatory analysis or revert to simple or analytical description to salvage the study. Even crude typologies in which types are defined but not related to one another represent movement from completely unordered data to more refined categories.

Validity and Reliability   Just as quantifying qualitative data and doing a content analysis can be questioned for their reliability and validity, so can analytical induction. Critics ask: "Can the observations made in one setting with one population be generalized to others?" "Do observations represent real differences, or are they merely the artifacts of the observer's biases?" "How honest and reliable are informants and respondents?"

When it comes to answering the first question about generalizability, the researcher must demonstrate that the case or cases studied are representative of the class of units to which he or she wants to generalize the findings. This is accomplished by carefully specifying the conceptual conditions under which the observations were made and the propositions were advanced. In answering the second objection, the investigator must introspectively examine his or her own perspective and indications in the data that it colored either what was seen or how data were interpreted. Anecdotes about PNs in the research report often emphasize these efforts. Finally, when you try to evaluate the credibility of informants, you can ask yourself some questions about them:

1. Do the informants have reason to lie or conceal what they think is the truth?

2. Does vanity or expediency lead them to misstate the facts?

3. Are they firsthand witnesses to the occurrence?

4. Are feelings about issues likely to lead to an alteration in the story line?

An alternative strategy for dealing with questions about credibility is to accept the philosophical position that an individual's statements and descriptions of events are indications of his or her personal reality and unique perspective and should be studied and interpreted as such. Here you view each datum as valuable in and of itself but with respect to different conclusions. For example, instead of learning what the quality of nursing care is like on a particular unit, you might find what people think good nursing care ought to consist of.

Discovering Grounded Theory

One of the most highly evolved and explicitly codified methods for developing categories and propositions about their relationships from qualitative data is called the *discovery of* **grounded theory**. According to Glaser (1978), one of the method's originators: "The grounded theory method offers a rigorous, orderly guide to theory development that at each stage is closely integrated with a method of social research. Generating theory and doing social research are two parts of the same process" (p. 2).

Basic Assumptions   Developing theory from qualitative data using Glaser and Strauss's discovery method (1967) rests on a set of basic assumptions:

1. *One goal of a theory or analytical explanation is that it have "grab." "Grab" means* that a theory is interesting and useful. To achieve this, theories must fit, be

relevant to, and work to explain, predict, and be modified by the social phenomena under study. Therefore, data are not forced or selected to fit preconceived theories. Instead of testing a few hypotheses deduced from existing theory, data are used to develop a rich, dense, and complex explanatory or analytical scheme.

2. *Unlike verificational research, in which data collection and analysis are viewed in a linear way—that is, as separate, consecutive steps—data collection and analysis go on simultaneously.* The concepts and propositions that emerge from the data direct subsequent data collection. Although this process is sometimes called "an inductive approach" because it starts with the more specific and moves to the more abstract, it actually reflects both inductive and deductive thinking at various points.

3. *The grounded theory method is transcending.* Substantive theory developed in one area of study always has the potential for transcending a particular setting and being extended to a wide variety of circumstances. An example is the discovery of a process like "fairing," used by nonprofessional staff members to manage their work in Soteria House, where conventional administrative controls were muted and denied. This process could be extended to analyze the distribution of labor in a family where sex-role stereotypes, job assignments, and the like were absent. The method is also transcending of other theories. The goal is not to confront or refute existing theories but to incorporate them as part of the data base for the analysis. It also transcends scholarly disciplines and can be as useful to nursing as to sociology. The possibilities, according to Glaser, are limited only by the analyst's capabilities.

4. *Despite the diversity that characterizes qualitative data, the grounded theory approach presumes the possibility of discovering fundamental patterns in all of social life.* These patterns are called core variables, or *basic social processes* (BSPs), and they account for most of the variations characterizing an interaction under study. Hutchinson found that, after spending months on three neonatal intensive care units, nurses had to cope with a social-psychological problem of the horror associated with the deformities, death, and even some of the treatments of the newborns. The BSP, or core variable, she explicated in her theory was called *creating meaning*. This variable addressed how, given the conditions and problems in such a unit, the nurses created meaning and obtained satisfaction from their work. When nurses failed to make some kind of meaning of their work world, they experienced burnout, depression, and low morale (Hutchinson 1984).

5. *Generating grounded theory takes time and the ability to think conceptually.* It takes time for ideas to develop about the data, and the analyst must be sensitive to pacing the study to provide for the creativity and energy it requires.

The final product of a grounded approach to qualitative analysis is a theoretical explanation that:

- fits the substantive area under study

- is sufficiently *dense* (accounts for a great deal of variation) and abstract to allow generalization to diverse situations

- allows for partial control over structures and processes in daily situations such as nursing practice

There are seven steps in developing a grounded theory: specifying the research problem, reviewing the literature, sampling, coding, memoing, discovering the overriding analytical scheme, and sorting memos to produce an outline.

Step 1: The Research Problem   For the purposes of writing a funding proposal or for a thesis or dissertation proposal review, the grounded theorist explains that the specific study problem will emerge from the data but that initially the research asks: "What are the basic social and psychological processes that explain interaction in a particular setting or under certain conditions?" This initial sensitizing question is supplanted with a grounded one in the final research report.

Unlike most deductive, theory-verifying research, a grounded theory begins without a highly focused research problem. A major requirement for a grounded theory is the discovery of a core variable, or BSP, that explains what is going on, but this conceptualization "earns its way" into the study by being grounded in the data. The analyst spends a considerable time in the field mapping out its relevant dimensions before a specific researchable problem is discovered. My experiences suggest that at least 50 hours of fieldwork precede one's ability to articulate a grounded study problem, the explanation of which becomes the core variable in the analysis. In my study of Soteria House, I began by asking the grounded theorist's initial questions:

1. What is it?

2. What are its properties?

3. How did it come to be and what is it becoming?

4. Under what conditions and with what strategies and consequences does it work?

5. What is the main story line here?

From data bearing on these questions I wrote the following TN:

> Soteria House has a noncontrol system as contrasted with the conventional system in mental hospitals. I've seen a conscious effort to mute and deny elaborate control structures like formal authority lines, a hierarchical division of labor, organizational ideology, schedules, therapies, medications, locked doors, uniforms, etc. An ethic that emphasizes freedom, spontaneity and individuality and opposes established psychiatric practices predominates. Doing away with traditional controls does not eliminate problems of social order [Wilson, unpublished field notes].

The specific research problem that emerged from these notes became: "In the absence of conventional, elaborate psychiatric control structures, *how are problems of social control solved?*" (Wilson 1982 p. 103).

Step 2: Reviewing the Literature The sociologist Anselm Strauss once commented, "Be aware of the wisdom of questioning received wisdom!" Theory-verifying and hypothesis-testing studies require that we read related literature to get the fullest coverage possible, from which we can then synthesize our theoretical framework, operationalize concepts, and perhaps import an existing measurement tool. We then collect data relevant to the concepts in our framework. In some cases, if the fit is poor, we make adjustments to fit the data to the framework as necessary.

When discovering grounded theory, you collect data in the field before reviewing literature. In Glaser's words, "It's hard enough to generate one's own ideas without the 'rich' detailment provided by literature in the same field" (1978 p. 31). Once the analytical scheme emerges, the grounded theorist reads other studies to discover how his or her work fits with existing research and what contribution it has made. Literature is reviewed to discover correspondence, conduct comparative analysis, and integrate a discipline's body of knowledge. The literature review is not a starting point or an attempt to gain scholarly fame. This attitude about reading is not meant to ignore the fact that ideas are built on other ideas or to be antiacademic and antischolarly. But protecting one's theoretical sensitivity and originality in interpreting data is of prime importance with this mode of inquiry.

Step 3: Sampling Again, grounded theory contrasts with theory-verifying research when it comes to sampling procedures. Instead of aiming at a predetermined probability (random) sample, the *grounded theorist uses a purposeful method called theoretical sampling.* Theoretical sampling reflects a rethinking of statistical sampling standards so that interactive research questions can be addressed. Theoretical samples are judged by the quality of the theory that emerges, whereas statistical samples are judged by their conformity to the rules of probability sampling theory. The analyst who uses theoretical sampling looks for variation, for situations that shed light on new properties of a process. See Table 13–4 for a comparison between theoretical sampling and statistical sampling.

Step 4: Coding Collecting, coding, and analyzing data go on simultaneously from the first day that a grounded theorist enters the field. Coding is the process of conceptualizing the underlying patterns in a set of empirical indicators. Instead of deciding on *operational definitions* of important concepts in advance of collecting data, the grounded theorist reads through each incident, phrase, line, paragraph, episode, anecdote, or statement in the data, line by line, and asks: "What concept is this datum an indicator of?" "What is actually happening in the data?" "What are these data a study of?" This is simply a more systematic and codified way of noticing the patterns in your clinical practice. Glaser calls it *concept specification* instead of concept definition.

TABLE 13–4 *Comparison of Theoretical Sampling and Statistical Sampling Approaches*

Item	Theoretical Sampling	Statistical Sampling
Purpose	To discover concepts, hypotheses, and their interrelationships—that is, theory. The magnitude of the relationships may be, but is not necessarily, part of the hypotheses	To obtain accurate evidence on distributions of people among categories to be used in descriptions or verifications
Adequacy	Judged on how wisely and diversely the analysts have chosen groups for insight into the full range of categories according to the type of theory—formal or substantive—they wish to develop. Inadequate sampling is characterized by a theory that is thin and not well integrated and by many obvious, unexplained exceptions	Judgment is based on techniques of random and stratified sampling used in relation to the social structure of a group or groups sampled
Closure	Must be learned. Data collection for a grounded theory study stops when new categories and their related aspects stop appearing in the data	Data collection must continue until the predetermined sample size is achieved

Three major types of code are substantive, selective, and theoretical.

Substantive, or *open*, *codes* are words that you find in the data that capture "what is going on." They are often words used by participants themselves. They are the terms used to describe:

1. dimensions

2. properties

3. conditions

4. strategies

5. consequences

Among the long list of substantive codes I wrote in the margins of my Soteria House study field notes were: *insulating, appeasing, being with*, and *low profiling* (see Appendix C). Substantive codes allow you to move from descriptive excerpts to a higher level of abstraction—concepts and constructs. In this way, substantive codes "earn their way" into your theory. The grounded theorist then does not assume the face value relevance of any conventional variable, such as sex, race, or social class, until it emerges as relevant in the data.

Open substantive coding both verifies and saturates individual codes. You can verify that patterns corresponding to your codes exist in the data by actively seeking variations and constantly comparing each incident with existing ones to become confident that your set of codes captures the major conceptual variations that exist under a certain set of circumstances. At this stage of your analysis it is important not to seek premature closure on your substantive codes. Acknowledge diverse codes as they appear, but always look for (1) their relationship to one another and (2) their relation to a possible core variable, or BSP.

Technically, the mechanics of substantive coding are:

1. Read through the data line by line, and write the code in the margin of the field note next to the indicator.

2. Construct a "laundry list" of substantive codes. In her study of men's role in contraception, Swanson found that men reported getting information about contraception in many ways. They:

    - read magazines

    - listened to the radio

    - watched television

    - talked to others

    - saw films

    - read pamphlets

Once her list stopped growing and codes were just being repeated, she moved on to the second type of coding operation, called selective coding.

Selective coding requires that the analyst note what is similar and what is different about the codes on the list and cluster codes to create *categories* that relate to one another. For example, one code in the list for how men get information about contraception was "talking to others." She then selectively coded data about talking with others into:

- public talking

- private talking

- professional talking

- same-sex talking

- cross-sex talking

Once possible variations on a core variable are identified, the analyst selectively codes for the full *range, variations*, and *properties* of the category. For example, for cross-sex talking, Swanson interviewed people who made only partial disclosures about contraception and people who had extensive conversations about it. These data allowed her to compare "truncated talk" with "full-range talk" by beginning the third type of coding, *theoretical coding.* The step of selective coding is necessary to move from the more concrete list of open codes to a more abstract, parsimonious set of categories. Once your process of theoretical sampling stops generating new categories, *saturation* has been reached. *Saturation of categories* means that the major recurring patterns have been discovered. Deciding when you have reached saturation requires that you know the difference between a new event on a descriptive level and a genuinely new conceptual dimension.

Theoretical coding involves figuring out how the substantive categories are related to one another. You accomplish this step by formulating propositions about relationships and actively verifying the proposed relationship in your data. The theoretical codes must "earn their way" into the analysis as well. Glaser (1978) identifies the following "families of theoretical codes":

1. the six Cs (causes, contexts, contingencies, consequences, covariances, and conditions)

2. process (stages, phases, passages, transitions, careers, orderings, trajectories, sequences, cycles)

3. degrees (limits, ranges, intensity, amount, boundaries, rank, averages, grades, criteria)

4. dimensions (elements, facets, properties, segments, aspects, sections)

5. types (kinds, styles, classes, genres)

6. strategies (tactics, mechanisms, techniques, ploys, procedures)

7. interactions (reciprocity, covariance, interdependency)

8. identity/self (self-image, self-concept, self-worth, self-evaluation, self-realization)

9. cutting points (boundaries, breaking points, benchmarks, tolerance levels, turning points)

10. culture (norms, values, beliefs, rules)

11. consensus (agreements, contracts, definitions of the situation, opinions, conformity)

12. mainline (social control, recruitment, socialization, status passage, stratification, social mobility)

13. ordering (temporal, conceptual)

14. units (group, nation, organization, social world, society, family, role, status)

In my study of conventional inpatient psychiatric treatment under the community mental health movement, I discovered a highly prescriptive structure of policy, regulations, and standards that transformed the old state hospital warehouse into a similarly bureaucratized *clearinghouse*. Here treatment consisted primarily of a *dispatching* process, in which patients were screened, patched together with medication, stamped with a diagnostic label, sorted into a legal category, and sent back to an unwelcoming community. Obviously the *dispatching* analysis is an example of relating categories as stages in a people-processing operation (Wilson 1985).

Step 5: Memoing   Writing up analytical memos of your ideas about how the data, codes, categories, and relationships will eventually be integrated into a core explanatory scheme is a critical component of the grounded theory method. The analyst's goal is to develop theoretical ideas about his or her data that, once sorted, provide the basis for writing up the final integrative scheme (see Appendix C). The source for memos is TNs written during the process of constantly comparing indicator with indicator, and then indicator with concept.

A memo can be a sentence, a paragraph, or a few pages. Memos help your developing theory in five ways:

1. They require that you begin thinking about the data at a conceptual level.

2. They summarize the properties of each category so that you can begin to construct operational definitions.

3. They summarize propositions about relationships between categories and their properties.

4. They begin to integrate categories with clusters of other categories.

5. They relate your analysis to other theories.

Memos allow you to escape the self-imposed tyranny of writing well at this stage and provide the freedom to capture ideas. Your objective is to get an idea down on paper and not worry about perfect prose.

Rules for memoing, according to Glaser (1978), include:

1. Keep memos separate from data, but cross-reference them to useful illustrations in the data.

2. Always interrupt data collection or coding to write a memo when an idea occurs to you.

3. Modify existing memos as your ideas are modified.

4. Keep a list of your substantive codes. Write memos on each one on the list.

5. If many memos on two different codes are similar, collapse the two codes into one.

6. Keep memos conceptual.

7. Write up one idea at a time and one idea per memo.

8. Keep memos flexible so that they can be sorted in a variety of sequences.

9. Label each memo with the code or codes it describes.

You will ultimately end up with hundreds of pages of memos, moving from specific codes to categories to relationships among categories and finally to a dense analytical scheme that accounts for all major patterns of behavior. A grounded theory is a molecular rather than a linear set of relationships. Most analysts try to diagram this complex set of interrelationships when they write up their final analysis (for an example, see Figure 13–1).

Step 6: Discovering the Overriding Analytical Scheme   Arriving at a final integrative scheme means that you have discovered, through the constant comparison method and the techniques described, a core category. This analytical scheme accounts for most of the patterns of behavior in the area under study and integrates and interrelates a dense array of other subcategories and propositions. You discover it by searching through your data, codes, and memos looking for the main theme, or "story line," that explains the problem reflected in the data. Here are some of the criteria suggested by Glaser (1978) for recognizing the core category in your analysis:

1. It must be central. You can easily relate all other codes, categories, and relationships to it.

2. It must recur frequently in the data—that is, be relatively stable and pervasive.

3. It must make sense to the people in the study setting.

4. It must allow for a "dense" explanation by incorporating a lot of descriptive variation.

5. It can be any one of the types of theoretical code.

Examples of core categories that were also BSPs include *cultivating*, *defaulting*, *centering*, *becoming*, *dispatching*, *infracontrolling*, *covering*, *balancing the mandates*, *protective governing*, *surviving on the brink*, and *reconnecting*.

Step 7: Sorting Memos to Produce an Outline   Sorting memos puts the data back together again in a coherent story. It integrates all the main ideas into a scheme. Technically, the analyst sorts all memos by codes:

1. specifying conditions, contexts, strategies, consequences, and interrelationships as recorded in the memo fund

2. linking illustrative examples from the analytical data files

3. incorporating relevant memos on related literature

The outcome of memo sorting is a theoretical outline on which the final research report is based. In my Soteria House study, it looked like this (Wilson 1982):

Infracontrolling: Social Order under Conditions of Freedom in an Antipsychiatric Community

I. "Presencing": Control of Resident Patients

   A. Mere presence
   B. Monitoring
   C. Intervening
      1. Active strategies
      2. Passive strategies

II. "Fairing": Management of Staff Work

   A. Establishing a fairing code
   B. Unfairing
   C. Restoring

III. Limiting Intrusion: Control of Outsiders

   A. Minimizing approachability
      1. Situational positioning
      2. Partial disclosure

   B. Deflecting
   C. Disengaging

Once memos are sorted, the grounded theorist writes the report, moving from the more general proposition to specific illustrations and including quotations and vignettes that make it plausible. The theory constitutes the study's "findings." Because it is grounded in data, it has relevance to the real world of nursing education, administration, and practice.

Evaluating the Credibility of a Grounded Theory

The aims and methods of discovering grounded theory are quite different from the aims and methods of theory-verification research. The criteria for critiquing a grounded theory and evaluating its credibility differ accordingly.

Some critics dismiss studies that use the methods described as invalid, unreliable, and too subjective. Others relegate this method to a form of "artistic" rather than "scientific" inquiring, based on a definition of scientific research as "inquiries that use formal instruments as the primary basis for data collection, transform the data collected into numerical indices of one kind or another, and attempt to generalize to some universe beyond itself" (Eisner 1981 p. 5).

The canons of quantitative analysis on such issues as sampling, coding, reliability, validity, indicators, frequency distributions, hypothesis construction, and presentation of evidence must be replaced by alternative criteria when one judges the credibility of qualitative research and grounded theory analysis.

Five Basic Criteria   Five criteria suggested by Glaser and Strauss (1966) represent the generic elements of the grounded theory method itself.

1. joint collection, coding, and analysis of data to promote maximum variation and verification in the data

2. systematic choice and study of several comparative groups that allow for the full generality and meaning of each category in the analysis.

3. trust in the researcher's own credible knowledge, based on having lived with partial analyses and tested them every step of the way and having had first-hand, face-to-face knowledge

4. a presentation of findings that includes clear statements of description to illustrate the analytical framework

5. confirmation by participants in the social world under investigation

Secondary Criteria   A good grounded theory, according to nurse scientists who work to develop them:

- results from formulating and discarding hypotheses if they are not supported by data

- has included a look for contradictory occurrences

- is based on a variety of *slices of data*, direct observations, interviews, and document analysis

- can transcend the substantive area and have broader relevance

- specifies the conditions under which it was developed and to which it can be generalized

- fits the data

- works to explain the variations in behavior in a given area and to predict what can occur when conditions change

- is relevant and comprehensible to people in the study setting

- is modifiable, dense, and integrated into a tight analytical framework

May (1986) suggests that the consumer ask the following questions when evaluating the credibility of a grounded theory.

1. *The research question.* Is it too narrow? Has the original question been supplanted with one grounded in data? Does it focus on exclusively psychological variables or social-interactional ones?

2. *Data sources*. Are multiple slices of data from a variety of sources (field notes, interviews, documents) used as the basis for analyses? Is the data base sufficient to capture all the range and variation in codes and categories?

3. *The literature*. Does the study include correspondence with, but not overreliance on, related literature?

4. *The analytical scheme*. Is it clear, plausible, and well integrated?

5. *Relevance to the real world of practice*. Will it make a difference?

Pitfalls of Grounded Theory It is obvious that developing a grounded theory is not a simple process. There are two primary pitfalls, premature closure and failure to find a core variable that integrates the analysis.

1. Premature closure refers to ending theoretical sampling and coding before the full range and variation for codes and categories have been discovered. This often occurs when an investigator is under the time constraints associated with a thesis or dissertation deadline.

2. A second significant pitfall occurs if a core variable, or BSP, does not surface. The question then becomes how to salvage the study. Writing the report as an analytical description is one option. The study may then be exploratory and descriptive but still offer directions for further research.

Phenomenological-Interpretive Analysis

Examining persons in context to understand processes of day-to-day living as well as significant, unique events can also employ a *phenomenological-interpretive* (or *hermeneutical*) research approach. The purpose of this method is to understand meanings and practices of people who function as cognitive, emotional, behavioral "whole beings" in their historical or background traditions.

Basic Assumptions Assumptions on which phenomenological studies are based derive from the philosophy of Heidegger. They reflect these ideas:

1. Situations are grasped as meaningful wholes by individuals who share common background meanings and language.

2. People must be studied in their cultural, social, and personal historical contexts.

3. Understanding one's world need not be conscious and fully cognitive.

4. Particular concerns shape human involvement in the world; concerns set up what is salient about situations and how people will act.

5. Language is the communication of one individual's mental representation of reality to another.

6. The task of a researcher is to uncover and understand meanings embedded in the practices and expressions of those under investigation.

7. To access "lived meanings" the researcher must study the pragmatic activity of daily life.

Research Questions in Phenomenological Research   Research questions in phenomenological studies reflect the preceding assumptions and are targeted toward grasping the lived experience and meanings connected to human events and processes. In a study of parental caregivers of young schizophrenics, Chesla (1988) posed the following questions for her interpretive phenomenological analysis:

1. What are the parents' explanatory models of schizophrenia?

2. What adaptive demands do schizophrenic illness behaviors place on parents and the family unit? Are there recurring themes across families?

3. How do personal background meanings and interpersonal concerns shape day-to-day stress and coping among parents caring for a schizophrenic child?

In another phenomenological nursing study of cancer survivors, Carter (1989) raised a similar set of researchable questions suited for interpretive methods of analysis.

1. What are the informants' understandings of cancer as an illness?

2. What common ways of being do informants share?

3. What themes and personal meanings are characteristic of informants?

4. What conflicts in interpretation between personal and cultural meanings emerged during their illness trajectory?

Data Analysis   Interpretive analysis or *hermeneutics* relies on analysis of *text* to understand human behavior and meanings. *Text* customarily refers to typed transcripts of observational notes and interviews. The researcher interrogates (analyzes) the text asking:

1. What practices occur (action/behavior)?

2. What are the situations/contexts of such practices?

3. What aspects of situations are salient from the informants' point of view?

4. What meanings do informants attach to their lived experience?

There are three approaches to analyzing and presenting studies that analyze text according to the preceding questions:

1. **Thematic analysis:** reading each informant's interview or observation text to identify prominent themes that appear across cases. Themes in Chesla's (1988) study of parental caregivers of a young schizophrenic family included: impact of illness on work, social life of caregivers, and personal meaning changes.

2. **Analysis of exemplars:** examining specific examples of events culled from interviews to generate rich descriptions of situations, actions, practices, and intentions in their complete form (Benner and Wrubel in press).

3. **Identification of paradigm cases:** finding resemblances between the paradigm case and other cases. Chesla (1988) used paradigms to formulate and name particular forms of care, such as "engaged care, self-care in tension with care of the other, care as specialized management, and care from a distance."

Credibility of Phenomenological Analysis.   It is no more appropriate to apply canons of scientific rigor from theory-verifying research to phenomenological, interpretive analysis than it is to apply them to grounded theory or analytical induction research. Sandelowski (1986), however, offers four areas of concern for rigor in interpretive studies:

1. *credibility* in that subjects themselves find that the interpretive story is "right"

2. *fittingness* in that readers other than study sample members can make sense of the findings in terms of their own experiences

3. *auditability* in that the investigator provides sufficient detail about analytical and other decisions throughout the study to allow another researcher to follow and judge those decisions

4. *confirmability* in that the researcher knows how his or her biases may have influenced the findings. Confirmability parallels the concern for neutrality in scientific work except that qualitative interpretive investigations seek engagement rather than detachment.

Ultimately it falls to the reader to judge the rigor and quality of interpretive research. However, Sandelowski identifies several strategies to produce a credible interpretive study.

■ Check for the representativeness of the data as a whole, of the coding categories, and of the examples used to analyze and present the data.

■ Triangulate across data sources and data-collection procedures to determine congruence of findings among them.

■ Check that descriptions contain both typical and atypical elements of data.

- Deliberately try to discount or disprove a conclusion drawn about the data.

- Obtain validation from the study subjects themselves.

These strategies are equally useful with all of the qualitative analysis approaches considered in this chapter.

Applications of Qualitative/Interpretive Research to Nursing Practice

Clinical nurses have only recently begun to rely significantly on reports of research findings to answer their questions. Heretofore they tended to rely on authority, tradition, and trial and error when deciding whether to warm an infant's formula or to oxygenate before, in between, or after suctioning (see Chapter 1). Much of nursing practice was a combination of folk healing traditions and technology. Nursing has operated at the "preparadigmatic" phase of developing theories in the discipline (Meleis et al 1980). As nursing's unique perspective has become clearer, Goldman's challenge has become more compelling: "It is up to us to accept strange and difficult ideas and to abandon the complacency of converting all that is novel into clichés of the familiar" (1980 p. 14).

The methods of qualitative analysis discussed in this chapter, and the discovery of grounded theory in particular, offer nursing one approach for developing much-needed middle-range theories for practice while capitalizing on the observational sensitivity of practicing nurses. Nursing also needs modes of inquiry and analysis that offer the freedom to explore the richness of human experience, with all its variation. Phenomenological interpretive studies hold promise for this goal. Nursing care requires an understanding of people in complex, changing social contexts. Its scope of practice encompasses people of all ages, social classes, developmental levels, and degrees of wellness and illness who are engaged in all sorts of psychological, physical, and social processes. Nurses apply and synthesize knowledge from physical, social, and medical sciences as well as the humanities. They recognize that theirs is a complex and diversified professional domain. They need research methods that are rigorous and that allow them to predict causes and outcomes. But they also need analytical methods that allow them to define, describe, and explain the real practice world of nursing to themselves and others. Grounded theory methods and phenomenological interpretation enable nurses to ask: "How can we become more sure of what we already know?" and "How can we know that which is not known?" instead of "How can we measure variables that we already know from a model or theoretical framework?"

Different research and analytical approaches need not compete with one another. No one entrenched philosophical stance or pet method in and of itself will lead to theoretical advances in nursing. True discoveries in nursing will probably come only from analytical pluralism. The qualitative methods and procedures described in this chapter represent one set of legitimate approaches for understanding certain kinds of research questions about everyday nursing practice. These questions are prompted by nurse scientists' world view and philosophy of science, and they represent one way of moving from observations to explanations and from practice to theory and understanding.

Guidelines for Critique

- What was the purpose of qualitative analysis in the study?

- What methods of qualitative analysis were applied to the data?

- Why were the analysis methods selected?

- If a content analysis was performed, what efforts were made to establish the validity and reliability of categories?

- If analytical induction was used, did the investigator make efforts to demonstrate that results are generalizable?

- If grounded theory methods were used, did the outcome theory meet standards for credibility?

- If phenomenological interpretation was used, did the investigator describe the process of arriving at the interpretation and provide adequate "thick" description to support findings?

SUMMARY OF KEY IDEAS AND TERMS

✓   *Analysis* is the separation of data into parts for the purpose of answering a research question.

✓   *Qualitative analysis* is the nonnumerical organization and interpretation of data in order to discover patterns, themes, forms, and qualities found in unstructured data.

✔   The philosophies of science on which qualitative research is based are called *symbolic interactionism* and *phenomenology*. Implications of these philosophies for research are:

- ■   Research should be conducted in the natural setting.

- ■   Reality and truth are emerging and relative, depending on the way people define them.

- ■   The research process itself is a source of data and analytical ideas.

✔   Four major purposes of qualitative analysis are:

- ■   exploration and description

- ■   accounting for and illustrating quantitative findings

- ■   discovery and explanation

- ■   extension of theory

✔   *Substantive theory* is a middle-range theory that explains something under a specific set of conditions.

✔   *Formal theory* or *grand theory* explains how something occurs under a great variety of circumstances.

✔   *Cognitive maps* are visual models or diagrams of categories and relationships in the analysis.

✔   *Straight description* uses categories imported from existing literature to organize data.

✔   *Analytical description* involves devising novel categories suggested to the analyst by "interrogating" the data to organize them.

✔   Preparing qualitative data for analysis involves duplicating field notes and interview transcripts, labeling them, and establishing organizational, methodological, and analytical files.

✔   Five major procedures for analyzing qualitative data are:

- ■   converting to quantitative data

- ■   doing a content analysis

- ■   using analytical induction

- discovering a grounded theory
- conducting a phenomenological interpretive analysis

✓ Six units of analysis for analytic induction are:

- acts
- activities
- meanings
- participation
- relationships
- setting

✓ *Grounded theories* begin with five questions:

- "What is it?"
- "What are its properties?"
- "How did it come to be, and what is it becoming?"
- "Under what conditions and with what strategies does it work?"
- "What is the main story line here?"

✓ Tasks in creating a grounded theory include:

- discovering the problem
- integrating literature
- theoretical sampling
- open coding
- selective coding
- theoretical coding
- memoing
- memo sorting
- discovering a core variable through constant comparisons
- developing an outline
- writing the theory

Some go on simultaneously.

✓   BSPs (basic social processes) serve as one type of core variable to explain most of the variations in behavior in the situation under study.

✓   *Saturation of codes and categories* occurs when no new conceptual patterns or properties emerge in the data. It tells you when to stop collecting data.

✓   Grounded theories must be evaluated for their credibility by research consumers who use alternative scientific canons.

✓   Phenomenological interpretive analysis seeks to describe and understand meanings and practices as "lived experiences."

✓   Phenomenological interpretation uses theme analysis, identification of exemplars, and paradigm cases to analyze text.

✓   The potential for nursing of qualitative analysis in general, and grounded theory and phenomenological interpretation in particular, is as an alternative to importing existing theory from other disciplines. The goal is to develop nursing theory from observations of nursing practice and human experience.

References

Bargagliotti LA, Trygstad LN: Differences in stress and coping findings: A reflection of social realities or methodologies? *Nurs Res* 1987; 0, 170–172.

Becker HS: Problems of inference and proof in participant observation. *Am Soc Rev* December 1958; 23:652–660.

Blumer H: *Symbolic Interactionism*. Englewood Cliffs, N.J.: Prentice-Hill, 1969.

Bowers BJ: Intergenerational caregiving: Adult caregivers and their aging parents. *Adv Nsg Sci* 1987; 9, 21–31.

Carter B: Cancer survivors. Doctoral Dissertation, University of California at San Francisco, School of Nursing, 1989.

Corbin J: Coding data. In *Qualitative Research in Nursing: From Practice to Grounded Theory*, Chenitz WC, Swanson J (editors). Menlo Park, Calif.: Addison-Wesley, 1986.

Chesla C: *Family Care of Schizophrenia: An Interpretive Study*. Doctoral Dissertation, University of California at San Francisco, School of Nursing, 1988.

Davis F: Professional socialization as subjective experience: The process of doctrinal conversion among student nurses, pp. 235–251 in *Institutions and Persons*, Becker H et al (editors). Chicago: Aldine, 1968.

DeGroot HA: Scientific inquiry in nursing: A model for a new age. ANS 1988; 10, 1–21.

Denzin NK: *The Research Act*. Chicago: Aldine, 1970.

Dickoff J, James P: A theory of theories. *Nurs Res* September/October 1968; 17:197–203.

Dreyfus HL: Being-in-the-world: A commentary on Heidegger's being and time, division I. Unpublished manuscript, Department of Philosophy, University of California at Berkeley, 1986.

Eisner E: On the differences between scientific and artistic approaches to qualitative research. *Educational Research* April 1981:5–9.

Fagerhaugh S: Getting around with emphysema. *Am J Nurs* January 1973; 73:94–99.

Glaser BG: *Theoretical Sensitivity*. Mill Valley, Calif.: Sociology Press, 1978.

Glaser BG, Strauss AL: The purpose and credibility of qualitative research. *Nurs Res* Winter 1966; 15:56:61.

Glaser BG, Strauss AL: The purpose and credibility of qualitative research. *Nurs Res* Winter 1966; 15:56–61.

Glaser BG, Strauss, AL: *Status Passage*. Chicago: Aldine, 1971.

Goldman I: Boas on the Kuakiutl: The ethnographic tradition. Sarah Lawrence College: Essays from the Faculty. 4:5–23, 1980.

Goodwin LA, Goodwin WL: Qualitative versus quantitative research or qualitative *and* quantitative research. *Nurs Res* 1984; 33, 378–380.

Gouldner A: Cosmopolitans and locals: Toward an analysis of latent social roles—2. *Admin Sci Q* March 1958; 2:444–480.

Haase JE: Components of courage in chronically ill adolescents: A phenomenologic study. *Adv Nsg Sci* 1987; 9, 54–63.

Hinds PS, Young KJ: A triangulation of methods to study nurse-given wellness care. *Nurs Res* 1987; 36, 195–198.

Hutchinson S: *Survival Practices of Rescue Workers: Hidden Dimensions of Watchful Readiness*. Lanham, MD.: University Press of America, 1983.

Hutchinson S: Creating meaning out of horror. *Nurs Outlook* 1984; 32:86–90.

Hutchinson, S: Chemically dependent nurses: the trajectory towards self-annihilation. *Nurs Res* 1986; 35, 196–201.

Jones E: Translation of quantitative measures for use in cross-cultural research. *Nurs Res* 1987; 36, 324–326.

Kelly HS: The meaning of current dance forms to adolescent girls: An exploratory study. *Nurs Res* November/December 1968; 17:513–519.

Leininger M (editor): *Qualitative Research Methods in Nursing*. New York: Grune & Stratton, 1985.

Lofland J: *Analyzing Social Settings*. Belmont, Calif.: Wadsworth, 1971.

May KA: A typology of detachment and involvement styles adopted during pregnancy by first time expectant fathers. *West J Nurs Res* 1980; 2:445–461.

May KA: Writing the grounded theory study. In *Qualitative Research in Nursing: From Practice to Grounded Theory*, Chenitz WC, Swanson J (editors) Menlo Park, Calif.: Addison-Wesley, 1986.

McCall G, Simmons JL (editors): *Issues in Participant Observation: A Text and Reader*. Reading, Mass.: Addison-Wesley, 1969.

Meleis A et al: Toward scholarliness in doctoral dissertations: An analytic model. *Res Nurs Health* 1980; 3:115–124.

Mosher LR, Menn A: Community residential treatment for schizophrenia: Two-year follow-up. *Hosp Comm Psychiatry* 1978; 29:715–723.

Norris CM: Restlessness: A nursing phenomenon in search of meaning. *Nurs Outlook* February 1975; 23:103–107.

Orsolits M, Morphy M: A depression algorithm for psychiatric emergencies. *J Psychiatric Treatment Eval* April 1982; 4:137–145.

Powers BA: Taking sides: A response to Goodwin and Goodwin. *Nurs Res* 1987; 36, 122–126.

Sandelawski M: (1986) The problem of rigor on qualitative research. *Adv Nsg Sci*, 8, 27–37.

Schatzman L, Strauss AL: *Field Research*. Englewood Cliffs, N.J.: Prentice-Hall, 1983.

Schutz A: *The Phenomenology of the Social World*. Evanston, Ill.: Northwestern University Press, 1967.

Searight MW et al: *Demonstration Study of a Second Step Nursing Program*. Rohnert Park, Calif.: Sonoma State University, unpublished report, 1978.

Standards of Psychiatric Nursing Practice and Professional Performance. Kansas City, Mo.: American Nurses' Association, 1982.

Swanson JM: *Men's Sexual and Contraceptive Work Biographies and the Management of Contraception*. Paper presented at the 108th annual meeting of the American Public Health Association, Detroit, October 21, 1980.

Weivers ME, Lenz ER: Relapse among exsmokers: An example of theory derivation. *Adv Nsg Sci* 1987; 9, 44–53.

Wilson HS: Limiting intrusion—Social control of outsiders in a healing community: An illustration of qualitative comparative analysis. *Nurs Res* March/April 1977; 26:103–111.

Wilson HS: *Deinstitutionalized Residential Care for the Mentally Disordered: The Soteria House Approach*. New York: Grune and Stratton, 1982.

Wilson HS: Dispatching: Usual Hospital Treatment in the USA's Community mental health system. In *Qualitative Researching Nursing: From Practice to Grounded Theory*, Chenitz WC, Swanson J (editors). Menlo Park, Calif.: Addison-Wesley, 1985.

Wilson HS: Presencing—social control of schizophrenics in an antipsychiatric community: Doing grounded theory. Pages 131–144 in Munhall P, Oiler CJ (editors), *Nursing Research: A Qualitative Perspective*. Norwalk, Conn.: Appleton-Century-Crofts, 1986.

Wilson HS: The process of family caregiving for a demented relative: Surviving on the brink. *Nurs Res*, in press.

14

Applying Statistics to Quantitative Analysis

HOLLY SKODOL WILSON ▪ SANDRA FERKETICH ▪ JOYCE VERRAN

Chapter Objectives

After reading this chapter, the student should be able to:

- comprehend the concept of scientific scales of measurement

- compare and contrast scales for nominal, ordinal, ratio, and interval data

- differentiate between descriptive and inferential statistics

- explain the processes for calculating frequency distributions; measures of central tendency, including the mode, median, and mean; measures of variability, including the range, the interquartile range, and the standard deviation; and measures of contingency and correlation

- interpret descriptive statistics from graphic presentations in research articles

- explain the logic and language associated with inferential statistics

- perform the four steps needed to test hypotheses using inferential statistics

- determine whether parametric or nonparametric statistics are appropriate in a nursing study

(Continued)

- compare and contrast appropriate use and interpretations of *t*-tests and analyses of variance (ANOVA)

- interpret an *F* ratio from an ANOVA summary table

- explain the logic of simple linear regression

- discuss nonparametric statistical procedures, particularly the chi-square

- apply the guidelines for choosing a statistical procedure in determining whether published nursing studies have employed statistics correctly and in planning one's own study

In This Chapter...

This chapter is an introduction to univariate statistical procedures commonly used in quantitative analysis. The next chapter continues the content with basic information on advanced statistical methods used in nursing research today. You may find that your needs are best met by using only parts of the content of each chapter. This text, however, is not meant as a substitute for a course in statistics or even as a substitute for a good statistical text. Instead, it presents the information you'll need as a responsible reader and conductor of nursing research.

Although the language of statistics may at first seem difficult we hope you will try to learn it. Statistics have become an important part of our daily lives. Annual rainfall, disease incidence, and the relationship between home sales and national growth affect us all. Furthermore, statistics are becoming an important part of nursing care. Does therapeutic touch affect perception of pain? If intravenous tubing is changed less frequently, will the incidence of infection and phlebitis change, and what will be the effect on patient comfort? How will the effect of an alteration in health policy be evaluated?

Research can be used to evaluate the quality of nursing care provided, to assess patients, and to answer critical patient-care questions. The term *cold*, when applied to statistics, probably connotes lack of feelings or sensitivity to the needs of the individual and society—numbers, not caring. Perhaps that is true in one sense, but it is up to us to use the numbers to our advantage. Statistics give us a rich source of information on which to base health care decisions, whether at the individual, family, or community level. To use statistics wisely, however, we need to understand the concepts underlying the analysis.

In both this chapter and the next, our aim is not to inform you of all the "how tos" of statistical tests. In this age of powerful personal computers and easily interpreted packaged analysis programs, you don't need complete mastery of complex derivations and computations.

It is, however, a good idea to engage the services of a statistical consultant early in the research process. A consultant can discuss various procedures you can use to address your research question. Once you select a test, the consultant can provide invaluable assistance in obtaining and organizing the data to make the analysis proceed smoothly.

Do not make the mistake, however, of confusing the consultant with the researcher. It is your project, and you are responsible for understanding the analysis and making critical decisions about the nature of that analysis. Simply dumping your data on the statistician's doorstep, though expedient, is not in your interests. In the long run, you will be hard pressed to explain your own research and understand that of others. If, however, you know whether a statistical technique was used appropriately, how to interpret the results, how to translate those results into words that others can understand, and how to arrive at logical conclusions, you will make statistics a valuable ally and servant.

Statistical concepts and operations are presented in the context of varied examples and are offered in the hope that being able to think statistically will sharpen your ability to think critically about nursing research. The kind of statistical knowledge that this chapter emphasizes will help you sustain a healthy skepticism when you read in the local newspaper that "a high proportion of women who take birth control pills have strokes" or that "compulsive jogging is just like anorexia nervosa." Furthermore, you will learn how to avoid inadvertently using statistics that mislead others.

Although reports of nursing research in recent years reflect a general trend toward increased statistical savvy, incidents of incorrect use of statistical tests, failure to meet statistical test assumptions, failure to attend to power analysis to determine an adequate sample size, misinterpretation of results, and what Reid (1983) calls "galloping alpha rates" still occur. If you, as a reader of research, are able to detect the misuse of statistics, you have gained important knowledge with which to decide if an investigator's conclusions are justified.

In the pages that follow, statistics are covered as both a collection of numerical facts expressed in terms that decribe and summarize quantitative data and as tools for speculation and prediction. Thus, both **descriptive statistics**, which organize, summarize, and present information in a usable, understandable form, and **inferential statistics**, which help us make inferences about populations based on samples taken from them, get full treatment.

We begin with the concept of measurement, which we've indirectly discussed in earlier chapters. A great deal about measurement is familiar to most of us—the number of milliliters in a vial, a patient's pulse rate or blood pressure reading, the amount of urine excreted over a 24-hour period. But nursing research is also concerned with less directly and precisely measureable phenomena. We will talk more about scales for measuring variables such as a patient's self-esteem, intelligence, stress response, disorientation, support system, and the like. The various ways of measuring and scales for levels of data provide a backdrop against which the major descriptive statistics, inferential statistics, and the concept of multivariate statistics are examined.

Some say that the element of *uncertainty* sets statistics apart from other areas of applied mathematics. In arithmetic, algebra, and geometry, conclusions can actually be proved. A **statistic**, however, is a numerical index determined from a subset (sample) of the population and describes the sample or is used to make inferences about the population. In all cases, however, we make judgments based on how likely or unlikely it is that this numerical index occurred by chance. Systematic knowledge about the likely outcomes of nursing interventions advances the scientific basis for practice far beyond trial and error or the authority of tradition. Statistics are valuable tools for analyzing numerical data to answer certain research questions relevant to nursing practice and building the knowledge base for the discipline.

Measurement Scales

Before doing your own research or even reading intelligently about research done by others, you need to understand the concept of *measurement*. We all engage in informal measuring every day. The well-baby clinic was busy that day, or it wasn't. The operating room schedule was full or pretty full. A patient's wound is healing quickly or slowly. **Measurement** in research, however, can be distinguished from casual day-to-day measuring by its planned, systematic nature. Research measurement occurs according to a well-specified, reasonable set of rules for the consistent assigning of numbers to represent the qualities or attributes being measured. The researcher attempts to make the measurement of an attribute correspond as precisely as possible to the reality being measured. However, much of the measurement used in scientific investigation only taps a small percentage of the possible data relevant to the attribute being measured. Scientific measurement can be summarized as

$$\text{Measurement} = \text{actual value} \pm \text{error}$$

The types of, sources of, and ways to minimize error are discussed in Chapter 6. This chapter's focus is on measurements that approach actual values of phenomena important in nursing studies.

Measurement involves the process of assigning numerical values to concepts under investigation. Statistics allow you to analyze those numerical values. (The major methods of analyzing *qualitative* data are explained in Chapter 13.) When an investigator spells out how something is to be quantitatively measured, he or she is in fact operationally defining and quantifying the study's key concepts or variables. Intelligence may be "a score" on a standard IQ test like the Stanford-Binet. A patient's preoccupation with body diseases might be measured using his or her score on some of the 550 items of the Minnesota Multiphasic Personality Inventory (MMPI). Postoperative recovery rate might be measured by the number of hours that elapse before a child returns to preoperative eating, sleeping, playing, and communicating patterns when split-screen videotapes of the child are shown to a panel of expert judges. These operations, called data collection, were considered in Chapters 10, 11, and 12. Most authorities are quick to point out, however, that it is not really possible to measure something itself. Rather, *one measures the attributes or qualities about something that vary.* You can't measure a female per se, but you can measure her height, weight, political attitudes, or self-esteem. These varying characteristics or attributes of something are called a study's variables. The clearer and more credible your process of transforming concepts or variables into measurements is, the more likely it is that your measurement reflects actual value rather than error.

Let's illustrate this process by imagining that we are interested in conducting a study of psychiatric nurses' beliefs about mental illness. We could collect data on this variable by interviewing a sample of nurses and use qualitative analysis methods; or we could administer the *Beliefs about Mental Illness Inventory*, which contains items like those depicted in Box 14–1. We could then transform our subjects' responses into scores or measures by developing a system of assigning numbers to the responses. Interpretation of the results would then have to be done according to the proper use of scales of measurement. The kind of scale used influences which statistical procedures can be used to analyze your data.

Defining a Scale of Measurement

A **scale** of measurement specifies all the possible values a given measurement might have. What really defines a scale of measurement is the complete set of potential measurement categories, not just the ones into which your subjects fall. Of course, measures can be crude or precise, ranging from only a few possible values to a larger number of them.

All measurement scales do have to have *at least two different possible measurement categories, or values.* In our example, for instance, we could score the psychiatric nurses who take our *Beliefs about Mental Illness Inventory* as simply "positive" or "negative." We could even score the intensity of the belief as "strong" or "weak." The actual system for scoring data generated with this instrument involves assigning

---

Box 14–1   Beliefs About Mental Illness Inventory Items

**Examples of a 2-Choice Scale
Beliefs About Mental Illness**

Positive .... or	Negative
(+)	(−)
Strong (1) .... or	Weak (0)

numbers to responses. Totals for various items are then added to determine whether or not the subject's dominant beliefs reflect the following:

- authoritarianism

- benevolence

- a mental hygiene ideology

- social restrictiveness

- interpersonal etiology orientation

Whatever the scale of measurement, it should, in addition to having at least two possible values, *be exhaustive*. This means that you can assign some number to each respondent in your study. For example, it would be inadequate to measure the clinical specialization backgrounds of Registry nurses in your city by specifying only *OB-Peds* and *Med-Surg* on your scale. You would at least have to add the category *Other* to be exhaustive.

Finally, measures along any scale of measurement should be *mutually exclusive*. If you are measuring the consciousness level of intensive care unit (ICU) patients, you can't put the same patient into both the "conscious" and the "unconscious" category at the same time. If you ever find yourself in doubt about the appropriate category, consider the possibility that your scale needs to be more precise and discriminating by providing, for example, a graded series of options between fully conscious and fully unconscious. Decisions about scaling must be made at a study's outset, however, so that all subjects will be measured with the same scale and according to the same measurement rules. Knowing from the start what scale you intend to use also influences which statistics you use to analyze your data. And knowing this keeps you straight about what kinds of question you will and will not be able to address in your study. Statistical procedures must be appropriate for a study's purpose and design, which includes the measurement scales for the study variables.

Levels of Measurement

Levels of measurement refer to the precision with which variables have been measured. Four hierarchical levels of measurement, defined originally by Stevens (1951), have been accepted as the traditional way to categorize measurement scales. These levels reflect the precision of the scales in measuring the attribute under study. Some analysts believe that the level of data resulting from using a particular measurement scale determines the kind of statistic that can be used. Not all accept this level of categorization as the prime determinant of statistical procedures and instead depend on the characteristics of the underlying distribution or on the way the attribute is viewed in reality. Even though there is controversy, the four levels of measurement provide a guide to help the beginner select appropriate statistical tests in planning quantitative data analysis. We will, therefore, discuss levels of data and refer to them later in conjunction with specific statistics.

Nominal   The most primitive and least precise level of measurement from a traditional scientific perspective is called a nominal scale—a scale for nominal data. **Nominal** level of measurement arbitrarily assigns some number to represent the categories into which an attribute or quality can be sorted. Measuring the sex of patients who develop lung cancer in the United States by labeling each as male or female and assigning numbers so that 1 = male and 2 = female is an example of a very simple nominal scale, or code, with two possible measurement categories. We use a nominal level of measurement when we sort patients according to their blood type or nursing diagnosis and assign numbers to a longer list of categories (see Box 14–2). The numbers themselves have no real meaning except as *a convenient code*. There is no implication of equal-sized steps between the numbers or of any inherent ordering of the categories in relation to one another. All we can conclude from nominal scales is that data sorted into different categories are nonequivalent. Nominal scales are nevertheless considered examples of scientific measurement, because two rules apply in the assignment of numbers: (1) all responses that are sorted into the same qualitative category are given the same number, and (2) no two categories can be assigned the same number.

The value of transforming qualitative, categorical data into nominal scales was covered in Chapter 13. Clearly you can perform cross-tabulations with other numerical data and calculate frequencies, if variables are expressed in numerical terms. The chi-square statistic, discussed later in this chapter, is also appropriate for nominal data. But don't be fooled into assuming that research results that have transformed qualitative categories into nominal scales have somehow invested the numbers themselves with any more meaning or order than that of convenient labels.

Ordinal   **Ordinal** levels of measurement rank order values. Numbers that are assigned to data according to ordinal scales have the characteristic of ordered cat-

---

Box 14–2   Nursing Diagnoses for Psychiatric Patients

1.00   Self-care limitations
1.10   Emotional stress or crisis
1.20   Emotional problems related to daily living
1.30   Physical symptoms which occur with altered psychic functioning
1.40   Alterations in thinking, perceiving, communications and decision-making abilities
1.50   Behaviors and mental states that indicate the client is a danger to self or others or gravely disabled

egories. We can't assume, however, that the numbers along the scale represent the same amount or change in the variable from one point to the next. Ordinal data are ranked "low," "medium," and "high," but the rank doesn't tell you anything about the distance between low and medium or medium and high. In short, although you can rate a variable on an ordinal scale, your measurement categories cannot be presented or treated as having equidistant intervals, even though the numbers you assign to the ratings might suggest it. You can ask parents, for example, to rate their hospitalized children on a 5-point scale where 1 = not at all regressed to 5 = extremely regressed. Even though the raters use the numbers from 1 to 5 to make the ratings, there is no guarantee that the intervals between the numbers are equidistant in the same way that measures of weight or time are. It might take only a few behavioral changes to alter a rating from 2 (slightly regressed) to 3 (moderately regressed), yet a dramatic change in activity might be necessary to alter the rating from 4 (very regressed) to 5 (extremely regressed) (see Figure 14–1). Because the numbers are assigned without the assurance of equidistant intervals, some experts believe that any statistical procedures that involve adding them, subtracting them, or taking their average are inappropriate. Frequency counts, percentages, and a few limited statistical operations explored later in this chapter can be used with ordinal scales.

What you *can* assume with ordinal data, for instance, is that 5 is more regressed than 4, that 4 is more regressed than 3, and so on. Therefore, ordinal data are more precise than nominal data. Obviously, saying that an attribute is different in degree and direction conveys more information than just saying that two attributes are in two different categories. Many nursing research studies that investigate attitudes use self-developed or standardized Likert scales. Traditionally, each item on these scales is considered to be at the ordinal level of measurement. However, in practice most researchers treat the summated scores from these scales as interval level data.

Scale for Interval Data **Interval scales** consist of potential measurement categories that, as in an ordinal scale, have an inherent order. In addition, however, the possible measures along an interval scale are *equidistant* from one another. This characteristic allows researchers to make statements about the *actual differences* between measures rather than just saying that something has more or less of an attribute than something else. Studies in the nursing literature concerned with the impact of preoperative care on postoperative patient outcomes might employ ordinal

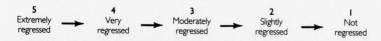

Figure 14–1 Example of ordinal scale for regression where 5 > 4 > 3 > 2 > 1.

scales that simply rate a patient's overall postoperative course as having "more" or "fewer" complications. An interval scale that plots temperature elevations indicative of infection clearly offers more precise information on the study question. Investigators, therefore, prefer to use interval scales whenever possible, because they not only provide more precise information but also permit the adding and subtracting of measures and the use of more sophisticated statistics that require taking a mean of measures. Many standardized psychological tests used in nursing research studies are based on interval scales. Blood pressure readings represent another example of an interval scale. A reading of $150/90$ is higher than a reading of $140/90$, and a reading of $140/90$ is higher than a reading of $120/90$. Furthermore, an interval scale assumes that the differences between systolic readings of 140 and 130 and 120 are essentially equivalent.

A final point on the subject of the interval scale is that, although it is considered to be a higher-level scale than either nominal or ordinal, it does not have *an absolute zero point*. Zero on interval scales is arbitrary. Almost all authors on this subject use the Fahrenheit and Celsius thermometers to illustrate this idea. Both are interval scales; the Celsius uses an arbitrary zero point of 0, and the Fahrenheit scale has an arbitrary zero point of 32. Neither point, however, really signifies the total lack of heat (see Figure 14–2). The lack of an absolute zero point prevents the researcher from making statements of magnitude, such as "an outside temperature of 100° F is twice as warm as a temperature of 50° F." This statement is false because there is some degree of warmth at 0° F that is not taken into account.

Ratio **Ratio scales** provide (1) rank ordering of measures, (2) equal intervals between measures, and (3) an absolute zero point. Ratio scales provide the most precise level of measurement for the purpose of applying statistical analysis procedures. These qualities allow the scale to communicate the maximum and most precise information and also make its data amenable to the most powerful and sophisticated statistical analyses. Examples of ratio scales used in nursing studies include time, length, and weight. Scores of zero on these measures really do represent the absence of the attribute being measured; therefore, statements of mag-

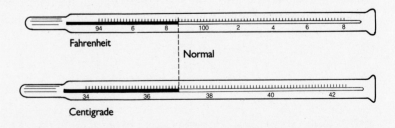

Figure 14–2 Illustration of two types of thermometers.

nitude are possible. Because the scales have an absolute zero, all mathematical operations are possible with them. In practice, the same statistics used with interval level data are used with ratio level data. The advantages of ratio scales are their increased precision and sensitivity in assigning a numerical value to an attribute. Ratio scales tend to dominate among the physical and biological measures and are seldom used when measuring more abstract psychosocial qualities. When psychosocial qualities are to be measured, interval scales are more common; however, some nurse reseachers are beginning to use a *magnitude estimation procedure* to develop ratio level scales for psychological qualities.

Quantitative Analysis Using Statistics

The researcher analyzing quantitative (or numerical) research data begins by recognizing measurements of variables under study as belonging to one of the four major levels. Knowing the level of measurement helps the researcher make decisions about which statistical procedures can be used to analyze the data and answer research questions.

Planning Ahead

A reseacher should plan how his or her data are to be analyzed. As should be clear from the discussion of scales, some statistical procedures require that data be collected in a particular way. Furthermore, some statistical tests work better when equal numbers in all groups of data are present (for example, equal numbers of control and experimental patients). It is probably wise to consult a statistician who can handle statistical questions, a computer analyst who can address questions related to a particular system or statistical package, or both early in your study planning phase to anticipate potential problems. Many experts urge that you actually think through your analysis to the extent of setting up dummy tables, or dummy analysis forms, to ensure that you will know how to handle the data once they are collected. A *dummy table* is simply a table without numbers. Figure 14–3 illustrates a sample dummy table for a study on postoperative infection. Once data have been collected, statistical analysis procedures constitute the tools initially used to interpret or make meaning out of the findings in relation to the study's theoretical framework and its specific research problem.

Specific analysis procedures depend not only on the research question and the type of data collected but also on the study design. Even if hypotheses are being tested, most investigators also attempt to analyze the data that may not relate just to the study hypotheses in the hope that some unanticipated insight may emerge. Most analysts also examine data on possible intervening variables. For example, in an outcome study of experimental and control patient groups where the indepen-

	Yes	No
Control group	N%	N%
Experimental group	N%	N%

Figure 14–3   Sample dummy table. Frequency of postoperative infection.

dent variable is *mode of teaching preoperative patients to cough, turn, and deep breathe* and the dependent variable is *the incidence of postoperative pneumonia*, analytic procedures would very probably include a comparison of the characteristics of the two study groups themselves to demonstrate that they were not significantly different to begin with, either physiologically or psychosocially.

Categories of Statistical Tests

The ultimate goal of analysis is to summarize your data in ways that will allow you to answer your research question. Although statistical procedures can be classified several ways, they are traditionally divided into two major categories: descriptive statistics, which are measures to summarize a large volume of data with individual numbers, and inferential statistics, which are measures that allow the researcher to make inferences about a larger group.

This chapter cannot cover all statistical tests used by researchers. New statistical tests continue to be developed, and some older tests are gaining in popularity. In the latter category are tests that were once difficult to perform or known by only a few researchers. Because of the ready access to computers and the increased sophistication of researchers, the use of advanced statistics has increased. The following discussion, although not exhaustive, introduces the reader to statistical procedures and may suggest avenues for further study.

An additional question is "Why are some procedures used when less complex ones might be used to address the same research question?" If the research can be designed so that only the variable under study is altered during the experiment and all other variables that might have an effect are controlled by sampling and design, then the simplest, least complicated statistical test is the best one. A simple analysis is easier to understand and easier to explain to other researchers and nurse clinicians. This is an important consideration for a practice-based profession, since clear communication between researchers and clinicians can make a difference in the practice of nursing.

Why, then, use complex procedures if simple ones will do? The main reason is that often we cannot control all other variables as we would like and sometimes we cannot even manipulate the variable whose effect we want to study. Certain complex procedures, therefore, have been used to handle some of these problems in the analytic phase of the research process. There is no substitute for good design, however. Do not be fooled into thinking that statistical tests can take care of all problems. If you need to review principles of design and sampling, please refer to the other sections of this text.

If you are using or reading about the statistics, what information do you need to evaluate the use of a particular statistical technique? First, you need a clear understanding of the test. Second, you need to be aware of the purpose, advantages, and disadvantages of various procedures and of the requirements, generally called assumptions, that must be met for a given procedure to yield stable, unbiased results. In other words, before you can trust the results of the test, you must perform it correctly with the appropriate data. If you keep these points in mind, you can make intelligent use of the statistical consultation that is available to you and understand the research results that you read.

Descriptive Statistics

Descriptive statistics are summary statistics and visual displays that describe the characteristics of the sample. Descriptive statistics include measures of central tendency, dispersion, and association. The term may also apply to tables and graphs used to display the results of these procedures.

Descriptive analysis includes a range of possible statistical operations from crude to precise methods of summarization for an entire data set. Descriptive statistics include measures of central tendency, dispersion and association. The terms may also apply to tables and graphs used to display the results of these procedures. The choice depends first, of course, on your study question and then on the level of measurement. Imagine that a school nurse has administered a battery of assessment tests (visual, hearing, intelligence, personality inventories, health histories, and physical exams) to a group of elementary schoolchildren. What strategies are available for putting this vast array of numerical data into some useful and meaningful form? She or he could:

1. rearrange the various scores by how often they occurred to get an overall picture of the data set

2. construct tables, graphs, and figures to visualize the data

3. convert raw scores to other types of scores such as percentile ranks, standard scores, or grades

4. calculate averages on each important variable to learn something about the typical status of the group

5. figure out the ranges or dispersion of scores and ratings in relation to the central point

6. look for relationships or correlations between two or more different measurements

All of the methods in the list above represent various kinds of descriptive statistics.

Visual Data Displays

A **frequency distribution** represents one way of organizing a mass of what might appear at first to be overwhelming and chaotic information. It involves systematically arranging numerical values from the lowest to the highest and then counting the number of times each value appeared in the data. A frequency distribution lets you quickly see what the lowest and highest scores were, where most of the scores tended to cluster, and, in fact, what the most commonly obtained score was (see Table 14–1). The construction of frequency distributions and frequency tables is really a rather simple process. If you are working with an extremely large number

TABLE 14–1   *Frequency Distribution of Test Scores (n = 55)*

Raw Score	Frequency
28	1
27	1
26	2
25	5
24	5
23	9
22	10
21	5
20	6
19	4
18	3
17	3
16	0
15	1

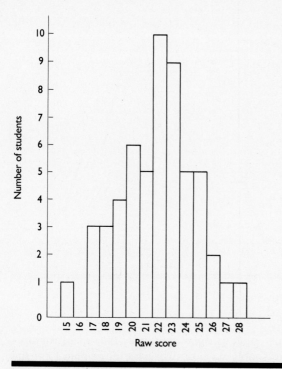

Figure 14—4 Histogram based on text scores from Table 14–1.

of measures, a computer program can construct frequency tables for you automatically. The steps for constructing a frequency distribution manually are as follows:

1. Find the lowest and highest scores or numbers in the data set for which you want to construct a frequency distribution.

2. Decide what the class interval will be and how many classes you will have. These are commonly called the Xs. Arrange them from lowest to highest value. Be sure that the classes of observation are mutually exclusive and exhaustive.

3. Construct a table that has columns for (a) each class, (b) the tally, or count, of how often the class appeared in the data, and (c) a frequency (a percentage).

4. Read through your raw data sequentially, and make a mark in the count column for each occurrence.

5. Add up all the frequencies, called the fs, and put the total number for each class in the *frequency* column. The sum of frequencies in that column ought to equal the total size of your sample ($\Sigma f = n$).

6. Complete the percentage column by dividing each frequency by the total number of data items and multiply by 100 ($\% = 100 \times f / n$).

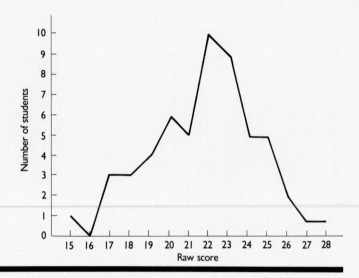

Figure 14–5 Frequency polygon based on test scores from Table 14–1.

Graphic Displays Many research studies display frequency data in **histograms** or **frequency polygons**. These are simply ways of displaying in graphic form the same information contained in a frequency table. In Figure 14–4, the vertical axis contains the frequency totals, with a zero at the bottom and the highest frequency at the top. The horizontal axis contains the classes of totals, with the lowest value on the left and the highest value on the right. Next, bars are drawn over each class of score with a height equal to the frequency of that particular class. Some researchers and consumers believe that such visual depictions of frequency information are easier and quicker to read than a table.

In the case of frequency polygons, dots connected by straight lines are used instead of bars to show the number of times that a class occurs. See Figure 14–5 for a frequency polygon based on hypothetical data.

The following example illustrates how you might organize and summarize measurements you've collected using the method of creating a frequency distribution.

Imagine that you have recently taken a position as a clinical nurse III in an educational facility for mentally retarded children. You intend to plan and implement a health teaching curriculum for the children in your care. You also believe that systematic assessment and clinical research are crucial to the development of your new role. You decide to begin by getting some assessment of the intellectual capacities of the center's resident population. According to the sampling principles presented in Chapter 8, you go to the records and pull out a random sample of 45 patients. You write down their IQ scores on a piece of paper and end up with results that look like those in Table 14–2.

TABLE 14–2 *IQ Scores of Educational Center Children (n = 45)*

x	f	x	f	x	f
104		81		79	
83		69		70	
66		53		69	
78		58		65	
35		50		67	
50		61		75	
55		80		79	
100		54		78	
68		85		77	
47		63		61	
60		62		61	
60		61		60	
55		60		55	
58		59		54	
61		58		50	

As you mull over these figures, it becomes obvious that you really can't make much sense out of them unless you organize them in some systematic way. You decide to list all the scores from lowest to highest and put a slash mark beside each score every time it occurs. The number of slash marks then represents the frequency of occurrence of each score. By this kind of grouping you can get a picture of the distribution of IQ scores for the retarded children you hope to teach (see Table 14–3). In this way you have achieved a manageable array of scores to help you target your health teaching curriculum to meet learner needs and abilities.

Frequency Distributions for Different Types of Data Scale If the data or scores you are working with are interval level and you have too many different scores or classes (usually more than 10) to make for a frequency table that is easy to read, you can combine measurements into bigger categories, because the measurements are ordered and equidistant.

If the data and scores you are working with are ordinal level, you can combine measurement categories into bigger classes but must not add raw scores together.

If you are constructing frequency distributions for nominal data, you can tabulate the number of subjects assigned to each class and the proportion of the total sample assigned to each category, so that you can compare one frequency distribution with another in a way that makes sense. The only difference is that you *cannot* place the classes or scale values in any order, because nominal data scales have no inherent order.

TABLE 14–3 *Frequency of IQ Scores of Educational Center Children*

x	f	x	f	x	f
104	|	65	|		
100	|	63	|		
85	|	62	|		
83	|	61	|||||		
81	|	60	||||		
80	|	59	|		
79	||	58	|||		
78	||	55	|||		
77	|	54	||		
75	|	53	|		
70	|	50	|||		
69	||	47	|		
68	|	35	|		
67	|				
66	|				

Measures of Central Tendency

Comparing whole frequency distributions is one way of making some sense of an array of numerical data. But it can also be somewhat awkward when you have to take several groups or conditions into account. In many cases, a group pattern is of less importance than some statistic that can summarize a whole distribution in a single number. Whenever a researcher is interested in questions like "What is a typical degree of nausea in the first trimester of pregnancy?" "What is the APGAR score of most babies born at home birth centers?" or "What is the average length of hospital stay for open heart surgery patients?" the researcher is raising questions of central tendency. There are several measures of central tendency, and deciding which one to use depends on:

1. the scale on which a variable was measured

2. the shape of the frequency distribution

3. the purpose for which you want to report it

Central refers to a middle value, and *tendency* refers to the general trend of the numbers. In other words, a measure of **central tendency** is a statistic that summarizes the data into one representative value.

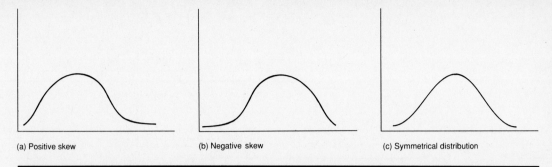

(a) Positive skew   (b) Negative skew   (c) Symmetrical distribution

Figure 14–6   Examples of skewed distributions

Distribution Shapes   Frequency distributions are usually characterized as either symmetrical or nonsymmetrical (also called skewed). **Symmetrical distributions** are shaped so that, if divided into halves, the halves could be folded over on each other and fit almost exactly. **Skewed distributions** have off-center peaks or humps and longer tails in one direction or another. If the longer tail points to the right, it is *positively skewed*; if the longer tail points to the left, it is *negatively skewed* (see Figure 14–6).

Frequency distributions can answer many different questions: "What is the most frequently occurring class of score?" "What is the distribution in a pattern of scores?" "How close does the distribution approximate a normal curve?"

An example of data that would appear as a skewed frequency distribution is the age at which American women complete menopause, because the majority of subjects are in the later half of life.

Distributions are also characterized by the modality of their shape. A **unimodal distribution** has only one high point, and a **bimodal** or **multimodal** shape has two or more (see Figure 14–7). The most common type of symmetrical, unimodal curve is called a **normal curve**, a bell-shaped curve with the greatest frequency at the

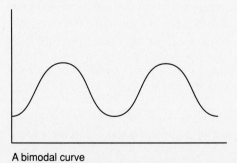

A bimodal curve

Figure 14–7   A bimodal curve

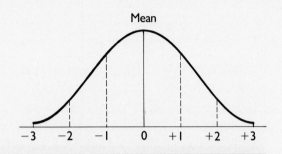

Figure 14—8 A normal, bell-shaped, curve

center. As you move away from the center, the frequencies become smaller and smaller (see Figure 14–8.)

The Mode For a frequency distribution of data from a nominal scale, the mode is the only measure of central tendency that makes sense. Calculations of the mean and median, discussed in the sections that follow, require equidistant categories or ordered categories. Neither of these, as you recall, is possible with a nominal scale. The **mode** is simply the category, or class, that has the highest frequency. In the case of a symmetrical distribution with a single peak, the mode is the same value as the median or the mean (if you can calculate them). Uses of modes in further statistical analyses are, however, very limited. You figure out a mode simply by looking at, or "inspecting," the frequency distribution into which you have ordered your data. Computer programs can also do this task for you.

The Median When your data are based on an ordinal scale, the median is an appropriate measure of central tendency. The **median** is the measure that corresponds to the middle score, because it lies at the midpoint of the distribution and divides the scores into halves. In other words, the median is the score at the 50th percentile. One major characteristic of the median is its insensitivity to extreme scores. This can work as a limitation or an advantage, depending on the study objectives of the researcher. In the set of scores 1, 3, 4, 11, 96, the median is 4. This is true even though the data set contains one extreme score of 96. It is important to understand that the median addresses the middle position of a distribution of numbers, not the value of the scores themselves.

The Mean The **mean** (*arithmetic mean*) of a set of measurements is simply the sum of the values divided by the total number of subjects. Stated in algebraic form, the mean is:

$$\overline{x} = \frac{x_1 + x_2 + \ldots + x_1}{n} = \frac{\Sigma\, x_1}{n}$$

Where x = the mean

$\qquad$ n = the number of scores

$\qquad$ Σ = the summation symbol, indicating the sum of all the measurements.

(Note: In general, lowercase letters denote sample specific statistics and values, whereas uppercase letters denote population specific statistics and values.)

This measure of central tendency, also called the *average*, is the most widely used one in statistical tests of significance. Most researchers attest that of all the measures of central tendency, *the mean is the most stable and unbiased.* If you calculate means of different samples drawn from the same population, they will fluctuate or vary less than modes or medians. However, the mean is also the least resistant measure of central tendency. In other words, the mean is sensitive to extreme values in a distribution and can be "pulled" in the direction of those extreme values. Because calculating the mean involves the addition of different values or categories, the categories must be ordered and equidistant; therefore, *the mean can be properly calculated only for interval or ratio data.* Whether the mean is necessarily the best statistic to describe intervally scaled measures depends on whether the frequency distribution is *symmetrical* and *unimodal.* In skewed distributions, the means lie below the distribution's peak, and in bimodal distributions, the means may fall between the two humps and not be very representative of actual values.

$\qquad$ Which measure of central tendency do you report in a study? The answer

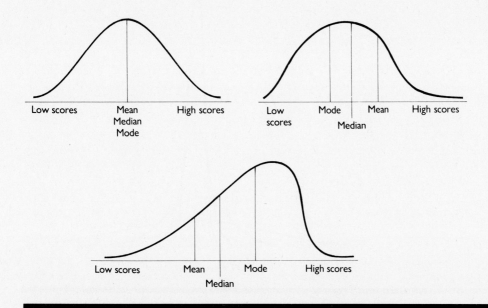

Figure 14–9 Measures of central tendency in normal and skewed distributions

depends on the level of measurement and the shape of the distribution of scores. It is often a good idea to report all three summaries to give the reader the most information possible. Of course, if you are using an inferential procedure to examine the difference between two groups on the basis of their median scores, you should always report the median. Similarly, if in your study you use statistics based on the mean, you should use the mean to describe the central tendency of the sample. (See Figure 14–9 for illustrations of measures of central tendency in normal and skewed distributions.)

Measures of Dispersion

The purpose of describing the central tendency of data is to describe how subjects are grouped. Measures of dispersion, in contrast, examine the variability of the scores. If the scores in a data set are very similar, there is very little dispersion. Two sets of data having symmetrical distributions, the same sample size, and the same value of central tendency could be very different in terms of the spread or dispersion of the measurements (see Figure 14–10).

Most authorities agree that, to describe a distribution of measures fully, you need to include measures of dispersion that reflect the extent to which scores are different from or similar to one another. Therefore, when a measure of central tendency is reported, the appropriate measure of dispersion should also be included.

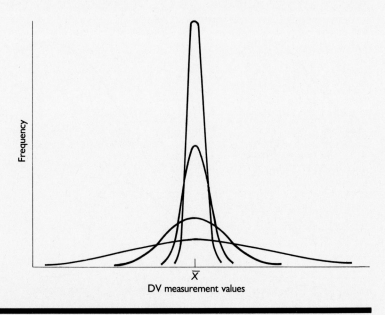

Figure 14–10 Symmetrical distributions. Four frequency distributions with the same mean and the same total sample size but different variabilities.

The most common measures of dispersion are the range, the interquartile range, the variance, and the standard deviation. These measures express the degree of dispersion of scores around the measures of central tendency. The variance and standard deviation are the most widely used measures of dispersion since they are associated with the mean and interval or ratio data. With nominal data, a frequency distribution as described earlier is used as an indicator of dispersion along with the mode as a measure of central tendency.

The Range   The **range** is the simplest measure of dispersion. It defines the difference between the smallest and largest numbers in the distribution. You compute it by subtracting the lowest score from the highest (Total range = the largest x − the smallest x). Table 14–4 lists a sample of hypothetical APGAR scores for newborn infants in a rural community hospital. Their range is $7 - 4 = 3$.

One of the obvious advantages of reporting the range is that it is easy to compute, but its disadvantages tend to outweigh this advantage. For one thing, it is considered a comparatively unstable statistic. One additional extreme score can change it. The APGAR score range of a second sample of babies born in the same rural community hospital, for example, might tend to fluctuate a lot. The range also doesn't take into account variations in scores between extremes and thus is customarily reported along with other measures of dispersion. If you relied exclusively on the range, a change in one individual score, the lowest or the highest, could alter the entire range figure drastically. To correct for this last problem the interquartile *range* or semiquartile *range* is often used as the measure of variability.

The Interquartile Range   The **interquartile range** is based on middle cases rather than extreme scores. It is more stable than just the range. It is found by

---

TABLE 14–4   *Sample of Hypothetical APGAR Scores for Newborn Infants in a Rural Community Hospital*

7	5	6
5	6	6
7	4	6
7	5	5
6	6	4
6	7	5
6	7	7
5	6	7
7	6	6
6	5	5

lining up the measurements in order of size and then dividing the array into quarters. The range of scores that includes the middle 50% of the scores is the interquartile range. Where Q is the symbol for quartile, the formula for obtaining the interquartile range is:

$$\text{Interquartile range} = Q_3 - Q_1$$

where Q_1 =   the value below which one-quarter of the scores fall
          Q_3 =   the value below which three-quarters of the scores fall

The **semi-interquartile range** is one-half of the range of scores within which 50% of the scores lie and is obtained by dividing the interquartile range by 2. The addition of deviant cases at either extreme leaves the interquartile (and semiquartile) range virtually unchanged. The range, interquartile range, and semi-interquartile range are the appropriate measures of dispersion to use with the median and ordinal data.

The Variance and Standard Deviation   The relationship of the variance to the standard deviation is analogous to the relationship between the interquartile range and the semi-interquartile range. Both reflect the deviation of scores from the mean. However, the standard deviation, which is the square root of the variance, is more easily interpretable. Therefore it is discussed in more detail here.

The **standard deviation** is an average of the deviations from the mean. *Standard* reflects the fact that the standard deviation indicates a group's average spread of scores or values around their mean. *Deviation* indicates how much each score is scattered from the mean. In reporting standard deviations for the sample, authors may use the abbreviation *sd* or *s*. When reporting the standard deviation for the total population, the Greek sigma (σ) is often used. The standard deviation is the most widely used measure of dispersion for interval or ratio levels of measurement.

The standard deviation is best understood by examining the normal distribution. The normal, or bell-shaped, curve (originally called the Gaussian curve after Carl Friedrich Gauss, its discoverer) is an important base for most statistical procedures. Four important characteristics about the shape of this curve are worth noting. These characteristics are easier to understand if we consider them in terms of the normal curve that has been transformed to a standard normal curve by changing all values to z scores. (If you are not familiar with z scores, you may wish to read that section of the chapter now.) On a standard normal distribution the mean is zero. Positive scores extend to the right of the zero line, and negative scores extend to the left. The four important characteristics of a standard normal distribution are:

- The scores cluster around the main vertical axis, the zero line.

- The curve is symmetrical and unimodal about the vertical axis.

- The size of the distribution is not limited, and positive and negative numbers can extend without limit toward infinity.

- The mean, median, and mode all have the same value, zero.

Furthermore, the following is true about the normal curve as well as the standard normal curve. Most of the values fall within approximately three standard deviations above and below the mean (68% of all values fall within one standard deviation on either side of the mean, 95% of all values fall within two standard deviations from the mean, and 99.87% fall within three standard deviations from the mean (see Figure 14–11). When you calculate the mean for a group of measures, you have the basis for calculating how much each individual measure deviates from the mean. One half of the deviations are positive, and one half are negative. By definition, when all deviations are summed, the result is zero. To deal with sums of deviations, it is useful to square the values to get rid of the negative signs before summing. Standard deviation of a *population* is found by the formula

$$SD = \sqrt{\frac{\Sigma(x_i - \bar{x}^2}{n - 1}}$$

Since the variance is not in the same units as the values of the random variable, it is customary to report the standard deviation, which adjusts for this disadvantage. The standard deviation, like the mean, takes into consideration all the scores or values in a distribution. It tells how variable the scores in a data set are. If, for example, we compared anxiety-scale scores for two samples of patients, each from a different culture, we might find that both distributions had a mean of 35. But when we calculated the standard deviation, we would discover that one had a standard deviation of 4 and the other a standard deviation of 9. We could immediately conclude that although the means were the same, the first sample was more homogeneous on the variable measured by anxiety score.

In summary, if you do not use a computer to calculate it, you can follow this step-by-step procedure to calculate a standard deviation:

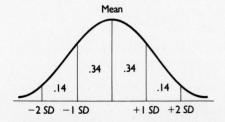

Figure 14–11   Bell-shaped curve and standard deviations.

1. Calculate the mean of all your measurements or scores.

2. Find the difference between each individual score value and the mean.

3. Square each deviation.

4. Add all the squared deviations, and divide by the total number of values to get the mean or averaged squared deviation. When the variance is being calculated for the sample, $n-1$ is used instead of N for an unbiased estimate of σ.

5. Take the square root of the average squared deviation to obtain the standard deviation.

Using the computer to accomplish such calculations, particularly when the number of scores or values in your data set is huge (for example, a national survey of all members of the American Nurses' Association), saves you time and eliminates arithmetic errors (see Chapter 16).

Standard scores, represented by the lowercase z, tell us how many standard deviations away from the mean a particular raw score is. Many intelligence and achievement tests use standard scores with a preestablished mean and standard deviation. The formula for computing the standard score is:

$$z = \frac{(x - \bar{x})}{sd}$$

where z = standard score
x = an individual score
$\bar{x}$ = mean score
sd = standard deviation

You can look up the z score in a table to find out how much of the distribution would lie below and above the corresponding raw score. In this way you can use the z score to determine the *percentile* of any particular raw score (for example, the percentage of values equal to or less than that score). When a researcher reports an individual test score, it is sometimes more meaningful to give a z score or a percentile than to give just the raw score. From a z score, it is possible to express one person's test performance in relation to that of the whole group. Another value of the z score is its ability to compare scores on two different tests.

Measures of Contingency and Correlation

Contingency Tables Many nursing studies are not just *factor-isolating*, or one-variable, studies. Most of the time we are asking more complicated questions about the interrelationships among variables. "Is there a difference in the morbidity rates of people from different socioeconomic backgrounds?" "Is there a relationship between the attitudes of health care workers toward AIDS patients and the incidence of AIDS in their community?" "Do men and women have different attitudes about receiving intimate bodily care from male nurses than they do from female nurses?" All of these questions have this in common:

1. They deal with two or more categories (usually nominal or ordinal scales with only a few levels, or ranks).

2. The data consist of frequency counts that are tabulated and slotted into the appropriate cells of a table.

3. Answers to the research questions require that we cross-tabulate frequencies of the two variables under investigation.

The method for answering such questions is to construct a **contingency table**, a two-dimensional frequency distribution in which the frequencies of two variables are cross-tabulated.

If you were trying to determine whether reminiscence or remotivation groups were selected at different rates by clients 70 years of age and older versus those less than 70 years old, you could construct a simple contingency table by placing one variable (*age*) along the vertical axis and the other (*type of support group*) along the horizontal axis. You would then tabulate the number of subjects belonging in each cell of the table and compute percentages (see Table 14–5). A reader can then see at a glance that patients 70 years or older preferred the reminiscence group and patients under the age of 70 preferred the remotivation group.

TABLE 14–5 *Sample Contingency Table for Age-Type Group Preference (n = 60)*

	Reminiscence Group	Percentage	Remotivation Group	Percentage
70 years or over	40	66	20	33
Under 70 years	20	33	40	66

Measures of Correlation   Many aspects of our daily lives are influenced by associations or correlations between variables. For example, if you are an obese, city-dwelling, unmarried, cigarette-smoking man with a family history of heart disease, you may pay more for health insurance no matter what your health record is. This typical policy is based on strong correlations between heart attack rates and these variables.

A correlation addresses the question of the extent to which two variables are related. For example: "To what extent is cigarette smoking related to the incidence of lung cancer or emphysema?" "To what extent is a diet high in saturated fat related to gallbladder disease?" "To what extent is a positive attitude toward labor and delivery related to the attitude of one's partner?" These questions are answered by calculating a statistic, or index, that expresses the magnitude or degree of a relationship. These statistics may also be termed measures of association.

Correlational Statistics—*correlation coefficients*—vary between $+1$ and -1. A correlation of 0 indicates no relationship, whereas correlations approaching ± 1 indicate strong relationships or perfect correlations. The plus or minus sign indicates whether the correlation is positive or negative. A positive, direct relationship indicates that as the values of one variable become larger or smaller, so do the values of the other. A negative, inverse relationship indicates that as the values of one variable become large, the values of the other tend to become small. Table 14–6 illustrates some examples of correlation coefficients. A correlation that is published without a plus or minus sign is usually interpreted as positive; that is, $r = .66$ means $r = +.66$.

It is important to remember that correlation coefficients reflect relationship, not cause and effect. A strong correlation does not mean that one variable caused the other variable to change. There are many controversies about causation, but they are not solved with simple correlation statistics. For example, in a temperate climate, there is a correlation between the number of leaves on a tree and the temperature. We cannot say that the number of leaves caused a certain temperature. Nor is it strictly correct to state that the temperature caused a change in the number of leaves. We understand that the number of hours of daylight causes the change in number of leaves. Needless to say, the issue of causation can be intricate.

TABLE 14–6 *Sample Correlation Coefficients*

$+.99, +.90 +.88$	High positive correlation
$+.33, +.29 +.39$	Low positive correlation
$+.00, +.12 -.01$	No systematic correlation
$-.19, -.33 -.25$	Low negative correlation
$-.93, -.77 -.80$	High negative correlation

Perfect correlations are rarely found in research, including nursing research. In a study involving psychosocial variables, correlations between $+.50$ and $+.70$ or between $-.50$ and $-.70$ may be considered quite strong. However, in studies with biophysical variables rather than psychosocial ones (see Chapters 9 and 10), correlations of less than $+.85$ or $-.85$ may be considered weak. The value attributed to any particular correlation coefficient is quite situation specific. There are ways, however, to determine if a particular coefficient could be considered different from zero, with a specified probability level. Once this has been done, the determination of the degree of substantive or clinical significance is made by the researcher and within the context of the work in the field.

Researchers frequently report a quantity called the *coefficient of determination* to help interpret the strength of the correlation. The correlation coefficient is squared, and the resulting quantity expresses the amount of shared variance between the two variables—that is, how much you would know about variable *x* if you knew about variable *y*. For example, if a researcher knows that the correlation between two variables is $-.70$, then the coefficient of determination is .49 or 49%. Therefore, if the correlation between self-esteem and depression is $-.70$, then 49% of the difference in depression among people in the sample is accounted for by the differences in their self-esteem scores.

The graphic, or visual, presentation of a correlation between two variables is called a **scatter diagram**, or **scatter plot**. Each dot, *x*, or point represents the position of a subject on the *x*- and *y*-axis variables. A scatter diagram can reflect both the direction (positive or negative) and the approximate magnitude of a correlation. The more the dots resemble a straight line, the higher the correlation. When you can know a person's position on one variable because you know his or her position on the second, the correlation is called *perfect*. A perfect correlation (negative or positive) is depicted on a scatter diagram by a sloped straight line (see Figure 14–12).

The two most common correlation statistics are the *Pearson product-moment correlation* (or Pearson *r*) and the *Spearman rho*. The first is a parametric technique that requires continuous data such as weight, height, and time. The second is a nonparametric technique that requires only rank-order scales. Because the Spearman

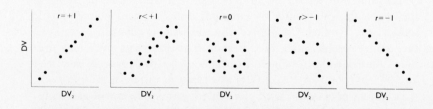

Figure 14–12   Sample scatter diagrams for different degrees of correlation between DVs.

correlation technique involves ranks, statisticians usually refer to it as the rank-order correlation technique. Both can be calculated with pencil and paper according to mathematical formulas, but most investigators use a computer to calculate and print these descriptive statistics (see Chapter 16).

Inferential Statistics

In the preceding section, you learned that one approach to analyzing quantitative data is to use descriptive statistics such as measures of central tendency, variation, and correlation to summarize the data set. Many nursing studies, however, are conducted for purposes that go beyond merely reporting characteristics of a particular sample of data. The investigators at the least want to report something about the descriptive characteristics of the population from which the sample was drawn. **Inferential statistics** are techniques that researchers use to generalize from the characteristics of a sample to the larger, unmeasured population from which that sample was drawn. We need to keep in mind that we don't know the "true" values from the population because we didn't measure all the subjects or values in the population. Rather, we are making a "best guess." The science of statistics helps us make the best guess and gives us a notion of how good a guess has been made. Estimation and hypothesis testing are the two basic types of inferential procedures. In the next chapter, we examine other advanced but related statistical tests, such as discriminant function analysis and factor analysis. These statistical procedures can be used in the context of either descriptive or experimental research investigations. (Certain correlational procedures are also used as inferential statistics when an alpha level is reported.)

Logic of Inferential Statistics

All inferential statistical tests are based on the assumption that chance is the only thing that produces variation among groups. Using a mathematical model, statisticians can calculate the probability that a statistic will assume a certain value if only chance is operating. Most tests are designed so that the larger the value of the statistic, the lower the probability of sampling error, chance, nonsystematic variation, or random error. So that researchers who use statistics don't have to keep recalculating the chance probabilities of different statistical tests over and over again, these values are available in tables. Most tables give probabilities such as 1 in 20 (.05), 1 in 100 (.01), or 1 in 1000 (.001) according to different sample sizes, because sample size is an important factor in calculating the accuracy of estimates. (See the section on power analysis in Chapter 8.)

Most inferential statistics let you reject the possibility that the results of a study are strictly due to chance whenever your statistical value is larger than the value you find in the tables (called the *critical value*). The *confidence level* listed in the table tells you how sure you can be rejecting that the difference between two groups was due to chance. Estimation and hypothesis testing are the two basic types of inferential procedures. These statistical procedures can be used in either descriptive or experimental research.

Inferring from a Sample to a Population

Suppose you want to know the average length of hospital stay for organ transplant patients in the United States. On the one hand, you could track every single patient admitted to an American hospital for this procedure, but your approach would be costly and time-consuming. If, on the other hand, you used the principles and procedures of inferential statistics, you could select a representative random sample from the population, calculate its mean length of hospital stay, and then make an inference about the mean length of hospital stay for the entire population. (See Chapter 8 to review the meaning of representative and random samples.) *Remember that inferential statistics are based on the assumption that the investigator has taken a random sample from the population.* You ought to find the sampling procedure reported in a journal article in one of the forms presented in Box 14–3.

Sampling Errors   Even when you infer characteristics of a population from a properly selected random and representative sample, there is always some chance that the actual mean of the population is slightly different from the means suggested in samples drawn from it. Remember that statistics are not about certainty but rather about likelihood of truth. If you calculate the mean for several different samples drawn from the same population, it is unlikely that they will all have identical means. The fluctuation of a statistic from one sample to another is called **sampling error**. Hypothetically, if you plot a frequency polygon of the means of all the

---

Box 14–3   Hypothetical Journal Excerpts Reporting on the Random Sampling Procedure

Twenty-five male and 25 female participants in prenatal classes were randomly selected from a population of 100 class members.

or

Twenty-five male and 25 female participants in a rural community health center's prenatal classes were randomly selected from a 100-member population by putting their names in an alphabetical list by first name, assigning consecutive numbers, and then selecting the sample using a table of random numbers.

possible samples that could be drawn from the population, you will end up with a *sampling distribution of the mean* and can then calculate the mean of the population based on the distribution of means in the frequency polygon. This notion, however, is really a theoretical one, because you would need to draw an infinite number of samples. Theoretically, though, statisticians tell us that the sampling distributions of means tend to follow a normal, or bell-shaped, curve. Therefore, you can calculate the standard deviation of a sampling distribution and reasonably assume that 68% of all the sample means fall between $+1$ and -1 standard deviations from the population's actual mean. The standard deviation of a theoretical frequency distribution of means of samples is called the **standard error of the mean**. The smaller the standard error, obviously, the more accurately a sample mean reflects a population mean.

Calculating the Standard Error of the Mean   Characteristics of a population can be inferred from just one random sample by using the following formula to calculate the standard error of the mean. The calculations can be done by hand calculator, but they are more often done by computer program.

$$s_{\bar{x}} = \frac{sd}{\sqrt{n}}$$

where sd =   the standard deviation of the sample
        n =   the sample size
        $s_{\bar{x}}$ =   the standard error of the mean

The important point about all this is that you can increase the accuracy of your estimate of a population's mean *by increasing the size of the sample* on which you calculate the standard deviation. When a small sample size is mentioned in a study critique or discussion of limitations, you know the criticism is justified because the accuracy of generalizing from the sample to the population is statistically questionable. There might be a point of "diminishing returns," however, in increasing the sample size to decrease the standard error of the mean. In the formula, $s_{\bar{x}}$ decreases in proportion to the square root of n. It is necessary to quadruple the size of the sample to decrease the standard error of the estimate by half. Other methods of decreasing the standard error of the mean estimate are linked to decreasing the standard deviation. This approach could be more profitable and cost-effective.

Estimation Procedures

Estimation procedures are used to find either *single value estimates* or **interval estimates** for population parameters. A **parameter** is a descriptive characteristic of a population, such as a mean or standard deviation. Some of these population parameters are analogous to the descriptive statistics previously discussed; in this case, however, the statistical term applies to the population, not the sample. It's important to examine these two estimates in more detail.

Point Estimation   First, **point estimation** is the use of a single value, determined from the sample, to approximate the population parameter. Two commonly used point estimates (parameter estimates) are the mean (a measure of central tendency) and the standard deviation (a measure of variability). As you recall, the formula for the standard deviation is slightly different when you are attempting to estimate the variability within the population.

Interval Estimation   Point estimators generally work well and are some of the most frequently cited research results. A word of caution, however: Point estimators fail to give some very useful information. The single number provides no information about the accuracy of the guess. Each random sample of the population probably contains different subsets of the larger population. The estimate of the mean, therefore, is likely to vary across these samples. The sampling distribution can be used to form an interval with a specified probability of containing the true value of the parameter. If we knew the interval within which our guess lies, we would know a great deal more about the guess itself. A large interval (in relation, of course, to the values in the sample) does not allow as good a guess as a small one. For example, if you're traveling between two cities, which of the two following statements about the duration of the flight gives more precise information?

1.   The average length of the flight is 5 hours. Over a number of flights, 95% fall within the range of 3 to 7 hours.

2.   The average length of the flight is 5 hours. Over a number of flights, 95% fall within the range of 4.5 to 5.5 hours.

Both airlines make the same guess or average about the population of flight times between city A and city B. Airline 1, however, is far less precise in its guess of how long it will take to fly between the two cities. All other things being equal, airline 2 is a better bet for getting you to city B in the time closest to 5 hours.

Consider another example. Suppose a researcher wants to report the amount of weight gained by premature infants in a given period of time. There are two groups of premature infants, ten infants in each group, each with a mean of 50 g gained (see Table 14–7). These are our best guesses of the population means based on these two samples. The group sizes have been kept small for ease of calculation, in case you want to check these figures. How accurate is the researcher with these two different groups? For purposes of this example, consider these two samples as two separate groups. Interval estimation gives information about the accuracy of the guess.

Interval estimation describes the use of a sample parameter to establish a range of values that will contain the true parameter of the population given a certain level

TABLE 14–7 *Confidence Interval Sample*

Weight gain for Group 1		Weight gain for Group 2	
Subject 1.1	65 g	Subject 2.1	42 g
Subject 1.2	35 g	Subject 2.2	45 g
Subject 1.3	68 g	Subject 2.3	46 g
Subject 1.4	32 g	Subject 2.4	47 g
Subject 1.5	44 g	Subject 2.5	49 g
Subject 1.6	61 g	Subject 2.6	51 g
Subject 1.7	56 g	Subject 2.7	53 g
Subject 1.8	58 g	Subject 2.8	54 g
Subject 1.9	42 g	Subject 2.9	55 g
Subject 1.10	39 g	Subject 2.10	58 g
$n = 10$		$n = 10$	
Mean $= 50$		Mean $= 50$	
sd $= 13.031$		sd $= 5.055$	
$s_x = \dfrac{13.031}{\sqrt{10}} = 4.137$		$s_x = \dfrac{5.055}{\sqrt{10}} = 1.599$	

of probability. The resultant range, with the upper and lower values specified, is a *confidence interval* (C.I.). These two extreme points are also known as the upper and lower bounds of the confidence interval. The term is appropriate because it provides a notion of how confident we can be that the proportion of correct statements, when the study is repeated many times, is equal to the probability level specified to establish the interval. The following example clarifies the notion of confidence intervals. Look at the elements of the confidence interval and then calculate two confidence intervals for the means of the groups in Table 14–7.

The confidence interval contains the following elements:

1. The point estimate of the sample parameter (in this case, the mean equals 50 for group 1).

2. The point estimate of the standard deviation of the sampling distribution (in this case, the standard error of the mean equals 4.137 for group 1).

3. The number of standard deviations in this distribution, containing the specified percent of the population

4. The sample size

5. Degree of confidence desired

These elements are put together in the following form, for our example.

$$P\left[\mu = \bar{x} \pm t\alpha_{(2),\nu}\, s_x\right] = 1 - \alpha$$

where μ = the population mean
$\bar{x}$ = the sample mean
α = the probability of a Type I error
ν = the degrees of freedom for the t value

(The t distribution is used for small samples from a normal distribution. If the sample is large, the standard normal distribution can be used.)

The numerical range inside the brackets is the **confidence interval** (C.I.). Although any confidence level can be used, it is common practice to use the 95% or 99% levels, just as is commonly done in hypothesis testing. The exact number of standard deviations in a t distribution with 9 degrees of freedom that contain 95% of the value is 2.262. For 99% of the values, 3.25 standard deviations are required.

Now fill in the values in the confidence interval statement for group 1, using the 95% level.

$$P\left[\mu = 50 \pm 2.262(4.137)\right] = 1 - .05$$

$$P[\mu = 50 \pm 9.36] = .95$$

To compute the lower bound:

$$L_B = 50 - 9.36 = 40.64$$

To compute the upper bound:

$$U_B = 50 + 9.36 = 59.36$$

Now you can state the whole range with a little manipulation of the formula. You can see, however, that it is just like the original statement, but now μ is placed in the center of the range.

$$P\left[\,40.64 < \mu < 59.36\,\right] = 95\%$$

For group 1, it can be said that, on repeated sampling, our estimate of μ will fall within the range of 40.64 and 59.36 95% of the time. Perhaps we want to eliminate some of the chance that we are wrong by setting a level of 99%. Use the same process but substitute 3.25 for 2.262:

$$P\left[\mu = 50 \pm 3.25(4.137)\right] = 1 - .01$$
$$P\left[\mu = 50 \pm 13.45\right] = .99$$
$$L_B: 50 - 13.45 = 36.55$$
$$U_B: 50 + 13.45 = 63.45$$

Now compare the 95% and 99% C.I. for groups 1 and 2. (You can do the arithmetic on your own; we provide only the final ranges.) The C.I.s for the 95% and 99% levels are $46.38 < \mu < 53.62$ and $44.80 < \mu < 55.20$, respectively. The second group has a much narrower confidence interval at both the 95% and 99% levels. If you were making a decision, you would probably feel more comfortable with the decision if group 2 were involved, even though the means are the same.

Your increased confidence reflects the fact that the interval has an inherent association with accuracy. Some of the elements in a C.I. are not changeable, but some definitely are. Sample size, standard deviation, and degree of confidence are key determinants of the length of the C.I. The three following relationships hold:

1. Variability and length of the C.I. are positively related.

2. Sample size and length of the C.I. are negatively related.

3. Level of confidence and length of the C.I. are positively related.

First, if variability is decreased by decreasing errors, for instance, in design, measurement, or sampling, the length of the C.I. also decreases. Second, as sample size increases, the length of the C.I. decreases. This becomes clear when you look at how the standard error is estimated. Try several examples in which you vary only the sample size. Third, if you accept a lower level of confidence about the statement and thereby incur a greater risk of error, the length of the confidence interval decreases. As you can see, there is no single way to proceed to obtain the smallest confidence interval. If you are really concerned with accuracy, you may be unwilling to lower your confidence level to achieve the smaller interval. You may instead want to investigate another strategy, such as decreasing measurement error, while keeping the confidence level high.

Hypotheses Tests

Estimating the parameters of a population is one major use of inferential statistics. *Testing hypotheses* is the other major use. Usually a researcher uses inferential statistics to compare two or more groups to find out if the corresponding populations are similar. For instance, Hathaway and Geden (1983), in a study of energy expenditure during three types of exercise program, used an inferential statistical procedure called analysis of variance (ANOVA) to demonstrate that groups were not similar in oxygen consumption and heart rate. In fact, for these variables, the isometric and active exercise programs were significantly more demanding than the passive or rest programs. Statistical procedures give investigators a way to decide whether a study's outcomes reflect true population differences or whether an apparent difference is due only to chance and not likely to happen again.

Hanson and Chater (1983) studied role selection by nurses, examining the relationship between interest in management roles and certain personality, demographic, and career background characteristics of 122 female nurses. The authors used a multivariate analysis of variance (MANOVA). Their analysis showed that, at a .05 confidence level, 7 of the 11 scales of the vocational preference inventory differentiated the management from nonmanagement groups (a distinction that was based on their scores on the business management scale of the Strong-Campbell Interest Inventory). Their findings allowed them to conclude that those who exhibited managerial interests were more practical minded, sociable, conforming, dominant, and expressive and had more occupational interests than those who did not exhibit such interest. Differences between the two groups on the 19 demographic and career background variables were not statistically significant.

Steps in Using Inferential Statistics to Test Hypotheses

Step 1: State the Null Hypothesis   The rules of statistical hypothesis testing are based on what might at first seem strange logic. They allow you to reject the idea that any difference you find between groups is due to chance or error, rather than allowing you to prove that there is a real relationship between the variables you are studying. The initial step in testing a hypothesis is to set up a null hypothesis. The **null hypothesis** is a statement that no difference exists between the populations being compared (see Chapter 8). This is essentially a statement that explains a study's results as being due *only* to chance factors or sampling error. The results of the statistical test are then stated in terms of the probability that the null hypothesis is false. The hypothesis, or opposite of the null hypothesis, is sometimes called the *alternate hypothesis* in research articles. If testing the null hypothesis shows that there is no difference, the hypothesis, or alternative hypothesis, indicates that there *is* a difference between groups being studied that is not due to chance alone.

In formulaic terms the null hypothesis (H_0) predicts that the population mean for one group $A(M_A)$ is the same as the population mean for group $B(M_B)$:

$$H_0 \, M_A = M_B$$

Using a stratified random sample of 130 patients from three hospital units, Nichols, Barstow, and Cooper (1983) tested the relationship between frequency of changing IV tubing and percutaneous sites and the incidence of phlebitis. They found that there were no significant differences in rates of phlebitis whether tubings were changed every 24 or 48 hours or whether sites were changed every 48 or 72 hours. Their null hypotheses were stated as follows:

Null Hypotheses:

There will be no difference in the incidence of phlebitis between the three treatment groups.

Group 1: IV tubing changed every 24 hours, percutaneous site changed every 48 hours.

Group 2: IV tubing changed every 24 hours, percutaneous site changed every 72 hours.

Group 3: IV tubing changed every 48 hours, percutaneous site changed every 72 hours.

Step 2: Select a Level of Significance   The level of significance is a probability that tells you how unlikely the sample data must be before you can reject the null hypothesis. In other words, when you reject a null hypothesis, you need to know what the chances are that you are making a mistake in doing so. You can make two kinds of mistakes: A **Type I error** (alpha error) is committed when you conclude that the null hypothesis is false when it is really true. That is, you conclude that the difference is not due to chance when in fact it is. Reid (1983) comments that the most prevalent statistical problems in the nursing literature that reflect the lack of protection against Type I errors are:

1. initial use of a *t*-test to compare more than one set of means

2. use of the *t*-test for comparison of Pearson correlation coefficients

3. use of univariate statistical tests when multivariate statistical procedures are more appropriate (see Chapter 15).

Type II (beta) errors occur when you conclude that the differences were due to chance when in fact they were not.

For most studies, a level of significance of $p = .05$ (a 1 in 20 chance of being wrong) is the maximum risk investigators are willing to accept for making a Type I error. A level of .01 (1 in 100 chance of being wrong) or .001 (1 in 1000 chance of being wrong) means that the likelihood that you are mistaken in rejecting the null hypothesis is lower. In journal articles, the level of statistical significance is sometimes called the *level of probability*. Finally, the .95 *level of confidence* refers to the same thing as the .05 level of significance, except it is stated backward. As should be clear from the preceding discussion, the harder a researcher tries to lower the risk of committing a Type I error, the greater the risk of committing a Type II error. In other words, if you use strict criteria to reject the null hypotheses, you increase the chance that you accept a false one. The best balance forces a thoughtful investigator to consider in advance all the important measurement, scaling, sampling, and statistical considerations important to this issue.

One more aspect of error levels must be taken into account. The experimentwise error is just as important as Type I and Type II errors. *Experimentwise* error refers to the level of the Type I error rate per group of related hypotheses per experiment, that is, the probability that at least one Type I error will occur among the set of related hypotheses. *Protecting the alpha* refers to maintaining a given probability of a Type I error (α) for the set of hypotheses per experiment. The particular level of α may be .05, .01, or some other predetermined level. Suppose you have three different groups in your experiment. In each comparison between group 1 and 2, group 1 and 3, and group 2 and 3, the Type I error rate (α) could be held at .05. However, when you consider the set of hypotheses, this rate no longer holds true. Special tables give exact probabilities for experimentwise error rates. A rough approximation based on the *Bonferroni inequality*, however, can be used:

$$\sum \alpha_i = \exp$$

In other words, the experimentwise error rate is roughly equivalent to the sum of the Type I error rates for the individual tests. In the example above, the experimentwise error rate is .15 (.05 + .05 + .05). If you do not want to use one of the multivariate statistics, you could protect your alpha by setting the experimentwise error rate at .05:

$$\sum \alpha_i = .05$$

Since there are three groups, the sum of the alphas ($\Sigma \alpha$) is

$$\frac{.05}{3} = \alpha$$
$$.0167 = \alpha$$

You could, of course, alter the alpha for any given hypothesis as long as you kept the sum at .05. See Reid (1983) for a discussion of this procedure.

Step 3: Look Up a Test's Significance in a Table In addition to knowing the name of the test performed, you need some information to look up the statistical significance or critical value of a calculated statistic in a table, be it a z table, t table, f table, or X^2 table. The first piece of information you need is the *degrees of freedom*. In general, degrees of freedom are based on the n used to calculate the statistic minus the number of restrictions placed on the observations to vary. For example, in a sample of ten cases with a specified mean, once the ninth case is determined, the tenth case can have only one value and cannot vary from that value. Therefore, $n - 1$ is the *df* in that case. The second piece of information needed is the confidence level (.01, .05, or .001) of the test statistic for whatever degree of freedom you decide on. The **critical value** for a specified degree of freedom and confidence level is the value of the test statistic that needs to be exceeded by the calculated statistic in order for the null hypothesis to be rejected. You find the critical value in statistical tables.

Step 4: Choose the Right Statistical Test Most statistical tests used in hypothesis testing by nurse researchers are classified into two types: **parametric statistics** and **nonparametric statistics**. Parametric tests have three important characteristics:

1. They involve the estimation of at least one parameter.

2. They require measurements on *at least an interval-level measurement scale.*

3. They involve the assumption that the variables are normally distributed (according to a bell-shaped curve) in the population, suggesting that *a sample size of at least 20 scores per cell is essential.* Given a normal distribution, parametric tests are considered more powerful than nonparametric ones, and therefore are preferred by most nurse researchers who are analyzing numerical data. *t*-tests and analysis of variance (ANOVA) are discussed in the pages that follow.

If the assumptions for parametric tests cannot be met, the second type of statistic is used. The nonparametric statistic is not based on the same assumptions, but instead it:

1. can be used with nominal and ordinal measurements

2. can be used when the sample size is small and there is no reason to assume that the scores follow a bell-shaped curve or normal distribution

---

Putt (1977) studied the effects of noise on fatigue in healthy middle-aged adults. The term *fatigue* was defined to include an identifiable set of body processes that underlie complex relations between the organism (person) and the environment, with an orientation toward demands of some sort being made on the organism. Putt studied a sample of 60 healthy adults to look at whether *rest* as a nursing intervention made any difference in perception of energy expenditure after performance of a psychomotor test. She also studied whether a noisy background made a difference. She used *t*-tests of group means for effects on each of the two variables under investigation. Although Donaldson (1977) presented a strong critique of some of the Putt study's conceptual underpinning, the study did illustrate the basic and most familiar parametric procedure for testing the differences in group means—the *t*-test. Most nurse researchers choose to use a computer to calculate *t*-tests on their data (see Chapter 16).

The *t*-Test

The ***t*-test** is designed to examine differences in two means. These may be means from two different groups, from one group at two different times, or from one group compared to a prespecified mean. If there are two groups involved, an important assumption is that the variances from these groups are equal. If the variances are not equal, you need to use a modified *t*-test, such as the Smith-Satterthwaite. On most computer printouts, pooled variances are given. If the variances are not equal, an unpooled variance test (e.g., Smith-Satterthwaite) must be used.

When you use *t*-tests, you have to decide whether you need to be sensitive to differences in either direction (greater or less). The *one-tailed t*-test is sensitive to differences in only one direction. When the direction of difference between populations is unknown to the researcher, it makes more sense to use a *two-tailed* test. For example, in testing a specific group intervention program against a placebo (or just a spontaneously informal group exchange), you wouldn't know which direction of difference was significant and therefore might choose a two-tailed test. When you want to reject the null hypothesis for any difference in means, be it positive or negative, you use a nondirectional two-tailed *t*-test.

t-Test for Paired Samples   In either a *within-subjects design* or a *matched-groups design*, a score in one situation can be paired with a score in another. In a within-subjects pretest and posttest design, you have a prescore and postscore for each respondent. You can then figure out the effect of a nursing intervention by testing whether you have statistically significant differences between the pretest and posttest mean scores. In a matched-groups design, a score in one situation can be paired with a score in another, and you can figure out the effect of intervention by estimating the difference for each pair. This statistic is often used in nursing studies that don't have control or experimental groups. Instead, the researchers compare values or scores of a sample before an intervention (biofeedback training, for instance) with scores after the intervention. The procedure involves comparing the pretest and posttest measures using an equation for paired-measure *t*-tests and then comparing the computed value of *t* with the *t* values in a table. For this kind of *t*-test, the degrees of freedom are equal to the number of pairs minus 1 ($df = n - 1$). Before you actually do the calculations, be sure you are using the correct *t* formula for the study. Find these formulas in a good statistics book, or get advice from a statistical consultant.

Advantages and Disadvantages of a One-Tailed t-Test   The major advantage of a one-tailed *t*-test is that a smaller difference between the means of two groups is statistically significant. But its disadvantage is that you have to redo the experiment to deal with the unexpected outcome of a large negative effect of the independent variable. You are not supposed to change your hypotheses after the fact to account for results that are the opposite of what you expected. Therefore, it makes sense to use one-tailed *t*-tests when you have good reason to expect the direction of a relationship or when you don't care about a result that goes in the opposite direction. Good reporting requires that you explain whether you've done a two-tailed or one-tailed test and give the rationale for doing so.

When the study involves a very small sample or the distribution of scores does not approximate a bell-shaped curve, a few nonparametric statistical tests can be used to calculate the differences between groups. Two of them are summarized in Table 14–8. If you are using computer software to test your hypotheses (see Chapter 16), you need only select the statistical operation and give the command.

TABLE 14–8 *Nonparametric Statistical Tests*

Name	Purpose	Rationale for Use
Mann-Whitney U test	Nonparametric test for determining difference between means of two samples Requires ordinal-level data and independent samples	Tends to be more powerful than others because it uses more aspects of the data
Wilcoxon matched pairs signed-rank test	Involves taking the difference between a pair of scores and ranking the absolute difference Requires ordinal level measures within and between groups	Is very simple to compute

Analysis of Variance

A one-way **analysis of variance** (abbreviated ANOVA) is an inferential statistical procedure that has about the same purpose as a *t*-test, that is, to compare the mean scores of two groups. The difference between an ANOVA and a *t*-test is that the *t*-test is used for comparing two groups, whereas a one-way ANOVA can be used to compare two or more groups. Because the ANOVA can be used with a greater number of groups, it is considered to be a more versatile statistical procedure. Also, because ANOVA alternative hypotheses do not state a direction, you don't have to worry about making one-tailed or two-tailed comparisons, as you do with the *t*-test. You do have to worry about the assumption of equal variances for each group. A commonly used statistic, Bartlett's test, examines the variances in each group and tests for equality. Furthermore, control of experimentwise error rate occurs within the context of an ANOVA and the subsequent post hoc tests.

Calculating the F Ratio   Using an ANOVA involves calculating the F ratio and then checking the value of that statistic against a table of F values for its statistical significance. Calculating an analysis of variance consists of obtaining two independent estimates of variance. One is based on the variability between groups (between-group variance, or s^2B), and the other is based on the variability within groups (within-group variance, or s^2W). If the between-group variance is large relative to the within-group variance, the F ratio is large, and the null hypothesis is rejected. If the between-group variance is small relative to the within-group variance, the F ratio is small, and the null hypothesis is more likely to be accepted.

A basic concept in calculating the F ratio in ANOVA is the *sum of squares*. The formula for analysis of variance divides the total sum of squares into the within-group sum of squares and the between-group sum of squares. To obtain variance estimates from these two numbers, you divide each by the appropriate degrees of freedom (usually $n - k$ and $k - 1$, where k = number of groups). The final operation with ANOVA is calculating the actual F ratio to determine whether the two or more variance estimates could have been drawn from the same population. If not, then you can conclude that the experimental treatments produced a significant difference between the means. The formula for the F ratio is the between-group variance estimate divided by the within-group variance estimate, or:

$$F = \frac{s^2 B}{s^2 W}$$

where: $F = F$ ratio
   $s^2 B$ = between-group sum of squares
   $s^2 W$ = within-group sum of squares.

When a study examines dependent variables from more than two conditions—for example, Norris and her colleagues' (1982) study of the effects of three nursing procedures (suctioning, repositioning, and a heel stick) on blood oxygen levels in premature infants—the researchers need some way to determine whether variation of the sample means was too large to be accounted for by repeated random sampling from one population. Rephrased in the opposite terms, researchers need some way of knowing if the independent variables, or experimental conditions, had differential effects on the dependent variable. In the Norris study the investigators wanted to know if the effects of the three routine nursing procedures differentially affected the blood oxygen levels in sick premature infants (DV = transcutaneous oxygen measured with a $TcpO_2$ monitor). They used an ANOVA to compare variances of the sample means with an estimate of the variance of the population of 25 babies who weighed less than or equal to 1900 g at birth and were diagnosed with respiratory distress syndrome in a neonatal intensive care unit.

The population variance is estimated by combining the variances of the individual samples. If the variance of the means is close in value to the estimated population variance, then the researchers assume that all the means come from samples of the same population. If the variance of the means is larger than the estimated population variance (as in the Norris study), then the researchers conclude that at least some of the means come from different populations. This finding indicates that the independent variables are having a real differential effect on the dependent variable. Norris and her associates found that $TcpO_2$ was decreased significantly during suctioning and repositioning of the babies but not during the heel stick and that the three nursing procedures had different degrees of change. Suctioning elicited the greatest decrease in $TcpO_2$, followed by repositioning and then heel stick. These results suggested that the type of procedure determined the sick infants' response. F ratios of $F = 27.01$, $p \leq .0001$, for suctioning and $F = 8.01$, $p \leq .001$, for positioning were calculated. ANOVA of the $TcpO_2$ trends during heel stick indicated that this condition did not differ significantly from the estimated population mean (p. 333).

TABLE 14–9 *ANOVA Summary Table for Experiment Comparing Different Item Arrangements*

Source	df	SS	MS	F
Test forms (IV)	2	16	8	4
Between group (error)	15	30	2	
Total	17	46		

Interpreting *F* Ratios from an ANOVA Summary Table It is harder to calculate *F* ratios than *t* values, and therefore most nurse researchers use computer programs to do the actual calculations. The results are usually presented in a summary table. To understand how ANOVA works and to get experience in reading ANOVA findings, practice with a hypothetical table.

Table 14–9 has five columns: *source, df, SS* (for sum of squares), *MS* (for mean square), and *F*. Under the first column are the names of the three rows. The first row is the name of the independent variable, in this case, *test forms for a nursing theory exam*. Another common name for the first row is *between-group*. The second row is usually labeled *within-group* or *error term*, and the third row is labeled *total*.

The numbers in the column labeled *df* (degrees of freedom) are computed by subtracting 1 from the number of different groups involved in the study. Like the Norris study of premature infants, this hypothetical study has three groups, so the test form source of the between-group row has 2 degrees of freedom. The degrees of freedom allow us to find the critical value for a test statistic in a table at a particular probability of the null hypothesis being true. To get the total *df*, simply subtract 1 from the total number of subjects, resulting in 17. To get the within-group *df*, simply subtract the *df* in the first row from the total, yielding $17 - 2$, or 15.

The various sums of squares (*SS*) are calculated using a relatively complex formula. But in reading a table like this or in constructing one, remember that the bottom number in the column, or total *SS*, should be equal to the sum of the other two *SS*. Most *SS* in reported nursing studies contain a decimal point, but whole numbers are used in the hypothetical table for ease of understanding.

The values in the column for the mean square (*MS*) are found by dividing the *SS* by the *df* found in the same row. There are only two values in the *MS* column, and if an author puts one in the *total* row, he or she has made a mistake.

The most important number is the single value in the *F* column, because it is this value, when compared with the critical values for *F* in a statistical table like the one simulated in Table 14–10, that permits you to reach a decision about accepting or rejecting a study's null hypothesis. The investigator looks up the between-group *df* (2) and the within-group *df* (15) at the approximate alpha level to find the critical value for *F*. If the *F* ratio that has been calculated is *larger* than the critical value at the appropriate place on the *F* table, then there is a statistically significant difference between the sample means. You can then conclude that the null hypothesis (that the groups are from the same population) should be rejected and that there is indeed a difference at a specified level of certainty that can be attributed to the different treatments, interventions, or procedures that make up the study's independent variable. Authors of research articles often emphasize this finding in their report by putting an asterisk next to the calculated *F* value in the summary table and indicate under the table the level of significance, for example, $p = .05$. Some *F* tables give critical values for two levels of significance in the same table by listing the higher level in parentheses or in a different size of type.

Follow-Up Multiple Comparison Tests   If you conduct a study using a one-way ANOVA to compare three groups and obtain an *F* ratio that is significant enough to reject the null hypothesis of equal means, you still don't know which of the means are different from the others. A number of statistical tests called *multiple comparisons*, or *post hoc comparisons*, help the investigator locate exactly where the significant differences lie after a significant overall *F* ratio has been obtained. These techniques are named after the people who developed them and include:

TABLE 14–10   *Critical Values for* F

df for Within-Groups	*df* for Between-Groups					
	2	**4**	**6**	**8**	**10**	**20**
5	5.89 (13.4)	5.29 (11.5)	5.05 (10.8)	4.92 (10.4)	4.87 (10.2)	4.66 (9.65)
10	4.20 (7.66)	3.58 (6.09)	3.32 (5.49)	3.17 (5.16)	3.07 (4.95)	2.87 (4.51)
15	3.78 (6.46)	3.16 (4.99)	2.89 (4.42)	2.74 (4.10)	2.65 (3.90)	2.43 (3.46)
20	3.59 (5.95)	2.97 (4.53)	2.70 (3.97)	2.55 (3.66)	2.45 (3.47)	2.22 (3.04)
40	3.33 (5.28)	2.71 (3.93)	2.44 (3.39)	2.28 (3.09)	2.17 (2.90)	1.94 (2.47)
120	3.17 (4.89)	2.55 (3.58)	2.28 (3.06)	2.12 (2.76)	2.00 (2.57)	1.75 (2.13)

- Fisher's LSD

- Duncan's new multiple range test

- Newman-Keuls

- Turkey's HSD

- Scheffe's test

Why Not Just Do Repeated t-Tests?   Although these multiple comparison procedures are a lot like applying several *t*-tests to the data following a significant *F* ratio, they differ in one important way—they control for *experimentwise* error rate. A *liberal* multiple comparison test will find a significant difference between means that are relatively close together. The Fisher's LSD is the most liberal of the tests mentioned above. A *conservative* comparison test will find differences only when the means are far apart. Of the comparison tests listed above, Scheffe's is the most conservative. Only Scheffe's test is appropriate for comparison of groups of unequal size. Those of you reading or writing about multiple comparison results may not find these reported in tables but rather will find the results of multiple comparisons reported in the text of a research article. There are a number of different ANOVA designs. The one-way ANOVA is the least complex. We review several others in Chapter 15.

Simple Linear Regression

Regression versus Correlation   The relationship of two variables to each other may be one of functional dependence. That is, the value of one variable is determined by the value of the other variable. For example, you may be interested in examining the relationship between number of weeks of prenatal care and weight of infants at birth. You could collect data on the two variables and use a Pearson correlation coefficient to describe that relationship. It might be reasonable, however, to consider birth weight a dependent variable. The expectation is that the weight of the infant at birth is a function of, or is partially determined by, the number of weeks of prenatal care. The opposite, of course, does not make sense; because, at least in this instance, there is a clear time order. A simple linear regression provides the tool for estimating the value of the dependent variable based on knowledge of the independent variable.

   The dependent relationship is termed the *regression*, and the term *simple* refers to the fact that only two variables are involved. In this procedure, there is a determination that one of these two variables is the dependent variable and the other is the independent variable. One can determine the value of the dependent variable from given values of the independent variable. If it is not reasonable to assume such dependency in the relationship, it is appropriate to use a correlational procedure.

   Linear regression describes a line of "best fit" that most closely defines the data points in the study. Think back to the scatter diagrams that accompanied the description of the Pearson correlation coefficient (see page 527). A straight line could be drawn through the clustered points so that the sum of the distances between any given observed point and the line was minimized. This minimization is called the concept of *least squares*. Obviously, many lines could be drawn through the data points; however, the one that minimizes the distances between the predicted point on the line and the observed point is the *"best fit" line*. If you were to overlay this line on the scatter diagram of observed points, as in Figure 14–13, you could make a judgment about how well the predictions fit the data. Figure 14–13A shows a scatter diagram and regression line with very poor fit. The distances between the observed points and the line are great, and summing those distances would yield a large error value. In Figure 14–13B, the fit is excellent. The observed points fall almost directly on the line, and summing those distances would yield a very small error term. In Figure 14–13C, a more realistic picture is shown of what regression lines normally do. Some observations are quite close to the prediction, and some are far away. The distances or error terms have a distribution. In Chapter 15, we review the assumptions underlying that distribution because they are important considerations in judging whether the statistic was used appropriately.

Of course, once this line is drawn, you must be able to describe its location very accurately. To do so, you use an equation for a straight line. This is the standard equation for describing the best-fit line in linear regression:

$$Y = a + bx + e$$

where a = estimate of alpha
        b = estimate of beta
        e = estimate of epsilon

Alpha (α), beta (β), and epsilon (ϵ) are population parameters. Of course, the only way to obtain these parameters is to have data on the entire population. Since

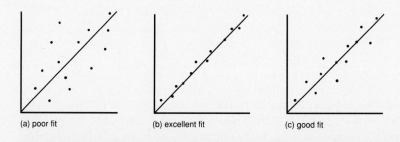

(a) poor fit   (b) excellent fit   (c) good fit

Figure 14–13   Placing the "best fit" line: (a) poor fit; (b) excellent fit; (c) good fit

this is not usually possible, estimates of these parameters are made based on the sample obtained for the study.

Alpha is called the *Y* intercept. Any of the many lines that could be drawn needs to start at a fixed point; otherwise, the line could not be uniquely described. In essence, this value for alpha anchors the line and is the constant in the equation. Although the *x* value varies by subject, the constant always remains the same, and each subject line starts there. It can be shown that the constant is the mean for the group. In other words, if we knew nothing else about the prenatal care, our best guess of an infant's weight would be the mean of the group.

Beta, or the regression coefficient, defines the slope of the line. This is the second important piece of information we need to define the line uniquely in space. Neither the constant nor the slope alone gives complete information; but with the two we can use this equation to predict birth weight from our knowledge of weeks of prenatal care. Epsilon stands for the population error terms, which should be equal to zero if the estimation is perfect. In most of our regression equations, there are error terms because there is a difference between the predicted value and the actual value. The term for the predicted value of the dependent variable is *Y hat*, $\hat{Y}$. The difference between the observed *Y* and $\hat{Y}$ equals the error term:

$$e_i = Y_i - \hat{Y}_i$$

The sum of the error terms is sometimes called the *residual sum of squares* or the *error sum of squares*.

Prediction   Now that we have all the pieces of information, what can we do with them? One thing we can do is predict an infant's weight. We can even know a bit about how accurate our prediction will be. The coefficient of determination, or explained variance, is also used in linear regression. We can interpret it by stating that an r^2 of a certain magnitude was obtained. A statistical procedure, the *F* test, determines whether the amount of explained variance is sufficiently greater than zero. We discuss this test in the section on ANOVA.

Furthermore, we can use the prediction equation to make predictions about other subjects from the population who were not included in the sample. This can be a powerful tool. With it, we could predict birth weights of babies whose mothers had very little prenatal care versus birth weights of babies whose mothers had much more. These statistics lend weight to, but don't prove, the argument that nursing interventions in the area of prenatal care are effective.

Cautions   Several words of caution are in order. First, it is unsafe to predict values outside the observed range. For example, if your sample includes only women who received prenatal care between 6 and 8 months of pregnancy, it is dangerous to extrapolate infant birth weights of babies born to mothers who received prenatal care at 4 months. In part, this is because we have based our estimation only on the range of observations in our sample. Beyond that sample the relationship might not even be linear; we cannot predict it.

Additionally, although we have assumed a mathematically dependent relationship, we have gathered no information about a cause-and-effect relationship. Causal relationships require more stringent assumptions and as such cannot be determined by statistical testing alone. Observed predictive relationships may be very useful in studying phenomena, but another variable altogether may be causing the observed change in the two variables in the regression.

Last, even if a regression function explains a relationship fairly well, it may still be an imperfect representation of the real world. This does not mean the regression is not useful, but we should not be lulled into complacency by finding a high R^2. The relationship may not be an adequate measure of reality. As an approximation, however, it may serve us well.

Nonparametric Statistical Tests

The statistical tests of inference that we have discussed thus far all rely on two important assumptions: (1) that the population distribution from which the samples were drawn conforms to a normal, or bell-shaped, probability curve and (2) that the data collected are interval- or ratio-level scales of measurement. Many nursing studies, however, focus on variables that don't conform to these two assumptions. A study that ranks patients in terms of their cooperativeness with a health care regimen is an example. The data would be ordinal, not interval or ratio, data and would not necessarily be distributed according to a bell-shaped curve. Clearly, parametric statistics would not apply, and the investigator would have to choose a statistical test appropriate to the data.

Nonparametric tests are those statistical tests that make no assumptions about the shape of the population distribution, and they are therefore called *distribution-free* tests. Different nonparametric statistical tests have been devised for few-category and many-category situations as well as for different designs. Some of the tests for ordinal data have a version for small samples (fewer than 20) and one for large samples. For analysis of data involving nominal, ordinal, or nonnormally distributed interval dependent variable scales, you'll need to refer to a good nonparametric statistics book. One classic is Siegal's (1956) *Nonparametric Statistics for the Behavioral Sciences*. Remember, when choosing a statistical test or when reading about the choice another researcher has made, that using parametric statistics when they don't apply can lead to mistaken conclusions. But using nonparametric statistics when parametric statistics are appropriate can mean that a less powerful test has been used, and the results may be an underestimation. Usually, the underestimation is not extreme.

Hints for Using Nonparametric Procedures   Saslow (1982) offers the following hints for doing nonparametric statistical tests.* These suggestions hold for parametric tests as well.

---

*Source: Based on C. A. Saslow, *Basic Research Methods*, New York: Random House, 1982, p. 246.

1. If you are unfamiliar with a particular test, read the introductory material carefully to see whether the test is right for your study.

2. If you decide to use the test, work through at least one example that is close to your study situation.

3. Be sure you understand the instructions for using a particular table for the test. There are many different formats for statistical tables, even for the same test.

4. Remember that selecting the correct statistical test for your data is more important than being able to do the actual calculations. These can be done by computer.

The Chi-Square for Nominal Data The **chi-square** (X^2) is a frequently used nonparametric statistic reported in the nursing research literature. This test can be used when your data are nominally scaled and you are interested in the number of responses, objects, or people that fall in two or more categories. The chi-square is calculated from the differences between observed frequencies and the frequencies expected under the conditions of the null hypothesis. Sometimes it has been called the "goodness of fit" statistic. *Goodness of fit* refers to whether a significant difference exists between an observed number and an expected number of classes or scores that fall into the nominal categories set out by the investigator. The expected number is what you would expect by chance or according to the null hypothesis. When the discrepancy is large between what turns up in your data and what you would expect to occur by chance, the chi-square statistic is large. If it exceeds the critical value in a chi-square table, taking into account its degrees of freedom, you can reject the null hypothesis and accept the alternative hypothesis.

The chi-square test is relatively easy to do, with only a few things to watch out for, according to Saslow (1982):*

1. Be sure to set up your null hypothesis correctly so that you know what you are rejecting. Whether you want a large or small difference depends on your research question.

2. If your sample size is too small, you might have to use a variation of the chi-square test (the smallest expected frequency must be 5 or more).

3. If your degrees of freedom are small (equal to 1), you will have to use a correction factor. (This involves subtracting one-half from each difference score before squaring.)

---

*Source: Based on C. A. Saslow, *Basic Research Methods*, New York: Random House, 1982.

The chi-square was used in a study of the effects of electrical surface stimulation on the prevention of atelectasis in experimental and control patients having abdominal surgery.

Menzel and Martinson (1977) focused on the effectiveness of electrical surface stimulation in controlling postoperative pain. But they were also interested in seeing whether the use of electrical stimulation near surgical wounds could alleviate the postoperative complication of atelectasis. A double-blind study of 27 adults who had had large abdominal incisions was conducted, and the patients were randomly assigned to experimental and control groups. The parameter of the presence or absence of atelectasis during the first 48 postoperative hours (nominal data) was included, based on the assumption that if patients were getting relief for their incisional pain from the electrical stimulation, they would then be better able to turn, cough, and hyperventilate, thereby preventing the accumulation of infiltrate in their lungs. Their findings on this parameter using the chi-square test showed that the day-1 and day-2 combined percentages for the experimental and control patient groups revealed no significant difference at the $p = .05$ level. Usually you determine that each group has a 50% chance of being in the category. After the observed numbers are obtained, a formula is used to calculate an χ^2 statistic, or you use a computer software package to calculate it for you.

To recapitulate:

- Chi-square is an inferential statistic that can be used with nominally scaled dependent variables (*yes* or *no, presence* or *absence*).

- A one-way chi-square test compares an observed frequency with the frequency expected by chance.

- The degrees of freedom for a one-way chi-square are the number of dependent variable categories minus 1.

- A two-way chi-square test can determine whether the frequency distributions of two variables are independent of each other.

- When there is only 1 degree of freedom for chi-square, a correction factor must be added to the chi-square formula.

- The chi-square test requires that there be a minimum expected frequency of 5 in any category. Meeting this requirement can involve combining categories or measuring larger samples.

- For repeated measures of the same subjects on the same dependent variable, a special variant of the chi-square test is needed, the McNemar or Cochran Q test (Siegal 1956 pp. 63, 161).

Guidelines for Choosing the Right Statistical Test

Choosing the correct descriptive or inferential statistical operation to use in your study involves knowing the answers to a few important questions:

1. You need to know on what level of scale the data for a dependent variable was measured.

2. You need to know whether you are working with a normal, or bell-shaped, distribution.

3. You need to know the details of your study design.

4. You need to understand your research question or hypotheses.

Saslow (1982) offers the decision tree in Figure 14–14 for choosing a statistical test correctly or for determining whether studies that you read in the research literature have employed statistical tools according to the rules. An investigator must sometimes consider using multivariate or more advanced and complex statistical procedures. This occurs when a study is intended to untangle relationships among three or more variables. These procedures include multiple correlation regressions (simultaneous, stepwise, and hierarchical), analysis of covariance, factor analysis, and discriminant analysis. These procedures are discussed in Chapter 15.

Guidelines for Critique

■ What is the level of measurement for the data collected? Are the statistical tests chosen to analyze the data appropriate to the level of measurement?

■ Are appropriate descriptive statistics reported for the data collected? Are there measures of dispersion reported for each variable and is it consistent for the measure of central tendency selected?

■ Are the statistical tests to be used in the research appropriately described with sufficient information to support their use?

■ Are the statistical tests used in the research consistent with the aims or hypotheses of the study?

■ Is the appropriate inferential statistic chosen for hypothesis testing?

■ If statistical hypothesis testing is used, were appropriate levels of significance stated?

■ Is the data presented in an easily understandable form? Do tables contain all information necessary to judge the validity of analysis?

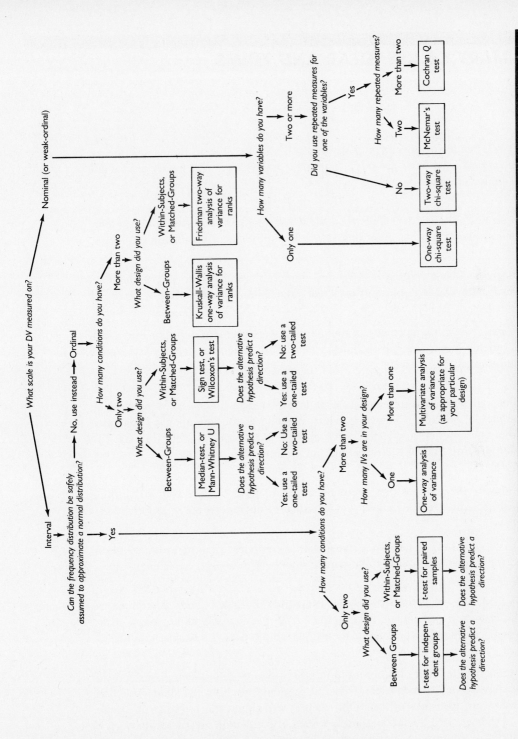

Figure 14–14   Decision tree for choosing a statistical test

SUMMARY OF KEY IDEAS AND TERMS

✔   If as a reader or doer of nursing research you are able to detect the misuse of *statistics*, you have gained an important knowledge with which to evaluate a study's findings.

✔   Statistics are analytical tools that allow you to show that something is more or less likely to occur according to the laws of chance or probability.

✔   *Measurement* is a process of assigning numerical values to concepts under investigation and is equivalent to actual value plus or minus error.

✔   A *measurement scale* specifies all the potential measurement divisions into which a variable might fall and includes at least two categories that are exhaustive and mutually exclusive.

✔   The types of measurement scale or levels of data are *nominal*, or naming; *ordinal*, or ordering; *interval*, in which possible measurements are equidistant from one another; and *ratio*, which is the highest level of scale for data with rank ordering, equal intervals, and an absolute zero point.

✔   Knowing the kind of measurement scale and level of data you are working with informs decisions about which statistical operations are appropriate.

✔   It is a good idea to consult a statistician, a computer analyst, or both early in a study's planning phase to anticipate how best to analyze your data.

✔   Statistical tests fall into two major categories. *Descriptive statistics* summarize the characteristics of data in a sample. *Inferential statistics* allow you to make inferences about a whole population from sample data and to test hypotheses.

✔   Frequency distributions presented in tables, figures called histograms and frequency polygons; measures of central tendency such as the mode, median, and mean; measures of variability such as the range, the interquartile range, and the standard deviation; and measures of correlation are the primary techniques of descriptive statistics that allow you to describe a data set.

✓   The formulas and assumptions about scale level for any statistical test should be looked up carefully in a statistics book.

✓   All inferential statistics are based on the assumption that the investigator has taken a random sample from the population, and you can improve the estimates about a population by increasing the sample size.

✓   The logic behind all inferential statistics is that chance is what produces variation among groups. The statistical test is designed to reject this assumption and conclude with a specified level of certainty that differences between dependent variables are due to the independent variable.

✓   The *critical value* is the size of a number in a statistical table that your calculated number must exceed to reject the explanation that differences are due to chance.

✓   The main steps in using inferential statistics to test hypotheses are:

   ■   State the null hypothesis (a statement that asserts that differences are due only to chance).

   ■   Select a level of statistical significance (the probability that tells you how unlikely the sample data must be to reject the null hypothesis).

   ■   Look up a test significance in the appropriate table to find the critical value for the degrees of freedom and confidence level you decide upon (.01, .05, 001).

   ■   Choose the right test for your study questions and type of data.

✓   If your sample size is larger than 20 scores per cell, if your variables are normally distributed (a bell-shaped curve), and if the measurement scale is at least an interval level, you can use more powerful parametric, rather than nonparametric, tests to test hypotheses.

✓   *Analysis of variance* (ANOVA) is an inferential statistical procedure that can be used to compare two or more groups by calculating what is called an F ratio.

✓   *Multiple comparison tests* are preferable to doing multiple t-tests, because the significance level need not be adjusted upward.

✓   The *chi-square* is one of the most frequently used nonparametric statistics for testing hypotheses with nominal data, but it must be modified if the sample size is small and the degrees of freedom are as low as 1.

References

Armstrong G: Parametric statistics and ordinal data: A pervasive misconception. *Nurs Res* 1981; 30, 60–62.

Donaldson SK: Critique: Effects of noise on fatigue in healthy middle-aged adults. *Commun Nurs Res* 1977; 8:35–40.

Hanson HA, Chater SS: Role selection by nurses: Managerial interests and personal attributes. *Nurs Res* January/February 1983; 32:48–52.

Hathaway D, Geden E: Energy expenditure during leg exercise programs. *Nurs Res* May/June 1983; 32:147–150.

Menzel NJ, Martinson IM: Effects of electrical surface stimulation on control of acute postoperative pain and prevention of atelectosis and ileus in patients having abdominal surgery. *Commun Nurs Res* 1977; 8:273–283.

Nichols EG et al: Relationship between incidence of phlebitis and frequency of changing IV tubing and percutaneous site. *Nurs Res* July/August 1983; 32:247–252.

Norris S et al: Nursing procedures and alterations in transcutaneous oxygen tension in premature infants. *Nurs Res* November/December 1982; 31:330–336.

Putt AM: Effects of noise on fatigue in healthy middle-aged adults. *Commun Nurs Res* 1977; 8:24–34.

Reid BJ: Potential sources of type I error and possible solutions to avoid a "galloping" alpha rate. *Nurs Res* May/June 1983; 32:190.

Saslow CA: *Basic Research Methods*. New York: Random House, 1982.

Siegal S: *Nonparametric Statistics for the Behavioral Sciences*. New York: McGraw-Hill, 1956.

Stevens SS: Mathematics, measurement, and psychophysics. In: Stevens SS (editor), *Handbook of Experimental Psychology*. New York: Wiley, 1951.

CHAPTER

15

Applying Multivariate Statistics to Quantitative Analysis

JOYCE A. VERRAN ▪ SANDRA FERKETICH

Chapter Objectives

After reading this chapter, the student should be able to:

- differentiate between univariate and multivariate statistics

- describe the logical use of multivariate statistics

- describe the similarities and differences between multiple regression, discriminant analysis, and canonical correlation

- compare and contrast various ways to examine differences between means

- describe the use of specific multifactorial ANOVAs such as two-way ANOVA, repeated measures ANOVA, and ANCOVA

- compare and contrast the use of a Hotelling's T^2 with a MANOVA

- describe the purposes of data reduction techniques such as factor analysis

- compare and contrast the two major extraction techniques of principal components and common factor analysis

- differentiate between orthogonal and oblique rotations

(Continued)

- describe the differences between varimax, equimax and quartimax rotations

- interpret the results of a factor analysis using prespecified criteria for factor loadings and eigenvalues

In This Chapter . . .

Research in nursing often deals with more than one outcome or anticipated effect of nursing care. Since nursing deals with the actual or potential responses of clients to a variety of health related stimuli, research into nursing interventions or the responses themselves cannot often be reduced to a single independent and dependent variable in each study. As our scientific knowledge grows, it becomes apparent that any intervention will affect clients in more than one way. Therefore, researchers measure each of the significant variables they expect to alter in a study.

By using multiple measures in a study, the researcher can obtain a more complete understanding of the phenomena under investigation. In addition, research is expensive to conduct. Initiating separate studies to investigate each potential response of clients to interventions or health related situations is costly in human and financial resources. In comparison, the cost of obtaining information on several variables in one study is relatively small.

Why Choose Multivariate Statistics?

Because many research studies involve multivariate questions that yield quantitative data, they should be analyzed with multivariate statistical procedures. Let's consider what such a study might involve. Imagine you are working on a surgical inpatient unit and you wish to know which of two types of preoperative instruction results in better surgical recovery. You know that recovery is a multidimensional concept that cannot be measured accurately with one variable. Therefore, you decide to use three measures of recovery from surgery: number of pain medications administered after surgery, number of postsurgical complications, and length of hospital stay. Your research hypothesis for this study is that patients who receive both written and verbal preoperative instructions will use less pain medication after surgery, will have fewer postoperative complications, and will have a shorter hospital stay than patients who receive only verbal information.

From the previous chapter, you know that the data collected for this hypothetical study could be analyzed with three *t*-tests for the difference in means of the two groups on each of the three variables indexing recovery. That's an obvious choice of analysis method, but it is not the best. Use of three univariate statistical tests in one study will result in an experimentwise error rate that is approximately three times greater than the α specified for each separate test.

The problem of multiple comparisons and their effect on Type I error is further discussed in Chapter 14, which addresses one way of handling the problem. The **Bonferroni inequality** or adjustment solves the difficulty of large experimentwise error rates very well as long as the researcher is satisfied with statistical answers that treat each variable one at a time. However, if the intent of the research is to provide a description and test that is closer to reality, then multivariate statistics are a must. We live in a multivariate world that cannot be addressed with univariate techniques, but instead must be considered as a whole.

Our hypothetical research study is an example of a common type of multiple comparison in research. Other situations requiring multiple comparisons are not this obvious. The repeated use of chi-square tests or Pearson correlation coefficients to examine significant relationships among a series of categorical or continuous variables constitutes another example frequently found in research literature. We address another less obvious situation of multiple comparisons when we discuss more complex analysis of variance (ANOVA) designs.

Definition of Multivariate Procedures

In general, **multivariate statistics** are applied to situations in which there is more than one dependent variable. (We are again using the terms *independent* and *dependent variable* in the statistical sense rather than in the sense of a manipulated or outcome variable). In the last example, there were three dependent variables: pain medication, postoperative complications, and length of hospital stay. We hypothesized that these measures were dependent or would vary with the type of preoperative instruction given to patients.

By this definition, many of the procedures we discuss in this chapter cannot be truly labeled "multivariate." For example, the techniques of multiple regression analysis and discriminant analysis deal with only one dependent or outcome variable but have more than one independent or predictor variable. These procedures are included in this chapter for two reasons. First, they are complex analysis procedures that require a level of sophistication and knowledge beyond the usual or more routine understanding of univariate analysis. Second, with the routine use of computers for data analysis, the use of complex or advanced statistics has become more common. For this reason, even the novice researcher should have a beginning knowledge of the purpose of these procedures.

For the purpose of this chapter, then, we consider multivariate statistics to include any procedure that involves more than one dependent and/or independent variable. As with univariate procedures, multivariate statistics have essentially two basic purposes: description and inference. However, the distinction between these two purposes is not as clear-cut as with the univariate procedures described in Chapter 14. Most of the techniques we describe in this chapter can be used for both descriptive and inferential purposes.

A more useful categorization of techniques is one based on the type of *research question being asked*. If the researcher is attempting to show a relationship among several variables or to predict the value of a variable on the basis of several others, then multivariate techniques of association and prediction are the appropriate choices. The statistics we discuss under this heading are multiple regression analysis, discriminant analysis, and canonical correlation.

If the research study involves the analysis of groups of individuals and the differences between them, procedures that deal with mean differences between and among groups are appropriate. In this section, we review two subcategories of statistical tests. The first subcategory involves more complex ANOVA designs than the one-way ANOVA discussed in Chapter 14. These designs include x-way ANOVAs, repeated measures ANOVA, and analysis of covariance (ANCOVA). In the second subcategory are the true multivariate tests of significance or those multiple analysis of variance designs (MANOVA) that deal with two or more groups and two or more dependent variables.

The third type of research question that can be handled with multivariate procedures is more complex than the two listed in the preceding paragraphs. In this case, the researcher is asking a descriptive question of whether data on a large number of variables can mathematically be reduced to smaller clusters or factors that are more easily interpreted and more theoretically parsimonious. We will discuss one family of data reduction techniques used to answer such research questions. These interrelated sets of procedures are considered under the heading of factor analysis.

Areas to Be Considered

In the statistics department of any university or college, a student could find several courses on multivariate analysis. Most of these courses deal with only a small number of the multivariate tests reviewed in this chapter. Therefore, our discussion of these procedures must be somewhat limited. Since the mathematics involved are quite complex, and since most procedures require the use of the computer, we do not attempt to review any formulas or computational procedures. Instead, we present material that allows you a conceptual grasp of each test. In other words, the point of this chapter is to give you a basic understanding of the most commonly used multivariate techniques. This information should help you to make informed judgments on whether the technique has been applied correctly, whether the appropriate information has been reported, and whether your research data should be subjected to multivariate, rather than univariate, statistical analysis.

Association and Prediction

In Chapter 14, you learned that a research question that examines the relationship between two variables measured in the same subject can be analyzed with a variety of correlational measures chosen on the basis of the measurement level for each of the two variables. In addition, questions of relationship were extended to questions of prediction, where the intent is to predict the value of one variable on the basis of another. In this case, bivariate regression is used to develop a prediction equation that contains a series of observations on a dependent variable, a constant intercept term, a constant regression coefficient that represents the slope of the regression line, a series of observations on an independent variable, and a series of computed error terms called *residuals*.

In this section, we review three techniques that are multivariate analogs of bivariate correlation and prediction statistics. The first two methods are used when the researcher has one dependent variable and more than one independent variable. The third type of analysis is useful when an investigator wishes to examine the relationship between one series of variables and another series. Statisticians usually use the term **vector** to refer to variables in a series. A **vector** contains a row or column of means, factor loadings, or other values.

In this chapter, multiple regression analysis is reviewed in greater detail than the other two techniques because multiple regression has become a popular technique in nursing research. Its popularity is due to its applicability to a number of nursing research questions and the ease with which it can be applied, given the widespread availability of packaged computer programs. In today's research market, it has become necessary, even for beginning researchers, to have at least a working knowledge of the values and problems of multiple regression analysis.

Multiple Regression

Imagine that you are employed in a long-term care facility. You notice that the morale of the residents varies greatly and seems to depend on (1) the amount of social interaction they have with other residents and (2) the duration of their stay in the facility. You suspect that (1) the more interaction the resident has, the better his or her morale and (2) the longer his or her stay in the facility, the lower his or her morale. Rather than basing your conclusions on unsystematic observation, you decide to conduct a study to examine your "hunch" more scientifically. You measure morale with an instrument that yields interval level data, and you time the durations of interactions of each subject in your study during a randomly selected week. In addition, you check subjects' records and record the number of days each has been hospitalized.

Your study data could be analyzed with two bivariate correlation coefficients. The results of these tests would tell you how each variable relates to morale individually; however, your original question had to do with how both interaction and length of stay relate to morale simultaneously. The appropriate statistic for this type of question is multiple regression, which allows you to look at how the best linear combination of the two independent variables is related to the dependent variable. The best linear combination of the two variables is determined mathematically using complex procedures. If you are interested in the mathematics of multiple regression, see, for example, Harris (1985).

Results of Analysis If you do a computer analysis of your data, you receive three major elements of a multiple regression analysis: the multiple correlation coefficient squared (R^2), which is also called the coefficient of determination; the regression coefficients, which are often called beta weights; and the multiple regression prediction equation.

The prediction equation is similar to that described in Chapter 14 in the discussion of bivariate regression. In this case, the equation is

$$\hat{Y}_i = a + b_i X_{1i} + b_2 X_{2i} + e_i$$

where $\hat{Y}_i$ indicates the value for morale achieved by each subject (i = subject 1 to subject N); a indicates the constant or slope of the regression line; b_1 and b_2 are the regression coefficients for the independent variables of interaction (X_{1i}) and length of stay (X_{2i}), respectively; and e_i indicates the residual error terms for each study subject. Using this equation, you can predict a person's morale score simply on the basis of scores on interaction and length of stay. The regression coefficients, or the bs, give each one of these variables a weighted value in the equation, while the constant term, or a, helps to standardize the measurement scale of the linear combination of independent variables to match that of the dependent variable.

Instead of reporting the regression coefficients, some researchers report beta weights. A **beta weight** is usually considered a standardized regression coefficient. In other words, it is the coefficient that would result if the independent and dependent variables were originally measured on the same scale. In an equation that uses beta weights (the symbol B is usually used for the beta weight) rather than regression coefficients, a constant term is not included since there is no need to equalize measurement scales when this has already been done with the weights. Obviously, if a person's score is to be predicted from the equation, unstandardized coefficients and a constant term should be used, since unstandardized raw scores on variables will be used for the computation.

Beta weights do have one advantage over regression coefficients. Because beta weights are computed with standardized variables, it is possible to determine which of the independent variables are better predictors of the dependent variable. Disregarding the sign of the beta weight, the variable that has the largest weight is a better predictor. Because beta weights allow this type of comparison across variables, most authors who are primarily interested in describing a multivariate relationship report standardized regression weights. Remember, however, that if the intent is to predict scores, the unstandardized regression coefficients and the constant term should be reported.

The regression equation and the regression coefficients are valuable pieces of information, but they do not tell the investigator how well the equation predicts the dependent variable of morale or how strong the relationship is between the linear combination of the independent variables and morale. To answer this question, the investigator needs to examine the R^2, or the coefficient of determination for the regression. The R^2 is the squared multiple correlation coefficient (R). An R may be interpreted as the correlation between the linear combination of independent variables and the dependent variable. The R^2 may be interpreted as the proportion of dependent variable variance explained by the linear combination of independent variables. An R^2 of .40 may be said to explain 40% of the variability in the dependent variable. Of course, the greater the proportion of variance explained, the better the prediction or association.

Key Decisions

Sample Size   Most multivariate procedures require fairly large sample sizes to yield unbiased results. In this sense, *bias* refers to the variation in results from sample to sample. When samples are very small, results of most statistical tests are unstable. In addition, with multivariate statistics, a certain sample size is necessary or the mathematics simply will not work. In the case of multiple regression, a minimum sample size of at least one more case than the number of variables in the regression equation is necessary. However, a sample size this small (for the hypothetical study, four subjects) would result in very unstable results. A rule of thumb is that the sample size for a regression analysis should be ten times greater than the number of variables in the equation plus an additional 50 cases (Thorndike 1978). In our hypothetical example, the sample would be 90 subjects. This rather conservative estimate of sample size, however, would afford more stable results.

Statistical Significance   Earlier, we described the basic elements of a regression equation and noted that it was possible to make decisions on how well each independent variable is associated with the dependent variable and how well the regression equation predicts the dependent variable. These decisions were based simply on the magnitude of the regression coefficients and the R^2. However, tests of significance can be used with these statistics.

When the researcher includes tests of significance, the multiple regression analysis is no longer simply descriptive but becomes inferential. Since inferential statistics are now in use, the researcher should preset the level of significance before starting the study. The null hypotheses being tested are that each of the regression coefficients is equal to zero and that the R^2 is equal to zero. If a regression coefficient is zero, the variable it relates to has no value in the regression equation and should not be included. If an R^2 is equal to zero, then the regression equation does not satisfactorily predict the dependent variable.

The statistic that is used to test for the significance of the regression coefficients and the R^2 is based on the F distribution and is termed an F-test. This test is similar to the one described in Chapter 14 for the one-way analysis of variance and is interpreted in the same way.

Entry of Variables   Most computer programs for multiple regression analysis allow the researcher to specify the way variables enter a regression equation. In the hypothetical study about morale in a long-term care facility, we suspected that both independent variables had an effect on morale so both were forced to enter the equation. This method of variable entry is usually called *forced entry*. No criteria

TABLE 15–1   *Methods of Hierarchical Entry of Variables into a Regression Equation*

Procedure Name	Description
Forward selection	Variables are entered one at a time into the regression equation based on a statistical criterion, such as the correlation between the variable and the independent variable. Variables are added sequentially until a prespecified level of significance is reached and the remaining variables are no longer significantly associated with the dependent variable. Should the regression coefficient for a variable in the equation become nonsignificant due to the entry of other variables, it remains in the equation.
Backward deletion	All variables specified are entered into the regression equation. Based on a preset statistical criterion, the variable having the lowest association with the dependent variable is deleted, and a new equation is computed. This continues until only the most significant variables remain in the equation. If the potential regression coefficient for a variable eliminated from the equation becomes significant due to the removal of other variables, it is not be reconsidered for entry.
Stepwise	This procedure is a combination of the forward selection and backward deletion procedures. Initially, the most significant variable is entered into the equation, followed by the second most significant. At this point the two variables in the equation are reconsidered. If one is no longer significant, it is eliminated. This procedure continues until the best set of predictors is found.

are invoked for when and how the variables become a part of the regression equation. They are simply added at the same time, and the best linear combination is determined.

Sometimes, a number of variables can potentially enter the regression equation. The intent of the research is not necessarily to determine how all of the variables affect the dependent variable but rather to determine which of the variables have a statistically significant impact. In this case, the investigator may choose to use one of many hierarchical types of variable entry into the regression equation. Some of these types of entry are described in Table 15–1.

Key Pitfalls

Multicollinearity   A major potential problem in multiple regression analysis is that independent variables can be highly correlated with each other. This problem, termed **multicollinearity**, results in biased regression estimates. Figure 15–1 shows the situation of two independent variables that correlate with each other as well as with the dependent variable. In this situation, some of the relationship of the second independent variable with the dependent variable is shared by the first independent variable. When one of these variables enters the regression equation,

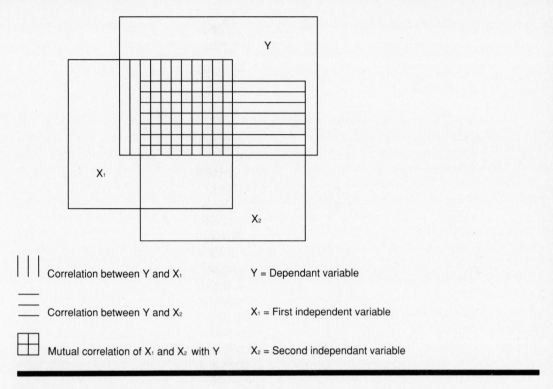

Figure 15–1   Multicollinearity among dependent variables in a regression equation

that variable alone accounts for all the relationship with the dependent variable, including that shared by the second variable. The second variable may not correlate sufficiently, once the shared association is removed to enter the equation at a statistically significant level. If it does enter, the regression coefficient reflects a smaller impact on the dependent variable than exists in reality.

Researchers should be aware of the problems caused by the interrelationships among independent variables and examine these relationships with a bivariate correlation matrix prior to using multiple regression. Most researchers look for correlations greater than .65 before they decide that multicollinearity exists; however, some authors, such as Gordon (1968), have cited problems when correlations occur at .80 or greater.

Violation of Statistical Assumptions   Like all statistical analysis techniques, multiple regression has some basic assumptions upon which the mathematics and significance tests are based. In multiple regression, assumptions relate to the error terms of the equation. These assumptions are that the error terms are independent of each other, are normally distributed, have a mean of zero and equal variance. Although multiple regression is robust to the violation of some of these assumptions, it does not perform well when several violations occur in combination. A set of procedures, called residual analysis, has been developed to test for violation of regression assumptions (Verran and Ferketich 1987). A researcher who is well versed in the use of multiple regression analysis should report the results of testing for violations of regression assumptions.

Reporting a Regression Analysis From reading the previous sections, you should have a fairly good idea of the kinds of things that a researcher using multiple regression techniques should report. Table 15–2 contains hypothetical data from the study on morale in long-term care facilities. We are assuming that the variables were entered using a stepwise procedure, hence an R^2 is given for each "step," or at each point a variable entered the equation. Note that the results of significance testing are also included in the table. In addition to reporting this tabular information, the investigator should address the results of the examination for multi-collinearity and for possible violation of assumptions. For an example of a study that uses multiple regression as the primary method of analysis, see "Finding Meaning: Antecedents of Uncertainty in Illness" (Mishel and Braden 1988).

Special Multiple Regression Problems

Categorical Variables   Usually, the variables in multiple regression problems call for interval level measurement. However, in some situations, the investigator may want to examine the effect of categorical variables, such as gender or marital status, along with the other independent variables measured at an interval level. It is possible to examine categorical variables in a regression equation by using a special coding technique called *dummy coding*. Pedhauzer (1982) discusses the purposes of dummy coding and the way it can be handled in a multiple regression analysis.

Path Analysis   Path analysis is a statistical technique for drawing causal inferences from nonexperimental data. Researchers testing a causal model, as Mishel and Bra-

TABLE 15–2   *Reporting the Results of Multiple Regression Analysis*

Dependent Variable	Independent Variable	b	B	p	R^2	p
Morale	Interation	1.55	.42	.02	.23	.03
	Length of stay	2.31	.29	.05	.32	.06
	Constant	6.14		.01		
$N = 143$						

den (1988) did, generally use this technique. Today, most path analysis is done using multiple regression. For further information, see the excellent chapter on the statistical analysis of causal models by Munro, Visintainer, and Page (1986).

Discriminant Analysis

Discriminant analysis is very similar to multiple regression with one exception. In this case, the researcher is still interested in prediction, but the variable being predicted is characterized by group membership. In other words, the dependent variable in a discriminant analysis problem is categorical. For example, suppose you conduct a study in an ambulatory care clinic with two groups of diabetic patients: those who comply with their medical regimen, and those who do not. You are interested in how social support, family stress, and hours of instruction predict compliance and noncompliance. When only two groups are to be predicted, the statistical technique is called *simple* discriminant function analysis. When more than two groups are to be predicted, the technique is called *multiple* discriminant function analysis.

Simple discriminant analysis is much like multiple regression except that the coefficients for the predictor variables are chosen for a different purpose. In this case, the coefficients are selected to maximize correct classification of subjects in one of two groups. The computer gives a critical cutoff score, which is compared against the predicted score calculated from the discriminant function equation. If the predicted score is above the cutoff point, the case is classified in the second group. In addition to the critical cutoff score and the discriminant function equation, a test of significance is given for the function. This *F*-test is used to determine whether use of the prediction equation results in better classification of people than would result from chance alone. By chance, such as by flipping a coin, we could classify people correctly 50% of the time. The *F*-test indicates whether the accuracy of prediction is significantly increased above the 50% chance level.

There are some significant differences in a multiple discriminant function analysis. First, a multivariate test of significance called *Wilk's Lambda* is done to examine whether the set of predictor variables can be used to differentiate among the groups. The null hypothesis is that the means of the predictor variables for each group are equal. In reporting this test, the researcher may refer to an *F*-test rather than a Wilk's Lambda. Often, the Wilk's Lambda is tranformed to an *F* statistic so that the more easily accessible *F* distribution may be used to test the null hypothesis.

The second major difference between simple and multiple discriminant function analysis involves the number of prediction equations obtained from the analysis. In multiple discriminant analysis, the maximum number of possible prediction equations is equal to one less than the number of criterion groups or one less than the number of predictor variables, whichever is smaller. Each person's predicted scores on each of the discriminant function equations are used in combination to predict the group to which the person should belong.

For further information on discriminant analysis, see Huck, Cormier, and Bounds (1974). For an example of how discriminant function analysis can be used in nursing research, see Champion (1987), who tested the hypothesis that the concepts of susceptibility, seriousness, benefits, barriers, health motivation, control, and knowledge would discriminate between groups on frequency of breast self-examination.

Canonical Correlation

Canonical correlation is a useful technique when the research study involves more than one interval level dependent variable and more than one interval level independent variable. Assume that you are working in the community with a group of hypertensive patients. You are interested in examining the relationship of a set of physical characteristics, such as body mass index and cholesterol level, to a set of psychological characteristics, such as locus of control, health value orientation, and life stress. You could run two multiple regression equations, with body mass index as the dependent variable for one and cholesterol level as the dependent variable for the other. However, this analysis does not show the true relationship between the two sets of variables. A better analysis technique for this problem is canonical correlation, which emphasizes the relationship aspect of the problem rather than attempting to predict each dependent variable from the independent variables.

In some respects, canonical correlation is like factor analysis, discussed later in this chapter. In factor analysis, the underlying structure of a set of variables is determined so that a reduced set of variable clusters or factors is obtained. *Canonical correlation* examines the correlation between a factor in the first set of variables and a related factor in the second set of variables. Therefore, there may be more than one canonical correlation coefficient in the analysis. However, there cannot be more correlation coefficients than there are variables in the smaller set. In our hypothetical study of hypertensive patients, the maximum number of correlation coefficients is two, since only two physical measures are under study.

A test based on Wilk's Lambda is computed for each of the canonical correlations. Unlike the R^2 used in multiple regression, the higher the Wilk's Lambda, the lower the variance accounted for in the factor derived from the dependent variable. In other words

$$1 - \text{lambda} = R^2$$

A test of statistical significance, called Bartlett's test, which is based on the chi-square statistic, is provided for each of the Wilk's Lambdas.

Most researchers using canonical correlation present a second type of statistic, called a *structure coefficient*, which represents the correlation between the weighted composite of the variables in a set with the original variables. These weighted composites are termed *canonical variates* and are new computed variables derived from the original variables. If the structure coefficients are high (above .30), the canonical variate represents the original variables in a meaningful manner. For more detailed information on canonical correlation, see Stevens (1986).

Mean Differences

In Chapter 14, we reviewed two general parametric procedures used to test whether groups are statistically different based on the mean scores of a dependent variable. In these tests, group membership served as the independent variable in the study, and the research hypothesis usually proposed that the value of the dependent variable depended on the group to which the subject belonged. The tests to be examined in this section are really extensions of the *t*-test and the one-way ANOVA described in Chapter 14. They are, however, used with more complex research questions that either involve more than one independent variable (*x*-way or multifactorial ANOVA), one dependent variable measured at more than one point in time (repeated measures ANOVA), or more than one dependent variable (Hotelling's T^2 and multiple analysis of variance or MANOVA). In addition, we will review a special analysis of variance procedure used to examine differences between groups after controlling for the effect of another variable (analysis of covariance or ANCOVA).

The multifactorial ANOVA, the repeated measures ANOVA, and the ANCOVA are simply extensions of univariate designs. It is only when the researcher uses a T^2 or MANOVA design that true multivariate statistics are employed in examining differences among means. This is true since T^2 and MANOVA designs involve more than one dependent variable, which is the basic definition of multivariate statistics. However, because of the complexity of multifactorial ANOVA, repeated measures ANOVA, and ANCOVA analyses, they are considered more advanced statistical techniques.

Extensions of Univariate Designs

Multifactorial ANOVA

Two-Way ANOVA   Suppose that you are working on a general medical unit of an acute care hospital. You have been asked to devise a self-medication program for three types of cardiac patients, those with angina, those with congestive heart failure, and those with myocardial infarction. You set up plans for teaching patients about self-medication. From the literature, you learn that there are a variety of ways to provide instruction. You decide to prepare both a slide-sound program and a booklet of information. You are interested in seeing which method of instruction

Main effect A

	Level 1	Level 2	Level 3
Main effect B			
Level 1	Cell 1	Cell 2	Cell 3
Level 2	Cell 4	Cell 5	Cell 6

Figure 15–2 A Two-Way ANOVA design

results in greater patient knowledge of medications and whether the diagnosis of the patient makes a difference in the degree of knowledge.

In this study, there is one continuous dependent variable: patient knowledge. There are, however, two independent variables: diagnosis and type of instruction. You could perform two one-way ANOVAs with this data, but by doing so, you would not only increase the experimentwise error rate of the study but also be unable to answer one very important question. You would not know whether the combination of instructional method and diagnosis made a difference in patient knowledge. It is possible that patients with congestive heart failure respond better to a slide-sound presentation, whereas patients with angina respond better to an instructional booklet. This type of question is termed an *interaction effect*, while the effect of each independent variable alone on knowledge is termed the *main effect*. The study design is diagramed in Figure 15–2 and is an example of a two-way multifactorial ANOVA with three levels on the first factor (diagnosis) and two levels on the second factor (instruction). Some researchers would term this ANOVA a 3 × 2 design, which indicates both that it is a two-way ANOVA and that the levels of the independent variable are three and two, respectively.

In a two-way ANOVA, three null hypotheses must be tested with F ratios. For our study, the three null hypotheses are: (1) there is no difference in mean knowledge scores among patients with angina, patients with congestive heart failure, and patients with myocardial infarction after each group of patients receives instruction; (2) there is no difference in mean knowledge scores between cardiac groups receiving instruction via a slide-sound program and those receiving instruction via an informational booklet; and (3) there is no interaction effect of diagnosis and instruction on mean knowledge scores.

When an ANOVA is calculated on research data, a special table should be included in the report of the results. In Chapter 14, you saw an example of such a table for the one-way ANOVA. Table 15–3 is an example of such a table for a two-way ANOVA.

TABLE 15–3   *Sample Table for a Two-Way ANOVA*

Source	SS	df	MS	F	p
Main effect A	6,611.34	2	3,305.67	67.37	.001
Main effect B	7,287.94	1	7.287.94	148.52	.001
Interaction	254.83	2	127.41	2.60	.074
Error	4,661.78	95	49.07		
Total	18,815.88	100			

As with the one-way ANOVA, if the *F*-test for one or both of the main effects is significant, follow-up tests should be done to determine the exact nature of the difference. Any of the follow-up procedures discussed in Chapter 14 can be used for this purpose. If a significant interaction effect is found in a two-way ANOVA, examination of main effects may be inappropriate. Instead of looking at overall means across the two independent variables, the researcher should concentrate on a comparison of means within each of the separate subgroups of the design. For a 3 × 2 ANOVA, there are six different groups of subjects, corresponding to the separate cells in Figure 15–2. In other words, the comparison of means to determine where the difference occurs must be done for each level of one independent variable in relation to each level of the other independent variable.

Three-Way ANOVA   A three-way ANOVA has three independent variables. Since three main effects are considered, there are many interaction effects in a three-way ANOVA. Consider a research study conducted by a group of nurse researchers to investigate the effects of respiratory rate (high and low), depth of respiration (deep and shallow), and mouth breathing (closed and open) on oral temperature measurement. In this 2 × 2 × 2 ANOVA, four interaction effects need to be examined: the interactions between rate and depth, between rate and mouth breathing, between depth and mouth breathing, and among rate, depth, and mouth breathing.

A 2 × 2 × 2 multifactorial ANOVA is diagramed in Figure 15–3. Note that there are eight different subject groups in this design. Each group corresponds to one of the small cubes in the large block.

In a three-way ANOVA, there are seven null hypotheses to be tested. Three hypotheses correspond to the three main effects, and four relate to the four interaction effects. Since the interpretation of interaction effects starts to get very complex when a three-way ANOVA is used, the ANOVA procedure is seldom used with more than three independent variables. If four or more independent variables are likely in a research study, another analysis procedure, such as multiple regression with dummy coding of the independent variables, is probably more appropriate.

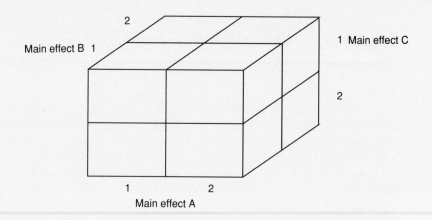

Figure 15–3 A Three-Way ANOVA

Repeated Measures ANOVA Suppose you again want to conduct a study on oral temperature, but this time you are primarily interested in the main effect of respiratory rates of 16, 20, and 24 respirations per minute. In addition, however, you want to see if the oral temperature changes with the length of time the subject breathes at these rates. Therefore, you decide to measure temperature after 5, 10, and 15 minutes. In this case, you have one independent variable, but the dependent variable is measured across time. This study could be analyzed with a two-way ANOVA. Unfortunately, the selection of an analysis method is not that simple.

When we measure the dependent variable several times in the same subjects, there is correlation between the measures. Each measure of temperature in the same subject is not independent of the next measure. It is likely that the higher the temperature reading is after five minutes, the higher it will be after ten minutes, without regard to the respiratory rate of the subject. The statistics used in a multifactorial analysis of variance do not take this relationship among measures into account. Correlation among measures will increase the error sum of squares (within group differences). Since the error sum of squares forms the denominator of the F-test, it would be more difficult to obtain a significant result if the usual ANOVA were used.

In a second example of repeated measures, the same subjects are exposed to all levels of a treatment. For example, a researcher might want to examine the effect of body position on intracranial pressure (ICP). To reduce the error that would result due to differences in patient condition, the investigator decides to expose all patients in the sample to each body position and measure ICP at each point. Since the same patients are being measured repeatedly, there is the likelihood of correlation among the measures.

In both of these cases, the researcher should use a special ANOVA procedure that takes the correlation among measures into account. As in the *x*-way ANOVA, more than one hypothesis is tested. Three *F*-tests result for the repeated measures over time. These tests examine the main effect of the independent or grouping variable, the main effect of time on the dependent variable, and the interaction betwen the independent variable and time. In the analysis of subjects exposed to the same treatment, two *F*-tests are performed. One examines the differences among the subjects in the study, and the other tests the difference in the treatments. The researcher is most interested in the last test; however, by calculating and testing the variation among subjects, the researcher removes this source of variation from the error term and reduces the chance of insignificant results.

Several problems are associated with a repeated measures ANOVA. Some of these relate to the design of the study and have to do with implementing safeguards against subjects becoming familiar with the measurement instruments in the repeated measures across time. When subjects are exposed to all treatments in a study, the researcher has to be aware that previous treatments may still be affecting the subject if sufficient time is not provided between the treatment levels.

In addition to posing these design problems, repeated measures ANOVA designs require more stringent assumptions about the data than do multifactorial ANOVA designs. One assumption is that the correlations and variances across treatments or times are equal. Munro, Visintainer, and Page (1986) describe this assumption in more detail and suggest other methods of analysis if the assumption is violated by the data.

Extensions of Repeated Measures Designs   It is possible to use a repeated measures design with more than one independent variable. For example, the three-way ANOVA example on temperature measurement could be extended to a repeated measure design by measuring oral temperature over time within the eight subject groups corresponding to the three independent variables. This would result in the performance of several more *F*-tests for the effect of time and the interaction of time with the independent variables in the study. For an example of a study using a multifactorial analysis of variance with repeated measures, see King, Norsen, Robertson, and Hicks (1987), who studied management of pain medication in post-surgical cardiac patients.

Analysis of Covariance   The analysis of covariance (ANCOVA) is a special ANOVA design that combines the power of multiple regression with an analysis of variance. The purpose of the ANCOVA is to reduce extraneous variation in the dependent variable due to the effect of separate variables on the groups being measured. Reducing or "controlling" this outside variation decreases the error sum of squares and increases the power of the test or the probability that a significant result will be found.

Assume you are interested in measuring the sleep patterns of two groups of hospitalized patients. For one group you implement a plan of care to improve patient sleep. The second group receives routine care. You learn from the literature that the age of the subject affects sleep patterns, and you wish to reduce this variation to obtain a more powerful comparison of your groups. Since age is a continuous measure, you can use an ANCOVA design with age as the covariate or the measure for which variance is being controlled.

Using the ANCOVA procedure, you first compute a regression analysis, with age as the independent variable and sleep pattern as the dependent variable. This regression is done without consideration for the group membership of the subjects. An F-test is calculated to determine whether the correlation between the two variables is significant. Once the regression is performed, the effect of age is removed from the dependent variable, and an analysis of variance is performed between the groups to determine if there are differences in mean scores not due to the age of the subject. In effect, you have conducted an analysis of variance between groups using the residual error terms of the regression equation. An F-test is then computed for the difference in mean scores.

Two new assumptions are associated with the analysis of covariance, in addition to those associated with the ANOVA model. The first is that the covariate and the dependent variable have a linear relationship. The second is that the direction (positive or negative) and magnitude of the relationship are alike in each of the groups being studied.

When an ANCOVA is performed, two F-tests result. A significant F-test for the covariate indicates a statistically significant relationship between the covariate and the dependent variable. A significant F-test for the difference between groups is interpreted just as it is for a regular ANOVA, and follow-up tests using multiple comparison techniques are in order.

Complex ANCOVA Designs   The analysis of covariance may be used with any of the previously discussed multifactorial and repeated measures ANOVA designs. Many investigators attempt to use the ANCOVA to equalize groups that have not been randomly assigned to treatments or to control for pretest differences even when there has been randomization. There is wide disagreement as to the value and accuracy of this form of equalization; however, such use of the technique is frequently reported in the literature.

True Multivariate Procedures

Hotelling's T^2   Imagine that you are working as a nurse counselor in a chemical abuse rehabilitation program. You are interested in examining the differences between two groups of clients: those who are in the program for drug abuse, and those in the program for alcohol abuse. The variables you are interested in examining are locus of control, self-efficacy, and ways of coping. Since you are looking at two groups it is possible to perform three independent t-tests, one for each variable. However, the potential for increasing the experimentwise error rate is the same in this type of study, in which you are examining the differences in two groups over several variables, as it is for multiple t-tests with more than two groups. In this case, there is an additional reason for avoiding univariate t-tests. It is likely that there will be correlations among the three variables for each group. Because of these correlations, the probability of a Type I error is increased, and the null hypothesis will be incorrectly rejected.

The use of multiple t-tests for several dependent variables in an investigation is a common data analysis error in research. Many researchers are not aware of the problems associated with this type of analysis and some research journals report studies in which the investigators used a series of t-tests. The fact of their publication does not make the analysis right.

The most appropriate test for analyzing a problem like the one above is the T^2, more often called Hotelling's T^2. In general, the T^2 compares two groups of subjects to determine whether there is a difference between them on one or more of the dependent variables after adjustments have been made for correlations and for the fact that more than one dependent variable is included in the analysis. The null hypothesis being tested is that the two groups of subjects have identical mean vectors. A significant T^2 indicates that the groups differ from each other on at least one of the dependent variables. In most studies, the calculated value for the test is reported as an F rather than a T^2, since the T^2 can be easily converted to an F-test, and the table of critical F values is readily available in most statistical texts.

A significant F ratio using Hotelling's T^2 tells the researcher only that there is a difference between the groups on at least one of the variables in the set of dependent measures. Follow-up tests are necessary to determine exactly which of the measures contributed to the overall significance. The two most common procedures used for these follow-up tests are discriminant analysis and simultaneous confidence intervals. We will not describe the use of simultaneous confidence intervals here. For a brief explanation of the procedure see Huck, Cromier, and Bounds (1974); for a more complex review, see Morrison (1976).

We discussed discriminant function analysis earlier. Although the analysis technique is the same as that described, the purpose is different when the technique is used to examine a significant T^2. Instead of trying to predict a dependent variable on the basis of several independent variables, we are now attempting to discover which dependent variables make the most difference in one independent variable (group membership). A comparison of the magnitude of the standard discriminant function coefficients answers this question. Essentially, the standard discriminant function coefficient is the standardized weight obtained for each of the dependent variables in the discriminant function equation.

So far, we have discussed a T^2 for independent samples. Just as with the univariate t-test, there are procedures to compute a T^2 for correlated groups. The interpretation of such a test is the same as that of a test done with two different groups.

Some special considerations apply when the T^2 is chosen as the analysis method for a research study. First, the test requires a larger sample size than is usual for univariate tests. The mathematics of the test will work as long as the number of subjects is greater by one than the number of dependent variables, but results will be less biased if there are ten or more subjects per variable. Second, two rather important assumptions underlie the T^2. These are analogous to those underlying the t-test (see Chapter 14). However, since we are dealing with multiple dependent variables, the assumptions have been extended: The sample data should come from multivariate normal populations, and these populations should have equal dispersion matrices. The investigator using the T^2 should address at least the second of these assumptions by reporting the results of a test that examines whether the variances on all dependent variables between the two groups were essentially equal. Several tests accomplish this purpose, depending on the computer program you use.

One-Way Multiple Analysis of Variance (MANOVA) Just as the *t*-test has a multivariate analog, so does the univariate ANOVA. This multivariate ANOVA analog can be used when there are more than two groups of subjects and more than one dependent variable. The null hypothesis being tested in a one-way MANOVA is that there is no difference in the mean vectors of the dependent variables among the groups of subjects.

Several alternative tests can be used in the MANOVA procedure to test the null hypothesis. The most commonly used is Wilk's Lambda. As with the T^2, the Wilk's Lambda is usually converted to an F value for use with the F table of critical values. Roy's largest root criterion and Hotelling's trace criterion can also be used to examine a MANOVA null hypothesis (Harris 1985).

As with the T^2, if a significant result is found with the MANOVA procedure, follow-up procedures are in order. The same procedures of discriminant function analysis and simultaneous equations are usually used.

Extensions of MANOVA Designs You can use the basic MANOVA procedure with multivariate data just as you can extend the basic one-way ANOVA to multifactorial designs and repeated measures or use it with a covariate. Thus, researchers may analyze their study data with two- or three-way MANOVA techniques or use a repeated measures MANOVA with a covariate. The interpretation and reporting of these procedures are highly complex. However, like many multivariate procedures, they are becoming more common in nursing research. For example, Gennaro (1988) used a three-way MANOVA to examine how the dependent variables of postpartal anxiety and depression were influenced by the independent grouping variables of gestational age, type of delivery, and parity. In addition, Gennaro used several other types of MANOVA designs to examine specific aspects of the data.

Data Reduction Techniques: Factor Analysis

Factor analysis refers to a variety of associated statistical techniques that are mathematically related to regression analysis. Equations that are linear combinations of a set are developed in both techniques. The basic underlying function of factor analysis, however, is to describe relationships among a large set of variables by reducing them to a smaller set of conceptually meaningful composite variables called *factors*. Unlike regression, with factor analysis, you do not specify a particular variable as dependent and others as independent. Furthermore, the use and interpretation of factor analytic results are complicated and open to subjectivity.

Since the general purpose of factor analysis is the derivation of a smaller number of variables or factors, the results provide a more parsimonious solution. Parsimony refers to the decision rule that, given two or more theoretically satisfactory explanations, the least complex solution with the fewest assumptions should be selected. For example, a researcher might have developed an instrument with 100 items measuring fatigue in patients with chronic illness. These items individually might measure fatigue very well. If the researcher could reduce the number of items to a subset that measured fatigue equally well, the measurement properties and clinical relevance of the instrument could be greatly increased.

Factor analysis also provides a means to develop composite scores that can alleviate the problem of multicollinearity among a set of variables when a regression approach has been selected. The factor analysis is performed first; the individual scores on instruments or variables can then be weighted according to the factor solution. One variable could then be used instead of a number of very related variables that could lead to problems with the regression solution. For example, a researcher might collect four measures of social support during a study. When preparing for the regression analysis, the researcher creates a correlation matrix and finds that these four measures are highly related. If all four are entered into the regression separately, the researcher will encounter problems due to multicollinearity. A linear combination of these variables, however, would obviate those problems.

Instrument validity can also be examined through factor analytic solutions. If a factor analysis solution supports the theory underlying the instrument, support for the construct validity of the instrument is also provided. The delineation of that structure and the interpretation of the results, which are rarely unequivocal, lend an air of subjectivity that is not often associated with quantitative analysis. The more complex the procedures, the more it is incumbent upon the researcher to have "thought it through." That is, a theory-driven approach and interpretation of results are more likely to be acceptable to the researcher and the scientific community.

The researcher who uses any of the factor analytic approaches must make a number of decisions to interpret the solution effectively. For a thorough discussion of each of these decisions, see Gorsuch (1983). Table 15–4 summarizes specific points at which decisions in factor analysis are crucial. Each point is discussed in greater detail in the following sections.

Confirmatory versus Exploratory Analysis

The researcher can approach factor analysis from one of two points of view. The first is that factors are to be discovered and underlying structure is to be discerned. In this, the exploratory approach, the researcher does not specify the number of

TABLE 15–4	*Major Decisions in Factor Analysis*
I	Confirmatory versus exploratory analysis
II	Preparation of the correlation matrix
III	Selection of the extraction procedure
IV	Selection of rotation procedures
V	Interpretation of factors

factors to be derived from the data before the beginning of the analysis. This approach can aid in the development of new theory and give insight into already established theory when no preexisting structure is specified.

In the second, or confirmatory, approach, the researcher has a notion, sometimes stated in the language of a research hypothesis, that there are x number of factors and further may state the composition of those factors and model constraints by theory. This approach can provide support for the underlying theory. Confirmatory factor analysis is a complex procedure and is one basis for covariance structure models. Long (1983) explains the differences between exploratory and confirmatory factor analysis.

In most factor analytic approaches, factors are unmeasured or latent variables derived from the data. As such, many researchers are reluctant to rely too heavily on the results of any one factor analysis. The solution is data specific and may be considered unstable between samples. The conservative analyst, therefore, uses the results of several factor analyses and examines them for stability over several samples. Furthermore, a large number of subjects is generally required for each item in the factor analysis. There is controversy about exactly how many subjects are necessary, but a sample size of ten subjects per variable is considered adequate under most circumstances.

Preparation of the Correlation Matrix

This procedure, like many other regression-related procedures, is performed on a correlation matrix. To find the best linear combination of variables that define a factor, the researcher applies matrix solutions. Although it is not necessary to understand the mathematics involved, you need to be aware that the contents of the matrix, particularly the main diagonal of the matrix, are of major interest. The elements of the main diagonal are critical because they are used in the matrix solution. Different researchers use different approaches to selecting main diagonal elements. As a beginning user of factor analysis, you are probably best served by selecting between the two major extraction routines, described later, and using the standard approaches to values placed on the main diagonal.

Selection of the Extraction Procedure

Two extraction procedures are most frequently reported in research journals. These procedures are principal components and common factor analysis. Within the common factor analysis model, there are several further approaches to extraction.

In principal components analysis, all variance is assumed to be common variance. All error is considered random and not reflective of any underlying structure. In principal component analysis, therefore, there is no attempt to discern an underlying structure. In a full component approach, there are as many factors as there are items. Some analysts use a truncated model in which only those factors (items) that are significant are retained (Gorsuch 1983). When trivial or nonsignificant factors have been dismissed, it should not be assumed that underlying structure is evidenced. Some analysts interpret only the unrotated factor solution, since it is consistent with the logic of the error assumptions of principal components analysis, whereas other rotate the factors. The advantage of a principal components solution is that the factors are derived from the "real" data and do not represent underlying unmeasured variables (Harris 1985, Nunnally 1978).

In *common factor analysis*, the analyst organizes the structure of the data by recognizing both random and systematic measurement error. The systematic measurement error is thought to be evidence of underlying theoretically sound structure. The danger, of course, is that the nature of that structure is open to misinterpretation. Common factor analysis can be approached through the extraction method of principal axes factoring, image factoring, alpha factoring, and general least squares approaches, to name only a few. For the novice factor analyst, the most common approach of principal axes factoring is probably best. This method is appealing in that it reflects the theoretical stance that systematic error is representative of underlying structure. The first factor variance is partitioned from the matrix, then the second factor is extracted, followed by subsequent factors. The advantage of this method, of course, is that underlying structure is discerned.

In summary, several extraction procedures can be selected. The extraction procedures are designed to maximize the independent sources of variance in the matrix. These procedures discern individual items or clusters of related items identified as factors. The factor matrix produced in this phase of the factor analysis is difficult to interpret. One more step is necessary, and that is factor rotation.

Selection of Rotation Procedures

Factor rotation is designed to meet the purpose of the second phase of the work: to delineate the factors clearly and cleanly so that they correspond to sets of interrelated variables (items). It may be helpful to visualize lines drawn in space and emanating from an origin. Each line can be rotated and the point at the origin held stable so that the line best "fits" the related data points. This is much like finding the best fit regression line. Depending on the type of rotation, however, certain requirements must be met. These requirements define the rotation procedures.

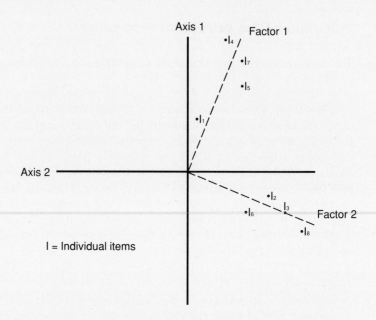

Figure 15–4 Orthogonal Rotation

Once again, we see two main types of rotations, orthogonal and oblique.

Within the orthogonal category, several rotations can be used. In *orthogonal rotation*, each factor must remain independent of all others. Thus, in our visualization of space, the lines emanating from the origin must be fit in such a way as to remain at a 90° angle to all others. Figure 15–4 illustrates this requirement with two factors. Only two are shown here because we are limited by the two-dimensionality of the page. In the hypothetical space we have visualized, however, we are not restricted to two dimensions and can have as many lines in as many dimensions as we like.

Once the decision to do an orthogonal rotation has been made, a choice among the different rotations must be selected. Three main types can be used. The goal of *varimax rotation* is to simplify the factors themselves. That is, an item is more likely to be very related to one and only one factor, but there may be more factors than with the other solutions. In *quartimax rotation*, the aim is to simplify the variables. That is, there is likely to be a smaller number of factors. In fact, quartimax rotation maximizes the relationship of the variables on the first factor extracted. The relationship of some of the variables, however, might be quite small. The final type, *equimax rotation*, is a hybrid of the prior two, and the goal is to simplify both factors and variables.

In *oblique rotations*, the requirement for independence is not maintained. Two lines could be drawn such that they are very close together and not at all at 90° angles. The underlying assumption is that the factors are indeed related and the rotation procedure should not impose an arbitrary requirement for noncorrelation. Interestingly, should an orthogonal rotation result, there is support for independence of the factors that orthogonal rotation alone cannot provide.

Criteria for Factors and Factor Loadings

Thus far, we have spoken in rather general terms about relationships of variables and factors. You need to master some specific language when interpreting the results of factor analysis. Once you understand these terms, you can understand and set criteria for interpreting the results.

Depending on the type of extraction procedure you select, you will interpret either an unrotated or a rotated factor matrix. The matrix is composed of factor coefficients (weights, loadings) for each variable in the original matrix relating to each factor extracted. Let's consider the number of factors extracted first. You can continue to extract factors until factors derived later seem trivial and make no sense. One criterion that can be employed is to examine the eigenvalues. **Eigenvalues** are the sum of the squared weights on each item for each factor. Many researchers use a long-established criterion of an eigenvalue being greater than or equal to 1.00. If the value is below that cutoff, the factor is not considered significant. Another way to examine the relative importance of a factor is to consider the amount of explained variance. There is no arbitrary cutoff as to how much variance should be accounted for by a particular factor. However, when the cumulative percentage of variance begins to change very little, then the retention of that factor in the solution adds little to the final interpretation.

Another test used to make a decision about the number of factors to be retained is the *scree test*. This involves a graphic representation of the eigenvalues. The eigenvalues are plotted on the vertical axis (see Figure 15–6), and the factors are plotted on the horizontal axis. The slope is quite sharp when the differences between the eigenvalues are high. As the slope begins to taper off or assume a more horizontal position, smaller differences in eigenvalues are indicated. Thus the factors, at this point, contribute little more to the overall explanation of the structure of the instrument.

Once the number of relevant factors has been determined, the investigator is interested in whether each item is appropriately placed in the factor. Table 15–5 gives an example of a rotated factor matrix. Each factor is noted, and the factor loadings or coefficients are placed under each factor. *Factor loadings* are the regression coefficients of the variables on each of the factors. The researcher is interested in discerning which loadings indicate that a variable explains enough variance within the factor to be meaningful. Again, there is no hard-and-fast rule about how to proceed in evaluating the appropriateness of each item being included in the factor. Some researchers accept a factor loading of .30 or .35 as evidence that the item belongs to the factor. Others require higher loadings. We have found that a modification of Thurstone's (1947) criteria is sufficiently stringent to provide items with clean loadings on one and only one factor. Each item must load on the appropriate

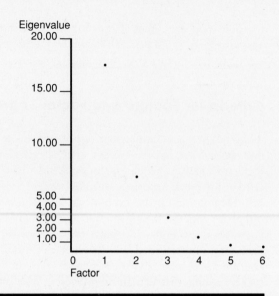

Figure 15–6 Scree test

factor at .50 or above, and there must be a .20 spread between that and the next loading. Items 1, 2, and 3 meet those criteria; items 4 and 5 do not.

Another aspect of the printout to be examined is the communality. The *communality* is the squared multiple regression coefficient for each variable across all factors. It is an estimate of the variance shared between that item (variable) and all extracted factors. The greater the communality, the greater the shared variance across the factors.

Interpretation of Factors

At this point, the theoretical expertise and logic of the researcher become the focal points. You have performed the mathematics, and now you must interpret the results. Interpretation should be completed in light of the original purpose of the analysis, the theory involved, and the orientation of the researcher to the process. The researcher has to be careful not to support preconceived notions without evidence. The researcher walks the fine line between being open to new solutions and alternate explanations while keeping in mind what is already known in the field.

Additionally, we must recognize that it is possible that a given solution can be an artifact of method and/or sample. Harris (1985) and Nunnally (1978) both suggest that several extraction routines and rotation methods should be used. Consistent

TABLE 15–5   *Rotated Factor Matrix*

Item/Variable	Factor 1	Factor 2	Factor 3	h^2
1	.78	.18	.29	.64
2	.64	.36	.07	.48
3	.53	.31	.04	.38
4	.46	.31	.15	.33
5	.30	.21	.36	.26

results with various methods are the most stable and may reduce the problem of method artifact. Replicated studies help reduce the problem of sample artifact.

We have given an overview of several of the multivariate statistics that are currently reported in nursing research. Although the novice researcher can use many statistical procedures without the assistance of a consultant, multivariate statistics do not fit that category. Good assistance in the early stages of your research is invaluable. No matter how good your consultant, you need to remember that it is you, the researcher, who has the ultimate responsibility for understanding and explaining the results of your analysis. Whenever you have a choice, select the simplest but most effective statistical technique with the least complex assumptions. This strategy makes it likely that you and those who read your work will understand your results.

Guidelines for Critique

- Is the study question appropriate to the selection of a multivariate statistical test? Is there more than one dependent variable? Is there more than one independent variable?

- Are the results of the multivariate statistical procedure presented clearly? Is enough information given in order to examine the validity of the analysis?

- Did the study have enough subjects to support the multivariate analysis?

- Is a reasonable explanation of the findings presented to the reader?

- If statistical hypothesis testing is used, were appropriate levels of significance stated?

- When decisions were made that did not have associated statistical probability levels, were acceptance or rejection criteria clearly stated?

SUMMARY OF KEY IDEAS AND TERMS

✔ Multivariate statistics are chosen for analysis of quantitative data to reduce experimentwise error rates and because multivariate questions need multivariate solutions.

✔ Multivariate statistics are defined as those that deal with situations in which there is more than one dependent variable.

✔ Many authors also consider techniques that deal with more than one independent variable as multivariate statistics.

✔ Multiple regression estimates the best linear combination of more than one independent variable as they are related to one dependent variable.

✔ A beta weight is a standardized regression coefficient which can be used to compare the relative importance of independent variables in a multiple regression equation.

✔ The R^2 is the squared multiple correlation coefficient and can be interpreted as the proportion of the variance in the dependent variable that is explained by the linear combination of independent variables.

✔ A researcher who uses multiple regression should report not only the results of the analysis but also the results of the examination for multicollinearity and possible violations of statistical assumptions.

✔ Discriminant analysis is similar to multiple regression except that the dependent variable is discrete.

✔ Canonical correlation is a procedure that examines the association between two vectors of variables.

✔ Multifactorial ANOVA is used to examine differences between groups when more than one independent variable is involved.

✔ Multiple Analysis of Variance (MANOVA) is a technique which examines the difference between more than two groups with more than one dependent variable.

✔ Factor analysis is a data-reduction technique used to determine the underlying structure of a number of variables.

✔ Factor analysis is frequently used in instrument testing.

✔ Common factor analysis and principal components analysis are two of the most frequently used factor analytic approaches.

References

Champion VL: The relationship of breast self-examination to health belief model variables. *Res Nurs Health* 1987; 10, 375–382.

Gennaro S: Postpartal anxiety and depression in mothers of term and preterm infants. *Nurs Res* 1988; 2, 82–85.

Harris RJ: *A Primer of Multivariate Statistics*. Orlando, Fla.: Academic Press, 1985.

Gordon RA: Issues in multiple regression. *Am J Sociol* 1968; 73, 592–616.

Gorsuch RL: *Factor Analysis*. Hillsdale, N.J.: Erlbaum, 1983.

Huck SW, Cormier WH, Bounds WG: *Reading Statistics and Research*. New York: Harper & Row, 1974.

King KB, Norsen LH, Robertson RK, Hicks GL: Patient management of pain medication after cardiac surgery. *Nurs Res* 1987; 36, 145–150.

Long JS: *Confirmatory Factor Analysis*. Beverly Hills: Sage Publications, 1983.

Mishel M, Braden C: Finding meaning: Antecedents of uncertainty in illness. *Nurs Res* 1988; 2, 98–103.

Morrison DF: *Multivariate Statistical Methods*. New York: McGraw-Hill, 1976.

Munro BH, Visintainer MA, Page EB: *Statistical Methods for Health Care Research*. Philadelphia: Lippincott, 1986.

Nunnally JC: *Psychometric Theory*. New York: McGraw-Hill, 1978.

Pedhauzer EJ: *Multiple Regression in Behavioral Research*. New York: Holt, Rinehart and Winston, 1982.

Stevens J: *Applied Multivariate Statistics for the Social Sciences*. Hillsdale, N.J.: Erlbaum, 1986.

Thorndike R: *Correlational Procedures for Research*. New York: Gardner Press, 1978.

Thurstone, LL: *Multiple Factor Analysis*. Chicago: University of Chicago Press, 1947.

Verran JA, Ferketich SL: Testing linear model assumptions: Residual Analysis. *Nurs Res* 1987; 36, 127–130.

C H A P T E R

16

Computers and Data Processing in Nursing Research

SANDRA L. SCHEETZ ▪ HOLLY SKODOL WILSON

Chapter Objectives

After reading this chapter, the student should be able to:

- Explain the most frequently used computer terminology

- Identify four characteristics that differentiate microcomputers from mainframes

- Collect information about local computer center resources and resource people that will be helpful in acquainting the student with the system

- List three input and three output devices

- Compare the options for inputting research data to the computer

- Describe three functions of a computer's central processing unit

- Identify one software program that can be used at each stage of the research process

- Name statistical procedures that can be carried out on research data using the SPSSx statistical package

In This Chapter . . .

This chapter introduces you to the equipment, people, and language you need to appreciate the power, fascination, and excitement that the computer can bring to nursing research. There are five good reasons for trying to become "computer literate" and avoiding computer phobia:

1. Computers are fast.
2. Computers rarely make mistakes.
3. Computers can do repetitious or tedious jobs.
4. Computers can help you manage the information deluge.
5. Computers can increase productivity and reduce costs.

The What and How of a Computer

The main use of a computer is to process large amounts of data rapidly. This function is the basis of the term **data processing**. Once data are processed, they are called *information*. Computers can process both *numerical data* such as age, weight, height, blood pressure, test scores, or diagnostic codes, and *alphanumeric data* such as letters, punctuation, names, and addresses. The time in which a computer can execute an instruction is usually measured in less than a *millisecond* (a thousandth of a second). Some computers can execute an instruction in *microseconds* (a millionth of a second), and the *nanosecond* (a billionth of a second) range is approachable.

A computer system consists of three areas designed to process data into usable information: *input*, *processing*, and *output*; they are backed by a fourth, *storage*, for keeping data. **Hardware** refers to the computer parts you can touch—the equipment in the system that stores, processes, and controls information. These units are related in the system as illustrated in Figure 16–1. **Software** is another word for the *programs* that instruct a computer what to do.

All computer chips are made of chips of silicon, a nonmetallic substance found in sand, rocks, and clay. A typical *silicon chip* is ⅛ of an inch square. Most chips easily fit on the head of a pin. A computer can accomplish the same work that 30 years ago required a 30-ton computer housed in a warehouse the size of a football field.

Silicon is used for chips because it is a semi-conductor; that is, it will conduct an electric current when chemicals are used to etch electronic circuits onto its lattice-like crystalline structure. Patterned on the silicon base are minuscule switches, joined by wires etched from thin films of metal. These are complete, or *integrated*,

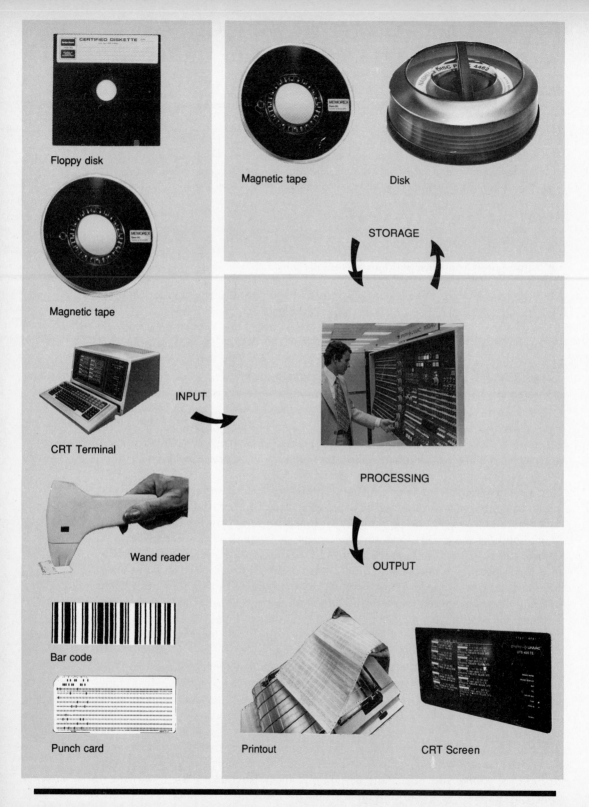

Floppy disk

Magnetic tape

Disk

STORAGE

Magnetic tape

INPUT

CRT Terminal

PROCESSING

Wand reader

OUTPUT

Bar code

Punch card

Printout

CRT Screen

Figure 16–1 A complete computer system.   Source: Capron, HL, Williams, BK: *Computers and Data Processing*, Menlo Park, California, Benjamin/Cummings, 1984.

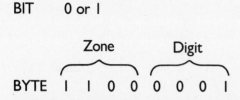

BYTE   I   I   0   0   0   0   0   I

Figure 16–2   The byte shows the letter "A" in computer code.

electronic *circuits*. Under a microscope, the chips's intricate terrain looks uncannily like the streets, plazas, and buildings of a giant metropolis viewed from miles up. The circuits (electrical switches) are turned off or on according to a **binary system**. The binary system is a yes-no "two-state system" that turns the circuit switches on or off through combinations of ones and zeros that represent data. One switch inside the circuit is called a *binary digit*, or **bit**. A single chip holds 3000 or 4000 bits. A group of eight bits that stands for a character (e.g., A, b, 2, $, etc.) is called a **byte** (see Figure 16–2). The eight bits on one byte can be arranged in 256 different ways to represent complicated data. Figure 16–3 illustrates how bits within a byte, by turning off and on like a lightbulb, represent the numerical code for the letter *A* to the computer. The number of combinations in one byte is more than enough to represent each letter, number, and punctuation mark in this chapter.

Most contemporary universities and hospitals (as well as banks and businesses) own or lease a large, million-dollar **mainframe** computer with terminals located in different places. These terminals are connected to the computer by telephone links. If you intend to use the computer center at your institution, the following information will help you get acquainted:

- The building, room number, and telephone number of computer locations
- Type and description of computer systems available to you
- Hours when computer center is open

I   I   0   0   0   0   0   I

Figure 16–3   The bit as a lightbulb flashing on and off.

- Staff members and consultants available

- Introductory computer courses, workshops, and contact persons

- Computer programs and packages available

- Location of terminals and microcomputer labs

- Availability and location of users' manuals

- Steps to get a user's I.D. number and computer account

- Places to pick up computer printouts

Most institutions also have **minicomputers** about the size of a refrigerator and a number of **microcomputers** (also called *personal* or *business computers*) sitting on desktops in offices and labs throughout the building. Each of these computers— the mainframe, the *minis*, and the *micros*, as they are called—basically perform the same functions. They store, retrieve, sort, compare, and process data. They perform arithmetic and statistical functions, and they do it very quickly. The main differences between the three main types of computer is their power as reflected in

1. speed

2. cost

3. amount of storage

4. number of users who can simultaneously share the machine

The mainframe is considered the fastest, with the most storage and the most multi-task and multi-user capabilities. It is usually the most expensive, while the least expensive microcomputer has the least speed, power, and storage capacity. However, with rapid advances in microchip technology and the introduction of superconducting chips, these distinctions have become blurred. Mainframes are now supercomputers, minis are comparable to mainframes, and it is no longer uncommon for personal desktop computers to have near-mainframe computing capacity. To understand what computers can do for the researcher, you need to know what computers do. A discussion of hardware and software is a good place to start.

Taking a Tour of the Hardware

Hardware refers to the electronic and mechanical parts in the computer system that store, process, control, and output information. The primary parts are input devices, the central processing unit, output devices, and external storage devices.

Input Devices **Input devices** put data into a form that the computer can recognize. The ways of entering data into a computer are:

1. a card reader, into which keypunch cards are put

2. the keyboard of a terminal, on which data are typed

3. a machine that reads data from floppy disks (explained later in the chapter)

4. a magnetic ink character reader (*MICR*) which reads (for example) numbers on a personal check

5. an **optical scanner**, which recognizes optical marks like those used on the answer sheet of a computer-scored test

6. a wand, which recognizes optical characters (for example, the wand attached to the cash register of a department store)

7. a light pen or touchscreen for altering data directly on a CRT (cathode ray tube) screen

8. bar code or magnetic stripe readers

9. a **mouse** (mechanical or optical) for pointing or drawing

The newest addition to this long list of input devices is the voice recognizer, a device that can take dictation and turn the spoken word into **ASCII** (the standard 7-bit code representing characters) files. As of early 1988 several of these devices, which combine hardware (an expansion board and microphone) with related software, were available. However, it will be some time before they are in widespread use.

Although most modern computer centers no longer use either card readers or keypunch machines to punch holes in computer cards, many concepts related to that way of entering data have been inherited from the long-time use of these machines. Therefore, we describe them briefly along with the most commonly used input device—the keyboard.

Keypunch cards contain small holes that represent data and can be read by a card reader. These cards contain 80 vertical columns and 12 rows. Each single column may contain a punch representing the numbers from zero to nine. Usually rows zero to nine are printed on the card, and the top few rows are used for identifying information. Data are coded on the card through a process called **keypunching**. A keypunch machine is a lot like a typewriter, except that it is used to punch holes in the columns of the card. After a deck has been keypunched, it can be taken to another machine, called a verifier, which checks that the holes in the cards are correct by comparing the data originally punched against rekeyed data.

Researchers prepare their data for inputting by plotting out a **code book** to designate which columns will contain which data (see Table 16–1). For instance, descriptive data on students enrolled in a nursing course can be translated into numbers that are punched in specific columns of a card. The system is called a *fixed-column format*, because the values for each variable you are studying are located in the same column for every case or subject. When the data for one subject require

---

TABLE 16–1 *Computer Codebook for Scoring the Social Relationship Scale (SRS) Subscale for Work*

Variable	Name	Column	# Columns	Scale/Description
1	ID#	1–3	3	3-digit subj code by site
2	WKNTWRKA	4	1	Work network total, time 1 (A) (Range = 0–8)
3	WKSORC1A	5	1	Work source for person #1
4	WKSORC2A	6	1	Work source for person #2
5	WKSORC3A	7	1	Work source for person #3
6	WKSORC4A	8	1	Work source for person #4
7	WKSORC5A	9	1	Work source for person #5
8	WKSORC6A	10	1	Work source for person #6
9	WKSORC7A	11	1	Work source for person #7
10	WKSORC8A	12	1	Work source for person #8
11	WKHELP1A	13	1	Subj. rating of helpfulness for 1st Name in Work List (Range = 1–7)
12	WKHELP2A	14	1	Helpfulness rating person #1
13	WKHELP3A	15	1	Helpfulness rating person #2
14	WKHELP4A	16	1	Helpfulness rating person #3
15	WKHELP5A	17	1	Helpfulness rating person #4
16	WKHELP6A	18	1	Helpfulness rating person #3
17	WKHELP7A	18	1	Helpfulness rating person #4
18	WKHELP8A	19	1	Helpfulness rating person #8
19	WRECIP1A	20	1	Reciprocity rating person #1 (1 = yes; 2 = no)
20	WRECIP2A	21	1	Reciprocity for person #2
21	WRECIP3A	22	1	Reciprocity for person #3
22	WRECIP4A	23	1	Reciprocity for person #4
23	WRECIP5A	24	1	Reciprocity for person #5
24	WRECIP6A	25	1	Reciprocity for person #6
25	WRECIP7A	26	1	Reciprocity for person #7
26	WRECIP8A	27	1	Reciprocity for person #8

more than one card, the variables must be entered on the same card for all members of the sample. For example, if David Bowie's age is punched in columns 6 and 7 of the third card, every other respondent's age would also occupy columns 6 and 7 of the third card in their case. There is no fixed limit to the number of cards a case may contain, and blank spaces need not be included between variables on a card. Blank spaces make it easier for you to read the cards, but the computer doesn't use them.

Once punched, the set of cards, or *deck*, is then placed into a *card reader*. This machine sends the data on the cards to the computer by translating the holes into electrical impulses. Key-to-tape and key-to-disk, also called key entry, have replaced keypunching and cards because of the former's increased speed, productivity, and accuracy. In these techniques, a magnetic spot is placed on a magnetized surface, such as a diskette or tape. The computer translates these spots into electrical impulses, just as the card reader translated holes in computer cards into electrical impulses, but now without that intermediate step.

Furthermore, the input format is not limited to the 80-column card image of keypunched data, although that format is still an option. The format need not be fixed. An unlimited number of columns can be used, although the format must be consistent for each observation or case within a particular data set. "Punching" in data, however, remains a manual process. If large amounts of data need to be input, most researchers hire a professional key-entry service that uses one of the above techniques. If resources are limited, it is not impossible to learn to enter your own data using a terminal or a standalone microcomputer as a data-entry device.

The keyboard of a computer terminal looks a lot like a typewriter's except that it has several extra keys. It allows you to type data directly into the computer for processing or storage. The computer also interacts with you, the user, by displaying instructions and responses on a screen called a *cathode ray tube* (CRT). This two-way communication between user and computer is referred to as the *interactive mode*. Keyboards can be used to type data onto tape or disks (also called diskettes and floppy disks). A **floppy disk** looks like a 45-rpm record encased in a heavy paper or hard plastic jacket.

Terminals are basically of two types. Those that can perform some processing are called a "smart" or intelligent terminal. The second is a "dumb" terminal, or a CRT, which merely allows data entry and has no processing capabilities. A microcomputer is an example of a "smart" terminal because it has its own CPU, whereas many of the keyboard-monitor combinations located near a mainframe computer center are dumb terminals. In the latter case, the processing is performed by the mainframe computer after data are entered and sent to it from the dumb terminal.

Output Devices   Output is data that have been transformed into information and can appear as printing on paper (printouts), spreadsheets (a particular form of printout), color graphics, electronic signals, and sounds. **Output devices** produce the results of computer processing.

A *printer* is a machine that produces *hard copy*, or printouts. (Soft copy, by comparison, is output displayed on the screen.) There are two types of printers. *Impact printers* work much like typewriters by physically striking paper. *Nonimpact printers* use heat, lasers, or sensitized paper. Impact printers include:

- *character printers*, which print character by character across the page from one margin to the other. The daisy wheel, consisting of a removable wheel with a set of spokes containing raised characters, is an example.

- *line printers*, which assemble all characters in a line at one time and print them out simultaneously. The printing can form a solid character of *letter-quality print*.

- *graphics printers*, which construct a character by activating a matrix of pins that produces the shape of the character. Dot-matrix printers are both faster and generally cheaper than letter-quality printers.

Furthermore, with advances in printer technology, the print quality of dot-matrix printers has improved, and many now have *near letter-quality* (NLQ) output. Some allow the user to switch from a draft mode, which produces output of lesser quality at a faster speed, to an NLQ mode, which produces output of higher quality at a slower speed. The speed of a printer is described in characters per second (cps). For a sample printout, see Figure 16–4.

Nonimpact printers have fewer moving parts and are quicker and faster. They include:

- *electrostatic printers*, which supply an electrical charge through the pens into the paper in the shape of the character. When passing through ink, the particles stick to the charged areas of the paper, producing a visible image.

- *electrothermal printers*, which essentially burn the images onto the paper. You may have to buy special paper for them, and in some cases the print fades from the page over time.

- *laser printers*, which are a lot like photocopiers. They involve electrical transfer onto a photoconductive surface, to which ink is then applied.

- *ink-jet printers*, which spray ink through an electronic field that deflects the ink and produces dot-matrix characters.

For on-line, real-time time transactions, when you are interacting with a computer, a computer *terminal*, or CRT, is best used for output as well as input. CRTs produce two major forms of output—alphanumeric and graphic. Alphanumeric terminals look like small television screens and display numbers and characters that include punctuation and special symbols. Graphics terminals display graphs, maps, and charts, sometimes in spectacular color. Most graphic terminals can also display alphanumeric data, but few alphanumeric terminals can also display graphics without the addition of special hardware.

As computer technology advances, more sophisticated forms of output become available. Other output devices include:

- computer output microfilm, called **microfiche**, which allows a lot of printed material to be presented in a small space

```
ANALYSIS OF NATIONAL PSYCHO-SOCIAL PROGRAM DESCRIPTION

FILE   NONAME    (CREATION DATE = 11/03/81)

NATFAC
                                    RELATIVE   ADJUSTED    CUM
                          ABSOLUTE    FREQ       FREQ      FREQ
CATEGORY LABEL      CODE    FREQ      (PCT)      (PCT)     (PCT)
CMHC                 1.       1        6.3        6.7       6.7
SMF                  2.       1        6.3        6.7      13.3
RESID RX FACIL       3.       3       18.8       20.0      33.3
HALF WAY HOUSE       4.       1        6.3        6.7      40.0
COMMUNAL GROUP HOME  6.       8       50.0       53.3      93.3
WORKING FARM         7.       1        6.3        6.7     100.0
                    99.       1        6.3      MISSING   100.0
                          ------     ------     ------
                   TOTAL      16      100.0      100.0
ANALYSIS OF NATIONAL PSYCHO-SOCIAL PROGRAM DESCRIPTION

FILE   NONAME    (CREATION DATE = 11/03/81)

NATFAC
      CODE
         I
    1. ****** (     1)
         I  CMHC
         I
         I
    2. ****** (     1)
         I  SMF
         I

    3. *************** (     3)
         I  RESID RX FACIL
         I
         I
    4. ****** (     1)
         I  HALF WAY HOUSE
         I
         I
    6. ***************************************** (     8)
         I  COMMUNAL GROUP HOME
         I
         I
    7. ****** (     1)
         I  WORKING FARM
         I
         I
     99.            (     1)
 (MISSING) I
         I
         I.........I.........I.........I.........I.........I
         0         2         4         6         8        10
         FREQUENCY

VALID CASES      15     MISSING CASES      1
ANALYSIS OF NATIONAL PSYCHO-SOCIAL PROGRAM DESCRIPTION

FILE   NONAME    (CREATION DATE = 11/03/81)
```

Figure 16–4 Sample printout.

■ graphics plotted on paper or transparency film, using either flatbed plotters or drum plotters

■ photographic graphics

■ robots

■ voice output devices

■ digital film recorders, which produce color slides and transparencies

The Central Processing Unit (CPU)   The **CPU** or **central processing unit** is the part of the computer that can be likened to the brain. Its function is to keep track of what is happening and execute a program that processes your data. It consists of three parts: (1) a **control unit**, which takes care of operating the electronic equipment; (2) an arithmetic-logic unit (ALU), which computes all the calculations that can be performed at hundreds of thousands per second by running an operating program; and (3) primary storage. The control unit acts as an orchestra leader directing other parts of the system to execute program instructions. The ALU controls arithmetical operations or mathematical calculations and logical operations.

Operations a computer can perform on your data include:

■ calculations. A computer can add, subtract, divide, or multiply one million problems in a second! These calculations are commonly called "number crunching."

■ rearrangements. A computer can put your data into alphabetical or numerical order.

■ reading input. A computer can read 100,000 characters each minute.

■ writing data onto an output unit. A computer can print out 260,000 characters each minute.

■ storage. A computer can store data in its own temporary memory or transfer it to an external storage device.

There are two types of processing. **Batch processing** of data, on the one hand, is a technique in which transactions are collected into groups, or batches, to be processed. One advantage of batch processing is that it is more efficient and thus usually less expensive than other types of processing. One disadvantage is that you have to wait for your data to be processed. **Direct-access** (also called interactive) **processing**, on the other hand, is a technique for processing transactions in any order they occur. *Real-time processing* is a common form of direct-access processing. It requires that your terminal be *on line*—that is, directly connected to the computer. The first advantage of real-time processing is that you don't have to wait. The second advantage is that you can continuously update your data. *Time sharing* is a system in which two or more computer users can share the use of a central computer and, because of the computer's speed, can receive simultaneous responses.

Storage   The *primary storage unit* is also called main storage, internal storage, or **random-access memory** (RAM), and it temporarily holds data and instructions for processing while a program is being run. RAM memory is active as long as the power supply to it is uninterrupted. However, when the computer loses electrical power, whatever was in memory is lost.

A *secondary storage device* allows data to be stored outside the computer on magnetic tape, magnetic disk, or mass storage. External, secondary storage is necessary because the storage inside the computer is only temporary. Auxiliary, or secondary, storage devices allow far more enduring, space-saving, and convenient data storage than volumes of files or shelves of boxes of keypunched card decks do. The ability to store a great deal of data in a small space is one of the computer's most impressive capabilities. Characteristics of secondary storage include:

1.   economy—because you save space and time in filing and retrieving data

2.   reliability—because others can't tamper with or remove your data

3.   convenience—because hours of searching through file cabinets and notebooks can be eliminated

The major types of secondary storage are (1) magnetic tape, (2) magnetic disk, and (3) mass storage.

Magnetic tape looks much like the tape used on reel-to-reel tape recorders. It's about ½ inch wide and is wound on a reel that's 10½ inches in diameter. The tape has an iron oxide coating that can be magnetized. The most common length of a reel of tape is 2400 feet, and the amount of data on the tape is the number of bytes per inch or characters per inch. A customary storage capacity or density is 1600 bits per inch (bpi). High-density tape is now 6250 bpi. A magnetic tape unit can either read data onto or retrieve data from the magnetic tape, using an electromagnet that reads the magnetized areas on the tape, converts them to electrical impulses, and sends them to the processor. Data on tape are stored sequentially. This means that your records are written onto the tape one after another. So, if you want to read case 33 of a data set, you must bypass all the preceding cases. Capron and Wiliams (1984) cite the following advantages of magnetic tape for storing your research data:

■   It is compact. One 2400-foot reel of tape at 1600 bpi can hold as much as 240 boxes of punched cards, and at 2000 cards per box these boxes would completely fill a closet!

■   It is reusable. Data on tape can be erased.

■   It is relatively inexpensive. A 2400-foot reel of tape costs less than $15.

Despite its advantages, it still has at least two drawbacks:

■   It is vulnerable to physical damage from heat, dust, stretching, and tearing.

■ It is sequentially organized, and you may have to read the contents of an entire file to add, delete, or revise one particular record.

Magnetic disk storage is a second form of external, or auxiliary, storage. A magnetic disk is a metal platter coated with ferrous oxide. The disk looks something like a long-playing stereo record but is usually 14 inches in diameter. Disks are grouped together in a disk pack that looks like stereo records on a spindle. Data can be retrieved much more quickly from a disk than from a tape, because the disk pack rotates over the read-write mechanism 40 times each second. Data are recorded as magnetic spots on the tracks on the surface of the disk. Disk capacity ranges from a low of 250,000 characters on a small, one-record disk to a high of 200 million on a modern disk pack. With disk storage you can go directly to the data you want at any point on the disk. This feature is called *direct-access storage*. The most obvious disadvantage of using disk storage is the cost. One disk pack typically costs $300 or more. The disk storage unit can cost thousands more. Also, confidentiality may be a problem, because unauthorized persons can access your data.

Because confidentiality of subjects' data is a primary concern to, and responsibility of, the researcher, every effort must be made to secure the data. A breach of confidentiality can be avoided by installing a system to lock either the disk or the power supply physically or to use an electronic lock, such as a password system, to keep the data from unauthorized persons. For a more general discussion of this topic, see Romano (1987).

A version of the magnetic disk for microcomputers is called a **hard disk**, *fixed disk*, or *hard card*. The disk diameter is much smaller, naturally, than that of a mainframe hard disk. A microcomputer hard disk is about the same size as the 5¼ inch floppy, with storage size ranging from 10 to 310 **megabytes** (MB), or 310 million characters. That is equivalent to 300,000 pages of information.

Diskettes, or **floppy disks**, are magnetically coded disks used in personal computers. They can be double-sided and hold up to one and a half million characters. One diskette can hold a 200–300-page term paper and costs as little as 75 cents.

Mass storage is the third form of secondary storage. It allows you to store large amounts of data that might have been collected, for example, in a national survey of health care needs or resources. Mass storage devices consist of honeycomblike structures that contain magnetic tapes, most commonly used in mainframes. When data are needed, a mechanical arm retrieves the cartridge from the cell and transfers the data on it to a magnetic disk. The whole process takes just 3 to 8 seconds. Some computer experts think the future of storage lies with bubble memory, because with these futuristic devices that consist of a chip coated with magnetic film, data do not disappear when the power goes off.

Hardware Summary

Mainframes, minicomputers, and microcomputers perform the same tasks of inputting, storing, retrieving, and processing vast amounts of data very quickly. They differ (from most to least, respectively) in cost, speed of processing, amount of primary and secondary storage, and number of tasks and users that can be accommodated at one time.

Data are input for processing by the CPU using any number of input devices, with the mouse becoming almost as common as the keyboard. The characters and numbers on the keyboard are one byte of data. The control unit of the CPU stores the bits of data and instructions until needed, then retrieves them to complete the processing you, the user, request. Other instructions awaiting processing by the CPU are held in RAM until needed. The resultant information is output by way of the monitor or CRT or to any number of other output devices, most commonly the printer, but also to a secondary storage device such as a floppy or hard disk for additional processing at a later time.

Software

A computer's hardware is no better than the software used with it. Software is the programs that make hardware do what you want it to do. The process of writing the series of instructions that tells the computer what to execute is called *programming*, and the person who does this job is called a *programmer*. In the early days of computers a program was entered directly by punching the programming code onto cards with a card punch. These were then read into the computer, using the same card reader that would read the deck of cards containing the data set. As technology improved, computer users began to transmit instructions to the computer using an interactive system that allowed them to carry on a dialog with the computer by typing at a terminal.

Software is classified into three major categories:

1. System programs

2. Programming languages

3. Application/software packages

Systems Programs   The program that runs all of the time in the background is the *operating system* (OS). In the microcomputer, the OS is commonly called the disk operating system or **DOS** (pronounced *doss*). It is the "traffic manager," directing the flow of all the electronic signals that enter or leave the computer. For example, it directs commands from the user at the keyboard to the control unit, the CPU, which then schedules the commands and directs the appropriate electronic signals to the monitor or printer. *Utility* programs are also a kind of system program, but in general they are used to manage files rather than hardware. Utility programs are used for repetitive housekeeping tasks, such as copying, erasing, and renaming files.

Programming Languages   At present there are about 150 programming languages in use for communicating with and instructing the computer. Some have colorful names, such as Hearsay and Jovial. The most commonly used ones, however, are **Fortran** (Formula Translation), **COBOL** (Common Business Oriented Language), PL1 (Programming Language One), and **BASIC** (Beginners' All-purpose Symbolic Instruction Code). Pascal (named after the mathematician Blaise Pascal) and C are two others. Languages are called lower level if they are more like the language the computer uses (the binary system of zeros and ones). Languages are called higher level if they are more like the languages people use.

Software Applications   In addition to the system programs and programming languages, there is another large category of software programs called software packages. These are also called application programs and run only when invoked by the computer user. They are designed to help the user complete tasks, solve problems, and produce specific output. There are thousands of specific packages for completing thousands of user tasks, from keeping track of names and addresses to managing a sophisticated research project. However, only general categories of software application programs that you might commonly use in the stages of the research process, described in Chapters 8 through 15, are discussed here. Examples are writing proposals and articles, completing an electronic literature search, keeping track of research subjects or grant budgets, analyzing data, and producing graphics for the final report or for presentations.

These programs are generally "user friendly" (easy to learn and use), although the instructions to the computer, which are not seen by the user, are written in a programming language. No longer does the user have to know programming. Instead, the user is provided with a way to make requests of the program. The options you as user must choose from are usually presented in one of three ways:

1. menu

2. template

3. command language

You can think of a computer menu as a restaurant menu with submenus. Your first choice is analogous to choosing from among "Appetizer," "Entrée," and "Dessert" menus—those three choices constitute the *main menu*. When you decide to have an appetizer, you must make another choice from that submenu. Using a template is like filling in a page with empty, labeled spaces or boxes. Command language structure requires learning what the specific commands mean to use them correctly. Usually the commands have user-friendly names, for example, "find" or "get," but they can also be very much like a programming language and thus, because of increased control, a very powerful tool for the user. More sophisticated software programs may allow you a choice: The new user may choose to use menus because they are more instructional, whereas the experienced user may choose the command level because it is faster since the user need not wait for a menu to appear on the screen.

Word Processing Programs   "Processing," to most writers, sounds at first like a nasty and uncreative thing to do to a word. But typing this chapter on a computer means you can simply delete mistakes electronically, add an idea you just thought of, move whole chunks of material to another part of the chapter with just a press of a few buttons, correct the spelling of a word throughout the whole chapter, run a thesaurus program that can provide half a dozen synonyms, check your spelling against a dictionary program, and do automatic footnoting and indexing. When finished writing, you press a few more buttons, and the printer prints the manuscript in less than one minute per page, with even margins and pages numbered.

A typical word processing program offers the following list of abilities:

- You can "word wrap." That means when you come to the end of a line, the next letter automatically begins at the start of the following line; words aren't hyphenated at the end of a line.

- You can search for and replace a name or misspelled word everywhere it appears.

- You can justify margins.

- You can move pieces of the text.

- You can type over existing text on screen.

- You can edit the portion of your paper that's displayed on the screen.

- You can view comprehensive instructions on the screen while running the program.

Less commonly available capabilities that would be useful for writing a journal article include:

- Footnoting for citations

- Printing hanging indentations in reference lists and bibliographies

- Providing two-line headers

- Outlining

- Checking spelling

Communication Software.   This specialty software is required, along with a piece of hardware called a **modem** (modulator-demodulator), for your computer to communicate over ordinary telephone lines with another computer. The software helps you set parameters for communications and allows you to make the necessary connections between the two computers. Two uses for communication software are (1) linking on-line information sources and (2) connecting your microcomputer to the mainframe.

On-line Information Retrieval.   You are certainly aware of the value of knowing how to use the library to search the literature related to your research project (see Chapter 8). You should also know about the benefits of using the computer to search the literature. Computerized literature searches represent another major application of technology in the research process. The most frequently used computerized bibliographic service among health professionals is **MEDLINE** (the National Library of Medicine's *Index Medicus* data base.) This system and **MEDLARS** (Medical Literature Analysis and Retrieval System) were initiated by the National Library of Medicine (NLM) in 1971. Over 2700 journals are indexed in these systems. A MEDLINE bibliography, for example, provides full journal citation including authors, article, title of journal, volume, issue, number of pages, and date. Nursing journals included in the *International Nursing Index* are available through this source.

To use the MEDLINE search you have to select search terms that are likely to yield references that are relevant to your topic. In most cases you will be able to request such a computerized literature search through your health science library for a fee of about $30. If you are ever ambitious enough to compile a comprehensive bibliography on a topic of interest or are assigned to do so in a course, the most conscientious and scholarly approach is to begin with a computerized search of the literature. Otherwise, it's tempting to make expedient and convenient rather than comprehensive choices (for example, including only those journals in your local school of nursing library), a practice not recommended to the readers of this text.

Besides the NLM data bases, a number of massive data bases are now available to the general public. For researchers, the electronic data base search is a powerful adjunct to our usual library searches, even with the assistance of a reference librarian. Although such services are not free—for example, you must pay for telephone connect time and purchase a subscription to the service, much as you would a magazine subscription—the process is really amazingly straightforward. Before, these resources were available only to major libraries. Today, dialing for data has the potential to improve the quality of research sustantially because it gives access to enormous bibliographic data bases (Garson 1987).

Knowledge Index is a service of DIALOG Information Services, Inc. It gives access to more than 35 of DIALOG's (over 200) most popular data bases at reduced rates during off-peak times. A one-time start-up fee of $35 (as of this writing) includes a user's workbook and two hours of free credit. The cost of access after the first two hours is $24 per hour of connect time. After two hours of practicing, you can make a thorough search of data bases with articles relevant to your research topic in as little as 30 minutes and for only $12. You can save the citations you have retrieved on a disk or the computer's buffer (RAM) at no additional cost.

Another popular information retrieval service is BRS/After Dark, a service of BRS Information Technologies. For a one-time fee of $75 and a monthly minimum of $12, you have access to over 90 separate data bases covering a multidisciplinary range of topics. Data bases are priced from $6 per hour, including the cost of connect time and telecommunications. Display charges per document are extra.

On a more limited basis, the NLM is now marketing an information retrieval software package called Grateful Med to search its extensive holdings. More than

20 data bases are included in the NLM system. Holdings include MEDLINE and MEDLARS, mentioned earlier. Grateful Med costs about $30 plus approximately $22 per hour for prime time connect time or $15 per hour for off-peak connect time.

CompuServe is the largest of several large, general-purpose information services that provide a limited number of bibliographical, text, and numeric data bases. It is also known for its electronic bulletin boards for computer users with a range of special interests, including nursing. Connect time is $15 per hour ($8 per hour off-peak), with some bulletin board services costing above the basic charge.

Database Management Systems (DBMS)   With research subjects to keep track of as well as hundreds of relevant references, how does one manage all of the information? One way is to use a **data base management system** designed to manage data in the form of records. Each item is called a *field*; a collection of fields is a *record*; and a collection of records containing the same kinds of data is a *file*. The user can design the equivalent of a blank form, organized to meet the needs of the task at hand. For example, you might want to keep track of subjects for a longitudinal study requiring sending three questionnaires over a period of six months. You need the subjects' names, addresses, telephone numbers, dates of entry into the study, and, possibly, the responses to each questionnaire, if it's not too complicated or lengthy. Once the data are entered, you can search the data base for those who entered at a certain time and are due to have a questionnaire sent. These programs can also generate mailing labels, quite a time saver. Even with only 25 subjects, you would need a minimum of 75 address labels, and typing each one would take considerable time. Many DBMS programs also have an electronic security procedure for encoding the file, thus denying access to unauthorized persons. This precaution ensures confidentiality of subject data, a primary concern of researchers.

Another special kind of DBMS program is designed to manage bibliographical or reference data. Some programs allow the user to set up such fields as *author*, *publisher*, and *journal* and to enter lengthy textual information, such as an abstract. Others have preset forms for entering all kinds of citations, from the standard journal article or book to less commonly cited sources, such as videotapes, music, and computer software. An example of the former program is Notebook II (Protem Software, Palo Alto, California), which retails for under $200. An example of the latter is Pro-Cite (Personal Bibliographic Software, University of Michigan, Ann Arbor), which sells for $395.

Electronic Spreadsheets.   Researchers also need to keep track of budget data, especially for formal proposals (see Chapter 17). A good way to keep track of budgets is to use an **electronic spreadsheet**. Think of rows of items and columns of figures to match, like the items in a household budget. Rows are labeled with numbers; columns with letters. A particular spreadsheet location, called a *cell*, is identified by the intersection of a row and column, e.g., A1, C12, DD200. Electronic spreadsheets, in addition to allowing you to input labels and numbers, also allow you to input formulas. For example, you can indicate that all the income items in cells B1 through B10 are to be added. You can also supply formulas to add all the expense items and subtract them from the total income, telling you how much money you have at the end of the month. Once you enter the formula, the program automatically makes the calculations regardless of the number of times the cell amounts are changed or corrected. The completed budget with its respective rows, columns, labels, and formulas is called a worksheet. One of the most popular spreadsheet programs is Lotus 1-2-3 (Lotus Development Corporation).

A program that combines a data base management program, a spreadsheet, and a third package we haven't discussed yet—graphics—is called an **integrated package**. Some integrated packages also have word processing and communications programs. Each of the components is designed to work easily and efficiently with the other components, and data entered in one part of the program can be used in the others. The Student Edition of Lotus 1-2-3 (Addison-Wesley and Benjamin/Cummings Publishing Companies, Inc., Reading, Massachusetts) is an example of such a program. The advantage of this educational version is that it is much less costly ($40) than the full version of Lotus 1-2-3 ($300). The limitation of this educational version is that you are limited to 256 rows and 64 columns. For the researcher who has a small sample size and a limited number of variables, the program is quite sufficient. Data entered in this program can also be transported to the mainframe and used by most of the major mainframe statistical packages as well as their microcomputer counterparts.

Statistical Programs.   Three prepackaged, or canned, statistical programs for analyzing quantitative data dominate the mainframe computing environment. These are: the *Statistical Analysis System* (SAS), the *Statistical Package for the Social Sciences* (SPSS), and the *Biomedical Statistical Software* (BMDP). Learning to use these mainframe packages is neither easy nor trivial. You not only have to learn how to use the packages and understand some statistics, but must also learn another program, such as the **Conversational Monitoring System (CMS)**, an interactive operating system needed to interact with the computer and statistical packages. Having some knowledge of a line editor program to input program lines (i.e., instructions for the statistical package) is also helpful. Line editors can be mainframe based, for example *Xedit*, or a microcomputer counterpart, *Kedit* (Mansfield Software Group, Storrs, Connecticut).

The features of each of these mainframe packages and their IBM Personal Computer (PC)–based counterparts are summarized in Table 16–2. These are summarized because of their widespread use. Microcomputer statistical packages are not limited to these; many more are generally available. See popular computer magazines, such as *MacWorld, PC World, PC Magazine, Byte, PC Tech Journal*, and *InfoWorld*, for reviews of such packages and information on where to buy them. See also several review articles of packages for both the IBM PC and the Macintosh computers (Fridlund 1986, Lehman 1987, Moad 1987).

Each mainframe environment is somewhat different. The best recommendation is to plan well in advance. Speak with faculty, classmates who have completed

TABLE 16–2 *Features of Mainframe and PC Statistical Programs*

Functions & Procedures	SPSSx	PC+	SAS	PC	BMDP	PC
			Programs Compared			
Data File Functions						
Data entry	x	x	x	x	x	x
Data verification and updating	x	?	x	x	?	?
Data management	x	x	x	x	x	x
File management	x	x	x	x	x	o
Transformations	x	x	x	x	x	x
Statistics						
Descriptive	x	x	x	x	x	x
Frequency distributions	x	x	x	x	x	x
Contingency tables	x	x	x	x	x	
Correlations and scatterplots	x	x	x	x	x	x
ANOVA/ANCOVA	x	x	x	x	x	x
Multiple regression	x	x	x	x	x	x
Factor analysis	x	x	x	x	x	x
Canonical correlations	x	x	x	x	x	x
Discriminant procedures	x	x	x	x	x	x
Clustering procedures	x	x	x	o	x	x
Survival analysis	x	o	x	o	x	x
Life tables	x	o	o	o	x	x
Analysis of additive scales	x	o	?	?	?	?
Nonparametrics	x	x	x	x	x	x
Log-linear models	x	x	x	o	x	x
Univariate and multivariate analyses	x	x	x	x	x	x
Box-Jenkins analysis of time series data	x	o	o	o	x	x
Repeated measures	o	o	x	x	x	x
Reports and Tables	x	x	x	x	x	x
Graphs/Charts	x	x	x	x	x	x
Special PC Functions						
Reads/writes ASCII files		x		x		x
Reads Lotus/dBase files		x		x		o

Key   x = Present   o = Absent   ? = Not Known

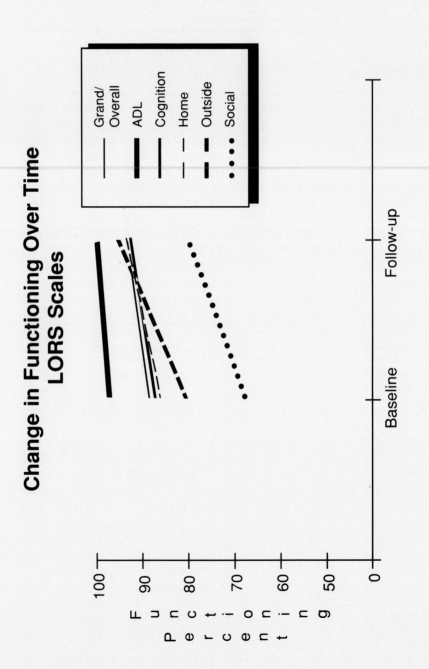

Figure 16–5   Line graph created using graphics package.

research, or a consultant to weigh the pros and cons of using the mainframe versus a microcomputer, especially if both are available to you. Visit your computer center. Identify what software is available and find out what classes you will need to take to plan the data entry and data analysis stages of your research using the mainframe.

Qualitative Analysis and Meta-Analysis   Two additional resources that allow alternative analysis of data deserve mention. The first is a program for the analysis of qualitative data, called the Ethnograph (Qualis Research Associates, Littleton, Colorado), priced at about $150. It is designed to manage field notes, transcripts, documents, and other types of text data collected and analyzed in ethnographic research, freeing the researcher to focus more attention on the interpretive aspects of the analysis. (See Chapter 13 for a more detailed discussion of qualitative analysis.)

The second is a package of 14 BASIC-language computer programs that perform a wide variety of meta-analytic procedures. **Meta-analysis** generally refers to the statistical integration of the results of independent studies. Mullen (1986) describes and reviews the package, identifying system requirements and the strengths and limitations of the programs.

Graphics.   Nothing is more satisfying than completing the research project and producing a finished product. A useful adjunct at this stage, in addition to a good word processing package, is a good graphics package. Graphics software is designed to help you produce quality tables, charts, and graphs for your written report or for presentation. With the right hardware—which might include a mouse or digitizing tablet for freehand drawing, a color graphics monitor for visualizing as you work, and either a good quality laserjet printer, a color printer, or a plotter for output— you are set to compete with the best of them. However, even without all of the bells and whistles, some programs work very well with just a keyboard, graphics monitor, and dot-matrix printer. So don't despair! Figure 16–5 is an example of a same-size line graph produced on a Macintosh computer using PageMaker, which is not even a full-fledged graphics program. The same chart was also plotted in six colors on mylar (transparency) and photographed to produce a slide for presentations.

The Student Edition of Lotus 1-2-3, mentioned earlier, is useful with regard to graphics. Data can be interchanged, that is, entered in the worksheet portion of the program and then used by the graphics module to create line, bar, stacked-bar, and XY graphs as well as pie charts. You can view the graphs you have created on the screen if you have a graphics monitor. If you have a color monitor, you can see them in color. If you can't view the graphs on the screen, you can create a file to print on a printer or plotter using the 1-2-3 PrintGraph program. You can convert ASCII files that you may have imported to a standard worksheet format and then graph them in the same way. This is a powerful tool for visualizing data input from other sources.

Many of the graphics packages reviewed by Seymour (1988) also import files from Lotus in what is called the ".WKS" or worksheet format. Some packages import files in ASCII, ".DIF", and ".SYLK" formats from data base management programs, other electronic spreadsheet programs, and even word processors. Transporting data from one program to another is an incredible time saver because you do not have to reenter data already keyed in once.

Mainframe versus Microcomputer   What are the relative advantages and disadvantages of using a microcomputer rather than a mainframe for data entry, data management, and statistical analyses, if the researcher has access to either a mainframe or microcomputer system *with the necessary statistical software*?

The major advantages of the mainframe over the microcomputer for statistical analysis, the most complex and computer-dependent phase of research, is the speed of processing and thus the time savings. Mainframe computers are especially superior for large-scale data and number-intensive studies. However, mainframe computing is costly, and access is less than ideal.

Although the strength of the microcomputer is really in word crunching and not number crunching, for smaller studies with no more than 250 variables and 2000 cases, the microcomputer is more than up to the task, working with amazing speed and accuracy. Because of its size, such a study, commonly completed by undergraduate and graduate students, does not require a mainframe. What you lose in speed you will gain in convenience, flexibility, control, and total freedom to explore your data and do additional analyses without worrying about running out of computer funds with "just one more" analysis to complete. For a more detailed discussion of "micros versus mainframes" with an emphasis on statistics, see Schrodt (1984).

Whether you use a mainframe or a microcomputer to analyze your data statistically, it is important to plan the analyses in advance and then determine whether the mainframe or a microcomputer has the most appropriate statistical programs to use. With the computers available today, you have a lot of flexibility because you can input data directly to the mainframe and then download and analyze them with a microcomputer statistical package, or vice versa. You can input data with any number of software packages that allow you to write ASCII, ".DIF", and even ".WKS" files (similar to graphics packages) from a word processor to a data base management package or even to a statistical package. The files are saved and then "uploaded" to the mainframe for statistical analyses.

Data Cleaning and Beyond

Before using a statistical package to analyze quantitative data, however, you should be sure that your data are "clean." **Data cleaning**, or finding the errors in your data, is one of the most unpopular parts of data analysis, because most people find it tedious and boring. But it can mean the difference between an otherwise fine study and disaster. Poor quality data yield poor quality results—thus the expression "garbage in, garbage out," or GIGO. The usual method for data cleaning is to run frequencies for all the scores on each item and then inspect them for the appearance of anything that is not plausible. For instance, if the possible range of scores is 1 to 5 and two cases have a 6, a keypunching error has probably been made. Once data are clean, the investigator usually asks the computer to obtain descriptive statistics or marginals on it, including measures of central tendency (mean, mode, and median) and measures of distribution (standard deviations, variance, and range) (see Chapters 14 and 15). In addition to descriptive statistics, most researchers ask for a list of all the data elements for each subject on a printout to be used for reference in the future (see Box 16–1)

Box 16–1   Scheetz Data File Listing—Demographics

Obs.	ID #	GROUP	AGE	SEX	MARITAL	EDLEVEL	ETHNIC
1	101	1	23	2	1	14	3
2	102	1	40	2	2	14	3
3	103	1	38	2	3	12	3
4	105	1	38	2	2	17	3
5	106	1	41	2	3	14	3
6	107	1	34	2	1	17	3
7	108	1	35	2	3	14	3
8	109	1	30	2	1	16	3
9	110	1	37	1	−9	16	2
10	112	1	28	2	1	17	3
11	113	1	41	2	3	16	3
12	114	1	20	1	1	12	3
13	115	1	37	2	1	16	3
14	116	1	26	2	1	16	3
15	201	2	37	1	1	16	3
16	202	2	35	1	3	15	3
17	203	2	26	1	2	14	3
18	204	2	40	1	3	17	1
19	206	2	27	1	2	11	2
20	207	2	35	1	1	15	3
21	208	2	24	1	1	13	2
22	209	2	31	1	1	15	4
23	210	2	31	2	2	14	3
24	211	2	38	2	1	12	3
25	212	2	40	2	1	18	2
26	213	2	39	1	3	16	3
27	214	2	43	1	3	18	3
28	215	2	36	1	1	13	3
29	216	2	32	1	1	11	3
30	217	2	29	2	1	14	3
31	218	2	39	1	2	11	3

Steps in Using a Computer on Data

Once data are cleaned, running any program or procedure on your research data involves six key steps:

1. Prepare your data for input into the computer, using a code book and either key entry or the keyboard (see Table 16–1).

2. Enter your data into the computer using your user ID and password.

3. Define your data to the statistical package you intend to use.

4. Transform your data to create any new variables that you want to study.

5. Run statistical procedures.

6. Store your data on tape, cards, or disk or transfer them to a diskette.

Buying Your Own Personal Computer

A decision to buy a personal computer (microprocessor) should be made cautiously. The fear of being left out in the cold or the desire to be the first among equals in your research class is propelling many of us into computer stores. But the new owner of a computer may find to his or her dismay that the aura of light that surrounds computer-equipped scientists in many of the magazine ads doesn't come with the machine! If you decide to buy a microcomputer, you'll probably want to get the following standard microcomputer components:

- A keyboard

- A computer processor

- A display screen

- At least two disk drives

- A 20 MB hard drive

- A dot-matrix or letter-quality printer

If you decide to shop for a computer, let the following rules guide you:

1. "Software dictates hardware." Find the software you want, usually in the form of a 5¼-inch floppy disk, and then study the machines that run it.

2. Never betray your primary use. If you have decided you can justify the price of a computer for a particular purpose—let's say word processing—don't be distracted by secondary uses like graphics.

3. Don't buy anything until you see it work. The road test you'd demand before buying a new car is doubly important here.

The new generation of true 16-bit personal computers is by and large a stunning rack of hardware. Each seems to have a particular and often unique capability. One is portable, and another is able to make the quality charts and graphs that heretofore only more costly machines could produce. Here are six factors to think about as you look for a personal computer.

Factors to Consider When Buying a Personal Computer

1. Memory   Remember, memory is measured in **kilobytes** (K) and **megabytes** (mb). We usually figure that one K contains 1000 bytes (actually there are 1024, but even computer buffs don't quibble over 24 bytes). In 1 mb, there are 1 million letters, or about a 420-page paperback. The size of your computer's memory limits what programs you can use. The internal memory of a computer has two phases—**read-only memory (ROM)** and **random-access memory (RAM)**. ROM is permanent memory and contains the computer's operating systems software and assembly language. The RAM loses its contents when the power is turned off, and so is called volatile working memory. When you load in a program, its instructions are dumped into the RAM. A complex statistical program requires considerable RAM capacity. Most experts suggest that you get a minimum of 640 K of RAM for analyzing research data.

2. External Memory or Storage   Storage of data outside the computer itself is usually done on tape cassettes, floppy disks, hard disks, or video disks. Storage is also measured in kilobytes or megabytes. Floppy disks file information as a series of magnetic traces. Their principal use is to store programs and feed them into your computer. You should be wary about using cassettes to store important data. Not only are they easily damaged, but they also operate serially, and so you must wind and rewind to locate specific files. Most desktop or personal computers come with a diskette drive that holds two floppy disks—a storage disk, and an applications program disk. One diskette can store about one million bytes, depending on size and quality.

3. Display   Display is what you see on your screen. It can be color or monochrome (usually green or amber), and its capacity is figured by the number of characters or columns per line. The **resolution** of your display (that is, how clear and easy it is to read) is determined by the number of picture elements (*pixels*) it has. The more pixels, the sharper the letters.

4. The Keyboard   You should choose your keyboard carefully. Some are springy, and some are spongy. Some keys don't move mechanically. Find one you like.

5. Interfaces   These are the places where you attach *peripherals* such as printers or disk drives to your computer through the input/output (I/O) ports. The more I/O ports your computer has, the more peripherals you can use.

6. Documentation   **Documentation** is the computer term for the manuals, instructions, and guides that come with your hardware and software. Read them carefully and try out some procedures before you buy. Instruction manuals that are difficult to understand can be a quick way of ruling out some computers.

Computer Costs for Research

If by choice, necessity, or virtue of the size of your data base you intend to use an institution's computer resources, you should anticipate the costs involved. Three primary sources of costs related to computer-based data analysis are:

1. data coding and input

2. analysis costs (CPU and consultant time)

3. data storage on a magnetic medium (Slichter, Hanson, and Gortner 1984)

Writing proposals to obtain funding for your research will be easier if you are familiar with these costs and include them in your budget (see Chapter 17). Discuss costs prospectively with your computer center consultants as part of planning your budget.

Computer People

Computer people include data entry people, computer operators, librarians, programmers, and system analysts. If you are a novice with no prior computer experience, you should turn to the experts for consultation and assistance.

- *Data entry people* put data on cards, disks, or tape for processing.

- *Computer operators* monitor the console, review procedures, and keep peripheral equipment such as printers running.

- *Librarians* are in charge of cataloging processed disks and tapes and keeping them secure.

- *Computer programmers* design, write, test, and implement programs.

- *System analysts* know about programming but have broader responsibilities that include planning and designing whole systems of programs, based on a clear understanding of users' requirements.

Computer-Aided Instruction (CAI) in Research

The computer is not only a tool you can use at every stage of the research process, it is also a learning aid that teaches you about the research process and statistical concepts. Special educational software may teach you basic terminology and concepts, problem identification, critiquing skills, and even how to construct tables and graphs. Learners acquire the knowledge and skills using computer tutorials, exercises, testing, and simulations. Here are some examples of these programs: Research Methodology and Statistical Concepts (Heshi Computing, Hitchcock, Texas); Nursing Research CAI (MOSBYSYSTEMS, St. Louis, Missouri); and the Clinical Research System for Personal Computers (International Medical Products, Minneapolis, Minnesota), which is more like a management system for a clinical research study. Prices for these packages range from $250 to as much as $3000 for the management system.

Guidelines for Critique

- What are the major differences between mainframes, minicomputers and microcomputers?

- What are the most common devices for data entry?

- What secondary storage devices are used primarily with microcomputers?

- How is the computer used as a tool in each stage of the research process?

- What are the primary statistical packages used for data analysis?

- What is one of the most important prerequisites to insure a quality research study?

- What features are important for a researcher to consider when planning the purchase of a microcomputer?

SUMMARY OF KEY IDEAS AND TERMS

✓   Mainframe computers are larger, faster, costlier and allow more users than microcomputers.

✓   Beginner's All-Purpose Symbolic Instruction Code (BASIC) is the most popular personal computer language. Some other languages include Pascal, C, FORTRAN (Formula Translation), and COBOL (Common Business Oriented Language).

✓   Control Program for Microcomputers (CPM) is a popular disk operating system for 8-bit machines.

✓   Disk Operating System (DOS) is a common disk operating system for 16-bit machines.

✓   The speed of a printer is measured in characters per second (cps).

✓   The cathode ray tube (CRT) is the screen on the computer, also called a monitor. The more pixels—individual points of light—it has, the easier it is on the eyes.

✓   *Documentation* is the printed information available for software and hardware. These manuals should be user-friendly—that is, easy to understand.

✓   The typefaces on a *dot-matrix printer* are composed of tiny dots. A *letter-quality printer* uses either a daisy wheel or thimble mechanism to make typewriterlike typefaces.

✓   Peripheral devices are external components of the computer that input to, and output from, the CPU. The most common peripherals are the keyboard and the printer. These are also called input-output (I/O) devices.

✓ A personal microcomputer that works as a stand-alone machine is an *intelligent terminal*. A dumb terminal is one of many terminals hooked up to a giant mainframe computer.

✓ A computer system consists of three areas: input, processing, and output; they are backed by a fourth area—storing data.

✓ Operations that a computer can perform on data include calculations, rearrangements, input, output, and storage.

✓ Statistical Analysis System (SAS), the Statistical Package for the Social Sciences (SPSS), and Biomedical Statistical Package (BMDP) are the major software programs used to compute statistical analyses of nursing research data.

✓ Finding errors in data by "data cleaning" can mean the difference between a good and poor analysis.

✓ Nurse researchers also use the computer to conduct literature searches.

✓ Software programs used in the research process range from word processing for writing and editing, data base programs for tracking subjects and managing data, statistical packages for analyzing, and graphics packages for creating charts and graphs.

✓ Security of data is enhanced using either physical or electronic locks on programs or the computer.

✓ Consultation with resource people in your computer center will help you achieve a realistic estimate of computer costs involved in conducting a research study.

✓ Buying a personal computer should be done thoughtfully, keeping in mind the purposes that it will serve.

Notes

Mention of specific software packages or hardware in this chapter is for illustrative purposes only, and does not constitute endorsement of any of the products by the authors. The following addresses of software manufacturers are provided for your convenience.

Addison-Wesley Publishing Co.
EMS Division
Lotus 1-2-3 Student Edition
Jacob Way
Reading, MA 01867

BMDP Statistical Software
1964 Westwood Blvd., Suite 202
Los Angeles, CA 90025
(213) 475-5700

BRS Information Technologies
555 East Lancaster Ave.
St. Davids, PA 19087
(215) 254-0233
(800) 468-0908

CompuServe
P.O. Box 20212
5000 Arlington Centre Blvd.
Columbus, OH 43220
(614) 457-0802
(800) 848-8199

DIALOG Information Services Inc.
3460 Hillview Ave.
Palo Alto, CA 94304
(800) 3-DIALOG
(415) 858-3785

Grateful Med
National Library of Medicine
MEDLARS Management Section
8600 Rockville Pike
Bethesda, MD 20894
(301) 496-6193 (within Maryland)
(800) 638-8480

Heshi Computing
P.O. Drawer M
Hitchcock, TX 77563

International Medical Products Corp.
4503 Moorland Ave.
Minneapolis, MN 55424
(612) 835-4018

KEDIT Mansfield Software Group
P.O. Box 532
Storrs, CT 06268
(203) 429-8402

Microsoft Corp.
16011 NE 36th Way
Box 97017
Redmond, WA 98073-9717
(206) 882-8080
(800) 426-9400

MOSBYSYSTEMS
11830 Westline Industrial Dr.
St. Louis, MO 63146
(800) 325-4177 (ext. 750)

Personal Bibliographic Software
P.O. Box 4250
Ann Arbor, MI 48106

SAS Institute, Inc.
Box 8000
Cary, NC 27511-8000

SPSS, Inc.
Suite 3000
444 North Michigan Ave.
Chicago, IL 60611
(312) 329-2400

The Ethnograph
Qualis Research Associates
611 E. Nichols Dr.
Littleton, CO 80122
(303) 795-6420
(303) 394-8664

References

Capron HL, Williams BK: *Computers and Data Processing.* Menlo Park, Benjamin/Cummings, 1984.

Fridlund AJ: Statistics software. *Infoworld* (September 1) 1986; 31–39.

Garson GD: *Academic Microcomputing: A Resource Guide.* Beverly Hills, Sage, 1987.

Lehman RS: Statistics on the Macintosh. *Byte* (July) 1987; 207–214.

Moad J: The new statistics. *PC World* (October) 1987; 252–255.

Mullen B: Session V. Statistical analysis on microcomputers. *Behav Res Meth Inst & Comput* 1986; 18, 165–167.

Romano C: Privacy, confidentiality, and security of computerized systems: The nursing responsibility. *Comput Nurs* 1987; 5, 99–104.

Schrodt PA: *Microcomputer Methods for Social Scientists.* Beverly Hills, Sage, 1984.

Seymour J: Business graphics software: At the top of the charts. *PC Magazine* (March 15) 1988; 93–139.

Slichter M, Hanson C, Gortner, S: Researchmanship: Computer costs for research grant planning. *West J Nurs Res* 1984; 6, 133–135.

P A R T

IV

Scholarly and Intellectual Craftsmanship in Nursing Research

17

Writing a Research Proposal

HOLLY SKODOL WILSON

Chapter Objectives

After reading this chapter, the student should be able to:

- Analyze circumstances that might influence what format a research proposal should take

- List the basic components of a research proposal that ought to be included, whatever the format may be

- Interpret the implications of (1) considering one's audience and writing for strangers, (2) making the proposal attractive, and (3) achieving a balance of detail and flexibility in planning the proposal

- Formulate a specific research proposal that reflects an effective synthesis of the six steps of proposal writing: (1) problem statement; (2) theoretical framework and literature review; (3) design, methods, and procedures; (4) timetable or work plan; (5) personnel, budget, facilities, and resources; and (6) abstract, title, and cover letter

- Evaluate one's own (or a colleague's) formal study proposal against conventional criteria for scientific merit

- Explain six strategies that are likely to increase one's chances of finding public or private funding for a proposed research project

(Continued)

- Describe the review process for the National Center for Nursing Research (NCNR)
- Appreciate the value of proposal-writing skills to the advancement of nursing education, nursing administration, and nursing clinical practice, as well as nursing science in the next decade

In This Chapter . . .

In the opinion of many authorities, the core of a research project is the soundness and coherence of its logic. You communicate this logic more or less effectively through a written research proposal. Here you have the chance to relate your study question to a scientific tradition or the problems of a professional discipline, describe and justify the methodology that you've selected, and reasonably project the importance of your possible conclusions. Like all other communication, proposal writing is part science and part art. In the words of Krathwohl (1977):

> Classes in painting can instruct an artist in the principles of shading, contrast and perspective, but it is the artist's creativity with these that is critical to success [p. 1].

This chapter presents the basic characteristics of a research proposal in a general way so as to be applicable to a wide range of study designs and methods. A section on "grantsmanship" and finding research funding offers both checklists for increasing your chances for success and information on why some proposals fail. Although no one set of standards or rules can hope to capture the variety of methods available for approaching the task of proposal writing, this chapter is intended to increase the likelihood that your research ideas are not rejected by research course faculty members, thesis or dissertation committees, or by funding agencies because they were poorly presented. A successful proposal is both logical and persuasive. This chapter guides you step by step through the process of planning research and communicating these plans effectively.

Purposes of Writing a Research Proposal

The reasons for writing a formal written research proposal vary:

- A proposal might be required by a thesis or dissertation committee or even for a nursing course as evidence that you not only are able to formulate researchable problems that have merit for nursing but also have the ability to plan systematically to address them.

- Most funding agencies, private or public, require submission of a research proposal.

- If you are hoping to convince a hospital, clinic, or other institution or group to allow you access and entry to collect data, it is usually a good idea to present the "official gatekeepers" with a study proposal (see Chapter 12).

- Institutional review boards (see Chapter 3) require an abbreviated proposal or prospectus before approving studies that involve human beings as research subjects, even when research is conducted as part of an educational experience.

- Investigators themselves often find that it is useful to synthesize and articulate the ideas and plans that have been evolving as they consider the specific topics of problem formulation, design, sampling, data collection, and analysis.

A well-written proposal should convince members of the scientific community that your research is significant and reflects mastery of background knowledge, methodological procedures, and the logic of inquiry necessary to conduct it. The proposal also addresses the expected significance of the results, the investigator's competence to conduct the study, and the availability of facilities and equipment necessary to the study.

Components of a Study Proposal

The exact format of research proposals and the extent of detail expected in them varies with the target review committee or funding agency. Some granting agencies provide their own guidelines, instructions, and proposal formats in an *application packet*. Such a packet, if available, is essential so that you can present your proposed study so that reviewers can compare it with other competing studies. Box 17–1 presents an illustration of instructions you would find in such a packet. A human subjects committee (or institutional review board) is interested in a brief prospectus that will enable the members to assess (1) the risk-benefit ratio of your proposed study and (2) your inclusion of adequate provisions for obtaining informed consent from prospective research subjects. A thesis or dissertation committee will probably be interested in the intricate details of your background knowledge, design, and methodology to ascertain that your study is feasible and has sufficient scientific merit. Most research faculty members believe that the clearer and more precise the original study proposal is, the smoother the conduct of the research project will be, because you will in effect be carrying out a previously designed plan that has received a thorough review and critique by a mentor.

Perhaps the major exception is field research. Field researchers inductively generate a conceptual analysis from qualitative, observational, and interview data (see Chapters 12 and 13). Such investigators make a conscious attempt to avoid

Box 17–1   Summary of Suggestions for Preparation of Research Proposals

Preliminary Informal Proposals

Prospective applicants normally find it desirable to submit a proposal in preliminary form as the basis for discussion before a formal request is prepared. This is usually in the form of a letter of a few pages which describes what the prospective applicant proposes to do, the rationale behind the proposed project, the personnel who would be involved, the expected outcome, and the nature and amount of support needed from the supporting agency, as well as support actually or potentially available from other sources.

It is suggested that the proposals be stapled on the upper left corner and include a cover sheet. A brief abstract or summary of the more important objectives and procedures contained in the formal proposal may be inserted following the summary sheet. Certain additional guidelines are generally furnished after program staff members have had an opportunity to review an informal and preliminary inquiry.

General Outline for Preparation of Proposals

1. *Cover page*: The cover page generally contains identifying information.

2. *Abstract*: The abstract generally occupies a single page, identifies a proposal, and summarizes the contents concisely and simply. The abstract must be written in language understandable by an informed layperson and give a clear, succinct summary of the proposed project. At the top of the abstract page the following items should appear on separate lines: title of project, principal investigator, contracting agency, amount of federal funds requested, and proposed beginning and ending dates. The summary portion of the abstract has three parts:

   a. a statement of the purposes, objectives, or nature of the project

   b. an indication of its expected contribution to nursing

   c. a compendium of the procedures or a description of what is to be done

3. *Narrative*: The narrative of the proposal communicates the principal investigator's (PI) plan and its probable effectiveness. It should be clear, concise, forthright, and complete. Within the body section, there are ordinarily four parts, which should be adapted as appropriate for the particular kind of proposed activity to be undertaken.

   a. *Problem and aims*—The first part tells *why* the proposed activity should be undertaken. It includes a statement of the problem or purposes, review of literature and related research, concise statement of objectives, or any other information necessary to establish a sound rationale.

   b. *Description of activities (procedures)*—This part tells *what* is to be done, *when* and *how*. It is the basis for determining the degree to which the

(Continued)

Box 17–1   Summary of Suggestions for Preparation of Research Proposals (Continued)

proposed activity can be expected to accomplish the aims or satisfy the needs set forth in the first part of the proposal narrative. It delineates procedures, outlines project arrangements, and describes findings to be produced. A time schedule for completion of the project is usually provided near the end of the proposal. The amount and kind of detailed information will vary according to the type of study.

c. *Relevance of the findings*—This part tells what new knowledge or contribution toward nursing can be expected and what steps should follow to build on the outcomes. This part tells how the results of the research may be disseminated or implemented.

d. *Personnel and facilities*—Personnel and facilities are a major determinant of capability. Personnel with major responsibilities are listed by name, position, title, experience, responsibilities within the project, percentage of time committed to the activity, and the extent to which this commitment has been assured. Consultants who have agreed to serve should be similarly identified (otherwise, the application should state the type of consultative assistance required). Facilities should be described, and the extent to which their use has been assured should be indicated.

4. *Budget*: The budget section of the proposal should make reasonable estimates, with enough detail to show careful analysis of expected costs and understanding of fiscal responsibilities in connection with conducting the proposed activity.

5. *Appended items*: Appended items should include:

   a. reports of pilot and related studies

   b. agreement with cooperating agencies

   c. data-gathering instruments

   d. prior approval

   e. clearance

   f. rights of human and animal research subjects information

---

premature closure on what exactly is important to study until they immerse themselves in the natural conditions of "the field" (see Chapter 12). Furthermore, the field researcher assumes an attitude of pragmatism about data-collection and analysis strategies rather than adhering strictly to a prefabricated plan, or blueprint. In short, the predominant attitude among this group of researchers is: If it works to advance the analysis (and it's ethical), try it!

For most other studies, however, the research proposal is regarded as a comprehensive summary of what you intend to do, how you will do it, and why it is important. An investigator who departs from the originally proposed plan is usually expected to report such deviations and explain why they occurred. Some institutions and agencies view the written research proposal as an actual *commitment on the part of the researcher to conduct the study in a specific way*, and the study itself must proceed as originally outlined. In this regard, a detailed, extremely precise proposal may be more constricting than helpful. Whether general or specific, the format for research proposals incorporates the sections listed in Box 17–2.

Later in this chapter we will take up each component of a research proposal and explain the decisions in detail. But first we look at some general hints for increasing the chances that your proposal will convince others of the merits of your research.

General Hints on Preparing a Proposal

Consider Your Audience, and Write for Strangers

Although *you* have no doubt devoted what might seem like an astounding amount of time to thinking through both your research topic and the approach you intend to take to it, remember that the readers and reviewers of your proposal may not be as well informed in your area of interest as you are. *Explain everything clearly and logically.* Avoid using jargon or abbreviations that may be commonplace in your nursing speciality area but "Greek" to a funding agency review committee. Readers who are unfamiliar with your subject will easily identify flaws in structure and internal consistency. Develop a chain of logic throughout your proposal that hangs together and has no weak links. For instance, objectives of the research must logically flow from the problem statement, and each hypothesis or objective must be addressed by a corresponding data-collection and data-analysis procedure. Choices of descriptive or inferential statistical methods must be consistent with the purpose of your study and the level of inquiry you are proposing. Check your proposal to be certain that you have not dropped objectives along the way or advanced certain data-collection plans without a corresponding plan for analyzing them. Good writing, like good speaking, uses visual aids. Make use of headings and subheadings, underlining, diagrams, flowcharts, and tables that tell the reader what the critical parts of your proposal are without requiring him or her to plow through endless pages of undifferentiated prose. On this point, however, keep Krathwohl's (1977 p. 21) admonition in mind: "The writer must also be careful to avoid the opposite extreme, jazzing the copy with . . . more gesture than sense. . . . Remember that research is essentially a scholarly activity."

Package Your Proposal So That It Is Attractive

In addition to not being well informed about your research interest, your reviewers and readers may also be less enthusiastic about the value or importance of your

---

Box 17–2   Components of a Research Proposal

1. a title

2. an abstract (or summary)

3. a statement of the study problem, purpose, and specific aims and their significance

4. the theoretical background and selective review of related research

5. hypotheses to be tested or research questions to be answered

6. the study setting

7. the design

8. the sampling procedure and characteristics

9. the data-collection strategies or instruments

10. the plans for storing, retrieving, and analyzing data

11. ethical considerations, such as provisions for informed consent and protection of human and animal rights

12. a timetable or work plan for the conduct of the study

13. a budget and statement of resources available or needed

14. a description of the qualifications of the investigator

15. references

16. appendixes

---

study than you are. It's up to you to convey not only what your project hopes to find out but also why doing it is important to the world, to nursing, or to the funding agency. As Polit and Hungler (1987) point out, "There's no need to brag or promise what cannot be accomplished but . . . it is not inappropriate to do a little selling" (p. 607).

Conveying a sense of enthusiasm for your project does not require Madison Avenue techniques. But making your proposal physically attractive is an effective strategy for increasing its appeal. Although fancy binding and printed covers may not only be overly expensive to produce and mail but also make your proposal cumbersome to circulate among readers, you should definitely pay attention to the following:

- Type the proposal or have it typed (using letter-quality or double-strike type if it's done on a word processor and printer).

- Proofread it, and proofread it again.

- Put it aside, and then reread it with some critical distance.

- Make revisions when necessary.

- Be sure to correct errors in spelling, grammar, and referencing. (The care you give to such details in your proposal often conveys something about your attention to the details of your research.)

- Number the pages.

- Make the required number of copies to be sent off, and keep at least two copies in different places for yourself.

- Check your proposal for consistent use of the future tense. (After all, you are proposing to do something in the future.)

- Follow the most recent guidelines and instructions for proposal submission that you can obtain from the agency or committee. (It's often an excellent idea to establish a relationship with a representative of the agency early in the proposal development phase to avoid going astray.)

Finally, your proposed research will be more attractive to a funding source or organization if you have taken the time to match the study it proposes with the organization's goals or fields of interest. Consulting agency publications, previously funded studies, or staff members is invaluable in acquiring this kind of information. Intramural funding for nursing research to improve patient care may receive a favorable review by the board of a private community hospital, but basic research dedicated exclusively to theory testing may not be within its institutional mission.

Balance Detail and Flexibility

A proposal should reflect a balance between sufficient detail, so that reviewers are convinced that the study is worthwhile and the investigator has the ability to conduct it, and sufficient flexibility. Writing such a plan is a craft that must be finely honed. The issue of length comes up here, and two general guidelines coexist: (1) When in doubt about including or excluding some piece of relevant information bearing on your proposed project, *it's better to include rather than exclude it*. (2) Page limitations are set for a purpose and should be respected. The solution to these seemingly incompatible guidelines is to *use appendixes to provide auxiliary information* and not try to crowd details into the main body of the proposal. Appendixes can give reviewers the benefit of the findings of a pilot study (see Chapter 1). They can also locate the proposed study within the context of a broader program of research. And they can incorporate the qualifications of the investigator. All these additional pieces of information may assist a reviewer in making a decision about your proposal but without unduly burdening someone who may, because of limited time, be reading a mass of proposals according to the "skip and skim" approach.

According to Krathwohl (1977), the typical sequence that many reviewers use is
something like this:

> Read and digest the summary or abstract. Skim enough of the first part of the problem
> statement to get a feel for it. Skim the literature review to figure out the unique
> features of this study. Skim the objectives and turn to the work plan and look over
> the flowchart, PERT diagram or timetable to get a detailed grasp of the study design.
> Check the qualifications of the investigator to see if the necessary competence seems
> present. Check the budget to be sure it's not out of line with the work proposed or
> not padded with equipment or travel that is unrelated to the research (or any other
> comparatively large budget items) [p. 22].

Some of the suggestions in the preceding general hints are clearly directed to
the experienced professional nurse who is seeking funding for his or her ongoing
research. But they are also applicable to undergraduate and graduate students who
must learn to develop research proposals either for specific course work or before
beginning master's theses or doctoral dissertations. Proposal writing is a relevant
skill for all nurses. In the following section, we give a realistic, step-by-step approach to writing one. The steps that follow specify communication tasks posed by
nearly all research proposals. Each proposal, however, demands its own unique
arrangement.

Steps in Writing a Research Proposal

Step 1: Introducing the Study: The Problem Statement

A meticulously crafted statement of the research problem usually begins a research
proposal. It must not only convince reviewers that the proposed study is important
but also reduce the scope of the problem to manageable terms by specifying a study
focus. If any specialized or esoteric concepts or terms are used in the problem
statement, they must be defined early and prominently so that reviewers don't base
their reading on any misconceptions. Many experts believe that this step is, in fact,
the art of research, because it requires creativity, perceptiveness, and imagination.
Although the study problem must not be too broad or grandiose, the potential
generalizability of the findings must also be explicitly stated. Funding decisions are
often strongly influenced by the clarity with which an investigator conveys how a
particular piece of research will contribute to theory or overall knowledge of general
or specific phenomena. Thus, *both the general statement of the purpose of the research
and the specific study question should be succinctly expressed and even underlined very early
in the proposal.* "The most common error in introducing research is failure to get
to the point—usually a consequence of engaging in grand generalizations" (Locke,
Spirduso, and Silverman 1987). Consider how each of the nurse researchers in the

following modified and adapted examples presented their study problems in early proposal drafts.

For the most part, the problem statements in the example below:

- introduce the central constructs

- precisely state the overall study question

- justify the problem as meriting study by providing the rationale

- admit of possible solution

- are intelligible to a reader who is generally sophisticated but may be relatively uninformed in the specific area of investigation

- formally state hypotheses or research objectives

It's not a bad idea to conclude the problem-statement section of a proposal with a sentence that begins: "Therefore, the specific problem for this investigation is . . ." It is surprisingly difficult to reduce all you want to discover to a single, unambiguous question.

EXAMPLE: Statements of Nursing Problems

Example 1   The concept of the hospice in the United States has evolved in the last decade. The research literature related to this kind of care is sparse. No one has systematically determined what hospice care givers actually do. Furthermore, no research has been conducted to ascertain from terminally ill persons and their families what it is that hospice care givers do that constitutes effective care. Therefore, the problem of this descriptive study is *to identify the effective and ineffective behaviors of hospice care givers in providing care to terminally ill persons and their families in a home setting* (Hehn, D. 1983).

Example 2   It is estimated that 3 million people suffer from a mental disorder annually. Of these, 1.7 million suffer prolonged, severe disability. These constitute the chronically mentally ill population, and the current overall estimate of how many of them have been deinstitutionalized into the community is as high as 800,000. Research on self-care in the basic aspects of living day to day for this population reveals a gap as to the influences of others on self-care practices. The proposed study investigates the influence of characteristics of social network on the performance of self-care by chronically mentally ill adults in the community (Scheetz S. 1984).

Example 3   Knowledge of one's state of health is a prerequisite for practicing self-care. A lack of knowledge has consequences that may seriously affect biological integrity and quality of cancer patients' lives when they are receiving radiation therapy. To date, no comprehensive anticipatory approach has been tried to help patients prevent or manage the side effects of radiation therapy before their development. *The problem for the proposed experimental study is to test the effectiveness of presenting side effect management techniques information before the occurrence of experienced side effects on care behaviors* (Dodd, M. J. 1982).

Example 4   The overall purpose of this descriptive study is to develop a valid and reliable instrument to describe and measure the phenomenon of fatigue in cancer patients (Piper, B. F. 1982).

Example 5   The problem for this study is to expand the body of knowledge about the experience of pain in adolescents. The long-range goal is to provide health professionals with information to enable them to deal more effectively with adolescents who are anticipating or experiencing pain. *The specific study question is, "Do adolescents hospitalized for acute or chronic illness describe the pain experience the same as nonhospitalized adolescents?"* (Savedra, M. 1982).

Source: Adapted from unpublished research proposals, University of California at San Francisco.

Remember that the intention of this first section of your proposal is to make the problem area of your study clear to a reader. Many proposal writers accomplish this by first presenting the larger context in which the problem is found and then narrowing down the big picture to the specific study that is being proposed. They demonstrate the relationship between the two and highlight why their study is important. The problem-statement section is often labeled "Introduction" and consists of three subheadings:

1. Statement of the Study Problem (including specific hypotheses or study questions and definitions of terms and variables to be studied)

2. Specific Aims of the Research (which specify the focus of the study and the contribution to knowledge it will make)

3. Significance of the Study (which addresses the background of the study problem and why it is important)

Although it is possible to reduce this section to a few seemingly simple parts, the art of creating a good statement of the problem in a research proposal is usually the product of vigorous intellectual effort.

Step 2: Theoretical Framework and Review of Related Literature

Both nursing research that is designed to solve practical clinical problems and studies that are conducted to test or yield knowledge for knowledge's sake must be placed in the context of what scientific work has gone before. Even Sir Isaac Newton paid tribute to his predecessors by commenting that he had been able to see some things that others had not because he had stood on the shoulders of giants. A review of relevant literature is included in a study proposal to accomplish several purposes:

1. It presents the theoretical basis, framework, or organizing scheme of which the proposed study is a part.

2. It offers not a mere bibliography but an analytical and critical appraisal of the important and recent substantive and methodological developments in your area of interest and indicates how your proposed study will refine, revise, extend, or transcend what is now known.

3. It informs and lends support to your assumptions, operational definitions, and even methodological procedures by demonstrating to your reader that the proposed study has profited from scholarly and scientific work that has preceded it.

TABLE 17–1 *Needs of the Chronically Mentally Ill Identified in the Literature*

Source	Material	Personal	Psychological
Bassuk & Gerson (1978)	Money Decent housing Transportation	Safety Guidance in coping with mechanics of daily living Adequate follow-up treatment Recreation	Vocational rehabilitation Sheltered employment or job referrals Activities and interaction with others
Paul & Lentz (1977)		Resocialization and assistance with ADL Reduction of bizarre behavior	Vocational/role performance or "salable" skills Sheltered employment or job referrals Supportive "roommate" in the community
Stein & Test (1978)	Money Food Housing Transportation	Freedom from a pathological, dependent relationship	Supportive other and motivation to persevere and to remain involved with life Coping skills Assertive support system

Source: Used with permission of Sandra L. Scheetz, RN, *The Influence of Social Networks on the Performance of Self Care by the Chronically Mentally Ill Adult in the Community.* Dissertation proposal, University of California at San Francisco, 1984.

Critics of this section of study proposals report that the single most obvious flaw is that authors tend to cite theory and prior research that have only the most tenuous connection with the study being proposed. As a result, this section has a disjointed quality, because it looks like a mere catalog or listing of marginally related work lacking a thoughtful, well-developed integration. Avoid statements that imply either that nothing has been done in your research area or that so much has been done that it is impossible for you to summarize. Statements of this sort are usually taken as indications that the investigator proposing the study does not really have a command of relevant literature and knowledge in his or her field. Tables 17–1 and 17–2 accompanied and summarized one research student's literature review.

Step 3: Preliminary (Pilot) Studies or Related Prior Work

In a *Nursing Research* guest editorial, Hayman (1987) commented on the merit of "programs of research" over single isolated studies. This section of a proposal describes the investigator's pilot and/or related research to:

1. Illustrate competence to pursue the proposed study

2. Outline contributions to knowledge in the topic area

3. Demonstrate how the proposed study evolved from prior work.

Step 4: Methods of Procedure

By this point in your proposal, you have presented the problems(s) you intend to study, the aims your research will accomplish, the importance and exact meaning of both of these, and the theoretical and empirical background of the present study. Now you must tell your readers or reviewers how you are going to bring about your results, that is, what activities you will conduct to accomplish your study objectives, test your study hypotheses, or generate theory.

Label the Design   Begin by labeling the general approach, or design, of your study (historical, survey, experimental, quasi-experimental, field study, case study, and so on). In effect, this general label allows you to quickly communicate your proposed procedure for inquiry and gives you an opportunity to anticipate questions about why you have selected the design that you have. In short, you should not only identify your plan but also substantiate the reasons for choosing it.

Discuss Confounding Variables   Confounding variables that might plague your study need to be addressed in your procedures section. You may eliminate some of them by using random sample selection and random assignment to comparative groups. Some may be addressed by your sample size or exclusion criteria. Others

TABLE 17–2   *Social Network Dimensions Differentiating Mentally Ill from Normals*

Dimension	Source
Size	Hammer (1978)
	Pattison (1975)
	Tolsdorf (1976)
	Sokolovsky et al. (1978)
Connectedness or density	Pattison (1975)
	Tolsdorf (1976)
	Sokolovsky et al. (1978)
Symmetry or reciprocity	Pattison (1975)
	Tolsdorf (1976)
	Sokolovsky et al. (1978)
Content or multiplexity	Tolsdorf (1976)
	Sokolovsky et al. (1978)
Frequency and/or amount of contact	Strauss & Carpenter (1972)
	Brown et al. (1972)
	Henderson et al. (1976)
	Vaughn & Leff (1976, 1981)
Network primarily kinship	Pattison (1975)
	Tolsdorf (1976)
	Turner (1979)
Orientation	Tolsdorf (1976)
Satisfaction	Hirsch (1979, 1980)
	[Note: With normals]

Souce: Used with permission of Sandra L. Sheetz; RN, *The Influence of Social Networks on the Performance of Self Care by the Chronically Mentally Ill Adult in the Community.* Dissertation proposal, University of California at San Francisco, 1984.

may be controlled for with certain statistical operations. But still others may be beyond any of these attempts to reduce their influence and must be identified as limitations of your study or constraints on the generalizability of your findings. Most authorities agree that it is preferable for you to acknowledge problems, errors in design, or limitations rather than attempting to ignore or disguise them. It is important to indicate that whatever compromises you have made with regard to the control of extraneous variables were given careful thought, that you are definitely aware of which variables need to be controlled to preserve the integrity of your study, that you have chosen not to control some, and why you believed it was not possible to do so. Krathwohl summarizes these points well (1977 p. 31):

> This is a place to demonstrate mastery of the problem. Probably nobody knows better than the researcher the multiple sources of contamination which might affect the study. Convincingly indicate the nature and basis of the particular compromise(s) being proposed and the reasons for accepting them. . . . Avoid expediency as a reason.

Most reviewers of research proposals are experienced scientists and scholars themselves, although they may not be experts on your specific study problem. They will recognize weaknesses and flaws in a study design such as lack of control or comparative groups, a Hawthorne effect, a regression effect, pretest effects, and a biased sample. Your design discussion ought to show how you have attempted to make your study as precise as you practically can.

Specify Data-Collection Approaches   You should state the exact steps you intend to take to answer every question or test every hypothesis proposed in your study. One organizational technique proposal writers use is to divide a sheet of paper into columns. Label the first column "Aim #1" or "Hypothesis #1," the second column "Method for #1," and the third "Evaluation or Analysis for #1." This strategy helps you to be certain that you indeed have a plan for dealing with all aspects of the problem that you have introduced and that you have set up a data-collection and analysis mechanism or procedure to address each of them. This section should:

- Report on the validity and reliability of data-collection instruments.

- Present information on the feasibility and appropriateness of the data-collection approach based on preliminary studies.

- Comments on the advantages of the proposed methods over alternatives.

If you expect to use published and previously tested tools for data collection, you need to tell your reader why you selected them and how they are appropriate to measure the variables that are important to your study question. The discussion of this relationship often appears in connection with the operational definition of each of your study variables. The measures that you elect to employ must not only be consistent with the variable's operational definition but also be supported by empirical evidence attesting to their validity, reliability, and objectivity. Assistance in evaluating certain instruments can be found in annual test reviews and compendia such as Oscar Buros's *Mental Measurement Yearbooks*, (1938–present) and others included in Chapter 10 of this text. If no instruments exist or are available to investigate the variables of interest to you, it is probably better to propose a methodological study to develop tools rather than to argue that instrument plans will be forthcoming. If "homemade" or "self-developed" instruments are to be used, be sure to justify them in terms of their fit with the operational definition of your study variables. Discuss the procedures you plan to use to develop them, and then establish their reliability and validity.

Describe the Study Setting Your methods of procedures section should also describe your research setting, if setting is a relevant consideration. In field studies, the investigator usually describes how entry to a setting will be acquired.

EXAMPLE: The Study Setting

The proposed study will be conducted at a 450-bed community hospital located in the greater Pittsburgh area. It has the only accredited cancer care program in the immediate area, and the investigator is currently the oncology clinical nurse specialist employed by this hospital. Furthermore, she is familiar with referring physicians.

Discuss Your Study Sampling You should discuss the nature and size of the sample and the rationale behind these decisions. The sampling procedure should be identified and explained in adequate detail *so that your study can be replicated and so that the extent of generalizability of your findings can be determined*. If statistical analysis is planned, the size of the sample is discussed with respect to a power analysis. If your sample members must meet specific criteria, these should be listed. For example, one pediatric nurse engaged in a descriptive study of adolescent cancer patients' experience of fatigue proposed the following sampling criteria:

Cancer patients ($n = 40$) will consist of adolescent leukemia patients admitted to any of three city hospital inpatient units or seen in these institutions' outpatient clinics. Furthermore, they must be able to read, write, and speak English as a primary language, be able to complete data-collection instruments, and be willing to maintain daily diary recordings. Finally, they must have confirmation of their cancer diagnosis. Exclusion criteria include patients who are (1) under psychiatric care; (2) taking antidepressants, sedatives, or thyroid medications; and (3) diagnosed as having diabetes, anemia, or thyroid disease.

You should also include the steps you will take to protect the rights of human and animal research subjects—such as informed consent procedures for the former and maintenance of care for the latter.

Present Your Analytic Procedures Finally, the methods or procedures section should present a method of analysis that is consistent with your study questions and aims. The assumptions of the statistics should fit the data that will be obtained. Most authorities agree that it is not always possible to anticipate every analysis procedure that will be used. It is to your advantage, however, to give your readers and reviewers evidence that you have thought through each step you will need to take to test every hypothesis or respond to every question in your study problem. Many advisers encourage you to generate mock tables that organize your data before you collect any, so that others know what you have in mind when it comes to analysis. For many proposal writers, that is a good time to consult a computer programmer or statistician who can make suggestions for your analysis plan or even your data-collection procedures. Table 17–3 represents yet another type of table frequently used in research proposals to demonstrate the structural organization of a study.

A careful plan and procedures section of your proposal need not prohibit discovery of serendipitous findings or inhibit your creativity. Instead, it must support your contention that you know how to answer the research question and possess the attributes of a serious scholar, at least with regard to using an approach that is consistent with systematic inquiry.

Step 5: Timetable or Work Plan

A work plan or timetable accomplishes two main aims:

1. It clarifies for the reader the overall flow of research-related activities. (This point is particularly important when the research project is very complex.)

2. It constitutes evidence that you have carefully and realistically considered exactly what you intend to do to carry out the proposed study.

TABLE 17–3   *Visual Illustration of Study Plan*

				Collection				Data Analysis			
Q/H	Instruments	Who Is the Sample	n	How	When	Where	By Whom	How	When	Where	By Whom
1											
2											
3											

Source: Prepared by James C. Stone and approved by the Academic Review Committee, Department of Education, University of California, Berkeley, January 30, 1979.

The timetable or work plan can be presented in a number of different formats, but in all cases, it must provide a clear, sequential statement of the operations that will be carried out in your study and must be consistent with the descriptive sections of your written proposal. Whether a table, graph, flowchart, PERT diagram or path analysis is used, the following information should be included:

1. the tasks or project activities

2. an estimate of the time required for each, and scheduled dates

3. personnel requirements for each activity

Accurately estimating the time and resources that will be needed to accomplish project tasks is difficult and often requires careful tracking during prior experiences. It is easy to underestimate, for example, the time that can be required to recruit and process project staff, the delays that can be associated with releasing funds to an organization, and the impact that peak times for other work (the beginning and end of the semester or fiscal year) can have on the progress of one's own work. Obviously, when unanticipated events delay the research progress, such accommodations as shifting of funds to hire temporary staff and work plan rearrangements become necessary. The simplest way to portray a work plan or timetable in a research proposal is to list research activities and associated dates or blocks of time. One oncology nurse represented her time schedule for the data-collection part of her research on fatigue in cancer patients in a table similar to Table 17–4.

TABLE 17–4 *Time Schedule for Data Collection*

	Pilot Study	**Descriptive Study**		
Time Period:	3/15/89–5/15/89	6/1/89–3/31/90		
Subjects:	$n = 18$ (9 students; 9 lung cancer patients	$n = 60$ (20 graduate students; 20 leukemia patients; 20 lung cancer patients)		
Data Collection:		Time 1 (Entry)	Time 2 (3 mos)	Time 3 (5 mos)
	Demographic data Medical history Fatigue diary (daily for 4 wks)	Demographic data Medical History Fatigue diary (daily for 4 wks)	Medical history Fatigue diary (daily for 2 wks)	Medical history Fatigue diary (daily for 2 wks)

Researchers employ a number of different formats for diagramming the schedule of work in a research project. One of the most familiar ones is the *program evaluation review technique*, or **PERT**. Many authorities believe that such diagrams or similarly constructed flowcharts are more informative than simple timetables, because they are a better way of indicating the interrelationships among work that goes on simultaneously or that overlaps. In the generic PERT diagram that appears in Figure 17–1, each arrow stands for a task, and circles indicate the beginning and end of each activity. Numbers in the circles refer to the list of activities. Events that the researcher considers particularly important can be designated by a square or rectangle. Where two or more lines of work meet, events can be marked with a triangle. The time line along the bottom shows the months during which the work is scheduled to take place. Clearly, it is easier to present your work plan or timetable with such a highly detailed approach if you can anticipate all the steps involved. Exploratory studies and field studies make this degree of specificity almost impossible, and a rougher rendition of the work plan or timetable would be expected.

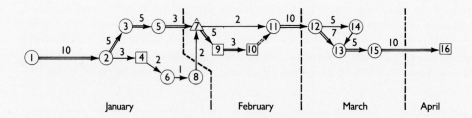

		January	February	March	April

PERT Activity List

Begin and End Events	Activity	Estimated Working Days	Symbol Code
1-2	Hire staff	10	◯ Begin or end event
2-3	Write questionnaire	5	▢ Milestone event
2-4	Develop sampling plan	3	△ Interface event
4-6	Procure mailing lists	7	→ Workdays for activity denoted by arrow
3-5	Pre-test questionnaire	5	
5-7	Revise questions and prepare for mailing	3	⇒ Critical path
6-8	Selection of the sample	1	
8-7	Prepare mailing envelopes	2	---- Constraint on arrowed activity by completion of or product form preceding activity
7-9	Prepare interim reports	5	
9-10	Clear questionnaire with sponsor and submit interim report	5	
7-11	Send questionnaire	3	
11-12	Wait returns	10	
12-13	Analyze intials returns	7	
12-14	Interview sample of non-respondents	5	
13-15	Integrate interview data in analysis	5	
15-16	Prepare final report	10	

Figure 17–1 Sample survey analyzed as a PERT diagram, time-scaled by months. (Adapted from D. R. Krathwohl, *How to Prepare a Research Proposal*, 2nd ed., Syracuse, N.Y.: Syracuse University Bookstore, 1977, p. 39. Reprinted with permission.)

Step 6: Sections on Personnel, Budget, Facilities, and Resources

Personnel This section of your proposal tells reviewers about the people who will be needed to conduct your study. It is, of course, crucial to identify the principal investigator, project director, or codirectors and to present their qualifications convincingly. Educational preparation, both formal and informal, professional experience, prior research positions in the field, and previous publications related to the proposed study all strengthen one's case. Although it may be expedient to include a "canned" biographical sketch already in your files, reviewers are more likely to be impressed by a presentation of project personnel, their "job descriptions," and background information *that has been carefully selected to highlight particular competencies relevant to this study*. A form for each participant's biographical sketch is often included in an application packet (see Figure 17–2). If you are proposing a large, complex study that will involve a lot of people, an organizational chart illustrating their relationship to one another is a good idea. Be alert to the fact that it is considered improper to list as consultants to your project people you have not first contacted. In fact, many agencies expect you to append letters of support or agreement from any consultants you intend to use. Researchers sometimes include the names of members of an advisory committee to attempt to add credibility to their proposal. Again, written consent to serve in such a capacity should be obtained in advance. Box 17–3 illustrates an excerpt from the personnel section of a nursing

Give the following information for key professional personnel, beginning with the Principal Investigator/Program Director. Photocopy this page for each person.		
NAME	TITLE	BIRTHDATE (*Mo., Day, Yr.*)
EDUCATION (*Begin with baccalaureate or other initial professional education and include postdoctoral training*)			
INSTITUTION AND LOCATION	DEGREE (*circle highest degree*)	YEAR CONFERRED	FIELD OF STUDY

Figure 17–2 Research and/or Professional Experience: Concluding with present position, list in chronological order previous employment, experience, and honors. Include present membership on any Federal Government Public Advisory Committee. List, in chronological order, the titles and complete references to all publications during the past three years and to representative earlier publications pertinent to this application. **DO NOT EXCEED TWO PAGES.**

Box 17–3   Hypothetical Nursing Research Grant Budget (Personnel Section)

NAME	TITLE OF POSITION	%/HRS.	SALARY	FRINGE BENEFITS	TOTAL
Holly S. Wilson	Principal Investigator	53%	$25,816	$6,841	$32,657
(Vacant)	Student Research Assistant	100%	$23,000	$1,190	$24,990
(Vacant)	Administrative Assistant II	100%	$26,884	$5,468	$35,352
(See continuation page for itemized list)					

(SUBTOTALS) $76,500 $16,499
ENTER TOTAL SALARY AMOUNTS PLUS FRINGE BENEFITS $92,999

education proposal submitted to a national health agency for funding.

Budget   Authors agree that the budget section of a proposal "states your project in monetary or financial terms." The total dollar amount is usually determined by the nature of the study you are proposing, the guidelines and policies of the funding agency, or both. The goal in preparing a budget is to make it realistic. If it is padded to include funds for desirable but not necessarily essential costs, such as extra travel or additional equipment, you risk being eliminated in competition with other proposals. If you have underbudgeted, you may not have sufficient resources to carry out your proposed plan of activities. The application kits provided by federal funding agencies include budget forms and detailed instructions for completing them. Foundations and private organizations may offer only general limits. Most grant applications, however, allow you to request funds in two categories: *direct costs* (the money that you spend to carry out the project tasks) and *indirect costs* (based on an established formula that your institution requires in exchange for serving as the institutional or administrative site for the grant). Indirect costs cover such things as providing heat and light to the building. They can be as low as 8% and as high as 40+% of the direct-cost base number. A written budget narrative should accompany the actual list of costs, to explain the reasons for requesting certain items and to link up the budget details with the project activities.

It is always a good idea to consult your institutional grants and contracts officers early in the process of preparing a research proposal budget. They not only review it for its agreement with institutional policies and salary schedules but can also give you the benefit of past experience with successful and unsuccessful requests. Although it may be time-consuming, it is better to telephone airlines, printers, the post office, secretarial services, computer resources, and the like to obtain at least general estimates of what various tasks and activities are going to cost rather than merely guessing. Even after all this initial effort, many budgets are renegotiated after a decision to support a project has been made and before funds are released. Prepare a realistic budget. Deliberate overbudgeting or underbudgeting often backfires. Reviewers evaluate the budget in relation to the aims and methods of the proposed project.

Facilities and Other Resources You should indicate the special facilities that are available to you in carrying out your proposed study. One customarily mentions the libraries (and their holdings), computer resources, special equipment or laboratories, office space, and secretarial support services. In many cases, institutions that have been successful in winning grants have this information already compiled and available to researchers who are preparing proposals. Although using such "canned" material can save time, be sure to edit it so that it is relevant to the research at hand. Astute reviewers will be more impressed with your proposal if you do.

If your study requires you to collect data in organizations or institutions other than your own setting, evidence of their willingness to cooperate with you, in the form of letters of agreement or contracts, should be attached. Many funding sources view an institution's willingness to allow you to use their facilities as added support for your proposal.

Step 7: Abstract, Title, and Cover Letter

Most proposals begin with a short (approximately 300-word) abstract, or summary. Even though it usually appears at the beginning of the document, most researchers write it last. The purpose of an abstract is to convey the essence of your proposed study to the reviewers. It not only introduces your study's importance to reviewers but may also be used as the basis for subsequent press releases or publications. An abstract may be used as the basis for entering your project into a computerized record-keeping system. For these reasons, your abstract should be composed carefully, accurately, and clearly. An abstract should include the most important points you wish to stress about your proposed research and should provide the maximum amount of pertinent information as concisely as possible. A well-written abstract not only presents the central idea of the study but also convinces the reader or reviewer that it is both interesting and important. It should whet the appetite and prepare the reader for the body of the proposal. The title serves similar purposes but in an even more abbreviated way. Try to avoid jargon and clichés in study titles. Instead, use key terms that will orient a reader to the nature of your study and *make sense.*

Finally, your cover or transmittal letter should indicate the agency, office, or grant competition for which your proposal is intended and may make reference to any contacts you may have had with agency staff during its preparation. Send the required number of copies by certified mail or an express service to ensure that your proposal meets the required deadline date.

Agencies' Criteria for Reviewing Proposals

All agencies, whether public or private, evaluate proposals that they receive according to sets of criteria. Knowing about such criteria helps you anticipate what will be scrutinized when your proposal is evaluated. Although some funding sources are more detailed in their criteria than others, common themes typically characterize proposal review checklists, and you should become familiar with them (see Box 17–4).

Acquiring Grant Support

Although this chapter has been developed as a resource for any nurse who must plan and formally prepare a research proposal, much of what has been presented is directed toward the challenges associated with obtaining money to support your studies. In some cases, of course, finding funding for proposed research is not a major problem. You may find yourself enrolled in a graduate or undergraduate course on the topic of, for example, constructing or testing data-collection instruments appropriate for nursing studies. As part of the course requirements you will become involved in selectively piloting the instrument with a small sample of subjects. In this case, any costs that may be associated with administering the instrument and coding or analyzing data acquired through its use may be subsumed under the operational budget for the course. In other instances, costs are sufficiently low for students to cover them simply as a school-related expense. Collaborative programs of research, in which student research is a "spinoff" of faculty research and therefore is funded under the overriding project, may minimize the necessity for students and novice investigators to make their own applications for funding.

In an era of fiscal austerity, however, and in the face of clear needs for studies that genuinely contribute to the knowledge base of nursing rather than merely demonstrating methodological mastery, skill in the art of "grantsmanship" is becoming increasingly valuable. It is helpful not only to nurse scientists but also to nurse educators, who must plan and systematically evaluate teaching programs; nurse executives, who must often rely on supplemental funds to implement an innovative demonstration project; and nurse clinicians, who seek scientific grounds

Box 17–4   Evaluation Checklists

I. **National Institutes of Health (Checklist of deficiencies)**

A. *The Problem*
- The problem is not of sufficient importance or is unlikely to produce any new or useful information.
- The proposed research is based on a hypothesis that rests on insufficient evidence, is doubtful, or is unsound.
- The problem is more complex than the investigator appears to realize.
- The problem has only local significance, is one of production or control, or otherwise fails to fall sufficiently clearly within the general field of interest to the prospective sponsor.
- The problem is scientifically premature and warrants, at most, only pilot study.
- The research as proposed is overly involved, with too many elements under simultaneous investigation.
- The description of the nature of the research and of its significance leaves the proposal nebulous and diffuse without clear research aim.

B. *The Approach*
- The proposed tests, methods, or scientific procedures are unsuited to the stated objective.
- The description of the approach is too nebulous, diffuse, and lacking in clarity to permit adequate evaluation.
- The overall design of the study has not been carefully thought out.
- The statistical aspects of the approach have not been given sufficient consideration.
- The approach lacks scientific imagination.
- Controls are either inadequately conceived or inadequately described.
- The material the investigator proposes to use is unsuited to the objectives of the study or is difficult to obtain.
- The number of observations is unsuitable.
- The equipment contemplated is outmoded or otherwise unsuitable.

II. **U.S. Office of Education (List of shortcomings)**

A. *Problem*
- Limited significance
- Local significance only
- Incomprehensible; not spelled out
- Not appropriate to this granting agency
- Overly ambitious objectives

(Continued)

Box 17–4   Evaluation Checklists (Continued)

B. *Procedures*
- Insufficient detail; vague
- Evaluation procedures inadequate
- Selection of subjects unclear, undefined and/or unrealistic
- Research design inadequate
- Variables uncontrolled
- Discrepancy between objectives and procedures
- No theoretical construct or rationale
- Research design overly complex; too many research components
- Statistical procedures unspecified
- Pilot study necessary
- Time schedule inappropriate

C. *Personnel and Facilities*
- Inadequate training and/or experience
- Time commitment inadequate or unspecified
- Consultants needed
- Personnel not specified
- Duties not specified
- Personnel specified but insufficient information provided

D. *Economic Efficiency*
- Budget too high for expected result
- Request for operational or support money

III. National Science Foundation

A review of the evaluation instructions provided to outside reviewers of National Science Foundation research proposals reveals concern about the same general areas noted above for the U.S. Office of Education and the National Institutes of Health. The instructional letter for one program area asks the review to comment on such points as the scientific merit of the research that is proposed and the qualifications of the applicant. It also requests a response to the following questions:
- Is the research well planned?
- Is the research important?
- Is the applicant aware of recent developments in the field?
- Is the applicant adequately trained to undertake the project?
- Is the support requested appropriate for the project?

The definitions of rating terms used by another NSF program may provide further insight into the criteria employed:

(Continued)

Box 17–4   Evaluation Checklists (Continued)

Excellent —The problem is very important and well defined in the proposal. The investigators are highly competent and fully capable of doing the job. Strongly deserves support.

Very Good —The problem is important and adequately defined in the proposal. The investigators are competent and the research will contribute to their growth. Deserves support.

Good —The problem may be important, but the research is not well defined. The approach is routine, but might contribute to graduate education or developing the potential of the principal investigator. The proposal is marginal in its present form.

Fair —The problem is probably unimportant or not well enough defined in the proposal to allow evaluation. The approach is questionable. The proposal is not deserving of support in its present form.

Poor —The problem is unimportant, subprofessional, or has been solved by others.

---

for their clinical decisions. Sexton (1982) identifies the following six steps in preparing a proposal for submission to a funding source.

Step 1: Establish Priorities

You must first identify projects that you need money for and studies that you wish you had money for. This step requires that you think about what you want to do, what kind of expenses and resources will be involved, and whether grant funds are in fact going to be necessary.

Step 2: Identify Funding Sources

Intramural Funding   Most academic institutions have research funds available on a competitive basis for seed money to conduct pilot projects or methodological studies—for example, increasing the likelihood that the investigator will be ultimately more competitive and successful when he or she applies for external funds.

Private Funding   Although public funding has predominated in nursing's past, more and more contemporary nurse researchers are approaching private foundations, of which there are over 25,000, or corporations that award grants for health-related projects. Many of the national voluntary health organizations, such as the American Cancer Society, support nursing research. Each February, the American Nurses' Foundation announces the availability of its competitive extramural grants program, which supports nursing research directed by registered nurses. The foundation specifically encourages proposals in the areas of clinical nursing and nursing administration. Many of the most distinguished doctoral dissertations conducted by nurses have been supported in whole or part by the ANF.* The deadline for submitting proposals to the ANF is July 1, and awards are announced by October 1 of each year. The maximum grant amount has been $2,500. Some private sources are summarized in Box 17–5.

The *Foundation Directory* contains program and funding information for at least 3,000 private funding agencies. Your reference librarian or grants officers can guide

---

Box 17–5   Private Sources for Nursing Research Funding

FUNDING AGENCY

American Nurses' Foundation
 2420 Pershing Rd.
 Kansas City, MO 64108
 (816) 474-5720

Kellogg Foundation
 400 North Ave.
 Battle Creek, MI 49016
 (616) 968-1611

Robert Wood Johnson Foundation
 P.O. Box 2316
 Princeton, NJ 08540
 (609) 452-8701

Sigma Theta Tau (National)
 National Honor Society of Nursing
 1200 Waterway Blvd.
 Indianapolis, IN 46202
 (317) 634-8171

---

*The ANF is a nonprofit corporation affiliated with the American Nurses' Association and located at 2420 Pershing Road, Kansas City, Missouri.

you to other resources that detail foundation funding, including lists and indexes of prior recipients and the topics of their projects.

Sexton (1982 p. 33) and others acknowledge that "less information is available about corporate philanthropy than about foundations." But she does list four useful sources of information on corporations:

- *Bank of America Corporation's Bibliography of Corporate Social Philanthropy*
- *Standard and Poor's Register of Corporations, Directors, and Executives*
- The Handbook of Corporate Social Philanthropy
- The Trade Association Directory

Physicians have been extraordinarily successful in acquiring funding for their research programs from drug companies. In fact, some critics believe that the quest for the commercial dollar threatens to tarnish the ethics of certain clinical research. But nurses of the future will be turning more in the direction of corporations for money. Because of their relationship to nurses or their public position on fostering health, companies may prove to be substantial investors in supporting nursing studies.

Public Funding The *Federal Register* (published Monday–Friday) informs the public of the missions, regulations, and grant-funds priorities of federal programs. The relationships of agencies under the Department of Health and Human Services (DHHS) is portrayed in Figure 17–3,A. The DHHS has been the largest source of funds for projects related to health. Many have "first" awards or small-grant programs. The *National Center for Nursing Research* (NCNR) was created as part of the National Institutes of Health in 1986. The mission of the NCNR is to support conduct and dissemination of information research related to nursing and patient care. The topics and mechanisms for support used by the NCNR appear in Figure 17–3,B.

Step 3: Compare Available Funds with Your Needs

Obtain the key information from these sources and compare the facts you acquire with your own potential projects and financial needs. Sexton (1982) alerts us that the following categories of information about any potential funding source are probably valuable.

- geographic distribution of awards
- types of project funded
- types of institution funded
- number of grants awarded
- amount of average award and range

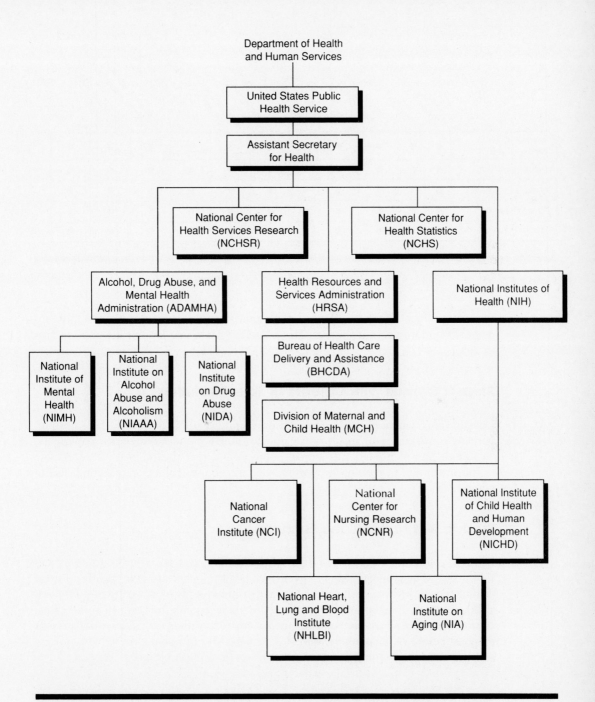

Figure 17—3A Relationships of agencies under the Department of Health and Human Services (DHHS)

	Research Project Grants	Program Project Grants	NRSA Individual Predoctoral Fellowship	NRSA Individual Postdoctoral Fellowship	NRSA Senior Fellowship	NRSA Institutional Training Grants	First Independent Research Support and Transition Awards	Small Business Innovation Research Awards	Academic Research Enhancement Awards	Academic Investigator Awards	Clinical Investigator Awards
Acute and Chronic Illness	●	●	●	●	●	●	●	●	●	●	●
Health Promotion	●	●	●	●	●	●	●	●	●	●	●
Disease Prevention	●	●	●	●	●	●	●	●	●	●	●
Nursing Systems	●	●	●	●	●	●	●	●	●	●	●
Special Programs	●	●	●	●	●	●	●	●	●	●	●

Figure 17–3B Topics and mechanisms for support used by the NCNR

Remember that priorities change often annually. For example. the NCNR announced a priority on nursing activities related to AIDS and low-birth-weight infants in 1987.

Step 4: Consult with Officers in Your Institution

Consult representatives of the research development office to ensure that your proposal is consistent with institutional policies about indirect cost rates, copyrights, and protection of human and animal subjects and that the proposal is acceptable to the institution in relation to matters such as the availability of space and use of equipment.

Step 5: Get to Know the Funders

Develop contacts with representatives of the funding agency before completing and submitting your proposal. Many executive staff personnel are able to offer a great deal of specific advice, such as to which department or division a particular proposal should best be directed and how to prepare an acceptable budget. In some cases, your contact person at the funding agency may be willing to read a draft of your proposal before its final submission. Learn what you can about the review process and the criteria according to which your research application will be reviewed.

Step 6: Follow the Rules

Write and rewrite the final grant application, conforming as closely as possible with the format, agency assurances, administrative approvals, number of copies, and deadline dates. Remember that the purpose of this final step is to persuade the funding agency that your study is worthwhile and merits being funded. Berthold's 1973 study of what influenced approval or disapproval of nursing research grant proposals in two national granting agencies revealed that

> approval or disapproval . . . is independent of investigator background variables [but] not of the judged adequacy of the investigative team to pursue and complete the specific project for which funding is requested. . . . In general funding is related to the judged adequacy of the proposal as submitted for peer group evaluation. Increased sophistication in asking relevant questions and in designing means for answering research questions in nursing should therefore yield a higher proportion of acceptable proposals [p. 298].

The Proposal Review Process

This chapter offers you a comprehensive guide to the challenging task of writing a formal study proposal, whether for funding or another purpose. What happens if, in fact, you do submit your proposal to a government funding agency such as the NCNR? It will be reviewed in a two-level process—first for scientific merit and second to determine if the project is relevant to the agency's program priorities (see Figure 17–4). A group of scientific peers called the "study section" reviews the proposal for its scientific merit. Their criteria include:

- scientific and technical significance and originality

- adequacy of the methodology to carry out the research

- qualifications of the principal investigator and staff

- availability of resources

- justification of the proposal budget and time frame

- protection of research subjects and issues such as biohazards

The study section then recommends (1) approval, (2) disapproval, or (3) deferral for additional information. The reviewers then assign a priority rating to each approved application, yielding a funding priority score. Finally, the National Advisory Council of the agency reviews the application's face sheet, the recommendations of the study section, the priority score, and the significance of the project based on current priorities. Final action rests with the director of the center or institute. You are notified of the review's final outcome within a few weeks of the National Advisory Council meeting. If your study is not approved, you can arrange with the staff representative to have the summary sheet of the reviewers sent to you. If your proposal is approved, you may enter into some negotiations about the budget and then finally receive an official *notice of grant award* that spells out terms

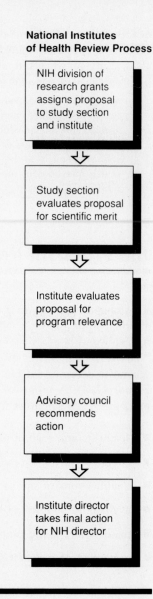

National Institutes of Health Review Process

NIH division of research grants assigns proposal to study section and institute

⇩

Study section evaluates proposal for scientific merit

⇩

Institute evaluates proposal for program relevance

⇩

Advisory council recommends action

⇩

Institute director takes final action for NIH director

Figure 17—4 National Institutes of Health Review Process

and conditions. Because most projects are funded on a three-year basis, it will not be long before you feel as if you must start the grant application process all over again. Fortunately, success breeds success, and surmounting the obstacles won't be quite as difficult the next time around, particularly if you learn from past experience.

Guidelines for Critique

- What is the purpose for writing the research proposal?

- Is the proposal complete and convincing?

- Is the proposal clearly and logically written, carefully presented, and sufficiently detailed without exceeding page limitations and other required conventions?

- Have all the steps outlined in this chapter been addressed in the proposal's preparation?

- Has the proposal been matched with a funding agency's mission and priorities?

- Is the principal investigator familiar with the targeted funding agency's grant submission packet and review process?

SUMMARY OF KEY IDEAS AND TERMS

✔   In an era when fiscal retrenchment coexists with nursing's goal of building a scientific basis for practice, writing research proposals that can relate a particular project to a scientific tradition, describe and justify the methodological procedures, and present the importance of possible conclusions is becoming acknowledged as an essential skill for all nurses.

✔   Because the exact format and guidelines for preparing a proposal may vary with the target review committee, it is essential to obtain an application packet or a set of guidelines from the agency, institution, or committee and conform to them as closely as possible when preparing a proposal.

✔   Some institutions and agencies view the written research proposal as a commitment on the part of the investigator to conduct the study in the way it was outlined and approved or else report and explain any deviations or changes.

✔   Regardless of the specific format of a research proposal, the following components are included in some way: a title; an abstract or summary; a statement of the study problem and purpose; the theoretical background and review of related research; the hypotheses to be tested or questions to be answered;

the study setting; the sampling procedures and sample characteristics; the data-collection strategies or instruments; the plans for storing, retrieving, and analyzing the data; ethical considerations of the study; a timetable or work plan; a budget statement that includes resources available and needed; a description of the qualifications of the investigator; and references.

✓   General hints for effective proposals: (1) Consider your audience and explain everything clearly and logically. (2) Package your proposal to generate interest in it, so that it is physically appealing and matches the mission or goals of the funding agency. (3) Balance detail and flexibility, and maximize the thoughtful use of appendixes to your proposal.

✓   The steps in writing a research proposal involve preparing (1) the problem statement; (2) the theoretical framework and review of related literature; (3) sections on pilot studies or related prior work; (4) the explanation of methods of procedure; (5) the timetable or work plan; (6) sections on personnel, budget, facilities, and resources; and (7) the abstract, title, and cover letter.

✓   The problem statement of a research proposal should include:

- a statement of the specific study problem, including hypotheses, study questions, and definitions of terms

- the specific purposes or objectives of the research

- the significance of or need for the study

✓   The theoretical rationale and review of related literature serves three purposes: (1) It presents the organizing scheme or theoretical framework of which the proposed study is a part. (2) It indicates your grasp of the important and recent developments in your area of interest and how your study will refine, revise, extend, or transform what is known. (3) It lends support to your assumptions, operational definitions, and methodological choices.

✓   A complete explanation of methods of procedure should consist of several parts:

- Label the general design.

- Discuss confounding variables.

- Specify data-collection and analysis approaches for each study question or hypothesis.

- Describe the study setting.

- Discuss the sampling procedure and sample characteristics.

- Present analysis procedures.

✔   A timetable or work plan should, either in a table or more detailed flowchart or PERT diagram, communicate the tasks or activities to be undertaken, an estimate of the amount of time required for each, scheduled dates, and the personnel requirements for each activity.

✔   The personnel section of a proposal should highlight the competencies specifically required to conduct the proposed study. The budget section includes direct and indirect costs and should be prepared in close consultation with your institution's financial officers so as to make it accurate, realistic, and congruent with institutional policies. Accompanying letters of agreement should reflect facilities and resources available for your project, and a statement of rationale should accompany requests that resources be provided by the funding agency.

✔   The abstract, or summary, should be written last. It should convey the essence of the proposed study in 300 words or less and convince readers that the study is interesting and worthwhile.

✔   Avoid jargon and clichés in study titles, and include a cover letter when submitting a proposal to a review group.

✔   Most review committees have similar criteria for evaluating the scientific merit of research proposals, and these should be considered carefully.

✔   Success in finding funding for your research from public or private sources will be more likely if you:

- Begin by identifying research projects that require grant funding.

- Next identify the funding available, using announcements, organizational publications, and your reference librarian.

- Identify relevant resources for learning about the missions, regulations, and grant priorities of various funding sources.

- Obtain key information from these sources, and match the facts you acquire with your potential research projects.

- Consult with staff members in your own institution's research development office.

- Develop contacts with representatives from your target funding agency before even beginning to write your proposal.

- Write and rewrite the final proposal, conforming as much as possible to the funding agency's format, guidelines, deadlines, and so on.

✓   The scientific study sections reviewing grant applications require that nurses increase their sophistication in developing concise, well-documented proposals for nursing research.

✓   One way of learning to improve your proposals is to request the summary sheet from your reviewers after a proposal is disapproved or assigned a low priority rating for funding.

References

Berthold JS: Nursing research grant proposals: What influenced their approval or disapproval in two national granting agencies? *Nurs Res* July/August 1973; 20:292–295.

Buros OK: *Mental Measurement Yearbooks*. Highland Park, N.J., 1938–present.

Hayman LL: Fatal flaws. *Nurs Res* 1987; 36, 267.

Krathwohl DR: *How to Prepare a Research Proposal*, 2nd ed. Syracuse, N.Y.: Syracuse University Bookstore, 1977.

Locke LF, Spirduso WW, Silverman SJ: *Proposals that Work: A Guide for Planning Dissertations and Grant Proposals*. Newbury Park, Calif.: Sage, 1987.

Merritt DH: The national center for nursing research. *Image* 1986; 18, 84–85.

Polit D, Hungler B: *Nursing Research: Principles and Methods*, 3rd ed. Philadelphia: Lippincott, 1987.

Sexton DL: Developing skills in grant writing. *Nurs Outlook* 1982; 30:31–38.

Stone JC: *Visual Illustration of a Study Plan*. Department of Education, University of California at Berkeley, 1979.

18

Disseminating Research Findings

HOLLY SKODOL WILSON

Objectives

After reading this chapter, the student should be able to:

- Compare and contrast oral presentations with journal writing or book writing as options for disseminating research findings

- Organize and execute journal articles, theses and dissertations, or speech scripts according to basic assumptions that promote a clear, readable style

- Choose words with precision, avoiding ambiguity, jargon, and unnecessary words

- Assemble essential writing aids

- Plan for effective use of visual aids in a professional speech

- Formulate strategies for effective speech delivery

- Anticipate techniques for fielding questions when giving a talk

- Evaluate his or her own oral presentations as well as those of others

- Design a focused and organized outline for a research paper

- Take steps to avoid rejection of an article by journal editors

- Write a good query letter

(Continued)

- Evaluate issues that arise when two or more authors collaborate

- Compose concise, specific, informative, and interesting article titles and leads

- Work quotations into manuscripts smoothly

- Differentiate plagiarism from paraphrasing

- Prepare tables and figures according to accepted guidelines

- Apply accepted criteria for writing the sections of a research report

- Discuss initial considerations in negotiating with a publisher to publish a book

- Advocate the value of disseminating research through writing and speaking

In This Chapter . . .

The only way the information produced through scientific work can contribute to the emerging body of knowledge in nursing or be used to make clinical decisions is to report your results, your methods, and your conclusions to others. You can do this by writing a thesis or dissertation, a book, a journal article, or a technical report or by giving a talk at a professional meeting. This chapter suggests rules, techniques, and illustrations for making scientific writing and speaking clearer and better. Preparing a formal speech and producing scholarly writing are not easy. Thinking effectively and clearly can be laborious. When you sit down to write, you may need an act of will to push yourself over the gap between you and the page. Having specific skills will certainly help you do that.

This chapter encourages you to view writing (including the preparation of a script for a speech) as a three-step process:

1. *prewriting*, when you gather together materials, take notes, and put your ideas into some beginning form or structure, such as a detailed outline

2. *writing*, when you sharpen the tone and style in which you express your thoughts by writing a first draft

3. *rewriting*, when you edit for coherent expression, keeping the development of your ideas clear and organized

The guidelines for writing and speaking put forth in this chapter are based on the simple premise that dealing with the theoretical or scientific in writing and speaking need not work against the goal of communicating your thoughts clearly. As Mirin (1981) suggests, the purpose of scientific writing is communication, not art, "but the basic principles of good writing apply to all writing" (p. 2).

This chapter takes you from start to finish through the steps and considerations involved in either preparing and publishing a manuscript based on research or planning and presenting a talk in a professional or other forum. It not only considers some of the subtleties of the psychology required in disseminating research findings but also addresses questions as specific as:

- How do I find potential outlets for my work?

- What makes a good query letter?

- What is the general format for a thesis? a scientific article?

- What goes into each section?

- How do I work quotations in smoothly?

- What are the characteristics of effective figures and tables?

- What makes for a good delivery in an oral presentation?

- What are the criteria for quality visual aids?

- What bugs journal editors?

- How do I go about getting a book published?

- What about authorship and copyrights?

When Styles (1978) was asked why nurses should write for publication, she replied, "Because the future of the profession depends on it" (p. 28). Unless nurses publish, the body of knowledge unique to nursing cannot grow and develop.

Options for Disseminating Research

Two major options exist for disseminating research results, procedures, and insights. You can write about them, or you can talk about them. Most of us realize that many scholars do both. Saslow (1982) points out that the advantage of speeches at professional or scientific meetings is that they *promptly inform* an audience about your work even while it's in progress and prompt others to tell you what they think. Articles, books, technical reports, theses, and the like are a *more permanent and complete record* of your work and are also *available to a wider audience*.

A talk obviously has the advantage of allowing you to obtain reactions from an interested audience. These reactions can stimulate your own thinking about your research. For example, long before I succeeded in having a paper published about bridging the gap between standard psychiatric diagnostic nomenclature and the nursing diagnosis movement, I had delivered numerous presentations and speeches on the topic. These talks helped me refine my emerging ideas. Talks can range from relatively informal presentations in classes for colleagues as part of a collo-

---

Box 18–1   American Nurses' Association Council of Nurse Researchers

Guide for Abstract Preparation

Abstracts are to be submitted in duplicate, typewritten and single-spaced on the forms provided. Both pages of the presentation application are to be completed.

Abstracts to be considered for paper presentations and symposia must be of completed research—completed as of the date the abstract is submitted. All abstracts for a specific symposium must be submitted together. Also, the organizer (moderator) for the symposium must submit a face sheet for the presentation application which includes the name, address, and telephone number of the symposium organizer, titles of all abstracts, and a brief summary (100 words) of the overall symposium. Poster presentations may be of either completed or ongoing research.

The summary of the research (250–300 words and must not exceed space provided in the presentation application) is to include:

1. the purpose of the study
2. the design
3. a description of the subjects, including sample size
4. methods of data collection
5. methods of data analysis
6. major findings
7. major conclusions

The investigator who is invited to present a paper at this nursing research meeting will be asked to provide one copy of the paper at ANA 30 days prior to the conference date.

Paper presentations will be limited to one presenter per paper although co-authors of the paper will be acknowledged in the conference program. Multiple authors may participate

in the poster presentations. All presenters will be expected to register for the conference in accordance with the registration procedures established for the conference. Presenters will *not* be reimbursed for expenses for attending the conference.

All paper presenters, primary poster presenters, and symposium organizers must be members of the ANA Council of Nurse Researchers.

Presentation applications should be sent to:
Research and Policy
   Analysis Department
American Nurses' Association
2420 Pershing Road
Kansas City,
   Missouri 64108

Source: American Nurses' Association, Council of Nurse Researchers, 1988.

---

quium series to formal presentations before a professional organization. In the latter case you must first locate a "call for abstracts" that gives you the guidelines and length limitations for an abstract (see Box 18–1). Next, you have to submit one. And finally, if your abstract is accepted by the program planning committee, you will be scheduled on the program for what is usually a 15- to 30-minute oral presentation.

Written reports of scientific work reach a much wider audience, but, because of the publication schedules of most professional journals, a year may pass before the findings are available to a nursing readership. Publishing a book or monograph based on your research takes even longer, approximately 10 months or so after you hand in the completed manuscript. Although the full-length research article is the most common outlet for published accounts of the work of nurse researchers, brief reports, letters to the editor, and abstracts also permit publication of aspects of your research that don't require a full-scale presentation. Of course, written accounts of your scientific work can also take the form of technical progress and final reports required by funding agencies. You may also write a thesis or dissertation, a scholarly treatise in which you present detailed evidence of scientific knowledge and expertise. (Sample guidelines appear in Box 18–2.) Before discussing the three main means for disseminating your ideas—the speech, the journal article, and the book— let's consider a few general assumptions basic to all writing or speaking about research.

Box 18–2   Dissertation/Thesis Guidelines

A. *Chapter Outline*

   1. Introduction: The study problem
     A. Introduction to problem and subproblems (What led you to choose this problem?)
     B. Statement of the problem
     C. Purpose(s) of the study
     D. Need for the study (significance)

   2. Literature review and conceptual framework
     A. Overview of relevant research directly related to your problem
     B. Conceptual or theoretical framework (discussion of theoretical framework underlying study and operational description of concepts) (A and B may be reversed)
     C. Assumptions
     D. Research questions and/or hypotheses
     E. Definition of terms

   3. Methodology
     A. Research design
     B. Description of research setting (if relevant)
     C. Sample
       1. Human subjects assurance
       2. Nature and size of sample
       3. Criteria for sample selection
     D. Data collection methods
       1. Techniques (observation, interview, instruments, chart audit)
       2. Instruments or apparatus
         a. Description
         b. Reliability and validity
     E. Procedure
     F. Data analysis

   4. Results
     A. Preliminary analyses, if relevant (sample characteristics, data-reduction techniques)
     B. Analysis of hypotheses or research questions
     C. Other findings

   5. Discussion
     A. Meaning of findings in relation to hypotheses or research questions
     B. Significance
     C. Limitations
     D. Implications for nursing
     E. Future research

(Continued)

Box 18–2   **Dissertation/Thesis Guidelines (Continued)**

B. *Standard Format for Dissertation Organization*
Every page must be numbered (including illustrative material) and appear in the order indicated below:

Title page	Not numbered
Copyright page (optional)	Not numbered
Abstract	Numbered with separate pagination (1, 2, 3)
Preliminary material (dedication, acknowledgments, table of contents, list of tables, list of figures)	Numbered with lower-case roman numerals (i, ii, iii, iv)
Main body of text (chapters with tables and figures incorporated at the appropriate point in the text)	Numbered with arabic numerals
References	Numbered with arabic numerals continued from text
Appendixes	Numbered with arabic numerals continued from references

Logical subcategories under each chapter heading should be developed, following the hierarchy for heading types outlined on page 32 of the APA Manual. Detailed guidelines for developing tables and figures are presented on pages 43–55 of the APA Manual.

C. *Format for Copyright Page and Abstract Page*

   1. Copyright page

TITLE OF DISSERTATION (ALL CAPS)

Copyright © 19xx (year)

by

(Your name as it appears on the title page)

   2. Abstract

TITLE OF DISSERTATION (ALL CAPS)

Jane Doe,

University of the United States, 19xx (year)

(triple space)

Text of abstract (double space) . . . . , etc.

General Guidelines for Presentations

Awareness of certain key principles is basic to preparing any written or oral presentation of your research.

1. Write for Strangers

Don't assume that your audience or readers know what you are talking about or that they will take the time or the energy to make sense of what you are saying. Writing *for* somebody (your audience), and *as* somebody (from a point of view), is what makes writing worth reading and speeches worth hearing. A writer who can achieve the appropriate relationship to his or her audience has mastered the art of creating the proper tone. Achieving an appropriate tone is a big step toward the clear and ordered thinking and writing that characterizes good scientific work. Remember that the worth of a talk or article is measured by what the audience or reader carries away, not by what the speaker or author puts out. Suppose you are presenting findings about nursing strategies that can decrease the pain associated with intramuscular injections to a general nursing audience. If you couch your findings in esoteric and obscure terms, you severely limit your study's usefulness to those who will read or hear your findings. In the case of a general nursing audience, "plain English has a lot to recommend it" (Saslow 1982 p. 325). If the audience is nurse researchers, be wary of making the tone condescending, overly emotional, or so technical that the important points are lost.

2. Get Off to a Good Start

Some writers and speakers find it easier to get started on a research report by getting some ideas on paper quickly, even in outline form, believing that they can always edit and polish the word choice and grammar later. Others construct their manuscripts or speeches like a brick wall, making one section perfect before building on it or developing it. Some authors schedule their writing projects in big blocks of intense time that might involve writing 3000 words or 15 pages or 15 hours each day. Others chip away at an article or speech in 2-hour time slots early in the morning before going to work, late into the night, or between children's naps. Olson (1972) offers these strategies for getting started:

1. Find a place in which to write, and guard it with your life. Words abhor crowds.

2. Write regularly; don't wait for the crack of the whip (or the pressure of an organization's or publisher's deadline).

3. Tell your story once, and tell it on paper.

4. Whenever possible, write about subjects that truly interest you. Bored writers produce bored readers.

5. Remember that getting started is half the battle.

3. Pay Attention to Writing Style

The aim of research reporting is to communicate fully, precisely, and clearly. A well-written manuscript should leave no doubt about what you did, why you did it, what you found, and what your findings imply. Most journals expect authors to use a standard outline format for research articles (see Box 18–3). One of the main reasons for this preference is so that readers can locate aspects of the article quickly and evaluate them without having to plow through all the details. Generally, poetic rhythms, stream of consciousness, personal or original use of words, and entertainment are not encouraged in scientific reporting. Writing according to the standards of scientific writing, however, does not mean that style and technique are irrelevant. They are just as important in scholarly and scientific writing as they are in creative writing. As Saslow (1982) says, "It takes a good deal of ingenuity to be clear and precise without being dull and repetitive" (p. 328). Although a number of authorities continue to preach that without exception scientific reports must use the third person and passive voice ("It was found by the investigators that . . ." instead of "We found that . . ."), this old rule is giving way. The so-called objective third person and passive voice are no guarantee that the research was objective and met the standards of validity and reliability. Lewis, former editor of *Nursing Outlook*, charges that the syndrome of pretentious prose in nursing literature puts unnecessary obstacles between the writer and the reader, makes readers dig for meaning, and impairs communication in a profession that needs a free and comprehensible exchange of ideas and findings on so many subjects. She illustrates her point by

---

Box 18–3   Typical Format for a Research Report

I. Front Matter
  A. Title page
    1. Title of study
    2. Authors' names
    3. Date

II. Table of Contents
  A. Chapters
  B. Bibliography
  C. Appendixes

III. Sections of the Paper
  A. The research problem
    1. Introduction to the problem
    2. Significance of the problem
    3. Purpose of the study
    4. Scope of the study
  B. Review of the literature (Divide into subheadings as necessary)

  C. Conceptual or theoretical framework (Divide into subheadings as necessary)
  D. Methodology
    1. Design
    2. Definition of variables
    3. Sampling
    4. Setting
    5. Extraneous variables
  E. Data collection
    1. Method and rationale
    2. Results of pilot study
    3. Reliability and validity
  F. Data analysis
    1. Method and rationale

  G. Results
    1. Presentation of tables and graphs or exemplars and themes
    2. Interpretation of results
  H. Discussion
    1. Summary
    2. Conclusions
    3. Implications for nursing
    4. Recommendations for further study and limitations

Appendixes
  Copy of consent form
  Copy of instruments
  Copy of tally or code sheets
  Correspondence

referring to an array of phrases scattered throughout nursing manuscripts, and we can add our own: a *burgeoning mandate*, a *plethora of logistics*, a *conceptually meaningful wholeness*, *finalization of the implementation of the program*, *operationalize*, *in terms of*, *with reference to*, *the fact of the matter is*, *as to whether*, and so on. Trust your own voice. Try to avoid affectations and hackneyed expressions. It's easy to fall into a formal, stilted style and forget that your real goal is *logical and lucid language*. Make your writing lean, direct, and specific.

4. Organize

Many novice writers, when they first sit down to write, take what some experts call "the buckshot approach." They scatter their presentation and ideas as diffusely as they can, hoping to hit some of the audience with some points, some of the time. The result is disjointed, incoherent writing. The way to avoid this approach is not necessarily, however, to report on a study in exactly the same time sequence as it was conducted, nor to rely on the old standby of "an introduction, a body, and a conclusion." Instead, first, let your thoughts dictate your words, and second, develop your paragraphs and sentences by looking backward and thinking of yourself as adding to what you've already done. This is called organizing your writing according to a *generative rhetoric*, in which you are clear about the focus of your paragraph and about developing and refining what has come before. Once a topic is introduced, subsequent sentences should make the logical support of or development of that topic clear. Subheadings take up space in a manuscript, but they help to keep the writer from wandering off the topic and are signposts that tell the reader where the writer is going. A well-organized speech or article should carry the listener or reader smoothly from one topic to another. This is usually handled by designing paragraphs that are neither too short nor long and rambling. Each paragraph should begin with a topic sentence that provides focus, and the rest of the paragraph should develop that topic. As you move from one paragraph to the next, you should provide your reader logical transitions.

5. Avoid Jargon

Because the goal of scientific speaking and writing is clear and precise communication, the words you choose should mean exactly what you intend. Colloquial expressions, pompous circumlocutions, ambiguity, and hackneyed clichés are rarely effective ways to convey meaning. Too much writing in nursing literature seems indifferent to meaning. Begin by omitting unnecessary, extraneous words. Strunk and White (1972) and others offer the following rules for vigorous, concise word usage:

- Choose a suitable design or format, and stick to it.

- Make the paragraph the unit of composition, and use it to keep the development of your ideas orderly.

Box 18–4   Examples of Writing Sparely

Wordy or Formal Usage	Concise Substitute	Wordy or Formal Usage	Concise Substitute
acquire	get	continue on	continue
add an additional	add	despite the fact that	although
any and all	any (or) all	during the course of	during
as to why	why	each and every one	each
at the present time	now	for the reason that	because
be acquainted with	know	in a manner similar to	like
commence	start	in all probability	probably

Source: Adapted from R. B. Ward, "Fog and How to Fight It," in *Practical Technical Writing*, New York: Knopf, 1968, pp. 27–28. Copyright © 1960 by Macmillan Publishing Company.

- Use the active voice rather than the passive voice.

- Put statements in a positive rather than negative form.

- Use definite, specific, concrete language.

- Omit needless words. See Box 18–4.

- Avoid the verb form *to be* and its variations, such as *there are* as much as possible. Select vivid, forceful verbs.

- Substitute a simple, familiar word for two complex, obscure ones.

Finally, remember that scientific writing requires an extraordinary attention to consistency and precision in the choice of words. Once a concept or variable is defined, substituting synonyms or approximations is less acceptable in research writing than in other expository forms. For example, in reporting a study of social support and self-care among the chronically mentally ill, it is not acceptable to casually substitute *social network* or *support system* for the concept *sources of social support* unless you defined them to mean precisely the same thing from the start.

6. Read Widely and Use Writing Aids

Most good writers and speakers like to read. They read for ideas, for style, for information, and to avoid duplicating the work of others. In Lewis's words, "In a profession constantly seeking new knowledge or at least seeking to build on and expand existing knowledge, we can't afford to keep on inventing or rediscovering the same old wheel." Reading keeps you informed of what others are doing in your area of research. Reading a journal alerts you to the publisher's preferences about length limitations, tone, placement of footnotes, references, use of illustrations and tables, and the characteristics of the readership. Reading can help you overcome obstacles presented by the need to include carefully and correctly prepared bibliographies, footnotes, tables, and figures. All writers and speakers should compile, read, and refer to the following writing aids.

- a good style manual, such as Turabian's (1973) *Manual for Writers*, that covers such subjects as spelling and punctuation, capitalization, underlining, quotations, footnotes, bibliographies, tables, illustrations, abbreviations, and numbers as well as the parts of term papers, theses, and dissertations. *Publication Manual* of the American Psychological Association (1983), Linton's (1972) *A Simplified Style Manual*, and the little classic on this subject, Strunk and White's (1972) *Elements of Style* are additional examples.

- a good general dictionary. Although there is no such thing as *the* dictionary, there is a difference between a dictionary that is newly compiled and kept up to date by experts working with a recent accumulation of recorded word usages and a dictionary that is patched together from older word books. The following ones are good choices: *American College Dictionary*, revised edition (Random House), *American Heritage Dictionary of the English Language* (Houghton Mifflin), *Random House Dictionary of the English Language*, *Webster's New World Dictionary of the American Language* (World), and *Webster's New Collegiate Dictionary* (Merriam).

- a historical dictionary. *The Oxford English Dictionary*, in 12 volumes and a supplement, is the greatest storehouse of information about English words. It traces the various forms of each word and its various senses, with dates and quotations from other writers to illustrate each sense. It is also available in compact paperback form.

- a specialized nursing dictionary. Look for the most recent one.

- indexes for locating health science literature and computerized data bases. Most good libraries provide a variety of services for locating information already available in health science literature. Your library may be able to obtain copies of articles or books through an interlibrary loan system when the source you seek is not in its collection. You may also find that your library has special collections and microfilm files and will conduct computer searches. *Consult your reference librarian regularly.*

- a medical dictionary. Taber's and Dorland's are two useful ones. They are revised regularly.

Reading for the pure joy of it is probably a habit for most writers. But reading manuscript and publication guidelines, articles and books that reflect the state of the art in your area of interest, and resources that represent helpful tools is a professional obligation. Reading does not guarantee that you will become a good writer any more than exposure to fine paintings means you will become an artist. But reading is probably the most valuable formative influence on a writer.

Giving a Talk at a Professional Meeting

Before you ever see your research in print, it's highly likely that you will present it in part or in full to an audience at a professional or scientific meeting.

Organization

The organization of a report of research findings in a journal customarily follows the format presented in Box 18–3, leaving results and discussion to the end. Many speakers, however, start their talk by calling attention to their findings and then follow with supporting evidence and essential methodological and statistical details. Beginning in this way catches the interest and attention of your audience, and including appropriate evidence convinces them that your research was carried out in a competent manner. At the end you can again summarize your findings. Ideas about your findings can be developed in a number of ways. Box 18–5 offers four possibilities.

Box 18–5   Ways of Developing Ideas

1. Conjunction (chronology; spatial description): "The stages of wound healing are as follows."

2. Disjunction (separation; mutually exclusive alternatives; comparison and contrast): "Group strategies that are helpful in fostering a client's ability to work through the death

of a parent differ for preschoolers and adolescents."

3. Concession (acknowledgment and additional line of thought): "Although the statistical significance of results in this research was inconclusive, the clinical significance

leads us to the following suggestions."

4. Condition (interdependent relations): "If the public image of nursing improves and becomes more realistic, we can expect the following shifts in third-party reimbursement policies."

Visual Aids

Most oral presentations benefit by the use of slides, overhead transparencies, and handouts. Here are some guidelines for preparing these materials.

1. Allow enough lead time to produce them.

2. Keep them simple. Seek advice from your institution's media resource department about how many lines can effectively go on a single slide or transparency.

3. Make sure that your audience can understand them. Remember that tables and graphs often contain printed headings or labels and that an audience must be able to read them from the back of the room. Don't try to cram too much information onto one visual, use extra-large type for labels, and be sure that any symbols or line drawings are clear and distinct.

Delivery

Here are some key guidelines:

1. Don't read your paper. Your audience will be bored. Often, you deliver too much information too fast, because you are unable while busily reading aloud to pick up visual cues that your audience isn't following or needs some elaboration or an illustration.

   On the other hand, don't count on being extemporaneously fluent. Write out, at minimum, a beginning and closing statement and a detailed outline on a set of notes. Refer to your notes if your mind goes blank due to performance anxiety. Keep to the sequence and order of your notes, glancing at them as you need to. Avoid the temptation to jump back to revisit an idea that you missed. Don't staple pages together. Flipping pages can distract your listeners.

2. If you have mistimed the length of your speech or paper and have to omit a section to keep within your allotted time, do so smoothly and unobtrusively without worrying out loud about "running out of time" or talking about all the sections you are leaving out. Making these blunders only costs you your stage presence, makes the audience feel cheated, and gives the impression that you were poorly organized or poorly prepared.

3. Never begin a speech or presentation by discrediting your qualifications on the subject at hand, your speaking ability, or your composure by saying, "I'm really nervous" or "I don't know why my work on this topic was selected" or "I despise speaking before audiences." Begin instead with an acknowledgment of the significance of the occasion, a clever anecdote, or some other opening line that piques the interest of the audience.

4. Always make notes on your script or outline to indicate the place where you intend to use transparencies or slides. This allows you to direct the audience's attention to a slide even if you can't see the screen from where you are speaking. It also allows you to ask the equipment operator to show the next slide. It's a good idea to have at least two copies of your referenced script so that your audio-visual assistant can read along with your presentation and anticipate technical matters.

5. Rehearse, preferably in front of a mirror and with a clock. Practicing your speech makes it familiar and smooth. Timing it allows you to be realistic about how long it takes to deliver various sections of it. A typed page generally takes 2 or 3 minutes to present, so a 30-minute speech should be around 12 pages without jokes or asides. Practice also decreases the likelihood that nervousness will cause you to make automatic gestures that may distract your audience. Practicing on the same day as your presentation is a particularly good idea.

6. Talk to your audience. Use eye contact, timing, and other speaking strategies such as inserted examples or asides to humanize your presentation. Look around the room at responsive members of the audience for signs of positive feedback, expressions of boredom and fatigue, or messages that you aren't being clear—or even heard. Knowing as much as possible about your audience's composition is always helpful in choosing the right tone and level.

7. Control the setting for your speech. Arrive in the room at least 30 to 45 minutes before your session to check out the functioning of your audio-visual equipment, to identify the presence of any unforeseen problems such as a fixed podium that's taller than you are, and to make other adjustments. Be certain that your transparency projector is properly focused and that the remote control for the slide projector is hooked up and works. Plan for someone to dim the house lights, and establish how you will cue him or her. If you find yourself in a highly formal convention center or hotel ballroom that seats 500 and only 30 people turn up for your presentation, anticipate strategies to decrease the distance and formality of your presentation. You might exchange your podium microphone for one that will allow you to move around, come down off the stage into the front of the room, and show your own transparencies or slides.

Fielding Questions

When the moment for your speech arrives, you may feel well organized, well prepared, and well rehearsed. But the prospect of fielding questions or criticisms from your audience—or of encountering total silence as a response to your paper—may be intimidating. You may fear having to think on your feet about new issues or being verbally attacked. A few hints to help you deal with these concerns follow:

1. Distribute index cards to those arriving for your speech, and ask them to identify one burning issue they would like to have discussed. Glancing through these suggestions can alert you to topics that might be raised during a question-and-answer period. These questions can also suggest material if your offer to respond to verbal questions is met with silence.

2. Plant a few relevant and significant questions with your associates and colleagues in the audience so as to break the ice and make it a bit easier for others to stand up and speak publicly if they wish to.

3. Repeat or paraphrase questions that are asked, so that everyone in the room can hear them, so that they will be picked up if your speech is being taped, and so that you will have a little extra time to organize your response.

4. If you are unable to answer a question, offer to send references or resource materials later or to talk personally with the questioner during a break.

Speaking is thinking out loud. It requires planning and practice. Because it is impossible to present as much detail in a typical talk as you can present in a research article or, certainly, in a thesis or dissertation, the success of a talk often depends on your ability to select the five or so major points that ought to be emphasized and developed. Saslow (1982) likens deciding what to include in a speech to getting ready for a backpacking trip. You lay out everything that is "essential" and then throw half of it away because otherwise your pack will be too heavy to carry. If you aren't selective about the ideas in your talk, you'll have too much extra baggage. Conveying too much information in a talk is a major pitfall to avoid. Another is assuming that the audience can understand aspects of the presentation that are overly complex or poorly presented.

Scientific Speeches

In any scientific presentation of research findings you should cover the following areas:

1. Describe the research subjects and the sampling procedures in enough detail to let your audience know how far your findings can be generalized.

2. If your design is at all complicated, be sure to make clear how many subjects were assigned to which group using which assignment method. (A handout or transparency can be useful here.)

3. Be sure that your audience has a clear idea of the amount and variety of data your findings are based on. For instance, in reporting a field study, be sure to say how many hours of participation you employed, how many interviews you conducted and with whom, and which documents you reviewed.

4. If you used statistical analysis procedures, specify the test used and other technical information, such as the level of significance.

5. Mention any limitations or assumptions that might have bearing on the interpretation of your findings, to assure the audience of your objectivity and honesty.

Guidelines for Evaluating a Talk

Saslow (1982) offers the following overall set of questions to use when evaluating any oral presentation, including your own:*

1. What were the major findings or conclusions? (They should have been mentioned at least twice.)

2. Were you given enough evidence to have faith in the conclusions?

   a. Did the speaker present enough of the method so that you understood approximately what was done?

   b. Were the results presented in a form you could readily grasp?

   c. Did the speaker report the statistical analysis necessary to establish that the results weren't due to chance factors?

   d. Did the speaker make a clear, logical argument why the results supported the conclusions?

3. Did the speaker give you the information that would allow you to generalize from the results, such as:

   a. type and number of subjects and other subject characteristics?

   b. duration of training of subjects (if appropriate)?

   c. any peculiar conditions of the setting for the study that might not be reproducible elsewhere?

   d. information about potential experimenter bias or subject attitude effects?

4. Did the speaker relate the findings to any wider field of research or application?

5. Did the speaker lose you at any point by:

   a. using jargon or self-defined terms?

   b. drowning you in detail?

   c. presenting information too rapidly?

---

*Source: Based on C. A. Saslow, *Basic Research Methods*, (New York: Random House, Inc., 1982), p. 377.

d. failing to emphasize the important points and distinguish them clearly from less important information?

e. distracting you with personal mannerisms?

6. Was the talk interesting?

Writing a Journal Article, Thesis, or Dissertation

Whether you are writing a book, a thesis, or dissertation, a technical report for a funding agency, or a journal article, you will go through a three-stage process: prewriting, writing, and rewriting. This section deals with how these stages apply to the writing of a journal article.

Prewriting

Prewriting is discovering what you have to say about your subject, finding the perspective from which to treat it, and doing all the organizational tasks required before making a deliberate effort to produce a first draft. For a scientific writer, it may include hours of brooding over the results of statistical analyses on computer print-outs. Or it may involve returning to the library to take more notes. It usually encompasses the following:

- targeting a journal or publishing house
- obtaining its instructions to authors
- sampling some previously published work
- sorting out issues of authorship
- drafting a letter of inquiry.

Prewriting also involves identifying your subject, deciding on a direction or purpose for your manuscript, and developing your purpose, intent, or direction into an outline of what you want to say about it. The framework of developmental questions in Box 18–6 offers an informal start for an outline of a research journal article. The typical format for a journal article in Box 18–3 and the criteria for a research critique in Chapter 6 are additional resources you can use in developing an outline.

A theoretical analysis or a methodological paper requires that you employ other strategies for developing a topic. These may be exploration, argumentation, or comparison and contrast. The questions in Box 18–7 can provide a start. Metaanalysis (studies to synthesize findings and research on a topic) is another growing category of published work (Schwartz et al 1987).

Box 18–6   **Questions That Your Outline Should Answer**

1. What is the general area of your research problem?

2. Why is studying this area important to nursing?

3. What previous work (theoretical and empirical) has been done that is related to your research?

4. What did prior literature suggest needed to be done next?

5. How does your work respond to this need?

6. What, specifically, did you do?

7. What were your results?

8. What did you expect?

9. What is the broader meaning of your investigation?

10. What needs to be done from here?

Choosing a Journal   It's always possible to write an article and then shop for an outlet for it. But journals differ in their length limitations, citation systems, audiences, and circulation. Most authorities agree, therefore, that it's a good idea to *think about where you might publish your manuscript before you even write it* to avoid having to make major revisions in tone, style, and format. It might surprise you to know that McCloskey's 1982 list of 50 American journals (excluding state nurses'

Box 18–7   **Questions That Aid in Developing a Paper**

1. What does my topic mean?

2. What are its characteristics or properties?

3. What are its parts, types, or forms?

4. How is it done?

5. What are the conditions for it or causes of it?

6. What are the outcomes or consequences of doing or using it?

7. How does it compare with something else?

8. What is the present status of knowledge about it?

9. What is its value?

10. What is my personal response to it?

11. What case or arguments can be made against it?

12. How can my topic be summarized?

association publications) that represented publishing opportunities in nursing had been put at 749 by Mirin (1981). Box 18–8 identifies major categories and examples of nursing journals.

Selecting a journal depends on the readership to whom you want to communicate your ideas. Before deciding on several and ranking them in order of your preferred outlet, be sure to read several issues of the journal to:

- get a sense of the tone and style its editors prefer

- get a feeling for the audience that reads it

- determine whether the time from submission to publication is acceptable to you

- judge whether your work will be timely and of interest to the editors

Reasons for Rejection   From the start, you should keep in mind that the chief reasons for rejection of manuscripts, either by journal editors, advisory boards, or official *referees* (anonymous peers who review your manuscript), are:

1. The subject of your manuscript is not relevant to the journal's readership.

2. The article is poorly written.

3. The central idea, or "little logic" (see Chapter 2), of your article is not unique.

Referees, reviewers, editorial board members, and editors use many criteria to eval-

---

Box 18–8   Major Categories of Nursing Journal

Journal Category	Example
General nursing	*American Journal of Nursing* *Nursing, 80's* *RN*
Speciality nursing	*Cardiovascular Nursing* *Heart & Lung* *Maternal and Child Nursing* *Supervisor Nurse* *Journal of Nursing Administration*
Research nursing	*Nursing Research* *Advances in Nursing Science* *Research in Nursing and Health* *Western Journal for Nursing Research*

uate an article for publication.

McCloskey (1982) further specifies the reasons that articles are rejected by nursing publishers:

1. The subject was recently covered or is already scheduled for a future issue.

2. The article is too technical for the journal.

3. The content is inaccurate or undocumented.

4. The work is based on a poor research design or faulty methodology.

5. Nursing concerns are not highlighted.

6. The content is unimportant.

7. The article is too much like a speech or term paper and would be difficult to change.

8. The conclusion is unwarranted by the data as presented.

9. The idea was previously published elsewhere.

10. The idea is badly presented.

Advice from Journal Editors   Nursing journal editors also offered prospective authors some words of advice in the McCloskey survey (1982):

- Manuscripts must be well organized, look neat, be double-spaced on good-quality bond paper, and have 1-inch margins throughout.

- Specifications for manuscripts are available from journals. Get them and follow them (see also Appendix E).

- Start with a literature review so that you won't reinvent the wheel.

- Outline before you write.

- If what you say is controversial, document your sources and recognize opposing points of view.

- Ask colleagues, mentors, and friends to critique your manuscript before you submit it.

- Write in a straightforward style, using the active voice when possible. Avoid sounding pompous or pedantic.

- Keep information concise, relevant, up to date, and accurate.

- Double-check all your figures and totals.

- Provide your name, title, credentials, address, phone number, and organizational affiliation.

Editorial Policies Most nursing journals include their editorial policy in each issue. From it you can learn exactly what kinds of article a journal wants to publish, what materials should accompany any submission (such as a short biographical sketch or a full résumé), how articles are to be prepared and submitted, and to whom. Some journals, such as the *American Journal of Nursing*, invite or solicit manuscripts from qualified experts. Others restrict acceptance of manuscripts to unsolicited ones that have been favorably reviewed by a panel of referees according to specific guidelines. Some journals include both. Understanding the editorial policy of a journal prepares you to write the kind of article the journal wants to receive and publish. Appendix E provides editorial guidelines for contributors for selected research journals. Kolin and Kolin (1980) differentiate most published nursing articles into five categories:

1. the case study

2. the research article

3. the article on procedures, processes, and techniques

4. the historical article

5. the article on a current topic

Matching the article you intend to write with the right outlet is an essential step toward success in getting published.

The Query Letter Whereas articles solicited by a journal editor have close to a 100% chance of being published, unsolicited manuscripts must be designed to compete to be seen in print. Writing a letter of inquiry (called a query letter) to the editor of the journal is one way to increase the likelihood that your unsolicited manuscript will be accepted.

In a query letter, you ask whether an editor of a journal is interested in reviewing your manuscript for publication consideration. Both editors and authors know that a well-written query letter can save them both time and effort, not to mention postage. Although a few journals discourage query letters, desiring instead to review the entire unsolicited manuscript, the majority prefer them.

It is proper to mail several query letters about the same piece of work to a number of different editors. If the responses are all encouraging, the author can then pick and choose. *But it is definitely not considered good etiquette to send out copies of full manuscripts to several editors simultaneously.* The unwritten code between editors and authors is that an author awaits a decision from one journal before trying another one. One way to alienate editors is to have them devote a great deal of time and effort to the review process and accept your manuscript, only to learn that you have agreed to have it appear somewhere else. Editors don't seem to object to what Mirin (1981 p. 10) calls "mass query mailing," but you must realize that if several journals indicate interest, it's only polite to write back to some of them to let them know that your paper is going elsewhere.

Box 18–9   Sample Query Letter

June 11, 1989

Dr. Shirley Smoyak, Editor
Journal of Psychosocial Nursing
SLACK Incorporated
6900 Grove Road
Thorofare, New Jersey 08086

Dear Dr. Smoyak:

Within a few years, "DRG's" and "Prospective Payment" are going to reshape the management of inpatient psychiatric care. In the May, 1984, issue of *Hospital and Community Psychiatry*, authorities in the field urged that psychiatry's extension be devoted to studying ways of estimating resource use and classifications of psychiatric clients. Nursing, whose unique contribution to the interdisciplinary mental health team is observation and management of basic needs among inpatients on a 24-hour-a-day basis, can offer an informed perspective on how psychiatry can participate in a prospective payment system without endangering the quality of patient care. Classification systems are needed to bridge the gap between standard psychiatric diagnostic categories (DSM-III-R) and what has become known as the "Nursing Diagnosis Movement."

Our article, *The Nursing Adaptation Evaluation* (NSGAE), offers a proposed VI Axis for DSM-IV and provides categories for a functional assessment of psychiatric patients useful to planning, documenting, and evaluating the effects of nursing care on hospitalized psychiatric clients. The computer processable numerical code system incorporates the patient's highest level of adaptive functioning in the areas of *Nutrition, Solitude and Social Interaction, Grooming (and Hygiene), Activity (and Rest)*, and *Elimination* in the past year, and his or her current overall level of adaptive functioning or self-care ability in separate ratings of adaptive functioning in the five basic need areas respectively. Our proposed Axis VI for DSM-IV is based on descriptive criteria, can provide practical guidelines for nursing and interdisciplinary treatment planning, and is currently being systematically evaluated in six clinical settings.

While the list of nursing diagnoses accepted for testing by the NANDA group very likely has an important future in the evaluation of a nursing diagnosis taxonomy, many psychosocial nurses attest to the need for a classification system that has interdisciplinary meaning and utility for the particular treatment planning requirements for psychiatric nursing care. We believe that our article introducing the Nursing Adaptation Evaluation (NSGAE) as a proposed Axis VI for DSM-IV responds to those needs and offers an empirical approach worthy of wider study.

If you are interested in receiving our manuscript for publication consideration, we can immediately send it to you for review upon notification.

(Continued)

Box 18–9   Sample Query Letter (Continued)

Sincerely,

Holly Skodol Wilson, RN,
PhD FAAN
Professor

cc: Eileen Morrison
     Lucy Fisher
     Patricia Underwood

HSW/b

Composing a query letter is part of the prewriting, developmental stage, because a note from the editor indicating interest in reviewing the manuscript may also contain some developmental suggestions that can save hours of revision time later. Another reason for writing your query letters early in the manuscript preparation process is that a publisher's or editor's interest in your work is a terrific source of motivation and inspiration, particularly when contrasted with the impact of spending months writing a long article only to have it repeatedly returned to you with a rejection slip.

Mirin (1981) recommends that a query letter have four parts:

1. a lead paragraph or two that catches the editor's interest and lures him or her into reading on

2. a paragraph that tells what the article will be about, what direction it will take, and what it will offer the reader

3. some facts, observations, or other citations that back up your basic premise and offer your credentials for writing the piece

4. two final paragraphs in which you make a strong statement designed to convince the editor that this is an article that he or she should publish and to ask if the editor is interested in reviewing the manuscript for publication consideration

A sample of a query letter appears in Box 18–9.

The Question of Authorship   Finding the right outlet for your journal article is certainly one of the most critical prewriting details. In the case of work that has multiple authors, determining from the start the order in which names should appear and what responsibilities each should assume is also important. Neither of these decisions should be made frivolously. The convention of resolving the decision of author sequence according to alphabetical order of last names is all but obsolete. If the article is chiefly your work, it will matter a lot to you later if you don't get the visibility, credit, and acknowledgment you deserve, especially because journal article publishing rarely involves any financial reward except for a token payment in relatively rare instances. McCloskey (1982) and others agree that the best and fairest way to allocate credit is giving most of the credit to the person who did most of the work.

Writing

Prewriting and writing overlap. Even so, certain considerations tend to present themselves in the context of composing your first draft. Keep in mind that even with the most careful job of prewriting, most well-written manuscripts go through several drafts before the content and organization represent the very best you can do with your topic in the time you have available. Several of the problems encountered in the writing phase are presented in the sections that follow.

Deciding on a Title Aim for a title that is concise, specific, and informative. The title should tell accurately and clearly what the paper is about. Linton (1972) points out that the title you choose may mean the difference between recognition and oblivion for your article: "You are providing the first index to your paper when you write its title, and the precision of your title may seriously affect the availability to science of your contribution" (p. 41). Although it's important to avoid unnecessary words that increase the length of your title without adding to descriptive accuracy and completeness, the APA *Publication Manual* (1983) acknowledges that as many as 15 words may be necessary to avoid being overly cryptic. Stay away from pretentiousness, triteness, clichés, and jargon. But a catchy title can generally be acceptable to the audience or readership of the journal if it still serves as an accurate guide to the work you are reporting. Box 18–10 shows some sample titles in poor and improved forms.

A good title should be short but explanatory. You can accomplish this goal by building key information, such as your study variables and subjects, into the title and avoiding unnecessary words. Avoid the tendency to select a title that merely represents one part of your article. Instead try for one that represents the focus and intention of the entire paper.

Writing the Lead Some journals require that you write a several-sentence lead section that can be boxed or put in boldface type at the opening of your article. In the absence of an official lead, consider your first sentences or paragraphs as the lead of your paper. Like your title, your lead section must engage the readers' attention and interest and inspire them to read on. A lead also sets the tone of the article and limits the article's scope so that the readers know from the beginning

Box 18–10   Sample Titles

Poor	Improved
Now They Can Choose: A Study of Health Beliefs Among Chinese-Americans Who Have Cancer	Health Beliefs About Treatment Among Chinese-American Cancer Patients (eliminates unnecessary words)
Pain Assessment: An Exploratory Study	Behavioral Indicators of Pain in Preschool Children During Burn Debridement (adds specificity and key features such as population and study conditions)
An Interpretative Study of the Nature of the Therapeutic Touch Process	Expectations, Beliefs, and Physical Sensations Experienced by Patients During Therapeutic Touch Treatments (increases specificity and clarity)
Prechemotherapy Patient Education: It's Affect on Patterns of Nausea and Vomitting	Prechemotherapy Patient Education: Its Effect on Patterns of Nausea and Vomiting (corrects misuse of *it's* for *its*, *affect* for *effect*, and corrects spelling error in *vomiting*)
Who Seeks Help: A Longitudinal Study	Arthritis in the Elderly: Patterns of Disability and Coping (incorporates key variables, increasing the chance of the articles being properly indexed)

what to expect. A lot of writers leave the composition of this very important part of an article until last. Once a manuscript is completed, you have a better idea of its tone and coverage anyway. Kolin and Kolin (1980) identify the following alternatives for leads, depending on the type of journal and, of course, the type of article you have written:

1.   a simple, clear, and straightforward statement of purpose, often used in scientific journals

2.   a dramatic, eye-catching use of statistics

3.   a client anecdote or history that engages human interest

4. a personal experience with which readers are likely to identify

5. a definition that orients readers to the topic

6. a question or several questions, with the implication that readers probably have or should have asked them of themselves

7. a comparison or contrast that whets the readers' appetite for more information

8. a historical summary to place the topic in context and interest the readers in getting more current information

Leads often must be written and rewritten many times before you are satisfied. Although you may not craft the opening sentences 50 times, as Plato supposedly did when he wrote *The Republic*, you should ideally attempt to write a lead or opening that evokes interest, is direct and concise, and makes promises that you fulfill in your article.

Writing Your Rough Draft   The following guidelines will help you get started on the first draft of your article:

1. Decide on an environment that is conducive to writing, preferably one where your resource materials are easily available, one that is free of tempting or annoying distractions, and one where you don't mind spending some concentrated time. Some writers who prepare their manuscripts on a word processor obviously write where their computer is located.

2. Fill up those white pages. Get something down on paper, and worry about editing and revising later. Follow the topics on your outline, and develop them.

3. Leave three spaces between lines, whether you write in longhand or type, so that you have room for changes and additions.

4. Number your pages and paragraphs so that you can move them around if doing so would improve your organization.

5. Decide what you intend to present in tables or graphs, and flag the pages on which you want them to appear. (Follow the guidelines presented later in this chapter for constructing tables and figures.)

6. Be prepared to cut and paste if you are not working on a word processor or to edit what you've written if you are. Both these strategies help you avoid having to rewrite or retype material when you reorganize it.

7. If at all possible set aside your first draft for at least a few days before rewriting it. A research paper for a course, a thesis, or an article should never be submitted "hot off the typewriter."

8. Ask a friend, colleague, or teacher to critique a later draft, and consider their suggestions before writing your final draft.

9. Proofread for typographical errors, spelling errors, missing words, awkward sentences, and redundancies.

10. Keep at least one copy for your own files.

It is beyond the scope of this chapter to discuss the technical aspects of grammar and style for scientific writing. For questions about tense, punctuation, parallel sentence construction, word usage, paragraphing, shaping sentences, and spelling, see Strunk and White's (1972) *The Elements of Style*, Linton's (1972) *A Simplified Style Manual*, Perrin and Ebbitt's (1972) *Writer's Guide and Index to English*, Kolin and Kolin's (1980) *Professional Writing for Nurses in Education, Practice and Research*, Mirin's (1981) *The Nurse's Guide to Writing for Publication*, or Tornquist's (1985) *From Proposal to Publication: The Nurse Researcher's Guide to Writing*. The following guidelines, however, will help you write your draft in a clear and organized way:

1. Eliminate all unnecessary, dull, and trite words.

2. Use active verb forms.

3. Check the order of paragraphs and sentences to be certain that each paragraph contains a topic sentence, that sentences build upon each other, that effective transitions move the reader between paragraphs, and that the order of ideas and the supporting evidence is clear and effective.

4. Consider your tone in light of your topic, your intended audience, and the type of journal to which you are submitting the article. Make sure your language is consistent with your intended tone.

5. Aim for versatility and variety in your writing. Don't overuse words or sentence structures. Without variety, your writing will be dull.

6. Above all, you must be clear. In Mirin's (1981) words, "Clarity doesn't make style but there can be no style without it and clarity means order. Without order, you cannot communicate" (p. 44).

Working Quotations in Smoothly   If you want your paper to read smoothly, you can't just drop quotations with a thud into your paragraph. You need to introduce a quotation with phrases such as:

- "As Lindsey discovered . . ."
- "In Hutchinson's words . . ."
- "According to Scheetz . . ."
- "Stotts observed that . . ."
- "Moody's work suggested . . ."

Generally speaking, extensive quotations aren't used in scientific articles. Three circumstances warrant the use of quotations:

1. The material is authoritative and convincing evidence in support of your thesis.

2. The statement is phrased exactly as it should be.

3. The idea is controversial, and you want to assure your readers about it.

Plagiarism and Paraphrasing   **Plagiarism** means to steal and pass off the work of another as one's own. It usually results from bad paraphrasing or improper referencing. Both paraphrasing that merely substitutes a few words for those of the original author and forgetting to use quotation marks and a reference citation are technically considered plagiarism, even if you somehow hypnotize yourself into thinking that those really were your own words to express your own ideas. The only safe way to paraphrase is to read the original over several times and then write your conception of what you've read *without looking at the original*. In other words, when paraphrasing, keep the source book closed.

Preparing Table and Figures   Complex results that involve numbers are often presented in tables and figures in a research article reporting findings. Descriptive statistics such as sample size, means, measures of variability, and the like are clearer and less cumbersome when presented this way. Keep in mind, however, that most journals will discourage excessive use of them and that tables and figures that are numbered separately should be on separate pages at the end of your manuscript. You should also note where you want them to appear, for example, *[insert Table 1 about here]*. An illustration that is not a table is called a figure. Pictures of equipment and graphs are examples of figures.

Good tables have the following characteristics:

1. All tables should have a clear, explanatory title and a number at the top.

2. A table should be comprehensible without any additional explanation. It should stand by itself.

3. A good table should not be overly complicated, and an intelligent reader should be able to figure it out without too much effort. If it's too complicated, put some of the information into a second table.

4. Tables shouldn't duplicate information presented in another form.

5. Tables should be cited by number in the text.

Good figures have these characteristics:

1. A figure should have its title or caption at the bottom instead of the top of the page.

2. Like tables, figures should not need additional explanation.

3. In the case of a graph, the axes (x = horizontal and y = vertical) should be labeled.

4. Figures should be used when you want to depict change over time visually or to make a more immediate and dramatic impact on the reader.

5. Like tables, figures should be referred to explicitly in the text of your article.

6. No more than four curves should appear on any given figure.

7. It's not necessary to give the total possible range on a grid if none of your data have extreme values.

8. The dependent variable is customarily plotted on the x axis, and the independent variable is plotted on the y axis.

9. Include a legend, or caption, that accompanies the figure and explains it.

10. Figures should not be larger than $8\frac{1}{2} \times 11$ inches when they are submitted for publication.

11. You must get permission to reprint a table or figure created by someone else. Consult one of the manuals of style for precise details on how to reference sources for tables and figures and on referencing in general.

Once you have written your first draft, you are ready to move into the final stage of composition, one in which you will pare and prune. Good writing springs not from formulas but from creative activity, clear thinking, personal commitment, and self-criticism.

Rewriting

When you've finished your first draft, put it aside for a while, ask someone else to look at it, and read it again with the proverbial blue editorial pencil in your hand. Use the four following sets of guidelines (Saslow 1982) to evaluate the sections of your research report and the quality of its style.*

Criteria for a Good Introduction   The title, lead, and introduction make an important first impression on your reader. Saslow suggests that the standards on which an introduction should be based include the following:

1. Is the general area of the research clearly introduced, and do you make a case for why more knowledge is needed in the area?

2. Have you summarized the present state of knowledge in the area?

3. Have you built a case for why your approach in the study is a reasonable one?

4. Are sources for facts, ideas, and speculations given and referenced?

---

*Source: Based on C. A. Saslow, *Basic Research Methods* (New York: Random House, Inc., 1982), pp. 344–359.

5. Is the specific study problem clearly stated before the methods section?

Criteria for a Good Methods Section

1. Is it clear who your subjects were and how many of them you used as data sources?

2. Are all the data-collection tools and instruments in your research described in enough detail so that someone else could replicate your study? Have you provided sources of any specific tests, figures to illustrate laboratory equipment, and the like?

3. Have you described your study design clearly, including the independent and dependent variables, the way subjects were assigned to groups, and so on?

4. Have you sufficiently described procedures, such as instructions to subjects, used to control extraneous variables so that your reader can evaluate any possible alternative explanations for your results?

Criteria for a Good Results Section

1. Have you described all the preliminary steps used to prepare your data for analysis?

2. Is the section well organized according to initial hypotheses or research questions?

3. Are descriptions and inferential statistics given to back up findings derived from quantitative data, and are analytic methods for qualitative data discussed? Is the statistical test named, and is it appropriate for the level of measurement and study question? Have you included the calculated test statistic, degrees of freedom, and significance level for inferential statistical tests?

4. Are the necessary tables and figures included? Are they in the proper format, clearly titled or captioned, easy to interpret, and able to stand alone?

Criteria for a Good Discussion Section

1. Are the results clearly summarized and emphasized?

2. Have you explained instances when your results differ from what you expected?

3. Have you discussed the relationship of your findings to the results of others?

4. Have you considered any effects that design or procedural limitations might have had on your findings?

5. Have you made your interpretations of your results clear?

6. Have you included any possible alternative interpretations?

7. Have you suggested ideas for future research or the application of your findings?

Box 18–11 offers you a final checklist for all research papers, whether they are reports of findings or other analytic, methodological, or conceptual essays.

Box 18–11   Final Checklist for Papers

1. Do you have a single, controlling idea you want to communicate? (To make your paper really clear, state this idea in the form of a thesis statement, and include it in your first or second paragraph.)

2. Does everything in your paper pertain to that idea? If something doesn't, either find a way to connect it clearly or omit it.

3. Have you organized your essay into clear sections and arranged them in the most logical and effective order?

4. Do you have plenty of supporting evidence to back up your ideas? Don't be afraid to draw upon your own experience; it's the most valid evidence of all. Be specific!

5. Are your paragraphs well developed? Most good paragraphs consist of at least five sentences that are themselves well focused and packed with essential information.

6. Are your paragraphs themselves well organized? Each paragraph should have some controlling idea, expressed in the topic sentence.

7. Are transitions between paragraphs and sentences smooth?

8. Do you have an interesting introduction, one that will grab your readers and make them want to read on?

9. Have you concluded your essay effectively?

10. Is your essay mechanically correct? Read your last draft and final version aloud; often you will catch errors that your eye might skim over.

11. Look up any words you're not sure how to spell; don't just guess and hope for the best. Also check the meaning of any word you're slightly unsure of.

12. Have you varied your sentence structure? Make sure your sentences aren't too short and choppy. Although an occasional short sentence is effective, more than a couple in a row have the stylistic interest of a Dick and Jane workbook. Practice joining sentences to connect ideas and establish logical relationships between them.

When you are ready to make that trip to the post office to submit your article, reread the journal's information to contributors. Doing so will ensure that you know:

- whether to double- or triple-space the manuscript

- how large the margins should be

- how many copies to send

- what information you should include about yourself

- whether you should include an abstract

- the name and correct address of the editor to whom you are sending your manuscript

- approximately how long it will take for your article to go through the review process

Postwriting

Reviewers or referees may take from two weeks to two months to make their recommendations about your manuscript to the journal editor. In the meantime, you'll probably receive a postcard acknowledging that your manuscript was received. After that postcard, patience is essential.

If your article is accepted, the editor will probably congratulate you in a letter and let you know when you can expect to receive proofs for proofreading. Be prepared for editors to expect you to be prompt with this task. Sometimes, acceptance for publication in a journal is conditional on making changes specified by the reviewers or editor. You as an author can always decline and send it elsewhere if you disagree with the changes requested. But if you do, you should officially withdraw it from the first journal.

If your manuscript is rejected, most editors will return it to you. The possibility of rejection always exists, and unless you can conclude with certainty that the editor is totally lacking in taste, sensitivity, and vision, you ought to try to determine why it was rejected and to grow from the experience. Editors do miss opportunities and make mistakes. Don't let a rejection from one journal keep you from submitting your article somewhere else if you still believe in its value.

Writing a Book

In most cases, authors of books, whether monographs presenting research findings in detail or textbooks like this one, are people who have established themselves as authors through their contributions to the professional literature. When you attempt to write a book, you must be equally clear about your idea, your audience, and the form in which you intend to present your work as when you write a journal article (Kolin and Kolin 1980). Writing a book, however, expands manyfold the amount of time and energy involved. Publishers estimate that it takes an author about 2 years to produce a text or reference book and then another 10 to 12 months to go through the production process. Figure 18–1 illustrates the phases of the book production process.

Approaching a Publisher: The Prospectus

Getting a book published requires that you form a partnership with a publishing company unless you intend to print, market, and distribute your book on your own

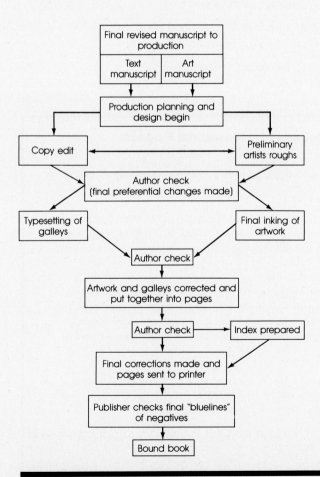

Figure 18–1   The production of a book.

(an idea that I'd discourage unless you have special resources, contacts, and expertise in the publishing enterprise). You approach a publisher with a **prospectus**, or *manuscript proposal*, that includes a detailed outline or table of contents and one or two sample chapters that you consider representative of the tone and writing style of the text. Box 18–12 outlines the components of a manuscript proposal. It's often a good idea to think of the prospectus as akin to your preface for the book, and as such it should at least address the following questions:

1. Why do you intend to write this book, and what need will it fill?
2. What is the level of the book, and what audience will be interested in it?
3. What are the main features of the contents and organization of the book?
4. How can the reader use the book to its best advantage?
5. Are there supplementary materials such as software or a student workbook?
6. If this is a revised edition of a previously published book, what is the essence of the revision, and what are the significant changes?
7. What acknowledgments do you intend to include?

Box 18–12   The Components of a Manuscript Proposal

PROSPECTUS: The prospectus should include a detailed discussion of the following points:

Rationale: Describe your reasons for writing the book and explain what you are attempting to accomplish. Discuss the current trends in the field and relate your book to the needs of the field (pedagogical, topical, and/or theoretical).

Market: Is this book designed to serve as:
1. a major textbook (which will normally be usable without supplementation)
2. a briefer "core" text (which will cover most traditionally required topics but would usually require supplementary reading in a full-semester course)
3. an originally written topical supplement covering a single topic or several topics

Subject and scope: What does the book cover or omit in terms of traditional topics, innovation, expansion, and/or improvement for this specific course(s)? Explain any unique features.

Approach: How is the subject treated in comparison/contrast to traditional approaches?

(Continued)

Box 18–12   The Components of a Manuscript Proposal (Continued)

Level: Is the book written for introductory or advanced students? Comment on the level and style of writing.

Physical appearance: What is the proposed length of the manuscript (total typewritten pages, double-spaced)? How many graphs, tables, figures, and photographs are to be included? (Please enumerate specific illustrative material.)

Ancillary items: Which of the following do you propose to accompany the text: instructor's manual (how extensive?), student guide, audio-visuals, computer material, etc.?

Competition: Compare/contrast your proposal with specific, major competitive titles in terms of approach, coverage, and features.

DETAILED OUTLINE: The outline should be complete for the entire text and detailed enough to give an accurate picture of the depth and breadth of coverage you plan. Reviewers cannot suggest deletions or additions to content unless they know exactly what you intend to discuss. It may be necessary in some cases to detail the outline to the third level of heads.

SAMPLE CHAPTER(S): These may be requested with the above material for initial review, or they may be requested after the detailed outline has been reviewed and perhaps revised—it depends on the nature of the project. Your editor would probably indicate which chapter should be completed after the initial review. As a rule, the sample should not be an introductory chapter, but one more representative of the text. It should include all features that you plan to include in the final text chapter (e.g., tables, figures, objectives, bibliography, suggested readings, etc.).

Negotiating a Publishing Contract

Once your idea, presentation, and competence have succeeded in capturing the interest of a publisher (or several), you must negotiate and sign a contract. You agree to deliver a completed manuscript by a specified date. The publisher agrees to produce the book, promote it, store it, sell it, and protect its copyright. The publisher also provides other assistance, such as obtaining in-progress reviews and locating a designer, production coordinator, illustrator, and indexer (if you don't want to do the index yourself). In return for your creative work as author, you are paid royalties (usually twice a year) that represent a percentage of the net sales revenue. A "standard contract" usually offers the author around 10% of net sales. In some cases, the royalty rate can include an escalation clause that increases the royalty percentage based on the number of copies sold per year, per edition, or per life of the book. Royalties for foreign sales are usually less than those for domestic sales.

Royalties are only one of the negotiable items in a publishing contract. Obviously, the financial success of a book is in the interest of both author and publisher. But as an author, you may also be interested in assurances about the developmental and editorial assistance that you can expect from the publisher. For example, will the publisher arrange for copy editing? What are the publisher's intentions about the physical appearance of the book (hardback or softcover, size, quality of paper)? What about the availability and amount of an advance against royalties that can help you offset costs of preparing the manuscript? Typing costs may total as much as $3000, and illustrations in many books cost even more. If you are working with a coauthor, you may need to offset costs of travel, long-distance phone calls, and so on. It's obviously preferable to be working on a project using the publisher's capital on an interest-free basis than to launch the venture with both your time and your out-of-pocket cash. Is there a possibility of receiving a grant that you would not have to pay back to the publisher out of your royalties? Will the publisher share some costs with you, such as for illustrations, permissions, or indexing?

Most important in deciding on a publisher, given comparable contract offers, is the quality of the company's work. Study the other books the publisher has developed and produced. Find out if the firm exhibits at important nursing meetings and advertises in prominent nursing journals. What do you think of its sales representatives? How professional are its brochures and fliers? Is the company known and respected in nursing? Does it strike you as having the kind of integrity you'd expect from any other business partner?

The Publisher's Precontract Review

Just as you will be investigating a potential publisher, the publishing company will be investigating the merit of your proposed book. This is usually done by sending out requests for precontract reviews by anonymous reviewers in whose judgment the publisher has confidence.

Writing the Book: Resources

Writing the manuscript for your book involves all the considerations of tone, style, organization, word choice, idea development, and mechanics that were discussed in the section on writing a journal article—and more. Seek out your publisher's guidelines for authors to get help with questions related to:

- setting up a filing system
- starting a permissions log

- punctuation, numbering, and alphabetizing
- indexing
- illustrations
- glossary
- supplements
- referencing
- reprints and new editions

About Copyright

A chapter on article and book writing wouldn't be complete without a word on the subject of copyright. **Copyright law** protects any author from having his or her material used without permission. It protects all kinds of original work, including illustrations, tables, diagrams, songs, and so on. Under the most recent copyright law (1978), any original work is automatically protected by copyright law when it is put on paper. The duration of a copyright consists of an author's lifetime plus 50 years. An author owns all rights to a work he or she creates unless those rights are transferred to the publisher of a journal or book. Publishers usually ask for these rights, but authors can stipulate the rights they want to keep and those they want to transfer to a publisher—for example, rights to publish the work in article form elsewhere. Some publishers won't accept an article or book manuscript for publication unless you transfer full copyright to them because of the benefits they can derive by control of all future uses of your work. Whether someone's work is protected by the copyright law or *in the public domain* (anything on which the copyright has expired), you should always acknowledge the source of materials and ideas that are not your own. The job of obtaining permissions or alerting a permissions assistant to the need for them is an important aspect of an author's responsibility, and a good publisher often assists.

Guidelines for Critique

- Have you considered general guidelines for presentations in preparation for a speech or a journal article?

- If you are doing a thesis or dissertation, have you reviewed the requisite guidelines carefully?

- Have you consulted a style manual and other writing aids to ensure that your final draft is a final, not a first, draft?

- If you are giving a talk about research at a professional meeting, have you considered all the ways you can be better prepared?

- Has your manuscript gone through prewriting, writing, and rewriting phases?

- Have you written a query letter to target journals?

- Have you given your work a catchy yet informative title, worked in quotations gracefully, and cited your sources carefully?

- Have you evaluated your manuscript against the final checklist in Box 18–11 before submitting it for publication?

- Are you well informed about the issues at stake in undertaking a book contract with a publisher?

SUMMARY OF KEY IDEAS AND TERMS

✓   The only way important information produced through your scientific work can contribute to the body of nursing knowledge or become part of the basis for clinical decision making is for you to report it to others.

✓   Disseminating research through speeches promptly informs a limited audience and gets early feedback for you; written reports make a more permanent and complete record of your work available to a wider audience.

✓   Dealing with scientific and theoretical subjects need not work against communicating clearly, specifically, directly, and in an organized, interesting style.

✓   Speaking is thinking out loud. It requires adequate planning and practice. The success of most talks depends on your ability to avoid information overload and to present well.

✓   All writing goes through the three-step process of (1) prewriting, (2) writing, and (3) rewriting.

✓   *Prewriting* involves identifying your subject, deciding on a direction and purpose, and outlining what you want to say.

✔ Study the journal that you intend to target for an article for the tone and style it prefers, its audience, the time gaps involved in the publishing process, and its interest in your topic.

✔ A *query letter* asks an editor of a journal if he or she is interested in reviewing a manuscript for publication consideration.

✔ When several authors collaborate on a manuscript, the order of authors' names should be settled from the start, preferably based on who did most of the work.

✔ A title should be concise, specific, and informative. It should catch a reader's interest and provide an accurate idea of its content.

✔ An article's lead, or opening paragraph, can take a number of forms but should be interesting, direct, and concise and should make promises you fulfill in your article.

✔ Always refer to a *style manual* for questions of tense, punctuation, word usage, spelling, and grammar.

✔ The safest way to paraphrase someone else's ideas and avoid plagiarism is to paraphrase with the source book closed.

✔ Creation of tables and figures (nonnumerical illustrations) should always follow conventional guidelines.

✔ A *research report* is usually written according to a customary format and should meet specified criteria.

✔ Never submit anything that's hot off the typewriter. Proofread, edit, and rewrite according to criteria for good writing style.

✔ A prospective book author should approach publishers with a *prospectus* for the book that includes certain essential details, a proposed table of contents, and one or two sample chapters.

✔ A *publishing contract* is an agreement between an author(s) and a publishing company about the details of a collaborative project. Pay attention to items such as royalties, advances, unrecoverable grants, editorial assistance, and sharing of costs, but also to the overall quality and integrity of a publisher's productions.

✔   A publisher is likely to obtain a number of *precontract reviews* from respected people in your area before offering you a publishing contract.

✔   *Copyright law* protects any author from having his or her written work used without permission. Many journal editors and book publishers require that you transfer copyrights to your work to them before they accept it for publication.

References

American Nurses' Association, Council of Nurse Researchers, Kansas City, Mo.: 1982.

American Psychological Association: *Publication Manual*, 3rd ed. Washington, D.C.: 1983.

Dorland's Illustrated Medical Dictionary, 26th ed. Philadelphia: W.B. Saunders, 1981.

Kolin PC, Kolin JL: *Professional Writing for Nurses in Education, Practice and Research*. St. Louis: CV Mosby, 1980.

Lewis EP: *Toward Getting Published: Guidelines for Nurses Who Want to Write*. New York: American Journal of Nursing Company, undated.

Linton M: *A Simplified Style Manual: For the Preparation of Journal Articles in Psychology, Social Sciences, Education and Literature*. Englewood Cliffs, N.J.: Prentice-Hall, 1972.

McCloskey JC, Swanson E: Publishing opportunities for nurses: A comparison of 100 journals. *Image* June 1982; 14:50–56.

McGraw-Hill: *Nursing Dictionary*. New York: McGraw Hill, 1979.

Mirin SK: *The Nurse's Guide to Writing for Publication*. Wakefield, Mass.: Nursing Resources, 1981.

Olson G: *Sweet Agony: A Writing Manual of Sorts*. Grants Pass, Ore.: Windyridge Press, 1972.

Perrin PG, Ebbitt WR: *Writer's Guide and Index to English*. Glenview, Ill.: Scott, Foresman, 1972.

Saslow CA: *Basic Research Methods*. New York: Random House, 1982.

Schwartz R, Moody L, Yarandi H, Anderson G: A metaanalysis of critical outcome variables in nonnutritive sucking in preterm infants. *Nurs Res* 1987; 36(5):292–295.

Strunk W, White EB: *The Elements of Style*. New York: Macmillan, 1972.

Styles MM: Why publish? *Image* June 1978; 10:28–32.

Taber CW: *Cyclopedic Medical Dictionary*, 14th ed. Philadelphia: FA Davis, 1981.

Tornquist EM: *From Proposal to Publication: The Nurse Researcher's Guide to Writing*. Menlo Park, Calif.: Addison-Wesley, 1985.

Turabian KL: *A Manual for Writers of Term Papers, Theses, and Dissertations*, 4th ed. Chicago: University of Chicago Press, 1973.

Ward RR: Fog and how to fight it. Pages 27–28 in: *Practical Technical Writing*. New York: Knopf, 1968.

APPENDIXES

A   Human Subjects Review Resources

B   Sample Abstract for Grant Applications

C   Qualitative Research Resources

D   Quantitative Research Resources

E   Contributors' Guidelines for Selected Research Journals

A-1   Sample Expedited Human Subjects Protocol

Submission date _____ 10/13/82 _____

Principal Investigator
(UCSF Faculty) _____ Professor Holly Wilson _____   University Title _____ Professor _____ Dept. Nursing–Mental Health

Co-Investigator
and Title _____ Sandra L. Scheetz, M.S., R.N., Doct. Cand. _____   Is principal investigator the sponsor/advisor only? Yes __X__ No _____

Mailing Address
(campus if possible) _____ N511E School of Nursing _____ Phone _____ 666-3903 _____

Project
Title _____ The Influence of Social Network Characteristics on the Performance of Self-care _____

_____ by the Chronically Mentally Ill in the Community _____

(A) *The point of this project is (Explain background, rationale, basic design, etc.):*

To investigate the influence of the characteristics of social network on the performance of self-care by the chronically mentally ill (CMI) in the community.

　　Much recent research has focused on the individual's primary group and the relationship to psychiatric epidemiology. More specific information is needed about the person's ability to function on a day-to-day basis, which is one aspect of the psychiatric disability. This is important because chronic mental illness is a major health problem today, and because one of the primary problems with this group is self-care. The proposed descriptive, longitudinal study would be an attempt to describe the social network of the CMI over time and the relationship of network characteristics to the performance of self-care in this population.

(B) *The subject population(s) will be selected (or excluded) on the following criteria (Consider how access will be gained as well as any problems relevant to special subject populations such as children, prisoners, etc.):*

One hundred twenty subjects who will be residing in the community will be solicited from in-patient psychiatric units. Criteria for inclusion are (1) adults ages 18–45; (2) voluntary admission to hospital; (3) English speaking; (4) diagnosis at discharge of schizophrenia, mood disorder, or borderline personality; (5) on, or approved for, Supplemental Security Income (SSI); (6) hospitalized one time in the past 5 years for at least 6 months OR hospitalized 2 or more times in the past 12 months; (7) must agree to participate in the study. Exclusion criteria are (1) physical deformities, physical injuries, and serious or chronic physical conditions; (2) organic psychoses; (3) primary diagnosis of substance abuse. Subjects will be asked to involve a friend or relative in a home visit follow-up.

(C) *The following procedures involving humans will be done for purposes of the study (If known, the expedited review category number from* Consent Forum, *issue 5 is 9) (If applicable, include interview themes and questionnaires if not commonly known):*

1. Charts reviewed by agency staff to determine eligibility.
2. Information Sheet (attached) will be given to potential subjects by agency staff.
3. Those interested in participating will be given the Informed Consent (attached) and the opportunity to discuss it with the investigator. They will be asked to sign the Consent.
4. Relative or friend named by subject will be contacted by investigator and invited to participate in

follow-up (Time 1 & Time 2). Informed Consent for Relative or Friend will be signed prior to administration of questionnaires at follow-up.

5. Consenting subjects (pts) will be given the following:
   a. Demographic Data Sheet—at Baseline.
   b. Modified Norbeck Support Questionnaire (Norbeck, Lindsey & Carrieri, 1981)—at Baseline, Time 1 & Time 2.
   c. Social Relationship Scale (McFarlane, 1980)—Baseline, Time 1 & Time 2.

6. Level of Rehabilitation Scale (Carey & Posavac, 1978)—rated by nurse at Baseline; rated by investigator at Time 1 & Time 2 by questioning relative or friend.

7. Katz Adjustment Scale (Katz & Lyerly, 1963) Forms S2 & S3 Subject and R2, R3 Relative all completed at Time 1 and Time 2 follow-up.

8. Consent to participate at Time 2 will be reviewed at Time 1 with Subject and Relative/Friend.

(D) *The risks involved in these procedures and the methods of minimizing the risks, inconveniences, or discomforts are (Include any potential for loss of privacy):*

It is possible that subjects will become frustrated or anxious while responding to the questionnaires. If the investigator or the subject determines that this is occurring, another appointment will be set up to complete the questionnaires.

The privacy of prospective subjects will be maintained by having agency staff do the initial screening for eligibility. Only the names of those who would like to participate will be given to the investigator. Subjects will be given a code number, and all identifying information will be separated from the responses. The code number will be retraceable only by the investigator for purposes of follow-up. Complete confidentiality of all information will be maintained.

Subjects' right to refuse to continue in the study or to withdraw at any time will be respected. It will be concluded that those who miss three follow-up appointments are "withdrawing" and will be dropped from the study.

All questionnaires will be filled out, and all appointments will be made at the subjects' convenience as to time and place.

(E) *Describe the anticipated benefits, if any, to subjects, and the importance of the knowledge that may reasonably be expected to result:*

There will be no immediate or direct benefit to subjects. This study has the potential to extend our theoretical knowledge about the network characteristics of the specific subpopulation of the chronically mentally ill over time, and knowing more about the relationship between network characteristics and performance of self-care by the chronically mentally ill is of clinical significance.

(F) *Describe the consent process and attach all consent documents. If waiver from use of written consent is requested, give the justification:*

Patients will be screened initially by agency staff. Those who meet the inclusion criteria will be given an Information Sheet for Prospective Participants (attached), which explains the study. Those who wish to participate will be given the Informed Consent (attached) and the opportunity to discuss the study with the investigator. The Informed Consent also includes a choice for the subject to participate in the 12-month follow-up. This aspect of the Consent will be reviewed with the subject at the one-month visit should the subject not wish to continue. Potential subjects will be asked to sign the Consent Form. Those who agree to participate will be given a copy of the consent and the Information Sheet to keep.

SOURCE: Used with permission of Sandra Scheetz, RN, MS, DNS candidate.
School of Nursing, University of California at San Francisco.

A-2   Information Sheet for Prospective Participants in a Research Study

Sandra Scheetz is a nurse and a doctoral student at the University of California, San Francisco. She is conducting a research study of persons, like yourself, who will be discharged from the psychiatric unit to return to the community to live. You are invited to participate in this study.

The following are answers to questions that people ask most often about the study.

1. What is the purpose of the study?

The main purpose of this community follow-up study is to help nurses and other mental health professionals learn more about how patients get along on a day-to-day basis after they leave the hospital.

2. What would be required of me?

Prior to leaving the hospital, you will be asked to fill out one personal information sheet and two paper-and-pencil questionnaires. These are *not* tests.

Also before discharge an appointment will be made to see you approximately 4–6 weeks after you leave the hospital. The follow-up visit will either be at your home or at the hospital, whichever is more convenient for you.

At the follow-up visit, you would be asked again to fill out three paper-and-pencil questionnaires.

You will also be asked to have a relative or close friend, someone you see on a daily basis, participate in the study by being present at the follow-up visit. You will choose this person to participate. This friend or relative will also be asked to fill out two short questionnaires and to answer some questions about how you are getting along.

3. What good will the study do me?

There will be no direct benefit to you. Perhaps you will get some satisfaction from knowing that, by answering the questionnaires, you have provided information that may help other patients returning to the community.

4. What will be done with the information I give about myself?

You are one of 120 people who are being studied in the community follow-up. All of the people are former patients like yourself. The information will be carefully studied by the researcher, who will write a report on the results of the study. These results may also be published in the professional journals where they can be read by other mental health professionals. Therefore, in the long run, the information you provide will be helpful for many people who are hospitalized, as you were, and helpful to the many professionals who give care to those patients.

Your name will not be used anywhere in the reports. Your answers will be given a special number to be used instead of your name. The information you provide will *not* be a part of your chart or treatment records, and will not be shared with the professionals who give you care.

5. Will filling out the questionnaires take a long time?

No. The average time for each set of questionnaires is 1 hour, once in the hospital and once at the follow-up visit, for a total of 2 hours. Some people may finish in 30 minutes, and others may take more than 1 hour. The time needed for your friend or relative to fill out the questionnaires and to answer questions is approximately 30 minutes.

6. What if I am unable to keep my follow-up appointment?

Please call Sandra Scheetz at 123-4567 or 890-1234 to let her know. If you need to call long distance, please call Mrs. Scheetz at 890-1234 and she will acccept a collect phone call. She will be glad to schedule another time for you that is more convenient.

7. How will I remember my follow-up appointment time?

About one week before the appointment time, you will receive a postcard in the mail to remind you.

8. Who will be present at the follow-up visit?

You and your relative or friend will be seen only by Sandra Scheetz or her research assistant.

9. Why do I have to ask a relative or friend to take part in the study?

Your relatives or friends who see you every day are the people who know most about how you are getting along. Of course you yourself will provide the most information, but another person will often notice things that you overlook. Research has already shown that a relative's report is a very useful source of information, even when the patient's own report about himself is also available.

10. What if I have other questions that haven't been answered here?

Please feel free to call Sandra Scheetz at 123-4567 (or leave a message). Or tell your nurse that you would like to speak to Mrs. Scheetz, and she will contact you on the unit the next time she is there.

What next?

If you would be willing to participate in this study, please fill in the information below, detach it, and give it to your nurse or to the research assistant on the unit. You will then be asked to sign a "Consent to Be a Research Subject" before filling out any questionnaires.

You may keep this information sheet for yourself and to share with your relative or friend.

Thank you for taking the time to read this!

SOURCE: Used with permission of Sandra Scheetz, RN, MS, DNS candidate. School of Nursing, University of California at San Francisco.

A-3 *Consent To Be a Research Subject*

Sandra Scheetz is a doctoral student in nursing studying psychiatric patients who return to live in the community and how they get along on a day-to-day basis after they leave the hospital.

If I agree to be in the study, I will fill out two questionnaires and a personal information sheet prior to leaving the hospital. I will also meet with Sandra Scheetz or her research assistant at my home or at the hospital approximately one month after discharge to fill out three additional questionnaires. I have agreed to have a relative or friend of my choosing participate in the home visit to answer additional questionnaires and additional questions.

I (AGREE) (DO NOT AGREE) (circle one) to be a participant in the 12-month follow-up study. Participating in this follow-up would require a second home visit with Sandra Scheetz or her research assistant. This second home visit would be like the first one and would be approximately 12 months after my discharge from the hospital.

Filling out the questionnaires may be an inconvenience to me and may take as long as 2 hours total. However, I may fill out the questionnaires at my convenience before leaving the hospital, and may also make the follow-up appointment at a time and place convenient to me. If I agree to participate in the 12-month follow-up, I will be contacted by phone or mail several times over the intervening 11-month period in order to find out if my address has changed and to make arrangements for the final home visit. This may be an intrusion on my privacy.

There will be no medical benefit to me, and I will not be paid for my participation. The study may produce information of use to medical health professionals in the future.

I have had the opportunity to talk with Sandra Scheetz or her research assistant about the study. If I have further questions, I may reach her at 123-4567 (or leave a message). If I have any comments about participating in this study, I should first talk with Mrs. Scheetz. If for some reason I don't want to do this, I may contact the Committee on Human Research, which is concerned with protection of volunteers in research projects. I may reach the committee between 8 A.M. and 5 P.M., Monday through Friday, by calling 890-1234.

I have been offered a copy of this form and an Information Sheet to keep.

I have the right to refuse to participate or withdraw from the study at any time. Refusing to participate will in no way affect my care at this medical center at any time.

Subject Signature

Date

SOURCE: Used with permission of Sandra Scheetz, RN, MS, DNS candidate. School of Nursing, University of California at San Francisco.

B Sample Abstract for Grant Application

DEPARTMENT OF HEALTH AND HUMAN SERVICES PUBLIC HEALTH SERVICE ABSTRACT OF RESEARCH PLAN	LEAVE BLANK
	PROJECT NUMBER

NAME AND ADDRESS OF APPLICANT ORGANIZATION (*Same as Item 11, page 1*)
School of Nursing, University of California, San Francisco, CA 94143

TITLE OF APPLICATION (*Same as Item 1, page 1*)
Geriatric Mental Health Academic Award

Name, Title, and Department of all professional personnel engaged on project, beginning with Principal Investigator/Program Director

Holly Skodol Wilson, R.N., Ph.D.   Principal Investigator/Awardee
Professor, Department of Mental Health and Community Nursing

ABSTRACT OF RESEARCH PLAN: Concisely describe the application's specific aims, methodology and long-term objectives, making reference to the scientific disciplines involved and the health-relatedness of the project. The abstract should be self-contained so that it can serve as a succinct and accurate description of the application when separated from it. DO NOT EXCEED THE SPACE PROVIDED.

The overall objective of this proposal is to secure funds that will enable me, over a three-year period, to undertake special supervised study and experiences that will prepare me to assume a leadership role in fostering programs of research and teaching among health science students and faculty at the University of California, San Francisco by becoming a professional resource person in the area of geriatric mental health. Special contributory objectives include the following:

1. To acquire knowledge, skills and competences in the field of aging health policy research and analysis.

2. To develop skill in the use of computer technology for applications to aging mental health policy research, including areas such as financing, manpower, program evaluation and efficiency of administrative structures for care delivered to the aged chronically mentally ill.

3. To build a network of professional and scientific associations with others conducting research in these areas, who may also become resources to other faculty and graduate students.

4. To develop strategies, resources, and structures for fostering the interest of other faculty and graduate students in research focused on geriatric mental health and their knowledge and use of research findings in related teaching and clinical work.

These aims will be addressed through a combination of formal course work in health policy and computer science, collegial mentorship and participation in research at UCSF's Aging Health Policy Center, attendance at scientific meetings and communications both formal and informal with faculty and students on committees, through presentations and my own publications.

LABORATORY ANIMALS INVOLVED. Identify by common names. If none, state "none."

C-1 Comparison Between Formal and Informal Interviewing

	Formal	Informal
Time	Agreed on and scheduled by investigator and interviewee	May be predetermined, but usually is not
Setting	Agreed on by investigator and interviewee; may occur in subject's natural setting or in formal setting such as an office or lab	May be predetermined, but usually is not; usually occurs in natural settings; researcher seeks out subjects as informants
Structure	Predetermined concepts, questions, and sequence, based on study purpose	Spontaneous and emergent, based on themes that appear
Role of Researcher	Unambiguous as information seeker	May be ambiguous: friend, colleague, participant
Questions	Use of a formal interview guide/schedule consistently with all respondents (e.g., questions are asked in same words and in same sequence)	General and may vary from interviewee to interviewee
Use of Probes	Based on responses; may be restricted so as to keep data collection consistent among subjects	Are used, especially early in project
Notes	Written or tape-recorded during interview	Not taken or recorded
Number of Interviews	Usually one or two; specified in study design	May require several to cover all content desired; will vary across respondents
Informed Consent	Official written consent	Oral consent; may get written consent; may provide information sheet
Interaction Between Researcher and Subject	Guided or deferred to beginning or ending interview by investigator	Encouraged and essential to developing informants

C-2 Sample Coded Field Notes

STRUCTURAL CONDITIONS
HAVE CONSEQ.
FOR ACTORS BEHAV.

RESOURCES FOR ATTENTION
   RATIO OF STAFF & PTS.

HIGH TOLERANCE FOR
BIZARRE BEHAVIOR
WHEN NOT SURVIVAL
ISSUE

MONITORING
INTERVENTION CONDITIONS

PROPERTY
INDIVIDUALIZED
NON-CODIFIED

PROPERTY
EMERGENT

CONSEQUENCE
STAFF CONFLICT
c̄ HOW MUCH CONTROL

COND.
DE-ELABORATE STRUCTURE
-PRIMITIVE STRUCTURE
WHEN PRES. ALONE FAILS

BUFFERING AND PROTECTING

TOLERANCE FOR PROFANITY
TUNED INTO IT
AS SIGNALING
CONDITION FOR PRESENCING
PRIVITIZED THERAPY TALK

TUNING IN
AWARENESS

PRESENCING
FOR ATTENTION

ON V. #12, p. 3

Mary (F. staff) tells me that she compares Soteria to Agnews State Hospital where there was a lot more out of control behavior because "everyone there is locked up and at least here residents can go around the corner to blow off steam. Also at Agnews there are a lot of patients and few staff while here people can get attention without blowing up to do it. Just the presence of a lot of staff and volunteers has something to do with it."

ON V. #12, p. 5

Paul (M. Resident) is standing upstairs in his doorway where he's been for many hours. I am told that he has sat in one place on the couch for 24 hours and stood in the doorway for 8. He stays there for the 8 hours that I am at the house. Sandy (F. staff) tells me that if he goes without eating or drinking for 3 days she or someone will try to get him to take something. He hasn't taken a bath for the month that he's been in the house, but when he goes without eating or drinking or going to the BR, they "take a very firm approach."

ON V. #10, p. 5

Mike (a visitor) asks Vaughn (M. staff) what would happen if some resident wouldn't eat. Vaughn answers "it's hard to say because how things get handled depends on the individuals involved. One time a resident wouldn't eat because he was paranoid. He started eating when a staff member fed himself one spoonful out of the dish and then one to the resident. Mike says what if it didn't work. Vaughn says he can't really say because people decide what to do as situations come up. Mike asks, "do you ever decide not to let someone do what they want to do?" Vaughn says "that's a real conflict area . . . how much to lay your trip on someone else. Everyone feels different about it, but like if someone was violent we'd try to stop him. We don't have any of the usual hospital equipment to do it . . . no locked doors, no drugs. A couple of times when people were really spaced out we'd put hooks and eyes at the tops of doors just so that if he started running out, he'd have to slow down to open the hook. We don't see our job as straightening people out. Instead we kind of buffer and protect him so he can have a place to go through his trip."

ON V. #7, p. 8

Tania is yelling and storming around the house. Says she needs a damn car because she has stuff to do, is sick of hassling with people when she wants to go somewhere. Hal stops doing the dishes and goes looking around the house for her. When he finds her they have a quiet private conversation which I can't hear.

Interview F. Staff (R.) p. 9

"Well for one thing, everybody recognized that he was in really heavy space. We've gone through enough here to become aware that they need attention at that time . . . on-going attention to protect them and to protect ourselves. With Joan a lot of times she'd get into really crazy space just because we weren't watching her and we were just lucky enough to catch her. When they're in that space you can't leave them be."

IN VIVO WORD
FOR PRESENCING =
"BEING WITH"

MONITORING
ANTICIPATING
ESTIMATING SUCCESS

CONTINUOUS COVERAGE
(VIGIL)

CONSEQUENCE

1. FEAR OF NEGLIGENCE
FROM PEERS

PERIODIC MONITORING

CONDIT. STAFF
RESOURCES

LIMIT SETTING

EX OF PERVASIVENESS
OF PRESENCING

Interview (M. staff G). p. 1

Q. (by Project Director) The things I am going to be asking you about are what we call "being with techniques." What are the techniques you use in instances of property damage, assaultiveness, fires, etc.?

A. With fires there's not too much to describe that. As we were sitting in the kitchen we smelled smoke and saw smoke pouring out of the back room so we just put it out and a couple of the people in the house stayed with the patients while the rest of us put it out. With Lonnie she was into breaking a lot of windows. You had to watch her constantly and be able to anticipate her. If you put your guard down and went to get a cup of coffee or something, she'd be gone and breaking a window. If I could I'd stop her. If I couldn't, like it was already broken by the time I got there, I tell her to go ahead and break the rest of it out."

Q. Tell me something about your experience of staying with people who are in dangerous or weird spaces for long periods of time . . . continuous coverage?

A. It scared me at first. Like the first night when Ellen thought I was death and I was going to rape her. I was really frightened that staff would come in saying what in hell are you doing. And I was concerned that she might call her parents or something and say she was getting raped. I had fears that I wasn't doing the right thing. Then I had doubts about what to do in these intense situations. Now having gone through them I know you don't ask anytime what you should do. You just work with the now. It has to do with the awareness and feeling for the situation at that time. It's not on a logical rational thinking level. It's on an emotional level . . . an intuitive level. You just allow them to be and protect when protecting is needed.

Interview (F. staff R.) p. 6

Q. What do you do when a person gets very withdrawn?

A. Take care of them. Feed them. Spot check on them. It depends if there's somebody else that's with the other residents. If there's a bunch of people then I can do a lot more. When Terry was in very heavy space, I would just stay with her, follow her around. The only time she ever did damage was when she was left alone . . . when she was lonely.

Q. How do you handle aggressive behavior in the house?

A. Well last week Terry picked up a catsup bottle and threw it against the plastic window. It had glanced a blow off Mary's head. Mary said, "Don't do that. I don't like it." And Terry turned and took off. I went after her and put my foot in the door she was trying to slam. At that point she said, "Can't anyone be alone?" and I said "No, I'm not going to leave you alone now. I want to talk about what's happening." When she's mad like that she can just talk about it. She obviously just wanted attention. I've never been involved when somebody's doing it in a heavy aggressive number.

PERSUADING
THERAPY TALK

SPECIALIZING
MULTIPLE PRES.
UNCERTAINTY
ACCUMULATED
STRATEGIES FOR
PREVENTION
(ANTICIPATION)
PRES. FOR RESTRAINT

CONSEQ. OF
CONTRADICTIONS

UNBALANCING
NEGATIVITY   ⟩ STAFF
CONFLICT

Interview (M. Staff V.) p. 49

Q. Could you tell a little bit about what you do when someone's into breaking things?

A. The first incident I got a call at home from Sandy that I should come over and help out because everyone was kind of scared. Paul was throwing glasses. I remember feeling confronted with a situation that I wasn't familiar with. At first there was a period of not knowing whether to grab him or stand back or what. Evidently there were several bottles on the table which now probably would have been taken off if that same situation would come up. People have been realizing to take glass and knives away when it's something like that. So what we finally did was actually restrain him.

Interview (F. Staff J.) p. 46

Q. What do you think about staff?

A. Things sometimes are so intense and heavy that it becomes a problem to keep myself in good balance. A lot of times we've gotten into such a negativity around here. It's kind of an ideal here that we would all live together in peace and harmony forever, which is just not so. When it doesn't happen it feels like a contradiction. There are so many undercurrents of things that aren't said. I think it's sometimes very upsetting and confusing from a resident's standpoint.

P.O.V. #12, p. 2

Mary and Frank tell me about the speeches they are preparing for a meeting in NYC. They are going to talk about "getting burned out" as a consequence of the strain of their work. Mary says she is really feeling like punching Terry because she just can't give her any more attention. "I'm sick of getting called while I'm at a party to come down here for her. I wish she'd leave. I'm really feeling burned out by her."

Interview with (F. staff R.) p. 13

Q. Anything else you want to say?

A. I think the most important thing that we do is nontherapy. Our letting-be process is beautiful and that's the most important thing we do here . . . non-manipulation. We are a family. We can do what a structured place can't which makes them feel okay about where they are. I don't think all people can go crazy in this setting but we're good for a lot of people though.

C-3   *Sample Outline of Codes in Qualitative Study*

An early process in analyzing qualitative field data is to develop substantive codes and then collapse the laundry list you've used to conceptualize the anecdotes and episodes grounded in your data. Codes from the Soteria study database included the following ones.

I. **Control of Residents**

A. Conditions:
High tolerance for certain kinds of deviant behavior
High nonresident-resident ratio
Circumscribed space (house rather than hospital)
Minimal control structures (no locks, restraints, chemicals)
Resident inclination to out-of-control behavior related to diagnosis of schizophrenia
Heavy and light times

B. Tactics:
Normalizing
Health-optimizing
Growth-optimizing
Conversion to staff values and behavior
Monitoring
Presencing
Spritualizing
Urging self-control
Anticipating; tuning-in

C. Consequences:
Contagion
Emulating staff
Property destruction
Contouring
Acting out

II. **Control of Staff**

A. Conditions:
Minimal structure (schedules)
Covering (time)
Limited shared socialization
Personal intimacy

B. Tactics:
Joking
Legitimizing own needs and limits
Monitoring
Cultivating
Muting of conventional controls
"Fairing" in management of work
Networking
Composure strategies
Peer consultation
Cohesion rituals
Confronting
Script innovating

C. Control problems:
Burning out
Bumming out
High staff conflict
High staff instability
Ripping off
Putting out

D. Consequences:
Getting by
Pulling out
Institution of structural controls

III. **Control of Outside Community**

A. Conditions:
Associated with NRI and NIMH (funded)
Heterogeneous, transitional neighborhood

B. Tactics:
Limited disclosure
Minimizing instrusion
Insulating
Accommodating
Privitizing

C-4 Sample Index Sheet for Grounded Theory Concept Indicators

An index allows the grounded theorist to link the analytical codes or concepts to specific indicators that can be located in field notes or interview transcripts. Descriptive indicators are used in the Findings Section to provide imagery for the concepts in the theory. This can also be achieved using a computer program like Ethnograph.

Conditions

Values of the House, pg. 1, 8, 42, 99
Freedom
Nonintervention
Health Optimizing
Staff control problems
Division of work, pg. 52, 77, 78, 88, 87, 91, 92
Strain, pg. 69, 81 (intrusive of staff personal life, pg. 106)
Cohesion maintenance, pg. 82

Staff Control Tactics

Staff specialization, pg. 51, 92
Joking, pg. 69
Fairing, pg. 77, 89
(Exemptions, pg. 77, 78)
Interest-oriented relating, pg. 81–82
(Cohesion-building)—Hospital imagery—rallying patient, pg. 110
Co-opting others for work, pg. 87

Control Related With Outsiders

Outsider control problems
Dependency of some residents, pg. 71–72
Misinterpreting, pg. 98, 102
Outrage, pg. 106
Intruding families, pg. 104
Outsider control tactics
Special allowances, pg. 108
Mediating between residents and outside, pg. 72, 94 (buffer)
Purposeful, goal-directed outings, pg. 90
Escorting, pg. 93–94
Insulating, pg. 97
Partial disclosure, pg. 98, 102
Appeasing, pg. 100, 104

Resident Control Tactics

(Variable conditions according to)

1. Situation with a precedent, pg. 49
2. Uncertainty about approach, pg. 50
3. Recognition of patterns, pg. 52
4. Estimating actual danger vs. attention getting, pg. 57

Presencing and multiple presencing, pg. 49, 71—variation escorting, pg. 94
Selective avoidance, pg. 50
Physical restraint, pg. 50, 55, 57, 60, 66
Therapy talk, pg. 54, 58, 62
Anticipatory prevention, pg. 56
Discounting or disguising, pg. 62
Interpreting by staff, pg. 60
Tolerating some out-of-control behavior, pg. 64, 67
Touching to establish contact
Joking, pg. 69
Verbal disapproval, pg. 70—verbal limit setting, pg. 96
Vigil, pg. 73—meds, pg. 84
Normalizing, pg. 75, 79–81 (excursions, pg. 82, 83, 89)
Monitoring, pg. 99
Tuning-in, pg. 109

Interview With Male Staff

Conditions

Ideology of freedom

Codes

Resident control problems

1. Physical assault, pg. 56, 57, 60, 70
Self-destructive behavior, pg. 59, 101

Destructive behavior (rampaging, breaking things) pg. 49, 50, 51
2. Verbal threats, pg. 54, 55
3. Sexual advances toward staff, pg. 61, 63 (crushes)
4. Variation—unintelligible or inappropriate language or communication, pg. 65

Regression, pg. 66, 70
Withdrawal, pg. 64
Unconventional conduct in public places, pg. 70, 94, 95, 96
5. AWOLs, pg. 97

C-5 Tentative Outline of Grounded Theory Based on Memo Sorting

An outline of sorted memos provides the final integrative scheme for a grounded theory. The following outline of memos contained the key ideas for the theory of infracontrolling at Soteria House.

TITLE: Theory of Infracontrol in a Psychiatric Residence

Preface   Relevance of questions of control in view of social trend away from total institutions and toward community treatment models

Purpose of the study related to concern for more rational and compassionate care. Provision of an explanation and basis for prediction through study of interaction, its contexts and consequences

Introduction of core analytical category of Primitive Infracontrol Structures and Processes. Use of this scheme to organize and integrate many events that might otherwise seem disconnected or paradoxical

Acknowledgments

Part I   Introduction

Chapter I   The Problem of Control within Psychiatry

Central idea is that people come to the attention of Psychiatry because of failure of self-control and labeling by others of such. Refer to Clausen's studies of families of mental patients and other research on pre-hospital career. Whether the focus is "custodial" or "treatment" centered, problems of control are central.

Chapter II   The Elaborate Codified Control Structures of Conventional Psychiatric Institutions

Identification of the Properties, Strategies and Consequences and Conditions of Elaborate Hospital control. Refer to Goffman's Asylums, Stanton and Schwartz, Strauss and Schatzman, Greenblatt, and other secondary sources for data

Part II   Types of Primitive Infracontrol Based on Its Properties

Chapter III   Properties of Primitive Infracontrol

> *Emergent*, based on extemporaneous innovation in face of immediate need
>
> *Primitive*, in the sense of operating at the survival level of food, sex, rest, shelter, and safety
>
> *Tacit*, in view of espoused values of freedom and nonintervention
>
> *Atheoretical*, in that persons do not all stand in some relation to any single theory or ideology. ideology
>
> *Temporary*, in that control structures do not persist over time and become codified but rather are abandoned when the need no longer is present
>
> *Reciprocal*, in that control is not exercised exclusively by one group on another

Chapter IV   Types of Infracontrol (to be developed via process of reduction from properties?)

Part III   Control Problems

Chapter V   Control of Staff

Conditions:	including absence of homogeneous educational experiences (no similar professional training or common pattern of socializing experience)
	Lack of elaborate structure for scheduling and assignments
	Implicit rule against criticism and no formal evaluation procedure for staff
Problems:	Maintenance of high group cohesiveness (good energy)
	Management of work equitably
	Control of ripping-off behaviors
Tactics:	Contouring of superficial behavior (appearance, language, diet, etc.)
	Cohesion maintenance rituals
	Fairing (implicit agreements about management of work)
	Confrontation through joking
Consequences:	Conflict between and among staff
	Exodus of factions of staff, yielding unstable associations over time
	Getting by

Chapter VI   Control of Residents

Conditions:	Relative absence of elaborate structural resources for control (no seclusion rooms, minimal tranquilizers, no ECT, no "therapies" in conventional sense)
	High risk; no locked doors, knives and other sharps available
	High tolerance for certain forms of out-of-control behavior (dirty, no sleep, etc.)
	Ratio of about 10 nonresidents (staff and volunteers) to 6 or fewer residents in the house
Control Problems:	Contagion of display symptoms among residents
	Violent behavior (breaking windows, fighting, self-destructive acts)
	Regressed behavior (refusal to eat, feces smearing, etc.)

D-1   Table of Random Numbers

71510	68311	48214	99929	64650	13229
36921	58733	13459	93488	21949	30920
23288	89515	58503	46185	00368	82604
02668	37444	50640	54968	11409	36148
82091	87298	41397	71112	00076	60029
47837	76717	09653	54466	87988	82363
17934	52793	17641	19502	31735	36901
92296	19293	57583	86043	69502	12601
00535	82698	04174	32342	66533	07875
54446	08795	63563	42296	74647	73120
96981	68729	21154	56182	71840	66135
52397	89724	96436	17871	21823	04027
76403	04655	87277	32593	17097	06913
05136	05115	25922	07123	31485	52166
07645	85123	20945	06370	70255	22806
32530	98883	19105	01769	20276	59402
60427	03316	41439	22012	00159	08461
51811	14651	45119	97921	08063	70820
01832	53295	66575	21384	75357	55888
83430	96917	73978	87884	13249	28870
00995	28829	15048	49573	65278	61493
44032	88720	73058	66010	55115	79227
27929	23392	06432	50201	39055	15529
53484	33973	10614	25190	52647	62580
51184	31339	60009	66595	64358	14985
31359	77470	58126	59192	23371	25190
37842	44387	92421	42965	09736	51873
94596	61368	82091	63835	86859	10678
58210	59820	24710	23225	45788	21426
63354	29875	51058	29958	61221	61200
79958	67599	74103	49824	39306	15069
56328	26905	34454	53965	66617	22137
72806	64421	58711	68436	60301	28620
91920	96081	01413	27281	19397	36231
05010	42003	99866	20924	76152	54090
88239	80732	20778	45726	41481	48277
45705	96458	13918	52375	57457	87884
64274	26236	61096	01309	48632	00431
63731	18917	21614	06412	71008	20255
39891	75337	89452	88092	61012	38072
26466	03735	39891	26362	86817	48193
33492	70485	77323	01016	97315	03944
04509	46144	88909	55261	73434	62538
63187	57352	91208	33555	75943	41669
64651	38741	86190	38197	99113	59694
46792	78975	01999	78892	16177	95747
78076	75002	51309	18791	34162	32258
05345	79268	75608	29916	37005	09213
10991	50452	02376	40372	45077	73706

Appendix D-2　The Standard Normal (z) Distribution

The Standard Normal (z) Distribution

z	.00	.01	.02	.03	.04	.05	.06	.07	.08	.09
0.0	.0000	.0040	.0080	.0120	.0160	.0199	.0239	.0279	.0319	.0359
0.1	.0398	.0438	.0478	.0517	.0557	.0596	.0636	.0675	.0714	.0753
0.2	.0793	.0832	.0871	.0910	.0948	.0987	.1026	.1064	.1103	.1141
0.3	.1179	.1217	.1255	.1293	.1331	.1368	.1406	.1443	.1480	.1517
0.4	.1554	.1591	.1628	.1664	.1700	.1736	.1772	.1808	.1844	.1879
0.5	.1915	.1950	.1985	.2019	.2054	.2088	.2123	.2157	.2190	.2224
0.6	.2257	.2291	.2324	.2357	.2389	.2422	.2454	.2486	.2517	.2549
0.7	.2580	.2611	.2642	.2673	.2704	.2734	.2764	.2794	.2823	.2852
0.8	.2881	.2910	.2939	.2967	.2995	.3023	.3051	.3078	.3106	.3133
0.9	.3159	.3186	.3212	.3238	.3264	.3289	.3315	.3340	.3365	.3389
1.0	.3413	.3438	.3461	.3485	.3508	.3531	.3554	.3577	.3599	.3621
1.1	.3643	.3665	.3686	.3708	.3729	.3749	.3770	.3790	.3810	.3830
1.2	.3849	.3869	.3888	.3907	.3925	.3944	.3962	.3980	.3997	.4015
1.3	.4032	.4049	.4066	.4082	.4099	.4115	.4131	.4147	.4162	.4177
1.4	.4192	.4207	.4222	.4236	.4251	.4265	.4279	.4292	.4306	.4319
1.5	.4332	.4345	.4357	.4370	.4382	.4394	.4406	.4418	.4429	.4441
1.6	.4452	.4463	.4474	.4484	.4495	.4505	.4515	.4525	.4535	.4545
1.7	.4554	.4564	.4573	.4582	.4591	.4599	.4608	.4616	.4625	.4633
1.8	.4641	.4649	.4656	.4664	.4671	.4678	.4686	.4693	.4699	.4706
1.9	.4713	.4719	.4726	.4732	.4738	.4744	.4750	.4756	.4761	.4767
2.0	.4772	.4778	.4783	.4788	.4793	.4798	.4803	.4808	.4812	.4817
2.1	.4821	.4826	.4830	.4834	.4838	.4842	.4846	.4850	.4854	.4857
2.2	.4861	.4864	.4868	.4871	.4875	.4878	.4881	.4884	.4887	.4890
2.3	.4893	.4896	.4898	.4901	.4904	.4906	.4909	.4911	.4913	.4916
2.4	.4918	.4920	.4922	.4925	.4927	.4929	.4931	.4932	.4934	.4936
2.5	.4938	.4940	.4941	.4943	.4945	.4946	.4948	.4949	.4951	.4952
2.6	.4953	.4955	.4956	.4957	.4959	.4960	.4961	.4962	.4963	.4964
2.7	.4965	.4966	.4967	.4968	.4969	.4970	.4971	.4972	.4973	.4974
2.8	.4974	.4975	.4976	.4977	.4977	.4978	.4979	.4979	.4980	.4981
2.9	.4981	.4982	.4982	.4983	.4984	.4984	.4985	.4985	.4986	.4986
3.0	.4987	.4987	.4987	.4988	.4988	.4989	.4989	.4989	.4990	.4990

Source: Frederick Mosteller and Robert E. K. Rourke, *Study Statistics* Table A1 (Reading, Mass.: Addison-Wesley, 1973). Reprinted with permission.

Appendix D-3 *t* Distribution

t Distribution

	α					
Degrees of freedom	.005 (one tail) .01 (two tails)	.01 (one tail) .02 (two tails)	.025 (one tail) .05 (two tails)	.05 (one tail) .10 (two tails)	.10 (one tail) .20 (two tails)	.25 (one tail) .50 (two tails)
1	63.657	31.821	12.706	6.314	3.078	1.000
2	9.925	6.965	4.303	2.920	1.886	.816
3	5.841	4.541	3.182	2.353	1.638	.765
4	4.604	3.747	2.776	2.132	1.533	.741
5	4.032	3.365	2.571	2.015	1.476	.727
6	3.707	3.143	2.447	1.943	1.440	.718
7	3.500	2.998	2.365	1.895	1.415	.711
8	3.355	2.896	2.306	1.860	1.397	.706
9	3.250	2.821	2.262	1.833	1.383	.703
10	3.169	2.764	2.228	1.812	1.372	.700
11	3.106	2.718	2.201	1.796	1.363	.697
12	3.054	2.681	2.179	1.782	1.356	.696
13	3.012	2.650	2.160	1.771	1.350	.694
14	2.977	2.625	2.145	1.761	1.345	.692
15	2.947	2.602	2.132	1.753	1.341	.691
16	2.921	2.584	2.120	1.746	1.337	.690
17	2.898	2.567	2.110	1.740	1.333	.689
18	2.878	2.552	2.101	1.734	1.330	.688
19	2.861	2.540	2.093	1.729	1.328	.688
20	2.845	2.528	2.086	1.725	1.325	.687
21	2.831	2.518	2.080	1.721	1.323	.686
22	2.819	2.508	2.074	1.717	1.321	.686
23	2.807	2.500	2.069	1.714	1.320	.685
24	2.797	2.492	2.064	1.711	1.318	.685
25	2.787	2.485	2.060	1.708	1.316	.684
26	2.779	2.479	2.056	1.706	1.315	.684
27	2.771	2.473	2.052	1.703	1.314	.684
28	2.763	2.467	2.048	1.701	1.313	.683
29	2.756	2.462	2.045	1.699	1.311	.683
Large	2.575	2.327	1.960	1.645	1.282	.675

Appendix D-4 Critical Values of the Chi-Square (χ^2) Distribution

Table 7 The Chi-Square (χ^2) Distribution

Degrees of freedom	α									
	0.995	0.99	0.975	0.95	0.90	0.10	0.05	0.025	0.01	0.005
1	—	—	0.001	0.004	0.016	2.706	3.841	5.024	6.635	7.879
2	0.010	0.020	0.051	0.103	0.211	4.605	5.991	7.378	9.210	10.597
3	0.072	0.115	0.216	0.352	0.584	6.251	7.815	9.348	11.345	12.838
4	0.207	0.297	0.484	0.711	1.064	7.779	9.488	11.143	13.277	14.860
5	0.412	0.554	0.831	1.145	1.610	9.236	11.071	12.833	15.086	16.750
6	0.676	0.872	1.237	1.635	2.204	10.645	12.592	14.449	16.812	18.548
7	0.989	1.239	1.690	2.167	2.833	12.017	14.067	16.013	18.475	20.278
8	1.344	1.646	2.180	2.733	3.490	13.362	15.507	17.535	20.090	21.955
9	1.735	2.088	2.700	3.325	4.168	14.684	16.919	19.023	21.666	23.589
10	2.156	2.558	3.247	3.940	4.865	15.987	18.307	20.483	23.209	25.188
11	2.603	3.053	3.816	4.575	5.578	17.275	19.675	21.920	24.725	26.757
12	3.074	3.571	4.404	5.226	6.304	18.549	21.026	23.337	26.217	28.299
13	3.565	4.107	5.009	5.892	7.042	19.812	22.362	24.736	27.688	29.819
14	4.075	4.660	5.629	6.571	7.790	21.064	23.685	26.119	29.141	31.319
15	4.601	5.229	6.262	7.261	8.547	22.307	24.996	27.488	30.578	32.801
16	5.142	5.812	6.908	7.962	9.312	23.542	26.296	28.845	32.000	34.267
17	5.697	6.408	7.564	8.672	10.085	24.769	27.587	30.191	33.409	35.718
18	6.265	7.015	8.231	9.390	10.865	25.989	28.869	31.526	34.805	37.156
19	6.844	7.633	8.907	10.117	11.651	27.204	30.144	32.852	36.191	38.582
20	7.434	8.260	9.591	10.851	12.443	28.412	31.410	34.170	37.566	39.997
21	8.034	8.897	10.283	11.591	13.240	29.615	32.671	35.479	38.932	41.401
22	8.643	9.542	10.982	12.338	14.042	30.813	33.924	36.781	40.289	42.796
23	9.260	10.196	11.689	13.091	14.848	32.007	35.172	38.076	41.638	44.181
24	9.886	10.856	12.401	13.848	15.659	33.196	36.415	39.364	42.980	45.559
25	10.520	11.524	13.120	14.611	16.473	34.382	37.652	40.646	44.314	46.928
26	11.160	12.198	13.844	15.379	17.292	35.563	38.885	41.923	45.642	48.290
27	11.808	12.879	14.573	16.151	18.114	36.741	40.113	43.194	46.963	49.645
28	12.461	13.565	15.308	16.928	18.939	37.916	41.337	44.461	48.278	50.993
29	13.121	14.257	16.047	17.708	19.768	39.087	42.557	45.722	49.588	52.336
30	13.787	14.954	16.791	18.493	20.599	40.256	43.773	46.979	50.892	53.672
40	20.707	22.164	24.433	26.509	29.051	51.805	55.758	59.342	63.691	66.766
50	27.991	29.707	32.357	34.764	37.689	63.167	67.505	71.420	76.154	79.490
60	35.534	37.485	40.482	43.188	46.459	74.397	79.082	83.298	88.379	91.952
70	43.275	45.442	48.758	51.739	55.329	85.527	90.531	95.023	100.425	104.215
80	51.172	53.540	57.153	60.391	64.278	96.578	101.879	106.629	112.329	116.321
90	59.196	61.754	65.647	69.126	73.291	107.565	113.145	118.136	124.116	128.299
100	67.328	70.065	74.222	77.929	82.358	118.498	124.342	129.561	135.807	140.169

Source: D. B. Owen, *Handbook of Statistical Tables*, © 1962, Addison-Wesley Publishing Company, Inc., Reading, Massachusetts. Attached tables. Reprinted with permission.

Appendix D-5 *Statistics Symbols*

x	value of a single score	β	probability of a type II error
f	frequency with which a value occurs	r	linear correlation coefficient
Σ	(capital sigma) summation	r^2	coefficient of determination
n	number of scores in a sample	r_s	Spearman's rank correlation coefficient
$n!$	factorial	m	slope of the straight line with equation $y = mx + b$
N	number of scores in a finite population		
$\bar{x}$	mean of the scores in a sample	b	y intercept of the straight line with equation $y = mx + b$
μ	(*mu*) mean of all scores in a population		
s	standard deviation of a set of sample values	y'	predicted value of y
		d	difference between two paired scores
σ	(lower case sigma) standard deviation of all values in a population	$\bar{d}$	mean of the differences d found from paired sample data
s^2	variance of a set of sample values	s_d	standard deviation of the differences d found from paired sample data
σ^2	variance of all values in a population		
z	standard score	s_e	standard error of estimate
$z(\alpha/2)$	critical value of z	T	rank sum used in Wilcoxon signed-rank test
t	t distribution		
$t(\alpha/2)$	critical value of t	H	Kruskal-Wallis test statistic
df	number of degrees of freedom	R	sum of the ranks for a sample; used in the Wilcoxon rank-sum test
F	F distribution		
χ^2	chi-square distribution	μ_R	expected mean rank; used in the Wilcoxon rank-sum test
χ^2_R	right-tailed critical value of chi-square		
χ^2_L	left-tailed critical value of chi-square	σ_R	expected standard deviation of ranks; used in the Wilcoxon rank-sum test
p	probability of an event or the population proportion		
		G	number of runs in runs test for randomness
q	probability or proportion equal to $1 - p$		
		μ_G	expected mean number of runs; used in runs test for randomness
p_s	sample proportion		
q_s	sample proportion equal to $1 - p_s$	σ_G	expected standard deviation for the number of runs; used in runs test for randomness
$\bar{p}$	proportion obtained by pooling two samples		
$\bar{q}$	proportion or probability equal to $1 - \bar{p}$	$\mu_{\bar{x}}$	mean of the population of all possible sample means $\bar{x}$
$P(A)$	probability of event A	$\sigma_{\bar{x}}$	standard deviation of the population of all possible sample means $\bar{x}$
$P(A/B)$	probability of event A assuming event B has occurred		
$\bar{A}$	complement of event A	E	maximum error of the estimate of a population parameter or expected value
H_o	null hypothesis		
H_1	alternative hypothesis	Q_1, Q_2, Q_3	quartiles
α	probability of a type 1 error or the area of the critical region	$D_1, D_2, \ldots, D_9$	deciles
		$P_1, P_2, \ldots, P_{99}$	percentiles

Appendix E–1   Advances in Nursing Science

Author's Guide

Purpose of the Journal

The primary purposes of *ADVANCES IN NURSING SCIENCE* (ANS) are to contribute to the development of nursing science and to promote the application of emerging theories and research findings to practice. Articles are sought which deal with any of the processes of science, including research, theory development, concept analysis, practical application of research and theory, and investigation of the values and ethics that influence the practice and research endeavors of nursing sciences. Projected topics for future publication are listed on the back of each issue and in the "Information for Authors" section of each issue; these topics should not limit submission of articles on other topics by prospective authors.

Article Preparation

Typing instructions

Type the article double spaced on 8½″ × 11″ nonerasable bond on one side of the sheet only. Leave a one-inch margin on all sides.

Include an abstract of 100 words or fewer. The abstract should briefly summarize the major issue, problem or topic being addressed, and the findings and/or conclusions of the article.

Type all headings on a separate line.

Number all article pages consecutively in the upper right-hand corner (text and references, followed by illustrations on separate pages).

Incorporate all corrections to the article where appropriate. If corrections are extensive, the article should be retyped. Any inserted pages can be numbered 1A, 1B, etc., to make renumbering the entire article unnecessary.

No identifying information (authors' names) should be included on the manuscript.

Tables

Type each table on a separate sheet, remember to double space. Do not submit tables as photographs. Number tables consecutively and supply a brief title for each. Give each column a short or abbreviated heading. Place explanatory matter in footnotes, not in the heading. Explain in footnotes all nonstandard abbreviations that are used in each table. For footnotes, use the following symbols, in this sequence: *, †, ‡, §, ‖, ¶, **, †† . . .

Identify statistical measures of variations such as standard deviation and standard error of the mean.

Do not use internal horizontal and vertical rules.

Cite each table in the text in consecutive order.

If you use data from another published or unpublished source, obtain permission and acknowledge fully.

The use of too many tables in relation to the length of the text may produce difficulties in the layout of the pages. Examine issues of the journal to which you plan to submit your manuscript to estimate how many tables can be used per 1,000 words of text.

Illustrations

Submit the required number of complete sets of figures. Figures should be professionally drawn and photographed; freehand or typewritten lettering is unacceptable. Typeset copy should be in Helvetica or other sans serif typeface. The first word of each label should have an initial capital letter; all other words should be lower case unless they are proper nouns.

Instead of *original* drawings, roentgenograms and other material, send sharp, glossy black-and-white photographic prints, usually 127 by 173 mm (5 by 7 in.) but no larger than 203 by 254 mm (8 by 10 in.). Letters, numbers, and symbols should be clear and even throughout, and of sufficient size that when reduced for publication each item will still be legible. Titles and detailed explanations belong in the legends for illustrations, not on the illustrations themselves.

When using a sample form (e.g., a sample requisition form for a particular hospital), provide a clean original copy of the form. Permission to use the form should accompany the form.

Each figure should have a label pasted on its back indicating the number of the figure, the names of the authors, and the top of the figure. Do not write on the back of the figures, mount them on cardboard, or scratch or mar them using paper clips. Do not bend figures.

If photographs of persons are used, either the subjects must not be identifiable or their pictures must be accompanied by written permission to use the photograph.

Cite each figure in the text in consecutive order. If a figure has been previously published—in part or in total—acknowledge the original source and submit written permission from the copyright holder to reproduce or adapt the material. Permission is required, *regardless of authorship or publisher*, except for documents in the public domain.

Legends for illustrations

Type all legends for illustrations double spaced, on a page separate, from the illustrations. When symbols, arrows, numbers, or letters are used to identify parts of the illustrations, identify and explain each one clearly in the legend.

Permissions

Authors must obtain permission for the following copyrighted material:

1. All direct quotes of 500 words or more from any full-length book (either a single quote or several shorter quotes from the same source).
2. All direct quotes of 50 words or more of a periodical article.
3. All excerpts from newspaper or other short articles.
4. Any passage from a play or song.
5. Two or more lines of poetry.
6. Any copyrighted table, figure, exhibit or illustration being reproduced exactly *or adapted* to fit the needs of the subject.
7. Any passage quoted *or adapted* from any abstract of another work. In general, you should not use abstracts in the preparation of your manuscript except as research tools.

When copyright holders grant permission they often request a specific credit line. Type the precise wording as given by the holder at the end of the reference item, table, etc. If no wording has been specified, include the following source line: "Reprinted with permission from (author, title of work, date of publication). Copyright (date, publisher." Copyright holders sometimes require that a fee be paid for permission to use material they hold the copyright to. It is the author's responsibility to pay this fee.

Adapting material from another source. Many authors do not want their work to be changed in any way. If you adapt material from another source (e.g., data from a table), we require written permission from the original author. The source line for the material should read: "Source: Adapted with permission from (author, title of work, date of publication). Copyright (date, publisher)."

References: AMA style

Text Citations. AMA style references are listed in numerical order at the end of the article, in the order that they appear in the text. *Each reference must be cited in the text in consecutive order.*

When more than two references are cited at a given place in the copy, use hyphens to join the first and last numbers of a closed series; use commas without space to separate other parts of a multiple citation.

As reported previously,[1,3-8,19]

If a quote is used, page numbers must be given in the citation. If the author wishes to cite different page numbers from a single reference source at different places in the text, the page numbers are included in the superscript citation and the source appears only once in the list of references.

Westman has reported . . .[5(pp3,5)]

Reference List Citations. References must be *typed double-spaced* with one-inch margins on all sides and included on a separate page at the end of the article.

References must follow AMA style.

Complete information on all sources must be given in the reference list. *Authors are responsible for the accuracy and completeness of their references. Make sure that all references include:*

a. At least 3 authors' and editors' names, followed by et al.
b. Complete title
c. Place of publication
d. Publisher's name
e. Date of publication
f. Page numbers, if needed
g. Volume numbers for journals
h. Month of publication for journals

Do not use ibid or op cit.
Try to avoid using the same reference over and over throughout the article.
Do not site more than 50 references.

Submission of Manuscripts

Three copies of the manuscript and abstract (one original and two copies), the article submission form (attached), and the copyright release (attached), and all related materials should be submitted to:

Editor, ANS
Aspen Publishers, Inc.
1600 Research Blvd.
Rockville, MD 20850

It is recommended that the author(s) submit manuscripts no more than four months in advance of the deadline date, but no later than the deadline, for submission of articles relative to the particular issue for which the article is to be considered. Please consult the list of forthcoming issues in the "Information for Authors" section of the latest issue of the journal for further information on the topics planned and the deadline dates for submission.

Appendix E-2   Applied Nursing Research (ANR)

Information for Contributors

Applied Nursing Research (ANR) is a refereed journal devoted to uniting the efforts of all professional nurses to advance nursing as a research-based profession. ANR will present nursing research in a clear, straightforward style to emphasize results and encourage readers to apply findings in their own practice.

Original Articles
Authors are asked to focus on research findings and how those findings can be applied to practice. The manuscript should convey the author's enthusiasm for the specific advances in clinical practice that are indicated by the research. Articles selected for publication will be those that avoid lengthy descriptions of research methods and statistical analysis. While it is necessary to document scientific merit, authors are asked to present material in a framework and style that highlight results and applications for nursing practice.

Manuscripts representing all clinical nursing specialties are invited. Studies related to nursing management, nursing roles, and professional development are also welcomed.

Manuscripts will be reviewed by two pairs of research-clinician referees. Publication decisions are based on the referees' evaluations.

Special Features

All professional nurses are invited to participate by contributing to *Applied Nursing Research*. Special features have been designed to promote a communication loop, fostering interchange among nurses primarily in practice, management, education, and research.

Ask An Expert

This feature provides practicing nurses an opportunity to voice their ideas on clinical problems, questions, or potential innovations which they would like to see studied by expert nurse researchers. Questions regarding basic clinical research techniques will also be published and answered.

Clinical Methods

In Clinical Methods, basic and effective techniques for conducting studies within clinical settings will be presented. Papers selected for publication will address methodological issues or techniques that are of concern to nurses conducting research.

Research Briefs

Abstracts of research in progress are invited. The emphasis should be on preliminary results and directions for continuing research.

Format

All manuscripts should be submitted in typed, double-spaced form. The cover sheet should include the title of the manuscript and the name, address, and telephone number of the author(s). Author identification should not appear elsewhere. Drawings or illustrations should be submitted camera-ready.

Manuscripts for original articles, special features, or clinical methods should be no less than 8 and no more than 12 double-spaced typewritten pages. Guidelines in the *Publication Manual of the American Psychological Association* (*APA*) should be used to format references.

Papers submitted for publication in the research briefs section should be no more than three double-spaced typewritten pages.

Query letters preceding manuscripts are welcome but not mandatory. Edited manuscripts are submitted to the first-named author for approval. Edited manuscripts become the property of *Applied Nursing Research*.

Please send five copies of each submitted manuscript to:

Joyce J. Fitzpatrick, PhD, FAAN, Editor
Applied Nursing Research
Case Western Reserve University
Frances Payne Bolton School of Nursing
2121 Abington Road
Cleveland, OH 44106

Appendix E-3 International Journal of Nursing Studies

Notes for Contributors

1. *Submission of manuscripts.* Manuscripts intended for publication in the Journal should be submitted in duplicate to: Professor Rosemary Crow, University of Surrey, Dept. of Biochemistry, Division of Nursing Studies, Guildford, Surrey, GU2 5XH, U.K. Manuscripts should be 4000–5000 words in length, plus tables and figures, and typed double-spaced. Authors of papers substantially longer than this are asked to make preliminary enquiries of the Editors before submitting the manuscript. Each manuscript will be assessed by at least one independent reviewer and constructive criticism may be forwarded to the authors of papers accepted for publication. The Editors reserve the right to the final decision regarding acceptance.

2. *Preparation of manuscripts.* As the Journal is distributed all over the world, and as English is a second language for many readers, authors are requested to use terminology which is internationally acceptable. In addition, the following points should be noted: (a) *Symbols.* Any Greek letters, or special symbols likely to be unfamiliar to the printer, should be identified in the margin the first time they occur on each page of the manuscript. (b) *Abbreviations.* Any abbreviations which authors intend to use should be written out in full and followed by the letters in brackets the first time they appear, thereafter only the letters without brackets should be used. (c) *Statistics.* Standard text book methods of presenting statistical material should be used. Authors are asked to avoid methods which may be acceptable locally but which could be confusing to non-native English speaking readers. (d) *References.* The Harvard System should be used in which the name of author followed by the year of publication in parentheses appears in the text, e.g. Jones (1981). If there are three or more authors the first author's name should appear followed by *et al.*, e.g. Jones *et al.* (1982). The list of references should be given at the end of the text with the authors' names in alphabetical order. For example:

> Overall, J. and Gorham, D. R. (1962). The brief psychiatric rating scale. *Psychol. Rep.* **10**, 799–812.
> Rosner, D. (1981). Breast Cancer. In *Cancer—Signals and Safeguards*. C. Murphy (Ed.), pp. 21–50. PSG Publishing Co., Boston.
> Seydel, H. Chait, A. and Gmelich, J. (1975). *Cancer of the Lung.* John Wiley, New York.

(e) *Abstract.* A 100-word Abstract, summarizing the contents of the paper, should be included.

3. *Biographical information.* In order to give readers an indication of the authority with which authors write on their chosen subjects, a brief biographical sketch of not more than 75 words should be submitted. This should be in narrative form, ready for printing. Authors should therefore select from their curricula vitae those items which they wish to have included.

4. *Reprints.* An order form will be sent out with the proofs. Twenty-five copies will be supplied free of charge to the first author and additional copies may be purchased.

5. No cash payment will be made for material published.

6. The original manuscript and diagrams will be discarded 1 month after publication, unless the Publisher is requested to return the original material to the author.

Appendix E-4 Nursing Research (NR)

Information for Authors

The Editor of NURSING RESEARCH welcomes manuscripts of relevance and interest to those concerned with the conduct or results of research in nursing. Manuscripts should be sent to Florence S. Downs, EdD, FAAN, Editor, NURSING RESEARCH, Associate Dean, School of Nursing, University of Pennsylvania, 420 Service Drive, S2, Philadelphia, PA 19104. It is understood that manuscripts submitted for consideration were prepared specifically and solely for NURSING RESEARCH, and that NURSING RESEARCH will have exclusive rights to the article and to its reproduction and sale in all countries. If aspects of this research are reported elsewhere, the author should include a copy of the publication(s).

Procedure. It is advisable to precede submission with a letter of inquiry to the Editor, describing the article. Manuscripts contributed to NURSING RESEARCH that are appropriate to the purpose of the journal are forwarded to members of a review panel who are experts in the subject matter of the particular study reported. The decision with regard to acceptance for publication is based on the evaluation of the referees. NURSING RESEARCH is concerned that the rights and dignity of all subjects involved in research be protected. No manuscript will be considered for publication unless it contains an explicit statement in this regard.

Preparing the Manuscript. The author should submit three double-spaced copies of the manuscript on 8½ × 11-inch paper using generous margins; 14–16 typewritten pages is a desirable length. Authors should use a good bond paper for the copy; do not use erasable paper. Because manuscripts are refereed anonymously, authors should list their names only on the title page. Accepted manuscripts become the property of NURSING RESEARCH and may be reproduced in other publications in whole or in part only with the permission of the Editor of NURSING RESEARCH. Rejected manuscripts will not be returned; therefore, authors should be sure to keep at least one copy for their files.

Style and Format.   Authors should follow the American Psychological Association *Publication Manual.* Format should correspond to that used in NURSING RESEARCH. Titles should be short and descriptive headings should be used to indicate the divisions of an article. Abbreviations should be spelled out the first time they are used, with the abbreviation placed in parentheses following the word. Greek letters or other special symbols should be identified in the margin the first time they are used. (This does not apply to the standard symbols used in statistical tests.) Addenda and appendixes are not used. The article should be accompanied by a 100- to 200-word factual abstract of the work presented.

Footnotes and References.   Incidental comments, qualifications, and the like, other than references to published sources, ordinarily are worked into the text. Personal communications and unpublished material should not be included in the references. If necessary to the article, they may be included in footnotes. Acknowledgements should be limited to persons making a substantial contribution to the author's work. For information regarding treatment of references, see the APA *Publication Manual.*

Tables and Figures.   Tables and figures are printed only when they express more, and do so more clearly and briefly, than can be done by words in the same amount of space. All tables and figures should be referred to in the text, but should be largely self-explanatory and should not duplicate the text. They should be typed double-spaced on separate sheets of 8½ × 11-inch paper and should be numbered consecutively, have descriptive titles, and indicate the source of the data. Any inconsistencies in marginal totals or other figures should be explained in a footnote. Charts and tables should be complete.

Reprints.   The authors will receive a few "tear sheets" of the article. Reprints may be ordered by the authors at a reasonable price. Order forms for reprints are sent routinely at the time of publication.

Appendix E-5   Research in Nursing & Health

Information for Authors

Research in Nursing & Health (RINAH)   invites research reports on nursing practice, education, and administration; on health issues relevant to nursing; and on applications of research findings in clinical settings. Papers on research methods and statistical techniques are desired. A theoretical paper is acceptable if research and knowledge are advanced; preference is given to papers that develop rather than review theories. Integrative reviews of the research literature may be accepted if gaps in knowledge are identified and directions for future research provided. Commentaries on or letters about published articles or research and theory issues are encouraged, as are brief reports of early pilot studies and initial instrument development.

Submission of manuscripts   Only unpublished work should be submitted. Manuscripts are accepted for blind review only with a signed copy of the copyright agreement included in each issue of RINAH. With research involving human subjects, the report should contain a statement that informed consent was obtained. Permission for identifying an institution should be forwarded with the manuscript. If aspects of the research are reported elsewhere, a copy of that publication also should be included. Authors are urged to seek colleague review prior to submission of manuscripts, including statistical consultation if indicated.

The manuscript should be typewritten, double-spaced on 8½ × 11-inch paper. Submit four copies (not carbons) of the complete paper, including the abstract and all tables and figures. Send manuscripts to: Margaret A. Williams, Ph.D., Editor, *Research in Nursing & Health*; School of Nursing, University of Wisconsin-Madison, 600 Highland Avenue, Madison, WI 53792.

Preparation of manuscripts

Papers must adhere to the style and format described in the *Publication Manual* (3rd ed.) of the American Psychological Association (APA), 1983. Authors should consult this Manual in preparing all details of their manuscripts. The text of an article typically ranges from 10 to 15 pages in length, with the pages headed and numbered consecutively from the title page through the last page submitted.

The general format for reporting empirical studies, review articles, or theoretical articles is discussed on pp. 21–22 in the manual. For guidelines in reporting qualitative research using an adapted APA format, see Knafl, K.A., and Howard, M.J. (1984). Interpreting and reporting qualitative research. *Research in Nursing & Health*, 7, 17–24.

Title Page.   The title page should include the following information: title, author(s) and their institutional affiliation(s), and running head (abbreviated title). The wording of the title should be useful for indexing and information retrieval. In addition, the following information should be included: degrees, positions, and departments of all authors; address and identifying information on financial support; acknowledgments; and address for reprint requests.

Abstract.   The summary of the paper should not exceed 100 words. The single paragraph must contain information on the problem, subjects, methods, findings, and conclusions.

Text.   Organize the text under the following headings: Introduction (not labeled); Method, with subsections on the sample, instruments or measures, and procedures; Results; and Discussion. The list of References, any Tables and Figures follow the text in that order. (Footnotes and Reference Notes are not used).

References.   Cite references in the text by the author's surname and year of publication in alphabetical order. If more than two authors, include all names the first time, and only the first author's surname with "et al." and date in subsequent citations. The references cited are listed alphabetically immediately after the text. Entries must include all authors of a publication with journal names spelled out. All references on the list must be cited in the text. Authors are responsible for the accuracy and completeness of all references cited and listed. The list should be double-spaced with a hanging indentation.

Tables.   Each table should be typed double-spaced on a separate sheet of paper and numbered with arabic numerals. The title should be brief, but the content of the table should be explained without the reader referring to the text. The content of a table should not duplicate material in the text. Table footnotes are indicated by lowercase letters, reserving asterisks for probability levels.

Figures.   The term figure refers to graphs, charts, illustrations, and halftones. All figures are numbered with arabic numerals, with title(s) listed on a separate page. Drawings should be prepared in black india ink, and photographs should be large glossy prints. Each figure should be identified on the back in pencil.

All manuscripts, submitted or solicited, are sent to three reviewers simultaneously. An effort is made to notify authors about the publication decision within about 2 months of receipt of the manuscript.

Appendix E-6 Western Journal of Nursing Research

The WESTERN JOURNAL OF NURSING RESEARCH is a quarterly journal devoted to the dissemination of research studies, book reviews, discussion and debate, and meeting calendars, all directed to a general nursing audience. Contributions are accepted from nurses both within and outside the United States. The views expressed in individual communications are those of the author and not the editorial board, the advisory board, or the publisher.

MANUSCRIPTS should be submitted in quadruplicate (keep a copy for your files) to Pamela J. Brink, R.N., Ph.D., F.A.A.N., Executive Editor, WESTERN JOURNAL OF NURSING RESEARCH, College of Nursing, The University of Iowa, Iowa City, IA 52242. Acceptable manuscript length varies and is dependent on subject and scope (maximum acceptable is 25 pages). Only manuscripts on 8½ × 11 white bond paper, typed double-spaced on one side of the paper, will be accepted for consideration. Manuscripts should be in accordance with the guidelines set forth by the American Psychological Association (APA). All identifying information about the author(s) should be on the title page only. The title page should include the article title, the name and academic degree(s) of each author, each author's institutional affiliation, and current mailing address. All source(s) of support such as grants should be designated as Footnote 1. For papers having multiple authors, one author should be designated as correspondent, and a complete mailing address and telephone number supplied. Author(s) will be listed in print as they appear on the manuscript title page.

INFORMATION EXCHANGE (such as book reviews, film reviews, computer software reviews) should be addressed to Frank McLaughlin, R.N., Ph.D., F.A.A.N., Department of Nursing, San Francisco State University, 1600 Holloway, San Francisco, CA 94132

Glossary

abstract   a section usually located at the beginning of a research article intended to summarize the entire study—includings its purpose, design, and findings—as briefly as possible.

abstracted empiricism   a research approach that focuses on facts in isolation from any theory.

accessible population   the population that is a feasible source of sample members.

accidental or convenience sampling   this type of sampling allows the use of any available group of research subjects.

alternate forms reliability   established by comparing scores from various versions of an instrument for equivalence.

analysis   refers to the separation of data into parts for the purpose of answering a research question.

analysis of exemplars   examining specific examples of events culled from interviews to generate rich descriptions of situations, actions, practices, and intentions in their complete form.

analysis of variance (ANOVA)   inferential statistical procedure that compares mean scores of two or more groups.

analytical description   a qualitative analysis method in which the researcher thinks up original classes or categories by inspecting and interrogating the data.

animal models   studies conducted on animals.

anonymous study   a study in which even the investigator cannot link a subject with the information reported.

applied research   research designed to solve practical problems.

ASCII (pronounced "as-key")   the American Standard Code Information Interchange, which uses seven bits to represent each character. Adopted as a standard by the U.S. government.

BASIC (Beginners' All-Purpose Symbolic Instruction Code)   a commonly used computer programming language.

basic research   research that aims to develop the state of knowledge for its own sake; also called pure research.

batch processing   a technique for conducting transactions with the computer by collecting data into groups to be processed together for efficiency.

before-after design   called the true or classic experiment in which subjects are measured before and after experimental treatment.

Belmont report   document published in 1978 that identifies respect for persons as one of the key principles in ethical research.

beta weight   refers to a standardized regression coefficient.

bimodal frequency   a frequency distribution with two high points.

binary system   an off/on two-state system that turns computer circuits on and off through combinations of ones and zeros, which represent data.

bit   one switch inside the computer circuit called a binary digit.

BMDP   (Biomedical Statistical Software Package) applications statistical package for analyzing research data.

bpi   refers to bits per inch as an indication of the secondary storage capacity or density of a magnetic tape.

byte   a group of eight bits that stand for a character in a computer.

case history   a qualitative research approach that provides highly readable imagery that can be explained by a theory.

case study   a study design that provides an in-depth analysis of a single subject for investigation, which may be an individual or group. Usually stimulates insight and suggests directions for further research. Sometimes viewed as synonymous with single subject descriptive research.

categorical variable   variables that represent unordered categories, groups, or classes.

cause and effect   a relationship that allows one to predict and explain. Requires that cause precede effect in time; requires evidence that the independent variable and dependent variable are associated, and rules out other factors as possible determining conditions.

Center for Nursing Research   the first national center for nursing research established in 1986 to serve as a clearinghouse and link among scientific organizations like the American Nurses' Foundation, the American Academy of Nursing, and the American Nurses' Association.

central tendency   a statistic that summarizes the data into one representative value.

chi-square   nonparametric statistical test used to determine whether a significant difference exists between an observed frequency and an expected frequency. Can be used with nominal level measurements.

clinical research   nursing research that generates knowledge to guide nursing practice. Identified by the ANA Commission on Nursing Research as having top priority in the 1980s.

cluster sampling   selecting a random sample of elements that have been grouped into clusters.

COBOL (Common Business-Oriented Language)   a commonly used computer programming language.

code book   a research tool used to designate which columns on a keypunched card contain which data.

concepts   abstractions that categorize observations based on commonalities and differences.

conceptual framework (conceptual model or paradigm)   a preliminary stage of a theory wherein interrelated concepts provide a structure for organizing phenomena of interest in nursing practice or research.

conceptual map   a diagrammatic representation of the variables in a theory.

confidentiality   the assurance that any information that a human subject divulges will not be made public or available to others.

confounding variable   other variables in addition to the independent variable that might affect the dependent variable. Can confuse the interpretation of a study's results if not controlled for in a study's design or procedures. Also called extraneous variable.

consent form   a written document reflecting an agreement between a researcher and subject concerning the subject's participation in a study.

construct   abstract concepts derived from a combination of existing theory and observations.

construct validity   an estimate of how well an instrument measures a theoretical construct as determined by hypothesis testing. For example, an instrument designed to measure creativity should differentiate creative and noncreative individuals.

content analysis method of analyzing qualitative data by counting the occurrence of specified units of analysis in the data. May refer to manifest content or inferred or latent content.

content area refers to the circumscribed area of content that an instrument measures.

content validity a systematic assessment (qualitative and quantitative) used to establish that an instrument adequately represents the entire content area/domain specified.

contingency table a two-dimensional frequency distribution in which the frequencies of two variables are cross-tabulated.

continuous variable variables that have a range of variability (e.g., weight).

control unit the part of a computer's central processing unit that takes care of operating the machinery.

Conversational Monitoring System (CMS) an interactive computer operating system that allows the user to give commands and get immediate responses or action.

correlation a statistic (called *r*) that shows the extent to which values of one variable are related to values of another variable.

CPU (Central Processing Unit) the "brain" of the computer, which keeps track of what's going on and executes programs that process data.

criterion measure an accepted measure of some variable.

criterion-related validity either concurrent or predictive. *Predictive* validity is a current instrument score that is used to predict future performance. *Concurrent* validity indicates an individual's current standing on a criterion measure related to the construct of interest.

critical value value of a statistic that needs to be exceeded by the calculated value in order for the research or alternate hypothesis to be accepted and the null hypothesis to be rejected.

critique a critical estimate of a piece of research involving a systematic appraisal according to specified criteria.

cross sectional survey a study design that looks at subjects who are at two different points in time with respect to an experience.

CRT (Cathode Ray Tube) screen or terminal resembling a television screen on which you can display computer keyboard type.

Cumulative Index to Nursing and Allied Health Literature (CINAHL) a resource for locating nursing journal articles.

CURN project a five-year Conduct and Use of Research in Nursing project, sponsored by the Michigan State Nurses' Association, which resulted in nine volumes focused on clinical research.

data the information an investigator collects from the subjects or participants in a research study.

data cleaning the process of trying to find errors in one's data set.

data processing the performance of functions on data that transform them into information.

Data Base Management System (DBMS) a software program that allows the user to keep a collection of records with similar data.

debriefing a process of disclosing to human subjects all information that was previously withheld in a study.

decision rule instruction established to ensure that unusual responses will be scored in the same way for all.

deductive approach emphasizes theory as a system of testable hypotheses arranged in a deductive logical sequence and research as a process for verifying or testing them. Moves from the abstract and general to the concrete and specific.

Delphi Survey of Research Priorities a 1974 survey conducted by the Western Commission on Higher Education for Nursing (WICHEN) and the Regional Program for Nursing Research Development that revealed 150 priority items in three areas, with an emphasis on patient welfare.

dependent variable (DV) the variable under study. Also called the criterion or outcome variable. Variability in the dependent variable depends on the preexisting conditions or factors that may be manipulated by the investigator.

description a qualitative analysis method in which the researcher finds classes in the data that correspond with a conceptual scheme or set of categories or concepts already existing in the literature.

descriptive statistics measures that summarize large volumes of data and are specific to the sample drawn from the larger population.

design the plan or blueprint used to get valid and reliable answers to research questions according to canons of science. Also called the protocol or program for a research study.

dichotomous variable variable with only two categories.

direct-access processing a technique of processing transactions in any order they may occur, without waiting for a batch of transactions.

directional hypothesis a testable proposition that specifies the expected direction of a relationship between concepts or variables.

direct relationship a positive correlation between two variables.

diskette also called a *floppy disk*. A magnetic medium external, or secondary, to a microcomputer, for electronically storing data.

documentation users' manuals and guides that contain instructions for employing software programs on a computer.

DOS the disk operating system for 16-bit machines; most common versions are PC DOS and MS-DOS, the former for the IBM PC, and the latter for IBM-compatible computers.

double blind a strategy to lessen effects of inaccurate ratings or responses in which neither the subject nor the data collector knows if subjects are members of the experimental or control group in a study.

dummy coding a special treatment of categorical variables for entry into a regression equation.

ecological validity the requirement that an experiment be sufficiently explicit, clear, and consistent to be replicated.

eigenvalues the sum of the squared factor loadings from each item for each factor.

electronic spreadsheet a software program designed to manage budget information in a row and column format; has computational capabilities.

empirical evidence refers to evidence derived through collection of data using one's senses—one of the characteristics of the scientific way of knowing.

epistemology the branch of philosophy concerned with how one determines what is true.

ethics a branch of philosophy concerned with what is good and bad and what one's moral obligations are.

ethnology the study of human beings as social and cultural organisms.

ethnography the systematic study of cultures, subcultures, and life-styles.

exemplars specific examples of events culled from phenomenological data to generate rich descriptions of situations in their complete form.

experiment study design in which the investigator can control or manipulate one independent variable, can randomly select sample members, and can randomly assign sample members to experimental and control groups.

expert sampling a type of purposive sampling that involves choosing experts in a given area because of their access to the information of relevance.

exploratory study type of study design used to gain familiarity or achieve insights about a phenomenon. Answers who and what questions. Also called factor-naming, factor-identifying, or factor-searching.

ex post facto a study in which researchers study something after the fact instead of manipulating an independent variable.

external criticism evaluation of historical studies for the genuineness or authenticity of their data sources.

external validity in an experimental design, the representativeness or generalizability of study results.

extraneous variable also called confounding variable, because it is a factor other than a study's independent variable that affects and confounds or confuses interpretation of a study's findings.

face validity subjective judgments by experts about the degree to which a test appears to measure the relevant construct.

facts derived from multiple congruent and similar observations of the same phenomena over time.

factorial design a design that matches subjects on a nominal variable that cannot be rank ordered before assigning them to experimental and control groups.

factor-isolating questions research questions that ask "what is this?" Also called factor-naming questions.

factor-relating questions research questions that ask how factors that have been identified relate to one another. Answers the question of "what is happening here?" Also called association testing.

field any social-psychological arena where an investigator gathers data relevant to the area of inquiry.

fieldwork data collection strategies that include observation, interviewing, case studies, and document review. Rely on firsthand knowing under natural conditions. Also called field methods.

fixed-column format keypunch system in which the variables and values for each and every subject are consistently located in the same columns.

floppy disks a magnetic storage device that resembles 45 rpm records encased in a heavy paper jacket and is used to store software and data. Also called diskettes.

focused interview an interview that begins with an outline of topics to be covered with every interviewee but allows freedom to deviate from the prepared agenda as well. Also called a partially structured or semistructured interview.

formative study evaluation study that occurs in process in order to provide ongoing feedback about a program.

Fortran (Formula Translation) a commonly used computer programming language.

frequency distribution an analysis method that involves determining how often scores or values appear in a data set.

frequency polygon graphic display of frequency table in which dots connected by straight lines are used instead of bars to show the number of times a class occurs.

goal-free evaluation evaluation study designed to include unanticipated consequences as well as data bearing on a program's goals or objectives.

grand theory an attempt to explain everything in a field, using global concepts that are often poorly defined and ambiguously related.

grounded theory a highly evolved and explicitly codified method for developing categories and propositions about their relationships from qualitative data. Closely integrated with a method of social research called "the constant comparative method."

halo effect an observer's tendency to rate certain subjects as consistently high or low on everything because of the overall impression the subject gives the rater.

hard disk a secondary storage device; a magnetic disk storage device that is usually fixed in place.

hardware the equipment in a computer system that you can touch.

Hawthorne effect changes that occur in people's behavior because they know they are being studied. Was first observed in the Hawthorne plant of the Western Electric Company.

Helsinki Declaration a guide issued in 1964 and revised in 1974 by the World Medical Association that differentiated between two types of research: (1) that which is essentially therapeutic, and (2) that which is directed toward generation of scientific knowledge and has no benefit to the subject. Served as one of the bases for H.S.S. guidelines.

hermeneutics an interpretive research approach that relies on analysis of text to understand human behavior and meanings.

histogram graphic display of a frequency table using rectangular bars with heights equal to the frequency in a particular class.

historical study type of study design intended to explain the present or anticipate the future using methods for collecting and evaluating evidence from the past.

hypothesis statement of relationship between two or more study concepts or variables.

independent variable (IV) the conditions or factors that precede measurement of the dependent variable or are manipulated by the investigator. Also called the input variable.

indirect relationship (inverse relationship) a negative correlation between two variables.

inductive approach a method that emphasizes data as the source for generating concepts and explanatory relationships. Moves from the concrete and specific to the general and abstract.

inferential statistics tests used to make inferences from a sample to the larger population.

informed consent the knowing consent of an individual or his/her legally authorized representative to decide whether or not to participate in a research project without undue inducement or any elements of force, fraud, deceit, duress, constraint, or coercion. The institutional review board (IRB) acts as a protective mechanism for human research subjects by reviewing protocols and risk-benefit ratios.

input devices parts of a computer system that allow data to be entered into and recognized by a computer.

726

internal consistency reliability   the statistical determination of how well each item on an instrument relates to all other items. Provides an indication of how consistently individuals respond to all items on an instrument.

internal criticism   evaluation of historical studies for the accuracy of the statements contained within the historical data sources used.

integrated package   a software program that allows from three to five software applications that might otherwise stand alone to interrelate and share data within a single program.

internal validity   in an experimental design, a determination that manipulation of the independent variable really makes a significant difference in the dependent variable.

interquartile range   a stable measure of variability based on excluding extreme scores and using only middle cases.

interrater reliability   reliability of measures across different raters.

interval estimation   uses a sample parameter to establish a range of values that are likely (given a certain level of probability) to contain the true population parameter.

interval scale   a measure of data that rank orders a variable with equal distance between points (e.g., Fahrenheit degrees).

instruments   devices or techniques an investigator employs to collect data. May include questionnaires, performance checklists, pencil-and-paper tests, biological devices, and so on.

instrumentation   process of using a device or combination of equipment for measurement.

invasive procedure   a medical intervention that involves penetration of the body for measurement.

keypunch cards   a form of computer input consisting of cardboard cards with 80 vertical columns and 12 rows.

keypunching   a process by which a machine that looks like a typewriter punches holes into the columns of a data card.

Kilobyte (K)   measure of memory for all modes of computer storage; refers to 1000 bytes; a kilobyte.

Likert scale   method of measurement in which respondents are presented with statements and asked how much they agree or disagree.

literature review   systematic search of published work to find out what is known about a research topic.

logging on   gaining access to a computer so that it can be used. Involves a user identification number and a password.

longitudinal survey   a study design that studies subjects over time, assessing their experiences at predetermined stages.

mainframe   a large, expensive computer with terminals located in different places throughout an organization.

materials   another term for the measurement devices used to collect data from study subjects.

mean   the measure of central tendency derived by dividing the sum of the values in a data set by the total number of values, scores, or subjects in it. Also called the average.

measurement   the actual value of a variable, plus or minus error.

measurement scale   the options on a psychosocial instrument to which subjects respond (e.g., strongly agree to strongly disagree). These options are usually assigned a numerical value for analysis.

median   the measure of central tendency that corresponds to the middle score.

MEDLINE/MEDLARS   the most frequently used computerized bibliographical services that access biomedical and nursing sources.

megabyte (MB)   one million bytes or characters.

mental measurements yearbook   a compendium that summarizes available information about an instrument and compares it with others in the field.

meta-analysis   the integration of the results of independent studies.

metaparadigm   the most global perspective of a discipline, which serves as an encapsulating unit, or framework, in which the more defined models, theories, or paradigms develop.

metatheory   a type of philosophical theory that studies the logical and methodological foundations of a discipline.

methodological notes (MN)   field notes that remind the researcher which methodological approaches might be fruitful.

methodological studies   designs that develop, validate, or evaluate research tools or techniques.

microcomputer   small desktop computer that is also called a personal or business computer.

microfiche   a computer output on microfilm that allows a lot of printed material to be presented in a small space.

middle-range theory   theory that examines a specific empirical area and at key variables in depth. Also called substantive theory.

minicomputer   a computer of medium size, smaller than a mainframe—although like it in design—and larger than a microcomputer.

minimal risk   an assessment that the risks anticipated to human subjects as a consequence of participating in the proposed research are not greater than those ordinarily encountered in daily life or during the performance of routine examinations or tests.

mode   the category or class that has the highest frequency. A measure of central tendency.

model   a structural, pictorial, diagrammatic, or mathematical likeness that represents some aspect of reality.

modem   modulator/demodulator; special piece of hardware that allows two computers to communicate via the telephone lines; may be internal or external.

mouse   a mechanical or optical input device used for pointing or drawing.

multicollinearity   occurs when an independent variable is a linear combination of one or more independent variables; e.g., there is a strong relation of one independent variable to another or to a series of independent variables.

multimodal frequency   a frequency distribution with more than two high points.

multivariate statistics   those statistics that test more than two variables.

necessary condition   a required condition if an event is to occur.

negative cases   anecdotes in qualitative data that run counter to the analyst's propositions.

network sampling   sampling in which the researcher uses informal networks to find subjects.

nominal scale   a scale that measures data by assignment of characteristics into categories.

nonequivalent pretest-posttest control group design   the most basic quasi-experimental design that uses comparative groups instead of random assignment to equivalent control and experimental groups.

noninvasive procedure procedure that does not involve penetration of the skin for measuring a parameter.

nonparametric statistics tests that can be used with nominal and ordinal data as well as when a sample size is too small to assume that a normal distribution exists in the population.

nonprobability sampling sampling that is not done according to the laws of probability theory. Includes various types of accidental and convenience sampling approaches.

normal curve a symmetrical, unimodal distribution curve with greatest frequency of values at the center. Also called bell-shaped curve.

Nuremberg Code (Articles) the first internationally accepted effort to set up formal ethical standards governing human research studies. Served as one of the bases for the H.S.S. guidelines.

nursing audit strategy for measuring the quality of nursing care after it has been given.

nursing research research into the processes and practice of nursing care.

null hypothesis statement that no relationship other than chance exists between or among a study's concepts or variables. Represents the study hypothesis stated in reverse.

numeric data consists of data expressed in numbers, such as age, weight, blood pressure, test scores, etc.

objectivity a characteristic of the scientific way of knowing that attempts to distance the approach to truth from the scientist's personal biases, beliefs, values, and attitudes.

observational notes (ON) descriptive, noninterpretive accounts of observations made in a field of study.

operational definition specifies what a researcher does to make a concept measurable.

ordinal scale a scale that measures data that rank orders a variable along some dimension.

paradigms include methods, laws, theory, and traditions that guide research in a discipline.

paradigm case findings in phenomenological research that reflect resemblances between several cases.

paradigm-transcending research scientific revolutions in which an existing paradigm in a discipline is significantly altered.

parameter a descriptive characteristic of a sample or population, such as the mean or standard deviation.

parametric statistics powerful statistical tests that are used with interval level data and normal distribution of a population.

parsimony the decision criterion that when two or more theoretically sound solutions exist, the least complex solution with the fewest assumptions should be selected.

patient log a data collection tool that is a diary or record of behavior.

personal notes (PN) field notes about one's own reactions and reflections related to observations in the field.

PERT (Program Evaluation Review Technique) a diagram of the scheduled work in a research project.

phenomenological (interpretive) research approach a research design and method with the purpose of understanding meanings and practices of people who function as whole beings within their historical or background traditions; a research approach for investigating "lived experience."

pilot study a small-scale practice run of a research project.

plagiarism stealing or passing off the work of another as one's own.

point estimation a single value determined from the sample that is thought to best approximate the population parameter.

polychotomous variable variables that have more than two categories (e.g., race).

population (N) the total possible membership of the group being studied.

population validity the determination that one can generalize from the actual sample to all possible sample members and likewise to the total population.

positivist a philosophy of science that asserts the similarity between the physical and psychosocial worlds and adheres to beliefs in obtaining objective data through measurement instruments.

posttest-only design after-only experimental design in which subjects are assigned to an experimental and control group, but data are collected only at the end of exposure to the independent variable. Considered the simplest experimental design.

power analysis a means of establishing that a study was conducted on a large enough number of sample members to justify results.

preexperimental study design study design with posttest only and no control group.

pretest sensitization a threat to external validity due to subjects being affected on the dependent variable by taking the pretest.

primary sources firsthand information used as data in historical studies. May include letters, diaries, photographs, eye-witness accounts, etc.

priority rating a number that indicates where an approved study proposal stands in relation to others as far as its priority for being funded.

privacy the assurance that one may behave and think without interference or the possibility that private behavior or thoughts may be used to embarrass or demean the person later.

probability sampling a procedure that requires every element in a population to have an equal chance of being included in a sample taken from it.

proposal written document that communicates the plan for, logic of, and importance of an intended research study. Also called a research prospectus or protocol.

proposition statement of relationship between two or more concepts.

prospectus proposal for a research study or manuscript that may be submitted to a funding agency, committee, or book publisher.

proxy measures measures of variables that cannot be measured directly.

purposive sampling judgmental sampling process in which the researcher intentionally selects sample members based on specified criteria.

psychometric properties refers to the validity and reliability of the instrument.

qualitative analysis the analysis of nonnumerical data. Often used in field research.

quality patient care scale (Qualpac) instrument to measure quality of nursing care while it is being given.

quasi-experimental study design study design used when it is not feasible to implement all the qualities of an experimental design.

quasi-statistics an analytic method to transform qualitative data into numerical frequencies and distributions.

query letter letter sent to journal editors to inquire about their interest in publishing a journal article.

quota sampling selecting a sample that may not be random and whose proportions may not be representative of the proportions in the population.

random-access memory (RAM) a term for primary storage that temporarily holds data and instructions for processing while a computer program is being run.

random sample a sample selected according to one of the procedures for probability sampling, ensuring that every element in a population has an equal chance of being included in the sample.

randomized block posttest design a variation on the after-only design which assigns subjects to the experimental and control groups after they have been ranked on some important variable.

range simplest measure of dispersion; represents the difference between the smallest and largest numbers in a distribution.

ranking technique similar to sorting in which respondents are asked to rank order objects or stimuli on the basis of some property.

ratio scale a scale for measuring data which has a true and meaningful zero point (e.g., weight) and in which there are equal distances between scores.

referees anonymous peers who review research proposals and manuscripts prior to approval for publication.

regression coefficient expresses the change in y that is, on the average, associated with a one unit change in x.

reliability a quality of a research instrument important in evaluating its worth. Means that the instrument produces consistent results or data on repeated use, usually because the investigator has standardized the process for using it. Also used to describe data or study design.

replication repeating prior scientific work to establish the limits of a study's findings and methodology.

representativeness a quality that usually refers to the extent to which a study sample represents the characteristics of a population.

research in nursing broad study of the nursing profession, including historical, ethical, and political studies.

research utilization implementation of research findings in practice.

researchable problem a question that can be investigated using the process of scientific research. Should be differentiated from a question of opinion or philosophy. Implies the possibility of empirical testing.

resolution a measure of clarity and ease of reading of a computer's display terminal, determined by the number of picture elements (called pixels) of the terminal.

reverse-scored items test items worded in the opposite way from the majority of items to avoid response set bias.

review the identification and summarization of the major features of a research study. Not synonymous with a critique.

risk of harm defined by the Department of Health and Human Services as exposure to the possibility of injury on the parts of human research subjects including physical, emotional, legal, financial, or social as a consequence of participating in a research-related activity.

risk-benefit ratio the balance between possible benefits to the individual or society of the proposed research in relation to the risk of harm to human subjects.

read-only memory (ROM) permanent memory that contains a computer's operating-system software and assembly language.

sample (*n*) a subset of the population selected as sources for data.

sampling error the fluctuation of a statistic from one sample to another drawn from the same population.

sampling frame all subjects in the population.

SAS (Statistical Analysis System) a statistical package of programs applicable to executing computations used in statistical analysis of quantitative data.

scale measuring instrument composed of several items that have a logical or empirical relationship to each other.

scatter diagram (scatterplot) a graphic presentation of the correlation between two variables.

scholarship contemplation in search of new insights.

scientific approach the systematic attempt to understand and comprehend the world, particularly its order.

scientific inquiry a process in which observable, verifiable data are systematically collected from the world through our senses so that we can describe, explain, and predict events.

secondary sources second- or third-hand accounts used as data sources in historical studies. The end products of studying primary sources. May include reference books, newspaper articles, etc.

semantic differential scale a psychosocial scale designed to quantify concepts in terms of their word meanings (semantic properties).

sensitizing concepts concepts used to focus and organize data initially. May be supplanted later with concepts grounded in observations.

Sigma Theta Tau the National Nurses' Honor Society, which sponsors regional conferences in order to promote research-based practice.

single-subject experimental design study that uses a single case but includes a reversal phase during which the intervention being tested is withheld while measures of the dependent variable continue.

situation-producing questions research questions that ask "How can I make something happen?" require knowledge of action that can change a sequence of events in a desirable direction. Knowledge of control. Also called situation-prescribing questions.

situation-relating questions research questions that ask "What will happen if . . .?" Often involve experimental or quasi-experimental designs.

skewed distribution frequency distribution with off-center peaks and longer tails in one direction.

Slater Nursing Competencies Rating Scale instrument designed to measure competencies displayed by a nurse.

snowball sampling a kind of accidental sampling that involves subjects suggesting other subjects to the researcher.

sociodemographic questionnaire a specialized instrument designed to obtain personal, social, and environmental data about subjects.

software the program applications that tell a computer what to do.

sorting a data-collection technique that asks respondents to sort cards into piles based on some specified dimension.

split-half reliability an indicator of the internal consistency of an instrument. It is determined by dividing an instrument in half, computing a score for each half, and correlating the two sets of scores.

SPSS (Statistical Package for the Social Sciences) an applications statistical package of programs used to analyze quantitative research data.

STAI (State-Trait Anxiety Inventory) a measure of anxiety.

standard deviation the most widely used measure of variability when a frequency distribution approximates a normal curve. It is the average of the deviations from the mean.

standard error of the mean the standard deviation of a theoretical frequency distribution of means of samples. The smaller it is, the more accurately a sample mean reflects a population mean.

standard score (z-score) the number of standard deviations between the mean and a particular raw score.

statement of purpose a statement that addresses the question, "why do a study?" conveys a study's overall aims, goals, or objectives.

statistics analytic tools that allow an investigator to determine that something is more or less likely to occur according to the laws of probability.

stratified random sampling selecting a random sample after categorizing the population elements into relevant strata or subpopulations.

sufficient condition a condition that is always followed by an event.

summative survey type of evaluation survey designed to address the effectiveness of the outcome of a plan or program.

survey research design that involves studying populations based on data gathered from a sample drawn from them. Generally serves the purpose of describing characteristics, opinions, attitudes, or behaviors.

symbolic interactionist a social-psychological scientific tradition, also called neo-idealist, that asserts that the differences between the physical and psychosocial worlds require different approaches.

symmetrical distribution frequency distribution with equal halves when folded in the middle.

systematic sampling drawing every nth element from a population to make up a sample.

systematic skimming the second level of reading, also called prereading.

test-retest reliability method for establishing reliability by administering an instrument on two or more occasions to the same respondents.

text typed transcripts of observational notes and interviews used as data in phenomenological research approaches.

thematic analysis an analysis approach to phenomenological research used to identify themes that appear across cases.

theoretical notes (TN) fieldwork notes in which the researcher attempts to derive meaning from observations of the field.

theoretical terms theory-specific terms that are not directly observable.

theory a set of interrelated constructs or propositions that present a systematic explanation of phenomena. A vision of truth or reality.

timetable part of a research proposal that clarifies the overall flow of activities in a sequential statement of operations. Also called a work plan.

time series design a study design that uses before-measures on a group as a baseline against which to measure the dependent variable.

triangulation the use of a variety of methods to collect data on the same concept.

t-test statistical test used to determine if the means of two groups are significantly different (e.g., not due to chance).

Type I error (alpha error) the conclusion that the null hypothesis is false when it is really true (e.g., that a difference is not due to chance when in fact it is).

Type II error (beta error) the conclusion that differences between groups were due to chance when in fact they were due to the effects of the IV.

unimodal frequency a frequency distribution with only one high point.

unstructured interview a fieldwork data-collection strategy that stresses the respondent's definition of the situation and encourages the interviewee to determine what is relevant.

validity the property/characteristic of a psychosocial instrument that means the instrument measures what it purports to measure (e.g., stress).

variable something that varies and has different values that can be measured. Results from operationally defining a concept.

variance a descriptive statistic that examines how scores or values in a data set are distributed.

vector a term used to refer to a row or column of numbers representing values on variables, parameter point estimates, and so on.

vulnerable subjects categories of subjects, such as children, fetuses, the mentally disabled, the elderly, captives, the sedated, and the unconcious, who may not be able to evaluate the risks of participating in a study by virtue of diminished capacity to give free and informed consent.

waveform a graphic representation of changes in a variable over time.

Index

Aamodt, A. M., 418
Abdellah, Fay, 16, 296-98
   list of nursing problems, 297
Abrams, R., 84
Abstract, 51-53, 112-13
Abstracted empiricism, 324-25
Accessible population, 256
Accidental sampling, 260
Active reading, 43-45
Activity and position, instrumentation
   and variables for, 383-88
Adler, Mortimer J., 43-45
Advances in Nursing Science, 54-55, 716-
   18
Affective instruments, 350-51
Agar, M. H., 419
Aged, sexual needs of, assessing, 437
Alcoholics Anonymous, 142
Alpert, Richard, 66
Alphanumeric data, 585
American Academy of Nursing (AAN),
   37
American Cancer Society, 645
American Journal of Nursing, 54, 675
American Medical Association, 70
American Nurses' Association
   Cabinet on Nursing Research, 27
   Commission on Nursing Research,
     40, 42-32, 108, 208
   Council of Nurse Researchers, 658
   Human Rights Guidelines for Nurs-
     ing in Clinical and Other Re-
     search, 69, 75-76
   Priorities for Nursing Research, 29
   social policy statement of, 5
American Nurses' Foundation (ANF),
   25, 37, 645
American Psychological Association,
   357, 665
American Sociological Society, Code
   of Professional Ethics of, 69,
   71-74
Analysis, 454. *See also* Qualitative
   analysis; Quantitative analysis
   content, 469-76
     reliability and validity of, 475-76
     steps in, 470-72
   descriptive, 511
   discriminant, 565-66
   path, 564-65
Analysis of covariance (ANCOVA),
   558, 571-72
Analysis of variance (ANOVA), 122,
   164, 534, 538, 540-44, 557
   multivariate, 535, 558, 567-69
   repeated measures, 570-71
Analytical files, 465
Analytical induction, 476
Analytic description, 458
Analytic reading, 44-45
   example of, 49-50
   guides to, 47-48

Andreoli, K. G., 169
Animal models, 399
Annual Review of Nursing Research, 53
Anonymity, right of, 84-85
Anthropology, 417
Application packet, 621
Applied Nursing Research, 56, 718-19
Applied research, 12, 291
Archaeology, 417
Archives of historical nursing docu-
   ments, 141
Arithmetic-logic unit (ALU), 594
Arithmetic mean, 518
Artificial language, 190-91
Artinian, B., 284
ASCII, 589
Atwood, J. R., 170, 211, 396
Autogenic 2000 Feedback Thermo-
   graph, 407
Autogenic 3400 Feedback Dermo-
   graph, 407
Awareness contexts, 422

Bacon, L. D., 355
Bafford, D. C., 408
Barhyte, D. Y., 355
Barnard, Kathryn E., 18, 39
Bartlett's test, 566
BASIC, 598
Basic research, 12, 291
Batch processing, 594
Bausell, R. B., 157
Becker, Howard S., 308, 357, 418,
   468
Beckstrand, J., 292
Before-after experimental design, 161
Behavioral instruments, 351
Beliefs About Mental Illness Inven-
   tory, 504
Belmont Report, 80
Benedict, Ruth, 418
Benoliel, Jeanne, 142
Berthold, J. S., 649
Beta weight, 560
Bias, 561
Bimodal distribution, 517
Binary system, 587
Binet, Alfred, 335
Biophysiological instruments, 369-71
   dependent variable and, 375-76
   independent variable and, 375
   selection of, guidelines for, 371-74
Biophysiological phenomena, measure-
   ment of, 376-77
Biophysiological variables
   measurement of, 374-75
   nursing research and, 409-10
Bit, 587
Blalock, H. M., Jr., 192
Blaus, P., 444
Blumer, Herbert, 421, 455
Bonferroni inequality, 557
Bounds, W. G., 111, 566
Bowers, B. J., 457
Boyer, D., 253
Braden, C., 564-65
Brammer, L. M., 442
Brickman, P., 308
Brink, Pamela J., 18, 55, 229-31, 243,
   261, 439, 445-46
Bronowski, J., 5

Brown, J. S., 336
Brown, Myrtle Irene, 307
Brown Report, 24
BRS/After Dark, 600
Bunge, Helen, 25
Buros, Oscar, 633
Bush, H., 281, 283-84
Byte, 587

Campbell, D. T., 157, 163, 168
Canonical correlation, 566-67
Canonical variates, 567
Capron, H. L., 595
Cardiac monitor, 370, 375
Card reader, 591
Carnegie, Elizabeth, 26
Carter, B., 491
Case history, field research and, 443-
   45
Case study, 142-45, 250-51
   advantages and disadvantages of,
     143-44
   field research and, 443-45
   steps in, 143
Castaneda, Carlos, 416
Cathode ray tube (CRT), 591
Causal hypothesis-testing research,
   288
Causal relationship, experimental de-
   sign and, 166
Central processing unit (CPU), 594
Central tendency, measures of, 516-20
Character printers, 592
Chater, S. S., 535
Chesla, C., 491-92
Chinn, P., 284
Chi-square distribution, critical values
   of, 714
Chi-square test, 548-49
Christy, T. E., 137, 139
Chulay, M., 387
Civilization, 417
Clarke, E., 390
Clayton, B. C., 322
Clinical interview, 437
Clinical research, 12-13
   priorities in, 40-43
Clinical Research System for Personal
   Computers, 611
Cluster sampling, 259-60
COBOL, 598
Code book, 589
Coding, grounded theory and, 482-86
Cohen, J. A., 267, 395, 401
Coles, Robert, 418
Common factor analysis, 577
Communality, 580
Communication software, 599
Comparative reading, 44-45
   guides to, 48
Comparative survey, 150
CompuServe, 601
Computer-aided instruction (CAI), 611
Computers, 585-608
   central processing unit of, 594-95
   data storage for, 595-96
   input devices for, 588-91
   output devices for, 591-94
   personal, 608-10
Computer searches, 51-53
Comte, Auguste, 417